ADAMS

16/16/FST/A7021

Instructional Course Lectures Trauma

Edited by
Paul Tornetta III, MD

Professor and Director of Trauma
Department of Orthopaedic Surgery
Boston University Medical Center
Boston, Massachusetts

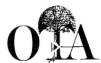

Developed with support from
Orthopaedic Trauma Association

Published by the
American Academy
of Orthopaedic Surgeons
6300 North River Road
Rosemont, IL 60018

American Academy of Orthopaedic Surgeons

First Edition
Copyright 2006 by the American Academy of Orthopaedic Surgeons
ISBN 10: 0-89203-397-5
ISBN 13: 978-0-89203-397-3

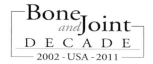

Editorial Board

Contributors

Arif Ali, MD
Orthopaedic Trauma Fellow
Orthopaedic Trauma Service
Hospital for Special Surgery
New York Presbyterian Hospital
New York, New York

Stanley E. Asnis, MD
Chairman
Department of Orthopaedic Surgery
North Shore University Hospital
Manhasset, New York

Michael R. Baumgaertner, MD, FACS
Associate Professor
Department of Orthopaedics and Rehabilitation
Yale University School of Medicine
New Haven, Connecticut

Judith F. Baumhauer, MD
Associate Professor of Orthopaedics
Chief Division of Foot and Ankle Surgery
Department of Orthopaedics
University of Rochester Medical Center
Rochester, New York

Daniel J. Berry, MD
Associate Professor of Orthopedics
Mayo Medical School
Consultant in Orthopedic Surgery
Department of Orthopedic Surgery
Mayo Clinic
Rochester, Minnesota

Mathias P.G. Bostrom, MD
Department of Orthopaedics
Hospital for Special Surgery
New York, New York

Andrew Burgess, MD
Academic Chairman
Orthopaedic Surgery
Orlando Regional Medical Center
Orlando, Florida

Mark S. Cohen, MD
Associate Professor
Director, Hand and Elbow Section
Director, Orthopaedic Education
Department of Orthopaedic Surgery
Rush-Presbyterian-St. Luke's Medical Center
Chicago, Illinois

William P. Cooney III, MD
Professor of Orthopedic Surgery
Mayo Medical School
Department of Orthopedic Surgery
Mayo Clinic
Rochester, Minnesota

Kenneth A. Egol, MD
Instructor, Orthopaedic Surgery
New York University School of Medicine
New York University Hospital for Joint Diseases
Department of Orthopaedic Surgery
New York, New York

Evan F. Ekman, MD
Director
Southern Orthopaedic Sports Medicine
Medical Director
Parkridge Surgery Center
Columbia, South Carolina

Diego L. Fernandez, MD
Associate Professor of Orthopedic Surgery
University of Berne, Switzerland
Orthopedic Department
Lindenhof Hospital
Berne, Switzerland

Christopher G. Finkemeier, MD, MBA
Associate Professor
Department of Orthopaedic Surgery
University of California
Davis Health Center
Sacramento, California

Alan E. Freeland, MD
Professor
Hand/Upper Extremity Surgery
Department of Orthopaedic Surgery
University of Mississippi Medical Center
Jackson, Mississippi

William B. Geissler, MD
Associate Professor, Orthopaedic Surgery
University Orthopaedics
University of Mississippi Medical Center
Jackson, Mississippi

Peter V. Giannoudis, MD
Consultant Trauma Surgeon
Department of Trauma
St. James University Hospital
Leeds, United Kingdon

Amit Gupta, MD, FRCS
Hand Surgeon
Christine M. Kleinert Institute for Hand & Microsurgery
Louisville, Kentucky

George J. Haidukewych, MD
Florida Orthopaedic Institute
Tampa, Florida

David L. Helfet, MD
Orthopaedic Trauma Service
Director, Orthopaedic Trauma Center
Hospital for Special Surgery
New York Presbyterian Hospital
New York, New York

Joseph P. Iannotti, MD, PhD
Professor and Chairman
Department of Orthopaedic Surgery
Cleveland Clinic Foundation
Cleveland Clinic Lerner School of Medicine
Cleveland, Ohio

Alan L. Jones, MD
Associate Professor and Vice Chairman
Department of Orthopaedic Surgery
University of Texas Southwestern Medical School
Dallas, Texas

Atul Joshi, MD, MCH (Orth), FRCS
JPS Health Network
Fort Worth, Texas

Jesse B. Jupiter, MD
Director, Orthopaedic Surgery
Massachusetts General Hospital
Professor, Orthopaedic Surgery
Harvard Medical School
Boston, Massachusetts

L. Andrew Koman, MD
Professor and Vice Chairman
Department of Orthopaedic Surgery
Wake Forest University School of Medicine
Winston-Salem, North Carolina

Kenneth J. Koval, MD
Chief, Division of Trauma
New York University Hospital for Joint Diseases
Department of Orthopaedics
Hospital for Joint Diseases
New York, New York

Joseph M. Lane, MD
Professor of Orthopaedic Surgery
Assistant Dean, Medical Students
Weill Medical College of Cornell University
New York, New York

Loren Latta, PE, PhD
Professor and Director of Research
Department of Orthopaedics and Rehabilitation
University of Miami
Miami, Florida

Sung-Rak Lee, MD
Attending Orthopaedic Surgeon
Department of Orthopaedics
Hallageneral Hospital, Jeju
Jeju, Republic of Korea

Ross K. Leighton, MD, FRCSC, FACS
Associate Professor of Surgery
Division of Orthopaedics
Dalhousie University
Halifax, Nova Scotia

L. Scott Levin, MD
Duke University Medical Center
Durham, North Carolina

David M. Lichtman, MD
Chairman
Department of Orthopaedics
JPS Health Network
Fort Worth, Texas

Julie T. Lin, MD
Fellow, Spine and Sports Medicine
Fellow, Metabolic Bone Disease
Department of Physiatry/Metabolic Bone Service
Hospital for Special Surgery
New York, New York

Ronald W. Lindsey, MD
Professor of Orthopaedic Surgery
Department of Orthopaedic Surgery
Baylor College of Medicine
Houston, Texas

Arthur L. Malkani, MD
Associate Professor
Chief, Adult Reconstruction
Department of Orthopaedic Surgery
University of Louisville
Louisville, Kentucky

Arthur Manoli II, MD
Director
Michigan International Foot & Ankle Center
St. Joseph Mercy Hospital, Oakland
Pontiac, Michigan

Joel M. Matta, MD
John P. Wilson, Jr. Chair of Orthopaedics
Good Samaritan Hospital
Los Angeles, California

Michael D. McKee, MD, FRCSC
Associate Professor
Division of Orthopaedic Surgery
Department of Surgery
St. Michael's Hospital and the University of Toronto
Toronto, Ontario, Canada

Dana C. Mears, MD, PhD
Professor and Chief
Division of Orthopaedic Surgery
Albany Medical Center
Albany, New York

Berton R. Moed, MD
Professor and Chairman
Department of Orthopaedic Surgery
St. Louis University School of Medicine
St. Louis, Missouri

Tom R. Norris, MD
Department of Orthopaedics
California-Pacific Medical Center
San Francisco, California

Shawn W. O'Driscoll, PhD, MD
Professor of Orthopedic Surgery
Department of Orthopedic Surgery
Mayo Foundation
Rochester, Minnesota

Steven A. Olson, MD, FACS
Chief, Orthopedic Trauma
Department of Surgery
Duke University Medical Center
Durham, North Carolina

Hans-Christoph Pape, MD
Professor
Department of Trauma Surgery and Orthopedics
Hanover Medical School
Hanover, Germany

Wesley P. Phipatanakul, MD
Department of Orthopaedics
California-Pacific Medical Center
San Francisco, California

Matthew L. Ramsey, MD
Assistant Professor of Orthopaedic Surgery
Shoulder and Elbow Service
Department of Orthopaedic Surgery
University of Pennsylvania
Philadelphia, Pennsylvania

William M. Ricci, MD
Associate Professor
Department of Orthopaedic Surgery
Washington University School of Medicine at Barnes-Jewish Hospital
St. Louis, Missouri

Jeffrey H. Richmond, MD
Chief Resident
Department of Orthopaedics
New York University Hospital for Joint Diseases
New York, New York

David Ring, MD
Department of Orthopaedic Surgery
Massachusetts General Hospital
Boston, Massachusetts

Craig S. Roberts, MD
Associate Professor
Residency Director
Department of Orthopaedic Surgery
University of Louisville
Louisville, Kentucky

Jorge L. Rodriguez
Professor
Department of General Surgery
University of Louisville
Lousiville, Kentucky

David S. Ruch, MD
Associate Professor
Department of Orthopaedic Surgery
Wake Forest University School of Medicine
Winston-Salem, North Carolina

Augusto Sarmiento, MD
Professor and Chairman Emeritus
University of Miami
Coral Gables, Florida

Luis R. Scheker, MD
Assistant Clinical Professor of Surgery (Plastic and Reconstructive)
Department of Surgery
University of Louisville
Louisville, Kentucky

Emil H. Schemitsch, MD, FRCSC
Head, Division of Orthopaedic Surgery
Professor of Surgery
St. Michael's Hospital
University of Toronto
Toronto, Ontario, Canada

Andrew H. Schmidt, MD
Assistant Professor
Department of Orthopedic Surgery
University of Minnesota
Faculty
Hennepin County Medical Center
Minneapolis, Minnesota

Russell A. Shatford, MD
Assistant Professor
University of Louisville
Christine M. Kleinert Instructor
Louisville, Kentucky

Tamara Simpson, MD
Orthopaedic Department
Hennepin County Medical Center
Minneapolis, Minnesota

Paul D. Sponseller, MD
Professor and Head
Pediatric Orthopaedics
Johns Hopkins University
Baltimore, Maryland

Andrew B. Stein, MD
Associate Professor
Department of Orthopaedic Surgery
Boston University Medical Center
Boston, Massachusetts

David J.G. Stephen, MD, FRCSC
Assistant Professor
Division of Orthopaedics
New York University/Hospital for Joint Diseases
New York, New York

Michael Suk, MD, JD, MPH
Orthopaedic Trauma Fellow
Hospital for Special Surgery
New York, New York

Nirmal Tejwani, MD
Assistant Professor of Clinical Orthopedics
Department of Orthopedics
New York University/Hospital for Joint Diseases
New York, New York

David C. Templeman, MD
Associate Professor
Department of Orthopaedic Surgery
University of Minnesota
Hennepin County Medical Center
Minneapolis, Minnesota

Karl-Göran Thorngren, MD, PhD, FRCSEd
Professor
Department of Orthopedics
Lund University Hospital
Lund, Sweden

Vernon T. Tolo, MD
John D. Wilson Jr. Professor of Orthopaedics
USC School of Medicine
Head, Division of Orthopaedics
Childrens Hospital, Los Angeles
Los Angeles, California

Paul Tornetta III, MD
Professor and Director of Trauma
Department of Orthopaedic Surgery
Boston University Medical Center
Boston, Massachusetts

Tsu-Min Tsai, MD
Clinical Professor of Orthopedic Surgery
University of Louisville School of Medicine
Christine M. Kleinert Institute
Louisville, Kentucky

John H. Velyvis, MD
Resident and Research Fellow
Division of Orthopaedic Surgery
Albany Medical Center
Albany, New York

James P. Waddell, MD, FRCSC
A.J. Latner Professor and Chairman
Department of Orthopaedic Surgery
University of Toronto
Toronto, Ontario, Canada

Jon J.P. Warner, MD
Chief
The Harvard Shoulder Service
Associate Professor of Orthopaedics
Harvard Medical School
Partners
Department of Orthopaedics
Massachusetts General and Brigham and Women's Hospitals
Boston, Massachusetts

Andrew J. Weiland, MD
Orthopaedic Surgeon
Hospital for Special Surgery
New York, New York

Arnold-Peter Weiss, MD
Professor of Orthopaedics
Brown University School of Medicine
Providence, Rhode Island

Gerald R. Williams, Jr, MD
Chief, Shoulder and Elbow Service
Associate Professor, Orthopaedic Surgery
University of Pennsylvania
Philadelphia, Pennsylvania

Scott W. Wolfe, MD
Professor, Orthopaedic Surgery
Weill Medical College of Cornell University
Department of Orthopaedics
Hospital for Special Surgery
New York, New York

Thomas W. Wolff, MD
Assistant Clinical Professor of Surgery
University of Louisville School of Medicine
Christine M. Kleinert Institute for Hand and Microsurgery
Louisville, Kentucky

Philip Wolinsky, MD
Department of Orthopedic Surgery
New York University/Hospital for Joint Diseases
New York, New York

Dedication

To my mother, Phyllis, who found the best in people, had compassion for all, and whose insight, guidance, and love have always made me believe that anything is possible.

Paul Tornetta III, MD

Preface

Injury is a leading cause of death in the United States in all age groups. Disability following injury is estimated to cost society more than 200 billion dollars annually. The treatment of injured persons is one of the most important areas of orthopaedic surgery from a societal perspective. Improving techniques in treating fractures gives patients the best opportunity to return to function, including work and personal activities. Even common fractures can lead to significant disability. Most orthopaedic surgeons treat patients with fractures on a regular basis. This volume of *Instructional Course Lectures* includes work in the areas of upper extremity trauma, lower extremity trauma, pelvic and acetabular trauma, and care of the trauma patient. The expert commentary provided by OTA members preceding the articles give insight into their importance. I hope that you enjoy this volume and that it adds to your current practices.

Paul Tornetta III, MD
President
Orthopaedic Trauma Association

Contents

Section 2 Lower Extremity Trauma

Section 3 Pelvic and Acetabular Trauma

Section 4 Care of the Trauma Patient

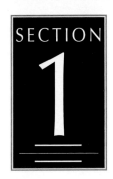

SECTION 1

Upper Extremity Trauma

Upper Extremity Trauma

The upper extremity provides one of our most important means for interacting with the external world and as such is often injured. Capable of generating great forces, as well as affording exquisite dexterity, the upper extremity is a highly adapted instrument of performance, sensation, and expression. For this reason, even relatively minor injuries can cause a period of significant disability, and more severe injuries can be life-changing events that can end careers or limit an individual's ability to live an independent life.

The treatment of upper extremity injuries continues to improve and mirrors advances in bone fixation and microsurgical techniques. We also better understand the need to minimize soft-tissue damage and start early range of motion under the direction of a trained physical therapist. Nevertheless, functional outcomes after even common injuries such as distal radius fractures are by no means uniform, and treatment recommendations continue to be refined.

The articles in this section are important because they summarize our best and most current understanding of how to manage a broad array of both routine and complex injuries involving the upper extremity. The expectation is that this information represents only a point on an ongoing trajectory of knowledge and that treatment recommendations will continue to evolve as we strive to improve functional outcomes and shorten periods of disability.

In the first article, Amit Gupta and associates present an excellent overview of managing the severely injured upper extremity. They outline the most current reconstructive ladder for managing complex bony and soft-tissue injuries, including the concept of immediate wound excision and one-stage reconstruction with emergency regional flaps or free tissue transfers. Despite continued skepticism from traditionalists, they provide compelling clinical evidence that this technique improves outcomes, minimizes morbidity, and reduces the period of hospitalization. The authors also explore the decision-making process, which is often more important than the actual surgical techniques used, and they correctly point out the need for innovation and imagination when managing these complex injuries.

The next article by Alan Freeland and associates outlines specific techniques of treating common hand fractures. They clearly elucidate that management of hand fractures should be based on general principles rather than on specific implants and that although function generally follows form, it should be achieved with the least amount of injury to the soft tissues. I agree with their assertion that Kirschner wires remain the cornerstone of fixation in the hand, and although plate fixation may be indicated in certain circumstances, it carries a higher risk of complications, primarily joint stiffness and loss of tendon excursion.

In their article on the treatment of distal radial fractures, David Ruch and associates present an excellent overview of a common topic in which a clear consensus regarding surgical management remains elusive. They point out that consensus is lacking largely because most of the expansive literature on this subject is scientifically flawed. Unstable fracture patterns currently are treated with open reduction and internal fixation using a variety of different internal fixation devices, despite the fact that no one device has proved to be superior to any other in a methodologically sound randomized or cohort study without a conflict of interest. I think it is too soon to throw out the external fixator, but I agree that the newer volar locking plates ultimately may prove to be a better routine treatment option. Ongoing multicenter studies comparing these two approaches hopefully will provide an answer in the near future.

Following this article, Jesse Jupiter and Diego Fernandez discuss the treatment of distal radial malunion, which is the most common complication of distal radius fracture. They assert that impaired function rather than radiographic deformity is the reason to treat a malunion, and they provide a sound management algorithm. However, since their article was published in 2002, there has been a shift toward performing corrective osteotomies through a volar rather than a dorsal approach, using a volar locking plate for fixation. I believe that this change is a significant advance because it eliminates the extensor tendon irritation seen with even low-profile dorsal implants. Recent studies also suggest that bone substitutes may eventually eliminate the need for autograft when performing these surgeries.

Jupiter and Fernandez also present an excellent algorithm for treating disorders of the distal radial ulnar joint (DRUJ) following distal radius malunion, and their discussion is expanded in the article by David Lichtman and Atul Joshi. Their article also reviews recent advances in our understanding of the anatomy and complex kinematics of the DRUJ. The authors suggest that injuries to the triangular fibrocartilage complex and DRUJ can be considered a single entity representing a spectrum of instability, and they present a logical plan for managing common pathologies.

William Cooney's article presents a comprehensive approach to managing scaphoid fractures. These fractures typically occur in young athletes and have the potential to result in prolonged disability in an active subset of patients. One recent trend has been to treat minimally or nondisplaced scaphoid fractures with percutaneous screw fixation; this approach can eliminate the need for casting and allow an earlier return to activities. I agree that this is an important concept, and orthopaedic surgeons should be familiar with these techniques, although I

personally favor a mini-open dorsal approach for fixation of most acute fractures.

The article on difficult elbow fractures by Shawn O'Driscoll and associates is a key chapter in this section because the elbow is critical to the overall function of the upper extremity. The elbow positions the hand in space and preserves a functional arc of motion and is therefore essential. Arthrodesis is consequently untenable, and although arthroplasty is an excellent salvage procedure for a serious traumatic elbow injury in a low-demand elderly patient, it is not a good option in a young patient. The authors provide excellent details on how to manage difficult fracture patterns, with cogent tips on methods of exposure and newer fixation techniques. They also describe the use of metallic radial head implants, which provide reliable lateral support to the elbow; these implants are a recent advance that allows relatively routine treatment of terrible triad injuries, which historically have had very poor outcomes.

In their article on diaphyseal humerus fractures, Augusto Sarmiento and associates discuss the biology of fracture healing and remind us that nonsurgical treatment is quite adequate for most of these fractures. The indications for surgery also are reviewed, as are the options for fixation. Although randomized controlled trials comparing plate fixation with intramedullary devices have

produced contradictory results, the authors make a sound argument as to why plate fixation remains the gold standard for open reduction and internal fixation of the humeral shaft.

In the article that follows, Joseph Iannotti and associates review the management of proximal humerus fractures. These authors recognize that most of these fractures also can be managed nonsurgically, but they include a discussion of surgical management of appropriate fracture patterns. The recent emphasis on minimally invasive techniques, which decrease the risk of vascular insult to the humeral head and minimize periarticular scarring, are given particular emphasis.

Dovetailing with this section is the brief article by Wesley Phipatanakul and Tom Norris on the indications for prosthetic replacement in proximal humerus fractures. Given that the outcome of late prosthetic reconstruction is inferior to early prosthetic management, appropriate initial decision making is critical. The authors describe the classic fracture patterns and patient factors best suited for hemiarthroplasty, emphasizing, as in the previous section, that a valgus impacted four-part fracture must be distinguished from a standard four-part fracture because the former is readily amenable to open reduction and internal fixation.

Trauma to the upper extremity is typically associated with significant disability. The goal of treatment, then, is to minimize the period of disability while providing for the most complete return of function. This collection of articles provides an excellent overview of how to assess, manage, and rehabilitate a broad range of common traumatic injuries to the upper extremity.

Nevertheless, despite the considerable advances that have been made in the treatment of these injuries, outcomes after even simple injuries are not consistently good. Future directions promise better fixation devices, biologic agents to improve fracture healing or reduce periarticular and peritendinous adhesions, and improved prosthetics for joints that previously could not be reconstructed. The goal of the surgeon who treats these injuries should be to stay abreast of these advances and thoughtfully integrate them into the care of patients.

Andrew B. Stein, MD
Assistant Professor
Department of Orthopaedic Surgery
Boston University Medical Center
Boston, Massachusetts

1

Treatment of the Severely Injured Upper Extremity

Amit Gupta, MD, FRCS
Russell A. Shatford, MD
Thomas W. Wolff, MD
Tsu-Min Tsai, MD
Luis R. Scheker, MD
L. Scott Levin, MD

The human hand is a supremely adaptable organ of prehension, sensation, expression, and communication. With its complex, integrated structures of skin, muscles, tendons, nerves, vessels, bones, and joints, the hand allows people to explore their environment, care for themselves, and earn a living. To watch a virtuoso pianist at work is to appreciate fully how the hand is capable of performing highly coordinated actions. The hand is so important as a tool and as a sensory organ that it could be claimed that the primary function of the upper extremity is to position the hand in space. Injuries of the upper extremity thus have a direct bearing on the function, sensation, and movement of the hand.

The upper extremity, our interface with the external world, is subjected to the forces of the world and is easily injured. Such injuries—industrial, agricultural, domestic, or vehicular—disrupt the fine, intricately balanced anatomy of the structurally complex and functionally adaptable hand and can devastate the life and livelihood of the injured person. For many patients, such as laborers, musicians, carpenters, surgeons, and dentists, loss of hand function means loss of a career. However, advances in the patho-physiology of tissue trauma, microsurgery, antibiotics, and bone and tendon fixation techniques have enabled reconstructive surgeons to achieve better outcomes that maximize function and minimize disability for patients who have a severe injury of the upper extremity.[1]

In this chapter, we present our concept of immediate comprehensive treatment of such injuries. Our discussion includes assessment of the patient, classification of injuries, provisional preoperative planning, wound excision, definitive decision making, structural repair techniques, soft-tissue coverage, operative innovation and imagination in reconstruction, rehabilitation, and determinants of outcome.

Assessment

The first step in the treatment of an injury of the upper extremity is the assessment of the patient's condition—that is, the extent, severity, and nature of the injury—and the hospital resources available for the patient's care. Before all else, an assessment of the patient's life-threatening injuries is imperative. There is always the danger of being sidetracked by a visually striking, bloody, and mangled upper extremity and thus overlooking potentially life-threatening conditions in the abdomen, chest, or head.[2] Other areas to keep in mind are the pelvis, spinal cord, and lower extremities, especially in the presence of open fractures. A trauma team and an appropriately equipped trauma room are needed to assess multiply-injured patients adequately and safely according to the principles of the advanced trauma life-support procedure published by the American College of Surgeons.[3]

Once life-threatening injuries have been expeditiously and conclusively ruled out, attention should be turned to the assessment of the patient's overall condition. This assessment should include a medical history, with medications, habits, allergies, and previous surgeries and other types of treatment recorded. The patient's gender, age, hand dominance, profession, hobbies, wishes, and aspirations should be noted as well. The history should also include when the patient last received the tetanus toxoid vaccination, the preinjury functional capability, and previous injuries of the upper extremity. The examiner should particularly look for diseases or habits that might (1) affect the peripheral capillary circulation (atherosclerosis, diabetes mellitus, smoking, and abuse of cocaine or another drug), (2) increase the risk of infection (immunosuppression such as with steroids, a history of transplantation, acquired immunodeficiency syndrome, and skin diseases), (3) influence the choice and dose of medication such as antibiotic prophylaxis (drug allergies and renal or liver diseases), (4) determine the feasibility and outcome of postoperative rehabilitation (psychiatric disorders, mental retardation, and drug abuse), and (5) increase the risk of postoperative bleeding, hematoma formation, or thrombosis (intake of aspirin or another anticoagulant medication and hypercoagulable states).

Present Injury

Once the medical history has been recorded, attention is turned to obtaining information about the present injury. This information includes the time, place, mechanism, and nature of the injury.

The time elapsed from the injury or from the onset of ischemia affects the functional outcome of any reconstruction. There is a direct association between the duration of ischemia and the potential for compartment syndrome, the risk and severity of infection, and the feasibility of macroreplantation.

The environment where the injury was sustained affects the risk of infection. Mutilating hand injuries that occur as a result of farming accidents, for example, are associated with a high risk of bacterial contamination. Extensive contamination is also seen in injuries resulting from motor vehicle collisions, snowblowers, woodworking tools, and industrial machinery such as a punch press.[4]

The mechanism of injury can be associated with a specific constellation or pattern of injuries. The type of tissue damage can be somewhat anticipated if the cause of the injury is known. The type of machine or equipment, with specific details regarding the machine blades, the distance between the blades, and the

number of blades or rollers, is essential information. The possibility of pressure injection, including the pressure rating and the chemicals that were injected, needs to be determined.

The nature of the injury defines the amount of tissue that was injured around the wound. A sharp, clean incision damages tissue only locally and around the area of ischemia, whereas an avulsion wound injures a much greater length of vessels or nerves. A crush injury produces varying degrees of damaged tissue according to the distance from the center of the wound. A thermal injury produces 3 concentric zones of dead or injured tissue: a central zone of coagulation, which is surrounded by a stasis zone, which in turn is surrounded by a zone of hyperemia.[5] A chemical injury, especially a pressure injection injury, produces extensive damage along spaces and compartments. A degloving injury tends to produce distally based flaps that are ischemic for a longer distance than usually is anticipated.

Calm and warm surroundings, compassionate and confident behavior on the part of the examiner, and concern for the stability and comfort of the patient allow for an extensive evaluation of an injured extremity. Liberal use of pain medications is indicated. Keeping pain to a minimum may sometimes mean deferring the complete evaluation until the patient is under anesthesia. Nevertheless, there is some benefit in gathering as much information as humanely possible in the emergency room if this can be done quickly and with relatively little discomfort. The examiner has to assess the circulation and sensibility of the extremity as well as basic functions that indicate whether major nerves are intact. This information along with a preliminary radiographic survey allows for proper preparation of the operating-room staff and for proper planning of the procedure.

The next step in the evaluation of an injured upper extremity is a clinical assessment of different factors determin-

ing outcome. The examiner should note active bleeding, which of course needs to be controlled but also indicates adequate perfusion and vascularity; the extent of devascularization, which in turn defines the extent of the debridement and the revascularization that is needed; the status of the skin, as any reconstruction will be threatened without a stable envelope and accompanying soft-issue coverage; the posture of the fingers, which may indicate tendon injuries needing repair and which directly affects the outcome and treatment plan; any deformities signifying fractures or dislocations, which necessitate appropriate preparation and operative planning; and the location and extent of the wound, which, together with the posture of the extremity during the injury, indicates the structures that were most probably injured.

Diagnostic Modalities

After the clinical assessment, there are several diagnostic modalities that can be helpful in the treatment of an injury of the upper extremity. These include radiographs of the extremity and the amputated parts, which provide information about osseous injuries of the extremity and the content and condition of bone in the amputated part; stress radiographs or fluoroscopy, which assist in the diagnosis of a ligamentous injury or even a rupture; and perfusion monitors (such as Doppler flow monitors) and compartment-pressure monitors, which can give valuable information about the patency of a vessel or the adequacy of perfusion of a certain anatomic area or compartment.

Classification of Injuries

The classification of injuries allows the surgeon to assess the potential for complications such as wound infection and to plan the necessary operative procedure. Rank and associates[6] classified wounds as tidy and untidy. The tidy wounds included a simple cut in the skin, a slicing injury with loss of soft tissue, a guillotine amputation, and an incised wound involving tendon or nerve injury.

Gustilo and associates[7] proposed the widely accepted fracture classification bearing Gustillo's name. In this system, type I indicates an open fracture with a clean wound that is less than 1cm long; type II, an open fracture with a wound that is more than 1 cm long without extensive soft-tissue damage; and type III, an open fracture with extensive soft-tissue damage. Type III injuries are subdivided into type IIIA (adequate soft-tissue coverage), type IIIB (periosteal stripping and exposure of bone, usually with massive contamination), and type IIIC (arterial injury necessitating repair). In this classification system, the importance of an adequate soft-tissue envelope and tissue perfusion is evident.

Büchler and Hastings[8] developed a different classification system that takes into consideration the so-called relevant structural systems of the upper extremity; these include bones, joints, extrinsic extensors, extrinsic flexors, intrinsic system, nerves, arterial blood supply, venous drainage, skin, and nails. They classified injuries as isolated (involving only 1 relevant structural system at a specific location) or combined (involving 2 or more relevant structural systems at a specific location). Combined injuries include crush injuries, volar combined injuries, extensive volar defects, dorsal combined injuries, and dorsal and volar combined injuries.

At our clinic, we modified this classification to include more details about the injury and to allow better communication between clinicians. Our classification system includes information on the location of the wound, with a letter indicating the location on the upper extremity (A indicates the arm; E, the elbow; F, the forearm; W, the wrist; H, the hand; and D, a digit) and a number (1 through 5) indicating the digit. The system also classifies the adequacy of the circulation (i indicates adequate and ii indicates

inadequate). The injuries are also defined as isolated (I), combined (II), or complete amputations (III). Isolated injuries can be closed (a) or open (b), and combined injuries can be dorsal (A), palmar (B), or dorsal and palmar (C). Thus, according to this classification system, a devascularized ring finger with flexor tendon and osseous injury would be classified as D4IIBii, a palmar laceration of the wrist with good circulation and cut flexor tendons and nerves would be classified as WIIBi, and an amputation of the forearm would be classified as FIII.

Provisional Preoperative Planning

It is important to have a thorough understanding of the soft-tissue injury when treating a mangled upper extremity. An evaluation that includes radiographs should be performed to assess the skeleton for injury patterns. When interpreting radiographs, the examiner should note the soft-tissue shadows to assess osseous devascularization. It is also necessary to assess bone loss, comminution of fracture fragments, dislocation, and whether there are injuries at multiple levels. The examiner must determine what implants should be selected and what functional loss might result from the destroyed joints and the amount of bone loss. All of these factors play a part in decisions about treatment.

Decisions with regard to anesthesia include whether to use regional block or general anesthesia. Regional anesthesia (axillary block) offers the specific advantages of vasodilation and postoperative pain control, but general anesthesia may be needed if the operative procedure is long, if the patient is uncooperative under regional anesthesia, if the regional block provides inadequate analgesia, or if an anesthesiologist who is experienced with axillary blocks is not available. Appropriate monitoring, such as with a Swan-Ganz catheter and an arterial line, should be used, particularly in elderly patients and for major limb injuries

where revascularization and blood shifts may cause hypotension, high lactate-acid loads, and cardiovascular stress.

When the operating room staff has been notified that a patient will be treated, the staff must be sure to have available the necessary equipment, such as an operating microscope, microsurgical instruments, fixation sets, and antibiotic bone spacers. Once the patient arrives in the operating room, appropriate communication with the operating room staff should include instructions regarding positioning of the table relative to the requirements for making radiographs, using operating microscopes, and performing fluoroscopy. Furthermore, the appropriate tourniquet should be applied to both the upper and the lower extremities, and the correct positioning should be determined by the type of free-tissue transfer that is needed. The patient is prepared and draped for the removal of vein grafts, nerve grafts, and skin grafts; for free tissue transfer; and for debridement of the extremity.

When amputation is a possibility, the operating team should be prepared for salvage of any structures from the amputated part, such as bone, skin, vessels, or nerves, that can be used not only to preserve the length of the injured upper extremity but also to provide material for grafts at other body sites in a patient who has sustained multiple injuries.

Wound Excision

Although every reconstructive surgeon has a clear concept of what is meant by thorough debridement, these concepts vary radically. There are, however, 2 basic strategies for debridement: serial debridement and wound excision (immediate debridement). Serial debridement removes only the tissue that is clearly dead. Wound excision, or immediate debridement, leaves only tissue that is clearly alive. A traditional serial debridement preserves questionably viable tissue in the hope that it is viable and will remain viable. However, serial debridement is the cause of many infections. A surgeon who uses this traditional and tentative approach endeavors to save a few strands of viable but probably functionless tissue at the risk of a devastating infection. Serial debridement also leaves open wounds that allow for desiccation of skin edges and bone ends. In addition, edema and granulation tissue can obscure the tissue planes and deeper structures, making a decision about their viability difficult. Furthermore, the wound resulting from a serial debridement may be even larger than that after a debridement performed on the day of the injury.

In contrast, immediate extensive debridement involves the removal of all doubtfully viable tissue and extension of the excision to live bleeding tissue. Immediate debridement is better than serial (delayed) debridement because tissue planes are visible when the wound is fresh. We therefore prefer the term wound excision, which has the connotation of tumor excision. When completed, the wound should look like the site of a surgical tumor extirpation.

Wound excision is the most important step in the treatment of a severely injured upper extremity. Without a thorough debridement, none of the complex reconstructions that we will describe are possible or advisable. Therefore, it is imperative that wound excision be supervised by a senior surgeon and not be left to the most junior member of the team. The process should be carried out under loupe magnification and with tourniquet control.

Traditionally, one of the techniques used to determine the adequacy of debridement margins has been bleeding. Traditionalists, therefore, decry the use of a tourniquet for debridement. However, without a tourniquet, bleeding may obscure the field, placing vital structures at risk. Furthermore, bleeding from adjacent live tissue may make it appear that devitalized tissue is bleeding and there-

fore alive. Also, bleeding is not the only indicator of injured tissue. With careful examination under loupe magnification, healthy tissue is usually easily distinguished from injured tissue. The only exception is healthy tissue with a destroyed arterial supply. Here, assessment of bleeding is a useful adjunct. After thorough debridement, the tourniquet can be released or it can be briefly released and then reinflated. This staged release of the tourniquet allows the viability of all structures to be examined and wound excision to proceed without torrential bleeding obscuring the surgeon's view.

Wound excision after a mutilating injury of the upper extremity involves several decisions. The surgeon must decide how much to debride, how to debride, and when debridement should be carried out again. Wound excision should be performed centripetally, starting at the periphery of the wound and working toward its center. Two millimeters of skin edge should be excised to obtain arterial dermal bleeding. We sharply excise crushed and contaminated skin to yield clear, vertical skin edges. Skin bridges, which may carry precious venous drainage, are preserved if possible, particularly during debridement of digits. However, if the skin bridge gets in the way or in any way hampers the debridement, it should be excised. All nonviable tissue, except blood vessels and nerves, is cut back to bleeding viable tissue. Subcutaneous tissue that is soiled should be debrided back to healthy fat. Fascia should be excised when it has been avulsed from overlying muscle and shows no sign of vascularity. Muscle is debrided to the level of healthy-appearing muscle. Devascularized and avulsed muscles are excised to bleeding tissue. Epineurium that is soiled can be removed, leaving fascicles behind. Nerves with ground in contamination are debrided under higher magnification. Structurally relevant bone fragments are

preserved. If a bone segment is crushed and contaminated, however, it should be excised, thus shortening the bone in preparation for internal fixation. All bone devoid of soft-tissue attachments should be removed.

The tourniquet is elevated again, the wound is excised further, and then the tourniquet is released. This process is repeated 2 or 3 times. Every hidden pocket is explored. Any thrombosed veins should be excised, and blood vessels should be preserved for reconstruction of vascular inflow.

Irrigation is used for the most part to keep tissues moist, but extensive pulsatile lavage should not be a substitute for appropriate debridement. Often, extensive pulsatile lavage insufflates tissue planes and can be destructive rather than therapeutic. Therefore, once the wound is completely excised, it is irrigated with Ringer's lactate solution, with use of a bulb syringe. Pressure irrigation is not necessary.

Some surgeons, however, place almost complete reliance on wound lavage, particularly pulsatile lavage, to perform the debridement and minimally excise only the most obviously dead tissue visualized without magnification. Lavage can be efficacious. In one study, lavage removed 70% of the silicone sand rubbed into experimental wounds.[9] Although impressive, this finding means that 30% of the particles were not removed. Such a wound debridement, which leaves heavy contamination and devitalized tissue or bone, or both, followed by an excessively tight closure of injured skin is associated with a high rate of complications. The results of surgeries performed in this manner should not be considered perspicuous evidence against immediate reconstruction; they simply demonstrate that immediate reconstruction will not be successful if debridement is inadequate.

If debridement is definitive—that is, if normal tissue planes are encountered at all levels—then reconstruction of bone, tendons, nerves, vessels, and skin coverage can proceed unimpaired. When, despite the surgeon's best efforts, the adequacy of the debridement is uncertain, such as in the treatment of crush injuries, infections, fasciitis, and contusion, then a return to the operating room within 24 to 48 hours should be considered. After wound excision, forearm and hand compartments are released as necessary. Carpal tunnel release is done if there are signs of nerve compression. Then the surgeon can proceed with further reconstruction.

Definitive Decision Making

After wound excision, the treatment of impaired arterial, venous, or arterial and venous circulation in a mutilated upper extremity must be considered. Most important, it is necessary to determine whether there is arterial damage or arterial insufficiency. Second, venous outflow of the wound may be impaired or insufficient, such as in patients with a large skin avulsion injury that has a distally based flap. Often, dermal perfusion and inflow are adequate but outflow will restrict ultimate inflow, resulting in necrosis of the flap. There are times when both the arterial and the venous systems need to be reestablished. In major limb revascularization, it is often desirable to reestablish arterial inflow before venous outflow because of the increased accumulation of metabolites, lactate, and cell breakdown products that can be hazardous to the patient if immediate venous flow is reestablished without purging of the revascularized part.

At times, temporary shunting is desirable to reestablish blood flow in the setting of major limb devascularization or replantation. In some patients, restoration of blood flow, even temporarily, should be done before excision of tissue if large amounts of muscle are devascularized and the duration of warm ischemia is long. (A devascularized part placed in plastic and then on ice will have

less metabolic damage than a warm ischemic part that is not placed on ice.) Temporary shunting can be achieved with heparinized feeding tubes, Sundt shunts, or heparinized intravenous tubes. Arterial shunts should be established as quickly as possible to avoid prolonged muscle ischemia. Once arterial inflow has been reestablished, outflow is observed through cutaneous and deep veins. The anesthesiologist and the operating team need to be prepared for rapid blood loss and must monitor the patient carefully.

After the shunt has been established, debridement and provisional or definitive osseous stabilization can be performed. While the debridement and the stabilization are being performed, a separate team should be removing an autogenous reverse saphenous vein graft, which is usually used in revascularization procedures. Shunting should be considered if the duration of ischemia is greater than 4 hours or if debridement and stabilization will take longer than several hours. For optimum use of an interpositional vein graft, the graft should not be made too loose or too tight and, whenever possible, it should be routed so that it is under a major muscle group rather than through a wound. If revascularization is completed and the vein graft can be hidden, there is no need for emergency coverage with a free tissue transfer. However, if the vein graft that is used to revascularize a threatened limb is exposed, then emergency free tissue transfer is strongly preferred to cover that graft and thus to prevent it from becoming desiccated or from rupturing. Occasionally, venous-venous interpositional grafts are used as well. Superficial veins may have to be reconstructed in major replantations because venae comitantes alone may not be sufficient to decrease postoperative edema.

Decisions about wound closure follow the reconstructive ladder: simple closure, skin grafts, local flaps, regional flaps, pedicled flaps, and, finally, free flaps. The

decision between temporary closure with antibiotic beads, Epigard, pigskin, or Xeroform and definitive closure with full-thickness or split-thickness grafts can be made at the time of the final wound closure.

Structural Repair Techniques
Planning of the Reconstruction

The surgeon should consider all of the reconstructive options, including amputation. Amputation should not be considered a failure but the first step in the reconstruction. The decision to amputate requires a judgment on the part of the surgeon. If adequate wound excision will remove so much tissue that functional reconstruction would be impossible, then an amputation should be performed.

Several injury-severity scores have been designed to try to make the decision to reconstruct or amputate more objective. The mangled extremity severity score (MESS), which was designed for the lower extremity, has been used for the upper extremity as well.[10] However, because the upper extremity has much different functional requirements, the score is inadequate for rating of the upper extremity.

Skeletal Reconstruction

Skeletal stability is the basis for all other reconstructions. The importance of definitive stable bone fixation must be emphasized because the vascular and functioning neuromuscular units that join with the skeleton to form a reconstructed extremity rely on a stable skeleton. Skeletal stabilization allows the surgeon to fix and forget the bone and concentrate on the rehabilitation of the patient.

Open reduction and internal fixation has been established as the so-called gold standard in the treatment of closed displaced unstable fractures of the upper extremity, with the possible exception of some humeral diaphyseal fractures, for which bracing still has a role. However,

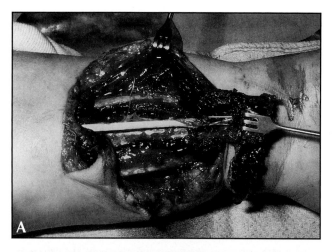
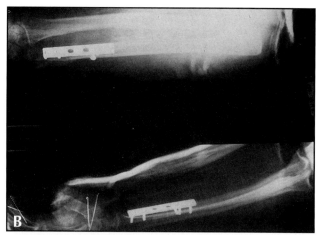
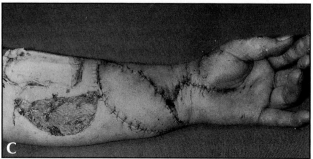
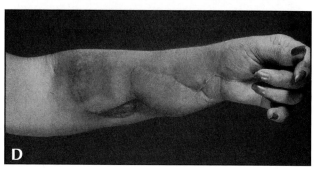
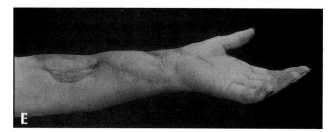

Fig. 1 A 43-year-old patient who sustained a fracture of the ulna with a large soft-tissue defect, muscle loss, injury of the radial artery, and exposure of the median nerve. **A,** Photograph showing the injured forearm. **B,** Radiographs showing plate fixation of the ulnar fracture. **C,** Photograph made after immediate coverage with a lateral arm flap. **D,** Photograph showing flexion. **E,** Photograph showing extension.

the treatment of open fractures is controversial.

The goals of treatment of open fractures include prevention of infection, stable fixation to allow early mobilization of joints and gliding of tendons, and achievement of union without deformity. The main impediment to treating open fractures in a manner similar to treating closed fractures stems from a fear of infection. Traditionally, the fear that devascularized, crushed, and contaminated bone fragments will lead to devastating infection and osteomyelitis has prompted the adoption of delayed primary closure, application of an external fixa-

tor, and delayed fracture treatment.

Fear of infection and nonunion after treatment of an open fracture is based on the experience with the lower extremity. In a series of 87 type III open fractures, Gustilo and associates[7,11] reported that 52% of the type IIIB fractures, 42% of the type IIIC fractures, and 4% of the type IIIA fractures were complicated by infection. Although the data of Gustilo and associates[7,11] included fractures of the upper extremity, there were only a few (only 5 radial and 3 ulnar type III fractures). Moed and associates[12] reported that 2 of 79 open fractures (3%) of the forearm were complicated by deep

wound infection. One of these fractures was type II and one was type III, as classified according to the system of Gustilo and Anderson.[11] Unpublished data from our center showed that, of 24 type III fractures (9 type IIIB and 15 type IIIC), none were complicated by deep infection or osteomyelitis (95% confidence interval, 0 to 11.7%) after treatment with open reduction, internal fixation, and immediate wound coverage (Fig. 1).

Nonunion is the other source of concern in the treatment of open fractures. Moed and associates[12] reported that nonunion occurred infrequently: only 7 of 79 fractures (3 of 19 type III fractures,

3 of 29 type II fractures (10%), and 1 of 31 type I fractures (3%)) went on to nonunion. In our unpublished series of 24 type III fractures of the forearm, 5 went on to nonunion (21%). Although no association was found between nonunion and the mechanism of injury, multifragmented fractures were prone to nonunion ($p < 0.0006$). There was also a trend toward more nonunions in the ulna than in the radius.

Even if external fixation is superior to internal fixation in the lower extremity, this does not mean that it is better in the upper extremity. The upper extremity differs from the lower extremity with regard to vascularity, functional requirements, and a greater ability to tolerate shortening. There are a number of disadvantages to using an external fixator in the upper extremity: the devices are bulky, they transfix muscles, they interfere with flap design and vascular access, and they cause joint stiffness. Moreover, it is difficult to use orthoses with external fixators. Also, in the forearm, it is extremely difficult to achieve and to maintain anatomic reduction of the radius and ulna, especially in the presence of comminuted or segmental fractures.

The other technique that we use extensively in the treatment of open fractures of the upper extremity is bone-shortening. Bone shortening, which the upper extremity is able to tolerate quite well, allows us to bypass a comminuted segment, thus avoiding complex internal fixation in crushed and devascularized segments. Moreover, by shortening bones, we can avoid vein grafts and nerve grafts in favor of end-to-end anastomoses of these structures. Meyer[13] pointed out that bone shortening was at least partially responsible for the overall good results of replantation in a combined series of patients from Shanghai, Louisville, and Zurich. This conclusion was reinforced by Axelrod and Büchler.[14] In our unpublished series of 24 type III fractures of the forearm, bone shortening was carried out

in 96% (23). The amount of bone shortening ranged from 0.5 to 2.5 cm, with an average of 1 cm.

Having outlined the rationale for our approach to open fractures of the upper extremity, we will discuss the bones individually because each bone possesses certain anatomic characteristics that require consideration before a surgery. If surgery for fixation is well reasoned and planned, the surgeon will encounter few setbacks; however, poorly planned fracture treatment with ad hoc intraoperative improvisations can prove frustrating and ineffective. All of our recommendations with regard to techniques are made with the assumption that adequate wound excision will be achieved first.

Humerus Treatment of the humerus involves several anatomic considerations. First, there is an intimate and integral association between the rotator cuff tendons and the proximal end of the humerus. Second, the distal fourth of the humerus is flattened anteroposteriorly, which greatly reduces the intramedullary diameter. Third, there are 4 major nerves (axillary, radial, ulnar, and musculocutaneous) associated with the humerus; the first 2 are vulnerable to injury during placement of locking screws. Fourth, there is a substantial soft-tissue envelope around the bone that increases the risk of pin-related problems if external fixation is used.

The first, second, and third considerations make the humerus anatomically unsuitable for locking intramedullary nailing. The third and fourth considerations increase the risk of complications associated with external fixation. The use of external fixators as a temporary measure is less than satisfactory because definitive fixation will require another procedure through a zone of injury with recently reconstructed nerves and vessels. Furthermore, if there is drainage about the pin tracks, a delay between removal of the fixator and definitive internal fixation is usually necessary.

In view of the problems and limita-

tions associated with the use of intramedullary devices and external fixators, our recommendation for the treatment of most diaphyseal humeral fractures in severely injured upper extremities is internal fixation with a 4.5-mm dynamic compression plate and screws. An extensile approach to the entire humerus is readily available and often facilitated by the soft-tissue injury. Open reduction and internal fixation of diaphyseal humeral fractures with a plate and screws allows debridement of crushed and devascularized bone segments and shortening in case of segmental bone loss. This protocol creates a simple fracture profile, sound rotational control, and stable interfragmentary fixation. The reconstruction of distal intra-articular fractures with interfragmentary compression and neutralizing reconstruction plates is unrivaled in terms of stability and restoration of anatomy, thereby facilitating early return of function.

Forearm Several anatomic considerations must be taken into account when treating the forearm. First, the radius and the ulna are 2 intimately linked bones, articulating with each other both proximally and distally and through the intervening interosseous membrane. The radius and the ulna are functionally interdependent. A structural or anatomic deficit of one is reflected by malfunction of the other. Accurate reduction of fractures of the forearm and subsequent maintenance with stable fixation are, therefore, vital in restoring rotation of the forearm.

Second, although the ulna is a relatively straight bone, the radius is not. Thus, stable internal fixation of the radius can be difficult if not impossible to achieve with intramedullary devices.

Third, there is an intimate relationship between the musculotendinous units and the underlying bones on the palmar and, especially, the dorsal surface of the distal part of the forearm. The tendons rub against or are trapped by pins

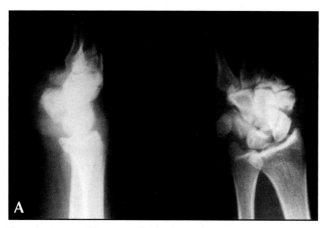 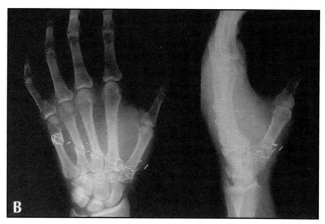

Fig. 2 A 30-year-old patient who had complete transmetacarpal amputation of all digits. **A,** Preoperative radiographs. **B,** Radiographs made after replantation, showing stable fixation of all metacarpals with 90-90 wiring.

used for external fixation. There are few problem-free areas in the soft tissue over the metaphysis of the distal part of the radius in which external pins can be placed safely.

The first and second considerations preclude the use of intramedullary devices in the forearm if the goal of treatment is early restoration of function without external splints. Furthermore, soft-tissue care in a severely injured limb is facilitated by the absence of external splints. The third consideration highlights the problems generated by external fixation. We think that external fixation has little place in the immediate treatment of fractures of the forearm except as a temporizing measure in patients with a single bone segmental defect for whom a delayed bone reconstruction is planned. The use of a 3.5-mm low-contact dynamic compression plate and screws gives predictable, accurate, stable, definitive fixation in patients with severe injuries and should be the fixation of choice for these difficult fractures. Sometimes, more than 1 plate may have to be used to stabilize segmental fractures.

Metacarpals The anatomic and biomechanical considerations in the treatment of metacarpals include the following. First, intact metacarpals lend stability to an adjacent broken one. The palmar sur-face does not lend itself to adequate exposure or the placement of a fixation device. Second, the dorsal surface is easily accessible but superficial. Bulky metal plates can be prominent and cause irritation of tendons. Third, some metacarpals have muscle and wrist tendon attachments that need careful protection to prevent entrapment. Fourth, accurate anatomic restoration of the mobile fourth and fifth metacarpal bases at the carpometacarpal joints is necessary to avoid a reduction of grip power. Fifth, during finger flexion, strong tensile forces act across the dorsal cortices of the metacarpals, generating, in turn, strong compressive forces on the palmar cortices of the metacarpals.

Stable fixation of diaphyseal fractures of the metacarpals is best achieved with plates and screws. In men and in women with large hands, 2.7- or 2.4-mm dynamic compression plates (dorsally placed because of the first, second, and fifth considerations) provide good, stable fixation. In small hands or in the treatment of uncomminuted fractures, 2.0-mm plates may suffice. Fractures of the bases of metacarpals can be treated effectively with interfragmentary screws supplemented with plates and screws. Occasionally, judiciously placed Kirschner wires (K-wires) will suffice.

In replantation, it is preferable not to undertake the extensive dissection necessary to place a plate and screws. Lister's method of wiring[15] or 90-90 wiring (placement of wires at 90° to each other) provides sufficient stability for early motion (Fig. 2).

Phalanges Treatment of the phalanges should be based on the following anatomic and biomechanical considerations. First, the extensor expansion is intimately related to the dorsum of the phalanx, thus allowing little room for metal plates or pins without interfering with tendon function. Second, metacarpophalangeal joints can be kept flexed for a few weeks without fear of joint stiffness because the eccentrically placed collateral ligaments are lengthened during flexion of the joint. Flexion of the metacarpophalangeal joint forms the basis for treatment of an unstable fracture of the proximal phalanx with the technique described by Belsky and associates.[16] Third, the collateral ligament attachment to the head of the proximal phalanx does not allow a great deal of error in the placement of a condylar plate or undue bulk of the plate. Fourth, there is no room for conventional dorsal plates in the middle phalanx because of the intimate relationship of the extensor mechanism. Fifth, the insertion of the extensor tendon to the base of the distal phalanx is close to the germinal matrix of the nail bed.

Displaced basal fractures of the proximal phalanx can be stabilized with the technique described by Belsky and associates;[16] with interfragmentary screws; or, in some situations, with a laterally placed condylar blade plate or a dorsal T-plate. Extensively comminuted segments should be excised and replaced with corticocancellous bone graft and a condylar blade-plate. Bone graft and a plate give immediate stability to the phalanx and allow for debridement of the crushed bone.

Displaced transverse fractures of the proximal phalanx without comminution can be firmly stabilized with sagittal interosseous wires (or 90-90 wires), supplemented, if necessary, with an oblique K-wire cut flush with the bone.[17] Spiral fractures of the proximal phalanx are best fixed with 1.5-mm interfragmentary screws. Fractures involving one condyle can be suitably stabilized with interfragmentary screws and an additional K-wire to control rotation. Bicondylar fractures are best treated with interfragmentary screws and a 1.5-mm condylar plate.

The treatment of fractures of the middle phalanx follows the same principles. If plate fixation is necessary, the plate should be placed laterally with minimum soft-tissue dissection. Early protected motion is essential. In replantations, extensive soft-tissue dissection is avoided, but stable bone fixation is carried out with the help of Lister's technique of wiring[15] or 90-90 wire. Terminal phalangeal fractures are stabilized with appropriately placed K-wires.

Joint Injuries

Major joint injuries are almost always more complex to reconstruct than are extra-articular fractures. Whereas bone from the iliac crest can be used to reconstruct the relatively small diaphyseal segments of the hand bones, joints are specialized tissue for which there are limited options, depending on the circumstances. Whichever option for joint reconstruction is chosen, it must be consistent with

the overall treatment of the extremity. The surgeon cannot plan to treat a severe intra-articular fracture of a metacarpophalangeal joint with early motion while at the same time planning to treat surrounding fractures of the same ray with immobilization. This is why the so-called balkanized treatment of injuries of the upper extremity, in which different services care for different structures, can lead to poor results. Optimum results are possible only if there is consideration of the rehabilitation needs of all structures by the entire team or if 1 person decides on the integrated management of the reconstruction.

Options for treatment of a joint injury include immobilization, open reduction and internal fixation, arthrodesis, soft-tissue arthroplasty, joint transfer, and prosthetic arthroplasty. Joint injuries with minimum displacement of the articular surface—especially those with minimum critical motion, such as the second carpometacarpal joint—are good candidates for consideration of immobilization. Unfortunately, immobilization of a severely injured upper extremity often leads to severe stiffness.

Open reduction and internal fixation is the best choice for a severely injured joint, as long as sufficient fragments are present (or replaceable) for reconstruction of the joint. Since immobilization of a joint, such as the metacarpophalangeal or proximal interphalangeal joint, is associated with increased morbidity, and since other injuries, such as those involving tendons, necessitate early motion, then joint fixation should be sufficiently stable to support early motion. In addition to the standard AO/ASIF armamentarium, absorbable K-wires placed through small cartilage or subchondral bone fragments, or both, allow for the anatomic reduction of articular surfaces without immobilization of the joint. Areas of pure cartilage loss cannot be reconstructed without obtaining cartilage-covered bone from another source.

However, if the subchondral bone remains bare, multiple small drill holes may lead to fibrocartilage filling in the gaps between the normal cartilage. Care must be taken to avoid burning the bone.

Sources of cartilage-covered bone for reconstruction include spare material such as a nonsalvageable digit. (This solution is less applicable to larger, more proximal joints such as the elbow.) If there is no appropriate spare material, sometimes a less critical joint, such as a toe joint, may be partially or completely removed to reconstruct a more critical joint. Khouri and associates[18] described the replacement of a proximal interphalangeal joint with a distal interphalangeal joint. Hastings and associates[19] used the dorsal lip of the hamate to reconstruct the volar lip of the proximal interphalangeal joint. Rib cartilage or subchondral bone has also been used to resurface joints.[20] As with any bone reconstruction, the field must be adequate for reconstruction. Once again, an impeccable debridement is the critical feature. Historically, bone fixation in the presence of inadequate debridement, particularly when coupled with a closure under tension of devitalized skin over devitalized contaminated tissue, has led to severe infections.

Arthrodesis is a useful technique, especially for joints that can lose motion without causing severe functional loss. The second and third carpometacarpal joints and, to a lesser extent, the distal interphalangeal joints are examples of joints that provide motion that is less critical to overall hand function, except in hands on which the highest demands are placed, such as those of a musician.

Soft-tissue arthroplasty is an option when the joint is not reconstructible, although better results can be expected in joints with lateral motion that is constrained by adjoining structures. An example is the metacarpophalangeal joints for which the other digits provide lateral stabilization. In joints without secondary stabilization, soft-tissue arthroplasty is more stable if a substantial portion of the joint remains intact, as is the case with an Eaton proximal interphalangeal joint arthroplasty.[21]

Joint transfer, such as the pedicled transfer of the distal interphalangeal joint to the proximal interphalangeal joint that was previously noted, can also be used to replace joints. Compatible joints from the foot are often transferred to the hand. Unfortunately, a good result of a transfer of a toe joint produces only 50% of normal motion. Such poor results differ little from those of an arthrodesis. Removal of the toe joint also creates an injury in a previously uninjured part of the body.

Complete joint transfers usually must be vascularized. Without vascularization, bone is eventually replaced by creeping substitution, but, until it is, the subchondral bone is unable to maintain the cartilage. Partial joint transfers, in contrast, allow some metabolic support of cartilage through joint fluid produced by the vascularized portion of the joint. Thus, we perform nonvascularized partial joint transfers but use vascularized complete joint transfers.

Prosthetic arthroplasty should be the solution for any joint injury that is not reconstructible. Unfortunately, prosthetic joints in the upper extremity are usually very poor options after injury. Although elbow prostheses continue to be improved and have some role in late reconstruction—particularly in an elbow on which low demands will be placed—they are far from ideal. Wrist prostheses have equivalent problems. Silicone metacarpophalangeal joint prostheses are an excellent short-term solution to the treatment of a hand on which an elderly rheumatoid patient will place low demands, but they are seldom satisfactory after an injury in a younger patient who will place high demands on the hand. Prostheses continue to be improved. An exciting development would be the availability of reliable off-the-shelf replacement parts.

Reconstruction of Blood Vessels

Whenever possible, we prefer to perform end-to-end vascular repair. However, when end-to-end arterial anastomosis is not possible, the next option is a vein graft. The radial and ulnar arteries can be reconstructed with use of a portion of the cephalic vein as a reversed vein graft, but only after it has been ensured that the vein has not been injured. Some surgeons have observed aneurysmal dilatations when arm veins have been used for reconstruction of major vessels. Aneurysmal dilatation occurs because these veins have thin walls. If aneurysmal dilatation is a real concern, then a reversed saphenous vein graft should be used. It is imperative that there is a good size match between the vessels. Sometimes, a flow-through free flap may be used to provide soft-tissue coverage and, at the same time, vascular inflow to the distal portion.

The superficial palmar arch is a challenge for reconstruction. There are a few options, including (1) the subscapular-thoracodorsal complex, which provides, through its many branches, an ingenious method of reconstructing the arch; (2) a reversed vein graft from the dorsal venous arch of the foot, although this should be avoided if a toe transfer may be used later; and (3) a reversed saphenous vein graft connected to either the radial or the ulnar artery, with the common digital arteries anastomosed, end to side, to the vein graft. If a flow-through vessel along with a long segment of bone is needed for reconstruction, the peroneal artery is an ideal graft (Fig. 3).

Tendon Reconstruction

The treatment of tendon injuries depends on multiple factors, some of which are interdependent. These factors include the location of the injury; whether the injury is to the flexor system, the extensor system, or both the flexors and the extensors; the nature and severity of the associated injuries; and the effect of these other injuries on the rehabilitation plan.

There are considerable anatomic differences between the flexor system and the extensor system. The extensor system is anatomically much more complex than the flexor system. Distal to the metacarpophalangeal joint, the extensor mechanism is an extremely complex system that allows multiple muscles to delicately balance 3 joints (the metacarpophalangeal, proximal interphalangeal, and distal interphalangeal joints), providing stability, strength, and motion. This complexity makes the extensor mechanism virtually impossible to reconstruct with current operative techniques. Nevertheless, dogma has it that almost all extensor repairs do well and that these repairs can be relegated to the most junior surgeon available. The actual results are not as uniformly excellent as this view holds;[22] however, the limited excursion of the extensor system and the power of the flexor system can yield imperfect results that satisfy some patients.

Conceptually, the flexor system is a simple cable between muscle and bone. However, the large amount of excursion that is required makes any dense scar tissue potentially disabling. Smooth tendon gliding is especially critical where the tolerances are very fine, as in zone II, thus making flexor tendon injuries difficult to treat. (The extensor tendons can have similar problems in zone VII, the extensor retinaculum.) In general, the more severe the injury of the tendon, the greater the importance of early motion. If there is a severe abrasion of the flexor tendon within zone II, early motion is critical to prevent dense scar tissue from forming throughout the sheath and virtually immobilizing the hand. This is even more critical when there are osseous injuries to the floor of the sheath as well.

Of all of the variables affecting the outcome of operative treatment of tendons, the level of the injury, the extent of the injury, and the associated injuries

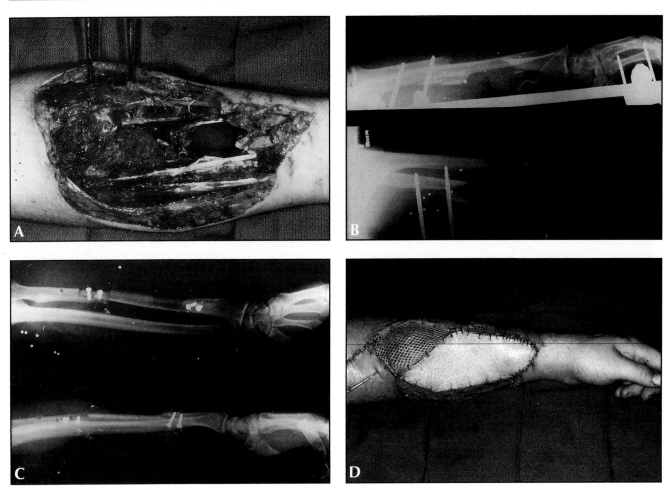

Fig. 3 A 22-year-old patient who was referred from another facility after a gunshot wound to the forearm. **A,** Photograph showing the injured forearm. There was extensive loss of skin and other soft tissues, including the radial artery and the median nerve. **B,** Radiograph showing a large segmental defect in the radius. **C,** Radiographs made after a flow-through free fibular graft was used to reconstruct the radius. The peroneal artery was used to reconstruct the segmental defect in the radial artery. **D,** Photograph showing a skin paddle with a fibular flap covering the soft-tissue defect.

probably have the greatest influence. Although the specific repair for each tendon at each level is outside the focus of this discussion, some generalizations can be made. The overall starting goal for tendon reconstruction is sturdy anatomic reconstruction with early motion. Tendon injuries necessitate early protected motion with dynamic splints. The more severe the injury, the greater the importance of early protected motion. Early motion is even more important after the treatment of flexor tendon injuries than it is after the treatment of extensor injuries.

Anatomic reconstruction of tendons is best accomplished with primary repair. If tendon substance has been lost, then a tendon graft can be used. Tendons from nonusable parts are the first choice if it is not more useful to preserve them for tendon transfers. If the tendon is going to be discarded anyway and a graft is needed, the tendon should be used. A tendon graft can also be obtained from standard sites for obtaining such grafts. The ipsilateral palmaris longus is the most commonly used donor tendon, although greater length is often needed and the ipsilateral palmaris longus may serve a

more important use later as a tendon transfer. Other sources of grafts include the contralateral palmaris longus and the plantaris and long extensors of the toes. Usually, we leave the great toe extensor because of its importance and only take the extensor digitorum longus from the toes that will extend through the extensor brevis—that is, the second, third, and fourth toes.

Tendon transfers, either primary or secondary, are another alternative. Despite our advocacy of primary reconstruction, tendon transfers should be done with caution in the period immediately after the injury. In general, we wait to reevaluate the patient until it becomes clearer what deficits will be present. Secondary tendon transfers can then be done.

In those rare cases in which early motion cannot be achieved because of other injuries, staged reconstruction with silicone tendon rods should be considered. This procedure is particularly beneficial in a patient who has a severe multiple-level injury involving the flexor tendons in zone II as well as other structures. In flexor tendon injuries in zone II, immobilized flexor tendons and sheaths fuse into one large scar mat. A late tenolysis would be of unlikely benefit and might harm other critical structures, such as nerves and arteries encased in the same scar.

Assuming that motion is possible, postoperative rehabilitation should include protection of the tendon repair with dynamic splinting to allow for motion but to minimize traction on the repair site. Splinting is more complex with combined extensor and flexor surface injuries. In patients with such injuries, the tendon repair that is the weakest and the one that would be most difficult to repair secondarily should receive the most protection. Usually, light extensor traction can be used, depending on the level of the injury.

Regardless of how the injury is treated, and even when the hand cannot be mobilized early, it is necessary to avoid the intrinsic minus position (extension of the metacarpophalangeal joints and flexion of the proximal and distal interphalangeal joints). This is particularly true if stiffness is inevitable, as it is following most severe injuries. The proximal interphalangeal joint has a propensity for flexion contracture, which, once fully developed, may be highly resistant to therapy. It is also preferable to maintain flexion of the metacarpophalangeal joints as extension contracture of these joints is often resistant to therapy.

Nerve Reconstruction

Of all of the facets of upper extremity reconstruction, nerve reconstruction is the most difficult. Although techniques for reconstruction of joints and tendons may be imperfect, excellent results are frequently achieved. In contrast, despite elegant research by many investigators, nerve reconstruction in adults virtually never restores preinjury function, even when the patient had a clean, sharp laceration, the most favorable of injuries. Severe traction injuries, with diffuse injury and a large nerve gap, have a much worse prognosis.

Wherever possible, nerve reconstruction is performed by simple neurorrhaphy (the nerve ends held together by 9-0 epineural sutures) if this can be done without excessive tension. In the special case of ulnar nerve injuries about the elbow, extra length can be gained by transposing the nerve. Short distances between nerves can be bridged by conduits, so-called artificial nerves such as inverted vein, silicone, and absorbable tubes.

The current standard option for the reconstruction of longer nerve gaps is with nerve grafts. Although vascularized nerve grafts can be used, there is no clear proof that they are superior. Nonvascularized grafts must be of relatively small diameter to allow for nutrition from the surrounding bed. Clearly, the surrounding bed must be capable of supplying that nutrition. Furthermore, removal of the nerve for the graft should leave a minimum deficit. Local sensory nerves such as the medial antebrachial cutaneous and lateral antebrachial cutaneous nerves can be used, especially if they have been lacerated proximally. The posterior interosseus nerve at the wrist can be removed with relative impunity, although the resulting graft is marginally sufficient to reconstruct a short segment of digital nerve. Sometimes, if use of a free flap such as the lateral arm flap is planned, sensory nerves that traverse the flap can be used as grafts. The sural nerve remains an excellent source for long fibers, and removal results in minimum disability.

Once again, the quality of debridement and the advantages of immediate reconstruction must be considered when deciding whether to perform an immediate reconstruction of nerves. If the wound is impeccable with a well vascularized bed, there is no deterrent to immediate nerve grafting. If there is a slight concern about the bed, the decision of whether to graft may depend on the source of the nerve graft. For instance, the surgeon may not wish to consume a virtually irreplaceable resource, such as the sural nerve, and may choose to delay the reconstruction. However, unless the wound bed is bleak, it is not reasonable to throw away badly needed nerve graft from a nonsalvageable finger.

Soft-Tissue Coverage

The goals of soft-tissue management are to protect vulnerable structures such as vessels (particularly grafts), vessel anastomoses, nerves, and tendons that may desiccate. Furthermore, that protection or coverage should not add to the disability by limiting hand function. Thus, soft-tissue coverage should provide maximum comfort and not restrict the range or power of motion as some burn scars do. Ideally, soft-tissue coverage should be sensate (this is less important proximally than distally) and cosmetically acceptable to the patient.

Although it is difficult to achieve all of these goals, a pragmatic approach is to choose the procedure that will result in the lowest morbidity and provide reasonable coverage with viable skin under reasonable tension. The reconstructive ladder helps to organize the treatment options into simple closure, skin grafts, local flaps, regional flaps, pedicled flaps, and free flaps.[23] Simple closure is the obvious choice whenever it can reasonably be done. However, when there is a severe injury of the upper extremity without bone shortening, primary closure is often impossible.

Skin grafts are the next simplest type of coverage. Traditionally, skin grafts are either split-thickness or full-thickness, with thinner grafts having more contraction. Contraction can often be desirable, as it shrinks the wound and pulls normal sensate skin in around the graft. However, grafts that are much thinner than 0.008 in (0.02 cm) are difficult to handle. Full-thickness grafts produce better-quality skin, but they have more difficulty surviving initially. They also produce a donor defect that requires closure. Thicker grafts are usually reserved for large defects of glabrous skin with an excellent bed.

Most grafts are meshed to prevent loss of the graft owing to the development of seromas. However, the graft can also be placed as a sheet graft with small holes, or so-called pie crusting, for drainage of seromas, although pie crusting is rarely as effective as meshing for drainage. Sheet grafts are considered more cosmetically pleasing, although some argue that the minor differences between an unstretched mesh graft and a sheet graft are unimportant in the upper extremity. It is universally agreed that a stretched mesh graft is cosmetically inferior to a sheet graft with equal take. This is particularly true as the mesh ratio increases beyond 1.5:1.

Since skin grafts require nutrition from the surrounding tissue, the underlying bed must be reasonably healthy. Skin grafts will not take over large areas of denuded bone or tendon. Skin grafts may bridge small (less than 1 cm wide) areas of denuded bone or tendon, but they do not always do so. In some cases, although the skin graft takes, coverage is suboptimum. Skin grafts provide limited protection. They can be used to cover vascular anastomoses, long vein grafts, and neurorrhaphy sites; however, they do not provide optimum coverage, especially if the plan is to excise the graft later.

Even if a graft takes by bridging prominent hardware, this will not provide a permanent solution. A skin graft is a particularly poor choice for coverage if secondary reconstruction such as tendon reconstruction, tendon transfer, or tenolysis will be performed.

Use of a local flap is the logical next step if a skin graft cannot be employed. Local flaps include, among others, the V-Y,[24] rotation, transposition, and cross-finger flaps; the flaps described by Moberg,[25] Foucher and associates,[26–28] Büchler and Frey,[29] Venkataswami and Subramanian[30] (and Evans and Martin[31]), and Quaba and Davison;[32] and their variations. Although these flaps are very useful in the treatment of injuries of the fingers, most are too small to be used in the treatment of more extensive injuries of the upper extremity.

Regional flaps have a greater role in the treatment of severe injuries of the upper extremity. The reversed radial forearm flap is the most commonly used regional flap and has the advantages of being thin and pliable. The disadvantage is loss of one of the 2 major arteries to the hand. Clearly, the reversed radial forearm flap would be a poor choice in a patient who had destruction of the ulnar artery, injury of the palmar arch, or an incomplete arch as shown by the Allen test. We rarely use the radial artery flap because we want to avoid damaging the circulation in an already damaged extremity. However, the radial forearm flap is the first choice of some hand surgeons.

The ulnar artery flap is the mirror flap of the reversed radial artery flap. Because the ulnar artery is considered the dominant vessel, the ulnar artery flap is much less commonly used. All of the prohibitions against using the reversed radial forearm flap apply to the ulnar artery flap.

The posterior interosseous flap[33] is pedicled on a reversed posterior interosseous vascular bundle with perfusion from a distal anastomosis between the posterior and anterior interosseous arteries. The flap described by Becker and Gilbert[34] is based on a distal ulnar artery perforator that is used to pivot distal forearm skin onto the hand. Both of these flaps have the advantage of sparing the radial and ulnar arteries. The radial artery and posterior interosseous flaps can also be used as free flaps.

Distant flaps, either pedicled or free, are used if none of the already described solutions are acceptable. The most frequently used pedicle flap is the groin flap, which is an axial pattern flap. However, random flaps from the abdomen or thorax can also be used. Because these flaps require 2 to 3 weeks for a new blood supply to develop from the skin into which they are inset, they have tended to be eclipsed by the use of free flaps. Certainly, there is a real potential for shoulder stiffness when pedicle flaps immobilize the extremity, particularly in an older patient who sustained even mild trauma to the shoulder at the time of the injury of the upper extremity. Other disadvantages of pedicled flaps include the obvious annoyance to the patient of having the hand attached to the body, the dependent position that the hand assumes, and the difficulty with performing therapy and allowing for early motion.

Nevertheless, pedicled flaps, either ipsilateral or contralateral to the injury, remain a very useful technique depending on the geography of the wound. The pedicled groin flap may be the initial choice for patients who have suboptimum vascular access in the extremity. The pedicled groin flap is an excellent fallback when free flaps have failed. Thus, the option of using the pedicled groin flap should be preserved, even when use of a free flap is planned. One condition under which the pedicled groin flap may be the preferred choice is when a toe-to-thumb transfer is planned at a later date. The pedicled groin flap does not consume vascular access, produces a good soft-tissue tube, and allows

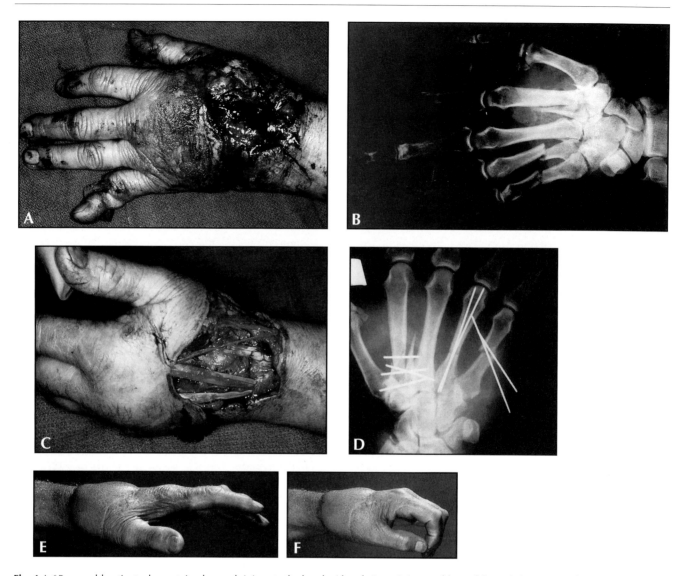

Fig. 4 A 65-year-old patient who sustained a crush injury to the hand with soft-tissue injury and loss of the radial artery. **A,** Photograph showing the injured hand. **B,** Radiograph showing multiple metacarpal fractures. **C,** Photograph showing the hand after debridement. **D,** Radiograph made after internal fixation. **E,** Photograph showing extension with a lateral arm flap covering the defect. **F,** Photograph showing flexion with a lateral arm flap covering the defect.

incisions to be made without having to compromise the incision to preserve the pedicle.

The list of possible free flaps for reconstruction of the upper extremity is long. However, from a practical standpoint, a few so-called standard flaps are used most of the time. These standard flaps vary from institution to institution and depend on local preference. In Louisville, the lateral arm, latissimus, and scapular flaps are mainly used, with the rectus, groin, and serratus flaps used less frequently.[35] Each flap has specific advantages and disadvantages in terms of position of removal, size, thickness, pedicle length, and donor defect. We most commonly use the lateral arm flap (Fig. 4). The site of removal can usually be closed if the width is less than 6 cm, and flaps of more than 20 cm in length can be obtained by extending the flap as much as 10 cm distal to the lateral epicondyle.

Immediate Reconstruction

Reconstruction can be performed in either a delayed or an immediate fashion. Traditional treatment consists of serial debridement and delayed reconstruction. Although this is a useful approach and is the fallback technique, immediate reconstruction combines debridement, reconstruction, and coverage into a single surgery. One-stage treatment, particularly in its most extreme form (the emergency free flap), is strongly rejected by traditionalists, who think that there is no advantage but considerable additional morbidity to such an approach.

It is true that, from a logical standpoint, serial debridement should result in the greatest conservation of tissue. If only the absolutely dead tissue is removed, marginal tissue has the chance to recover and be saved. Serial debridement also allows time for quantitative results of cultures, although there is no proved advantage to these cultures.[36] Serial debridement leaves vital structures exposed, leading to desiccation of vulnerable tendons, nerves, and vessels. Surrounding these vulnerable structures with viable healthy tissue as soon as possible may contribute to the survival of marginal critical structures.[37]

The perception of increased morbidity associated with immediate reconstruction is historically based on experience almost solely with the lower extremity. However, beliefs regarding treatment of the lower extremity, whether accurate or not, cannot be blindly transferred to the upper extremity. The upper extremity has entirely different functional requirements, in terms of power, motion, stability, and sensibility, than the lower extremity.

Traditional treatment also is steeped in wartime traditions. On the battlefield, where an unlimited number of casualties can be expected, it is not possible to commit all available resources to 1 patient. Le Maitre, who is responsible for the modern conception of excisional debridement, noted that thorough debridement could be done only between battles.[38] The circumstances surrounding the injury also play a role. For example, in World War I, debilitated soldiers, lying wounded for many hours in the manure-impregnated battlefields of Flanders and then managed with inadequate debridement and tight closure of nonviable skin, invariably had severe wound infections. This experience from The Great War developed into a prohibition against immediate reconstruction and coverage.

Flying in the face of this prohibition is replantation. A replant is a devascularized open fracture with tendon, nerve, and arterial injury, yet the treatment is thorough debridement, osteosynthesis, tendon repair, revascularization, nerve repair, and closure. In reality, a replant is nothing more than a badly obtained contaminated composite free flap with a long duration of ischemia.

The perception of increased morbidity from immediate reconstruction is refuted by data from multiple reports showing that emergency free flaps can be done with a high success rate and low morbidity. Furthermore, immediate reconstruction reduces the number of surgeries, rehabilitation time, and overall cost.[39]

In the mid 1980s, Godina[40] reported the results of free-flap procedures that had been done within 72 hours (usually within 24 hours) and compared them with the results of delayed reconstruction. He reported a failure after 0.7% (1) of 134 free flap procedures done within 72 hours, 12.0% (20) of 167 done between 72 hours and 3 months, and 9.5% (22) of 231 done after more than 3 months. An infection developed after 1.5% (2) of the flap procedures done within 72 hours, 17.4% (29) of those done between 72 hours and 3 months, and 6.1% (14) of those done after more than 3 months. The number of surgeries and the duration of the hospital stay were dramatically reduced for the group that had the immediate flap procedure.

The initial results of emergency free flap procedures performed in Louisville were reported in 1988.[41] Thirty-one emergency free flap procedures were done within 24 hours after the injury, and the only complications were 2 infections (6%) and 1 loss of a flap due to infection. Similar results have been obtained in China[42] and Austria.[43]

Since the published 1988 study, we have tracked the results of emergency free flap procedures at our clinic. In a sample of 95 emergency free flaps used in

a group that included 40 severe open fractures, 8 flaps were reexplored for thrombosis and 2 were lost (a 98% rate of survival). The average duration of hospitalization was 11 days (range, 4 to 50 days), and an average of 1.7 procedures were performed. There were 14 infections, although the definition of infection was not uniform. Seven of the infections followed the treatment of open fractures. There was no osteomyelitis and no limb loss from infection.

Despite these good results reported from multiple centers, immediate reconstruction in general and immediate free flaps in particular remain underused. Anecdotes of disastrous consequences of coverage of contaminated wounds are recounted as the reason to avoid emergency free flaps. However, many of the procedures described in these anecdotes were not performed with the precepts defined here; that is, they were done without thorough debridement and tension-free closure of healthy skin.

Our conviction is that most severe injuries benefit greatly from immediate reconstruction (Fig. 5). Immediate reconstruction offers the best chance for the least residual functional deficit by allowing for early motion. Even for those who remain unconvinced by the evidence in favor of early motion, the low morbidity, decreased duration of hospitalization, and lower costs should be important considerations.

However, immediate reconstruction is not indicated for all patients in all places under all circumstances. Serial debridement with delayed reconstruction has its place. The surgeon must be highly skilled to perform single-stage debridement and reconstruction, whereas serial debridement requires much less skill. Furthermore, adequate human resources must be available for immediate reconstruction. It is possible to start an extensive reconstruction with a free flap at midnight in a clinic with many staff surgeons and a large fellowship pro-

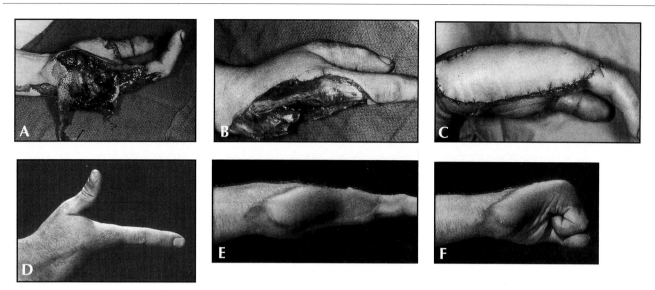

Fig. 5 A 21-year-old patient who fell asleep with the hand on a train track. **A,** Photograph showing the injured hand. **B,** Photograph made after debridement. **C,** Photograph made after immediate coverage with a lateral arm flap. **D,** Photograph showing the result of the procedure. **E,** Photograph showing extension. **F,** Photograph showing flexion.

gram, but this is much less realistic for the solo practitioner in a small hospital that needs its operating room available for other emergencies.

In addition, the patient must be a good candidate for the procedure. Severe multiple injuries often preclude a single, long reconstruction of less vital structures because the risks associated with anticoagulation are high. Although free flap procedures can be performed without anticoagulation, it is certainly helpful to have the option of anticoagulation in case problems with the free flap develop.

Immediate reconstruction is also a poor choice for certain types of wounds. Although almost all wounds can be debrided until they are clean, certain types of wounds, such as severe electrical burns and a large number of contaminated puncture wounds, sometimes cannot be adequately debrided. Immediate reconstruction also is not appropriate for infected wounds or for wounds for which amputation is the strongly preferred treatment.

Surgical Imagination and Innovation in Reconstruction

Much of the decision making with regard to reconstruction can be organized into a systematic approach. The first step is to determine whether a single-stage or multistage debridement will be performed. Second, if an adequate single-stage debridement has been performed, the surgeon should evaluate what structures are present, what structures were lost, and what structures are needed. Third, the reconstructive approach must be chosen, a decision that is greatly aided by surgical experience (either direct experience or that gathered from indirect sources such as mentors, texts, or the medical literature) and by knowledge of what kind of results can be expected from specific reconstructive procedures.

Although such a formal, organized approach is the key to obtaining the best possible results, the surgeon's imagination and innovation also are integral parts of decision making with regard to reconstruction. The need for imagination and

innovation is especially great when multiple structures are being reconstructed simultaneously or so that the use of material that would otherwise be discarded (from nonsalvageable digits, for example) can be maximized (Fig. 6).

Innovative problem solving cannot be formalized into a strict algorithm. However, innovative solutions often share some common features. First, the surgeon should consider a wide variety of options, ranging from the most intricate reconstruction to the most extreme ablative solution, primary amputation. The option that is chosen must provide the most function and the least disability. Second, any material that would otherwise be discarded should be carefully considered for possible uses, either for individual structures or for composite structures, either vascularized or nonvascularized (Fig. 7). Such material should be discarded only with the greatest miserly reluctance.

Third, the reconstruction should dovetail with the rehabilitative plan.

Although innovative thinking is cur-

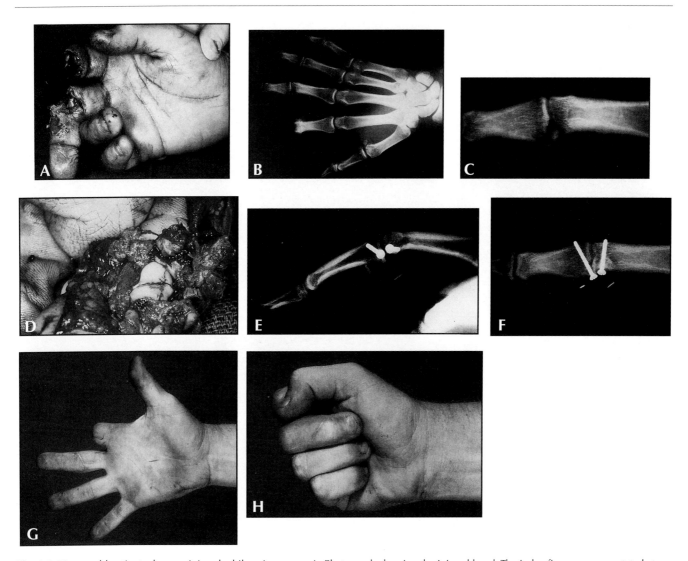

Fig. 6 A 30-year-old patient who was injured while using a saw. **A,** Photograph showing the injured hand. The index finger was amputated at the proximal interphalangeal joint; the amputated part was not replantable. The long finger was partially amputated with preservation of the ulnar digital artery and nerve. **B,** Radiograph showing the injured hand. **C,** Radiograph providing a close-up view of the proximal interphalangeal joint of the long finger, showing loss of the radial segment of the joint. **D,** Photograph made after the distal interphalangeal joint from the amputated index finger was used as a nonvascularized osteochondral graft to reconstruct the proximal interphalangeal joint of the long finger. **E and F,** Lateral and anteroposterior radiographs showing the completed reconstruction. **G and H,** Photographs showing excellent function after the reconstruction.

rently of great value for reconstruction after mutilating injuries of the upper extremity, future clinical breakthroughs may greatly simplify reconstruction if transplantation can be done with an acceptable rate of morbidity.

Rehabilitation

Decisions about rehabilitation are based on the extent of the injury, the stability of the osseous platform, and the structures that were repaired. Rehabilitation starts immediately in the operating room by the surgeon elevating the limb, placing the hand in the position of function, and optimizing the safe position of the hand. The principle is to do as much as possible as early as possible, but the motor-tendon units, joints, and fractures need to be monitored so that the fixation of these structures is not affected. Late reconstructive decisions, made months or even as long as a year after a mutilating injury, are based on the need for additional bone grafts, tendon transfers, tenolysis, provision of more stable coverage, neural grafts, and improving function. There is also a role for aesthetic aftercare with the use of tissue expanders and scar revisions that may be important to patients, partic-

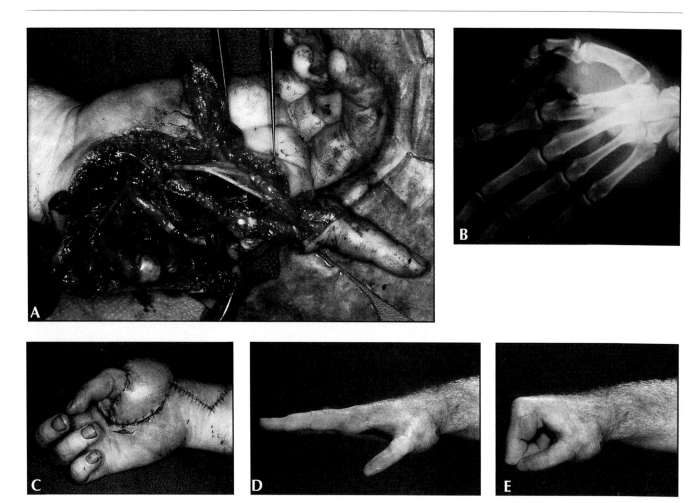

Fig. 7 A 41-year-old patient who sustained a punch-press injury to the hand. **A,** Photograph showing the injured hand. **B,** Radiograph showing the injured hand. **C,** Photograph showing the hand after surgery. The intact distal part of the index ray was pollicized, and the soft-tissue defect was covered with a lateral arm flap. **D,** Photograph showing extension. **E,** Photograph showing flexion.

ularly adolescent girls whose body image has been changed by a traumatic injury.

The extensive reconstruction that we described will surely fail unless it is matched by an efficient and structured rehabilitation program consisting of bracing, physical therapy, and occupational therapy. Each rehabilitation program must be individualized to the patient, the injury, and the reconstruction. The goal is early motion to ensure tendon-gliding and joint movement, which, in turn, reduces edema and subsequent stiffness.

For rehabilitation after combined palmar injuries, we use a modified version of the dynamic brace that was originally proposed by Kleinert and associates[44] and

modified by Werntz and associates.[45] If there is a distal ulnar-nerve lesion, however, this brace is contraindicated. In that situation, we consider a brace with a light extension assist and an active and assisted passive flexor protocol. For rehabilitation after combined dorsal lesions, we attempt to protect and to assist the extensor mechanism with an extension outrigger splint allowing for full active flexion. The extension outrigger can provide passive extension at the metacarpophalangeal or interphalangeal joint. When a patient has combined dorsal and palmar injuries, the extension outrigger is modified to provide both passive extension and early active flexion.

Early use of transcutaneous electrical nerve stimulation helps to prevent the onset of reflex sympathetic dystrophy in susceptible individuals. We also use external muscle stimulation before reinnervation of muscles and early strengthening programs to optimize the patient's return to work.

It is essential to note that patients do not block out severe trauma but remember the incident in great detail, returning to the moment of injury again and again in their minds. Patients grieve for missing parts and often suffer depression.[46] Many patients even remember the anniversary of the injury, reliving the event and often amplifying it in their minds. These patients need psychological assistance to help them let go of the constant preoccupation with the injury experience.

Determinants of Outcome
In our experience, the most important determinants of outcome have included the nature and severity of the injury, the reconstruction technique (with immediate reconstruction providing better results than multistage reconstruction[39]), the rehabilitation technique, and the patient's compliance.

Pitfalls and Complications of Treatment
The most important pitfall is improper assessment of the patient's general condition. Another important pitfall is poor judgment. A good treatment decision, such as a timely amputation, can quickly put a patient on the path to rehabilitation. However, it is easy to commit a patient to years of fruitless, frustrating, and expensive reconstruction. Inadequate wound excision is the major cause of complications such as deep infection leading to loss of a flap or to osteomyelitis.

Logistical support in terms of equipment and personnel, sophisticated training, and meticulous technique are important prerequisites for undertaking the reconstruction that we described. If these conditions cannot be met, such complex reconstruction should not be attempted. After stabilization, the patient should be transferred to a facility where the reconstruction can be carried out properly. Alternatively, the route of staged reconstruction could be chosen, albeit with the cost of lost function.

Adequate postoperative pain relief ensures the patient's cooperation with early mobilization programs. Moreover, pain relief reduces the likelihood of reflex sympathetic dystrophy developing. It is important to realize that poor rehabilitation affects the result of even the most brilliant reconstruction. The patient's compliance can be ensured with information, education, and compassion.

Overview
It is crucial to stress that the treatment protocol that we described is inherently a team approach with the surgeon as the team leader. It is the responsibility of the reconstructive surgeon to use so-called orthoplastic techniques—that is, state-of-the-art techniques of orthopaedic and plastic surgery—for structural restoration. Similarly, it is the surgeon's responsibility to make sure that the whole process, from the initial assessment of the patient to the final rehabilitation, is handled smoothly and professionally. All of the treatment decisions that were discussed in this chapter must be included in the surgeon's analysis, not weeks after, but at the time of, the mutilating injury.

Acknowledgment
The authors thank Stan Goldman, PhD, for his assistance in preparing this chapter for publication.

References
1. Scheker LR: Salvage of a mutilated hand, in Cohen M (ed): *Mastery of Plastic and Reconstructive Surgery.* Boston, MA, Little, Brown, 1994, vol 3, pp 1658–1681

2. Gupta A, Kleinert HE: Evaluating the injured hand. *Hand Clin* 1993;9:195–212.

3. Committee on Trauma of the American College of Surgeons: *Resources for the Optimal Care of the Injured Patient.* Chicago, IL, American College of Surgeons, 1990.

4. Gupta A, Wolff TW: Management of the mangled hand and forearm. *J Am Acad Orthop Surg* 1995;3:226–236.

5. Jackson DMG.: The diagnosis of the depth of burning. *Br J Surg* 1953;40:588–596.

6. Rank BK, Wakefield AR, Hueston JT: *Surgery of Repair as Applied to Hand Injuries,* ed 3. Edinburgh, Scotland, Churchill Livingstone, 1968, pp 3–14.

7. Gustilo RB, Mendoza RM, Williams DN: Problems in the management of type III (severe) open fractures: A new classification of type III open fractures. *J Trauma* 1984;24: 742–746.

8. Büchler U, Hastings H II: Combined injuries, in Green DP, Hotchkiss RN (eds): *Operative Hand Surgery,* ed 3. New York, NY, Churchill Livingstone, 1993, pp 1563–1585.

9. Nichter LS, Williams J: Ultrasonic wound debridement. *J Hand Surg* 1988;13A:142–146.

10. Johansen K, Daines M, Howey T, Helfet D, Hansen ST Jr: Objective criteria accurately predict amputation following lower extremity trauma. *J Trauma* 1990;30:568–573.

11. Gustilo RB, Anderson JT: Prevention of infection in the treatment of one thousand and twenty-five open fractures of long bones: Retrospective and prospective analyses. *J Bone Joint Surg* 1976;58A:453–458.

12. Moed BR, Kellam JF, Foster RJ, Tile M, Hansen ST Jr: Immediate internal fixation of open fractures of the diaphysis of the forearm. *J Bone Joint Surg* 1986;68A:1008–1017.

13. Meyer VE: Hand amputations proximal but close to the wrist joint: Prime candidates for reattachment (long-term functional results). *J Hand Surg* 1985;10A:989–991.

14. Axelrod TS, Büchler U: Severe complex injuries to the upper extremity: Revascularization and reimplantation. *J Hand Surg* 1991;16A:574–584.

15. Lister G: Interosseous wiring of the digital skeleton. *J Hand Surg* 1978;3:427–435.

16. Belsky MR, Eaton RG, Lane LB: Closed reduction and internal fixation of proximal phalangeal fractures. *J Hand Surg* 1984;9A:725–729.

17. Zimmerman NB, Weiland AJ: Ninety-ninety intraosseous wiring for internal fixation of the digital skeleton. *Orthopedics* 1989;12:99–104.

18. Khouri RK, Orbay JL, Badia A, Foucher G: PIP joint reconstruction with homodigital DIP joint transfer. Read at the Annual Meeting of the American Society for Surgery of the Hand, Denver, Colorado, Sept. 12, 1997.

19. Hastings H II, Capo JT, Steinberg B, Stern P: Hemicondylar hamate replacement arthroplasty (HHRA) for PIP fracture/dislocation. Read at the Annual Meeting of the American Society for Surgery of the Hand, Boston, Massachusetts, Sept. 3, 1999.

20. Takayama S, Nakao Y, Horiuchi Y, Itoh Y: Arthroplasty of MP and PIP joints using a chondroperichondrial graft. *Tech Hand Upper Extrem Surg* 1998;2:115–118.

21. Eaton RG, Malerich MM: Volar plate arthroplasty of the proximal interphalangeal joint: A review of ten years' experience. *J Hand Surg* 1980;5A:260–268.

22. Newport ML, Blair WF, Steyers CM Jr: Long-term results of extensor tendon repair. *J Hand Surg* 1990;15A:961–966.

23. Scheker LR: Soft-tissue defects of the upper limb, in Soutar DS (ed): *Microvascular Surgery and Free Tissue Transfer.* London, England, Edward Arnold, 1993, pp 63–77.

24. Atasoy E: Reversed cross-finger subcutaneous flap. *J Hand Surg* 1982;7:481–483.

25. Moberg E: Aspects of sensation in reconstructive surgery of the upper extremity. *J Bone Joint Surg* 1964;46A:817–825.

26. Foucher G, Braun JB: A new island flap transfer from the dorsum of the index to the thumb. *Plast Reconstr Surg* 1979;63:344–349.

27. Foucher G, Smith D, Pempinello C, Braun FM, Citron N: Homodigital neurovascular island flaps for digital pulp loss. *J Hand Surg* 1989;14B:204–208.

28. Foucher G, Citron N: The role of microvascular surgery in acute hand injuries, in Soutar DS (ed): *Microvascular Surgery and Free Tissue Transfer.* London, England, Edward Arnold, 1993, pp 54–62.

29. Büchler U, Frey HP: The dorsal middle phalangeal finger flap, in Gilbert A, Masquelet AC, Henetz VR (eds): *Pedicle Flaps of the Upper Limb: Vascular Anatomy, Surgical Technique and Current Indications.* Boston, MA, Little, Brown, & Company, 1992, pp 147–153.

30. Venkataswami R, Subramanian N: Oblique triangular flap: A new method of repair for oblique amputations of the fingertip and thumb. *Plast Reconstr Surg* 1980;66:296–300.

31. Evans DM, Martin DL: Step-advancement island flap for fingertip reconstruction. *Br J Plast Surg* 1988;41:105–111.

32. Quaba AA, Davison PM: The distally-based dorsal hand flap. *Br J Plast Surg* 1990;43:28–39.

33. Masquelet AC, Penteado CV: The posterior interosseous flap, in Gilbert A, Masquelet AC, Hentz VR (ed): *Pedicle Flaps of the Upper Limb: Vascular Anatomy, Surgical Technique and Current Indications.* Boston, MA, Little, Brown, & Company, 1992, pp 111–118.

34. Becker C, Gilbert A: The dorsal ulnar artery flap, in Gilbert A, Masquelet AC, Henetz VR (eds): *Pedicle Flaps of the Upper Limb: Vascular Anatomy, Surgical Technique and Current Indications.* Boston, MA, Little, Brown, & Company, 1992, pp 129–134.

35. Scheker LR, Kleinert HE, Hanel DP: Lateral arm composite tissue transfer to ipsilateral hand defects. *J Hand Surg* 1987;12A:665–672.

36. Breidenbach WC III: Emergency free tissue transfer for reconstruction of acute upper extremity wounds. *Clin Plast Surg* 1989;16:505–514.

37. Lukash FN, Zingaro EA, Salig J: The survival of free nonvascularized bone grafts in irradiated areas by wrapping in muscle flaps. *Plast Reconstr Surg* 1984;74:783–786.

38. Fackler ML: Misinterpretations concerning Larrey's methods of wound treatment. *Surg Gynecol Obstet* 1989;168:280–282.

39. Sundine M, Scheker LR: A comparison of immediate and staged reconstruction of the dorsum of the hand. *J Hand Surg* 1996;21B:216–221.

40. Godina M: Early microsurgical reconstruction of complex trauma of the extremities. *Plast Reconstr Surg* 1986;78:285–292.

41. Lister G, Scheker L: Emergency free flaps to the upper extremity. *J Hand Surg* 1988;13A:22–28.

42. Chen SH, Wei FC, Chen HC, Chuang CC, Noordhoff MS: Emergency free-flap transfer for reconstruction of acute complex extremity wounds. *Plast Reconstr Surg* 1992;89:882-888.

43. Ninkovic M, Deetjen H, Ohler K, Anderl H: Emergency free tissue transfer for severe upper extremity injuries. *J Hand Surg* 1995;20B:53–58.

44. Kleinert HE, Kutz JE, Ashbell TS: Primary repair of lacerated flexor tendons in "no man's land." *. Bone Joint Sur* 1967;49A:577.

45. Werntz JR, Chesher SP, Breidenbach WC, Kleinert HE, Bissonnette MA: A new dynamic splint for postoperative treatment of flexor tendon injury. *J Hand Surg* 1989;14A:559–566.

46. Kashani JH, Frank RG, Kashani SR, Wonderlich SA, Reid JC: Depression among amputees. *J Clin Psychiat* 1983;44:256–258.

Surgical Treatment of Common Displaced and Unstable Fractures of the Hand

Alan E. Freeland, MD

William B. Geissler, MD

Arnold-Peter C. Weiss, MD

The hand is an instrument of performance and protection. Whether at war, work, competition, or recreation, an individual's reflexes routinely place the hand in harm's way to protect the head and body. Accidents inevitably occur, resulting in fractures of the metacarpals and phalanges and other injuries. This chapter addresses, in particular, the craft of reduction and stabilization of displaced, irreducible, and unstable fractures of the hand as an integral part of reestablishing skeletal integrity and refined digital function. The goals of treatment include returning manual laborers to their work or to the practice of their special skills, professionals to their tasks, students to their classrooms, writers to their pens, musicians to their instruments, artists to their brushes and easels, athletes to their contests, parents to their families, children to life's enjoyments, and increasing numbers of the world's population to a variety of digital keyboards and computers.

Fracture management should be principle-driven. These principles include the attainment of anatomic (or near-anatomic) position, adequate stability to allow both fracture healing and early active digital motion, and minimization of additional soft-tissue damage when fixation of the fracture is required.[1]

Function follows form. Although there is some tolerance for deformity, excessive angulation or rotation of a fractured digit may obstruct the motion and function of an adjacent digit and, consequently, the hand. Bone angulation, shortening, or a combination of the two affects muscle-tendon tension, leading to digital deformity as well as to loss of motion, strength, power, and endurance.

While the prevalence, rate of development, and severity of posttraumatic arthritis and pain in the joints of the hand may be less than those in larger joints, particularly weight-bearing joints, there should be no complacency in the pursuit to reestablish joint congruity when repairing an intra-articular fracture.[2-4] A single millimeter of incongruity may be acceptable, but an effort should always be made to correct an offset of 2 mm or more, especially if it is accompanied by joint subluxation.

Fracture stability need not be rigid but must be reliable. The method or the implant or implants selected do not necessarily have to be the strongest available, but a threshold of stabilizing force that will reliably allow fracture healing in concert with early rehabilitation must be achieved. Fracture fixation only needs to be strong enough to immobilize the fracture until the strength of the healing callus surpasses that of the fixation. Although stability may not hasten healing, it ensures the process by protecting tissue revascularization during repair. Fracture stability may also inhibit infection.

Surgical incision, especially when it is accompanied by periosteal violation and particularly when flexor-tendon zone II is involved,[5] carries the risk of functionally limiting scar formation. The physician must balance the potential benefit of the increased biomechanical stability that may be gained through surgical treatment against the risk of consequent digital stiffness.

Anatomic reduction and fracture stability help to control and minimize pain and are instrumental in permitting the early active range of motion exercises that are the cornerstone of rehabilitation and recovery. Placement of the hand and wrist in a functional or "safe" ("rehabilitation-ready") position neutralizes and balances the muscle forces acting at the fracture site. (In a rehabilitation-ready position, the wrist is extended 15° to 20°, the metacarpophalangeal joints are flexed 70° or more, and the proximal interphalangeal joints are in 0° to 10° of flexion.) This position also places the digital joint ligaments at maximal length to prevent permanent contracture and is particu-larly important in reduced fractures that are considered stable without the application of implants. A functional hand and wrist position also is instrumental in placing the extrinsic and intrinsic muscles at or near their resting tension, at which point they can generate the maximal strength and power that are so critical for the recovery of digital motion. Once motion is regained, further muscle strength, power, and endurance follow more easily. The treatment of edema and the promotion of softening, mobilization, and desensitization of integumentary scar tissue may proceed concurrently.

Plain radiographs alone are almost always adequate for the evaluation of hand fractures. Metacarpal fractures may be difficult to evaluate in the lateral plane because of overlap of adjacent metacarpals. Oblique radiographs with the hand pronated or supinated (or both) at 30° to 45° are helpful. Oblique radiographs also are helpful in the evaluation of intra-articular fractures. Avulsion fractures of the proximal, dorsal, and palmar lips of the phalanges, as well as their extent and degree of displacement, sometimes may be seen and fully appreciated only on true lateral radiographs. The true extent of the angulation of an extra-articular proximal phalangeal fracture near a joint often may be accurately assessed only on a true lateral radiograph.[6] Oblique radiographs may create an optical illusion of less angulation than truly exists, which may lead the surgeon into the complacency of accepting angulation that should actually be corrected. A CT scan occasionally may be useful, especially in the assessment of an intra-articular fracture, par-

ticularly when there is intra-articular comminution.

Most hand fractures are closed, simple, and stable. They are unlikely to move from the position that they are in when they are initially seen, even during the process of rehabilitation of the digits. Radiographs demonstrate minimal displacement (less than 1 to 2 mm of translation and less than 10° to 20° of angulation) or no displacement. These fractures may not be associated with any apparent clinical deformity on visual inspection. A digital or wrist block may allow the physician to recognize the presence of functional deformity or instability. These fractures require only a brief period of static or dynamic splinting or even buddy-taping to an adjacent finger, and a short period of rehabilitation.[7-14] Some comparable but displaced fractures may be stable following closed manipulative reduction, and they may be treated similarly. They should be monitored during the first few weeks after reduction until fracture callus is visualized on radiographs, as loss of reduction may occur. The course of treatment typically is uncomplicated, and the functional outcomes are commonly good.

More severe fractures may be displaced and may be associated with visible deformities because of their configuration, periosteal disruption, and unbalanced muscle forces. If these fractures are unstable following reduction, they will require fixation with an implant to maintain anatomic position during fracture healing and to allow simultaneous rehabilitation. A digital nerve block with local anesthesia followed by observation of digital motion or by stress-testing may assist the physician in determining whether the fracture is stable and whether fixation is necessary.

Most reducible but unstable closed simple fractures may be reliably treated with transcutaneous Kirschner-wire (K-wire) fixation. This type of treatment has been termed closed reduction and inter-

nal fixation (CRIF).[15,16] Soft-tissue damage from insertion of this type of implant is usually minimal.

While CRIF can be performed with use of ordinary radiographic control, C-arm fluoroscopy substantially simplifies the procedure by allowing instantaneous adjustments of the fracture reduction and of the insertion site, angle, and depth of the wire in two planes or more. A pointed reduction forceps is instrumental in achieving and maintaining fracture reduction. If the reduction forceps is cannulated, wire insertion is further simplified. An assistant holds and stabilizes the hand or finger while the surgeon drills the wire into the proper position.

Open reduction usually is required for fractures that are irreducible because of swelling, soft-tissue interposition, or interlocking of the fragments. Following open reduction, internal fixation usually is indicated because of fracture instability. It also may be prudent to allow earlier and more intensive rehabilitation in these situations in which more than ordinary scar tissue formation is anticipated. This type of treatment is designated as open reduction and internal fixation (ORIF). Other relative indications for ORIF include open fractures (especially those associated with bone loss or other complex injuries); intra-articular, periarticular, comminuted, and multiple fractures; fractures that have occurred in association with other fractures in the same extremity; and fractures in multiply injured or noncompliant patients. ORIF with K-wires may be necessary in certain situations in which CRIF would ordinarily have been done with radiographic assistance. Widgerow and associates,[17] for example, reported that ORIF was successfully performed in the absence of radiographic capability in a third-world country. This technique may also be important when radiographic equipment is unavailable, broken down, or malfunctioning or when there is a power failure. Meticulous attention to surgical detail may overcome an absence or failure of technical equipment in some situations. Miniscrews have been inserted through small "portal-sized" 1- to 2-mm incisions. This procedure is termed limited open reduction and internal fixation.

Open reduction and mini-internal fixation in the hand is less controversial for the treatment of nonunion or malunion, for early arthrodesis of an irreparable intra-articular fracture, and for later arthrodesis in a hand with symptomatic posttraumatic arthritis than it is for the treatment of acute fractures. Strong, reliable long-term fixation is needed to support bone grafts, osteotomy sites, and arthrodesis sites, which may need a longer healing time because of the extensive osseous defects and the extensive dissection associated with these procedures. Additionally, firm fixation is required so that early and intensive therapy may be applied to inhibit or prevent adjacent tendon and joint adhesions, especially when tenolysis or capsulotomy has been performed concurrently.

Implants

K-wires are the cornerstone of hand-fracture fixation.[7-18] They can be inserted either transcutaneously after closed reduction of a fracture or following open reduction. They do not compress but internally splint the bone while the fracture heals. The fracture reduction should be as precise as possible prior to the insertion of the wires in order to ensure optimal stability of the fracture-implant construct.

K-wires are inexpensive and almost universally available. They require little additional instrumentation, can be inserted with either hand or power-driven drills, and create little additional soft-tissue trauma. They may form an integral component of other open wiring techniques, such as figure-of-8 tension-band wiring and circumferential wiring. They can also be used adjunctively to enhance the stability of almost any other form of internal or external fixation. An oblique

K-wire may add substantial additional stability to a construct that is less than adequately stable. These wires are generally left in place until fracture callus or healing is visible on radiographs or for as long as they are tolerated. Fracture healing usually is sufficiently advanced at 3 to 4 weeks after insertion so that the K-wires can be removed.

K-wires with a 0.045-in (1.1-mm) diameter may be used almost universally in the hand. Occasionally, for larger bones, such as the metacarpal or the proximal phalanx, K-wires with a 0.062-in (1.6-mm) diameter may be selected. For children and for smaller bones, such as the middle or distal phalanges, wires with a 0.035-in (0.9-mm) diameter may be the best choice.

K-wires or their equivalents can be inserted into the medullary canal of metacarpals and phalanges for fracture fixation.[15,16,19,20] When used in this fashion, these devices can be left in place temporarily or permanently. The principal difficulties include a lack of rotational control and delayed union or nonunion. Fracture collapse may occur when K-wires are removed prematurely, which may result in nonunion or malunion of the fracture and consequent digital stiffness. This risk increases with fracture comminution.[21] Miniscrews, and even miniplates, may obviate this risk.

Miniscrews, miniplates, and the instruments necessary to apply them are relatively expensive compared with K-wires and other wiring systems. Their insertion is technically more demanding than that of K-wires, and there is less margin for error. Specialized training and surgical experience are definite advantages that enhance an individual's proficiency in their use. A sterile operating environment is mandatory. Good lighting, experienced personnel, and reliable radiographic support often are critical to obtain a successful result. The advantages of these implants are the added stability provided by fracture compression and

the resultant or independent neutralization of bending, rotational, and shear forces acting upon the fracture site. These features help to ensure timely fracture healing and to allow earlier and more intensive digital rehabilitation.

A miniscrew is little more than a K-wire with threads and a head. Insertion of a miniscrew is associated with little if any additional soft-tissue trauma compared with that associated with insertion of a K-wire.[22] Drilling the proximal cortex to the same diameter as the screw threads creates a "gliding hole" through which the miniscrew slides without resistance until it engages the "core hole" that has been drilled in the opposite cortex. The "core hole" has the same diameter as the core of the miniscrew. This creates a lag effect, resulting in compression at the fracture site.

Miniplates must be used judiciously, especially on phalanges, since the dissection necessary for their application may disrupt periosteal circulation at the fracture site and may stimulate substantial fibroplasia (scar formation).[10,12,14] Miniplates are particularly useful for the treatment of open fractures associated with bone loss and extensive comminution. Miniplates have generic anatomic or descriptive names; examples of those devices include straight tubular and limited-contact miniplates, minicondylar plates, mini-T or mini-L plates, and angled miniplates. Mini-H plates have been designed to facilitate digital replantations. Physiologically, these miniplates stabilize fractures by compression, neutralization, or buttressing. In some instances they may compress the fracture and neutralize the external forces acting on it, and in others they may buttress the fracture and neutralize the external forces acting on it. Compression and buttressing cannot take place concurrently because they are diametrically opposed forces.

When a miniplate is applied to compress a fracture, the fracture must first be

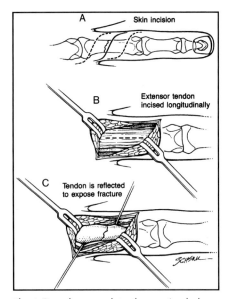

Fig. 1 Dorsal approach to the proximal phalanx. (Reproduced with permission from Pratt DR: Exposing fractures of the proximal phalanx of the finger longitudinally through the dorsal extensor apparatus. *Clin Orthop* 1959;15:24.)

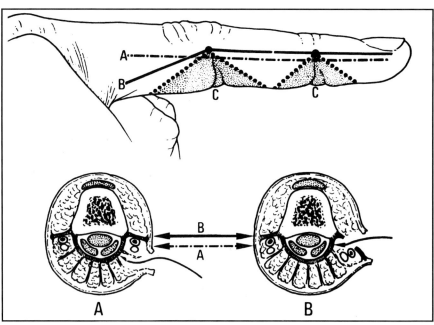

Fig. 2 Midaxial approach to the proximal phalanx. Line A indicates the midlateral line; line B, the midaxial line; and line C, the interphalangeal joint flexion crease. (Reproduced with permission from Littler JW, Cramer LM, Smith JW (eds): *Symposium on Reconstructive Hand Surgery*. St. Louis, MO, CV Mosby, 1974, p 90.)

accurately reduced. The miniplate is then stabilized on one side of the fracture with miniscrews. On the other side of the fracture, a hole is drilled eccentrically through the plate hole most distant from the fracture. When the miniscrew is inserted into this hole and the screw head engages the plate hole, it pulls the miniplate and the attached fragment toward the screw, placing the fracture under compression. This is called the "spherical gliding principle" of screw-head engagement of the plate hole.[1] The fracture is placed under compression while the miniplate is placed under an equal amount of tension. Thus, this construct is called a "compression plate" or a "tension-band plate." The terms are synonymous. The bone will not move until and unless the compressive force of this "preload" is exceeded.

The Pratt incision (or a variation of it) has been the classic dorsal utilitarian approach for fractures of the proximal phalanx[23] (Fig. 1). A midaxial incision may be preferable for some fractures in an effort to move the zone of injury away from the extensor mechanism and to minimize the risk of adhesions to this tendon[24,25] (Fig. 2). Metacarpals can be approached through a direct longitudinal incision. If two adjacent metacarpals are fractured, they usually can be approached through a single incision made between them[26,27] (Fig. 3). The fracture is exposed by subperiosteal dissection initiated from the lateral side in an effort to protect the gliding tissue on either side of the extensor tendon.

Miniexternal fixators can be used to treat a variety of hand fractures. While their advantages include minimal or no exposure of the fracture site and adequate stability, they have no compelling advantage over K-wires in the treatment of simple closed fractures of the hand. Conversely, they may be especially useful for comminuted intra-articular fractures; for the initial provisional and, sometimes, permanent definitive fixation of severe open fractures; and for mutilating injuries associated with soiling, comminution, bone loss, and full-thickness skin loss.[28]

Ideally, a minimum of two threaded or smooth half-pins are inserted on either side of the fracture. Pins with a 0.062-in (1.6-mm) diameter are ordinarily used for smaller adult bones such as the middle and distal phalanges and for children, whereas pins with a 0.08-in (2.0-mm) diameter are used for adult metacarpals and proximal phalanges. K-wires with similar diameters can be substituted for half-pins. Smooth pins are sufficient for short-term application (4 to 6 weeks). They are further stabilized when a mini-external fixator compresses or distracts the fracture. Threaded pins provide more stability than smooth pins, especially when a mini-external fixator is applied for long-term (6 to 10 week) definitive fixation of a fracture with a defect that requires bone grafting. Ancillary K-wires or miniscrews can be used in conjunction with a mini-external fixator to secure larger fracture fragments. Occasionally, a mini-external fixator may be used to support a miniplate that spans but does not independently secure a fracture.

Extensor tendon transfixion is more easily avoided in metacarpal applications than in phalangeal applications. A longitudinal incision of approximately 1 cm in the dorsal apparatus may avoid irritation and allow limited motion of the digit. Pin sites are a source of risk for infection and require daily wound care (cleaning and antiseptic application). The prevalence of nonunion is related to the size and severity of the bone defect while the prevalence of infection is related to the size and severity of the wound and the degree of initial contamination.

Bone grafting may be indicated when there is a cortical defect at the site of fixation of a miniplate, comminution, a bone defect, or atrophic nonunion.[1] Cancellous bone from the proximal part of the ipsilateral ulna, the distal part of the ipsilateral radius, or the ilium is the mainstay for bone grafting of defects in the hand. Cancellous bone can be placed in the barrel of a syringe and compressed by the plunger.[29] The compacted cancellous bone can then be disengaged from the barrel with use of a long spinal needle inserted through the barrel outlet. This dense cancellous bone then can be inserted to provide additional structural support at the site of the defect. If there are any viable cells in the cancellous bone, compacting increases their numbers per unit of volume. Although not scientifically confirmed to date, it is our impression that revascularization and incorporation occur more rapidly in compacted than in noncompacted cancellous bone graft.

Unicortical bone grafts from the ilium, the proximal part of the ipsilateral ulna, the distal part of the ipsilateral radius, or tricortical bone grafts from the iliac crest can be sculpted to fit larger defects (1.5 cm in length or greater) or can be used when the stability afforded by cortical bone is needed. Ball-and-

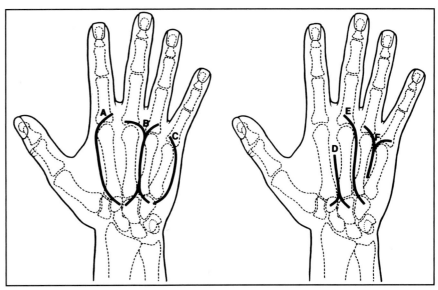

Fig. 3 Approaches to the metacarpals. A, Radial approach to the second (index) metacarpal. B, Approach to the third and fourth metacarpal shafts through a single incision. C, Ulnar approach to the fifth metacarpal. D, Approach to the bases of the second and third metacarpals through a single incision. E, Approach to the head of the third metacarpal and the base of the fourth metacarpal through a single incision. F, Approach to the heads of the fourth and fifth metacarpals through a single incision. (Reproduced with permission from Freeland AE, Geissler WB: Plate fixation of metacarpal shaft fractures, in Blair WF, Steyers CM (eds): *Techniques in Hand Surgery*. Baltimore, MD, Williams & Wilkins, 1996, p 257.)

socket or mortise articulations at the bone graft-fracture junctions reestablish bone length, alignment, and stability while providing a large cancellous interface area for healing. Donor-site defects can be packed with synthetic bone graft to minimize the risk of later fracture at that site.

Metacarpal Fractures

The unbalanced pull of the interosseous muscles and extrinsic digital flexors on the distal fragment may cause dorsal angulation of metacarpal fractures.[30,31] Dorsal angulation of as much as 10° more than the motion afforded at the carpometacarpal joints does not ordinarily cause a functional deficit.[26,27] Compensatory carpometacarpal motion allows accommodation of the metacarpal head in the palm of the hand in slightly angulated fractures and prevents painful pressure from a palmarly displaced metacarpal head when tools and implements

with a handle are grasped and used. The intermetacarpal ligaments prevent more than 3 to 4 mm of shortening.[32] The second and fifth metacarpals are more likely to shorten since they have the suspensory effect of only one intermetacarpal ligament. Approximately 7° of extensor lag develops in the fingers for each 2 mm of residual metacarpal shortening after fracture healing.[33] In any case, angulation of more than 30°, shortening of more than 4 mm, or a combination of these findings interferes with normal intrinsic muscle-tension dynamics and may cause weakness, loss of endurance, cramping, and clawing, each of which should be prevented by correction of the deformity[30-34] (Fig. 4). The metacarpals are very intolerant of malrotation. As little as 5° of malrotation may translate into 1.5 cm of digital overlap during finger flexion.[27,35]

Metacarpal shaft fractures can be classified by pattern. Simple fractures may be

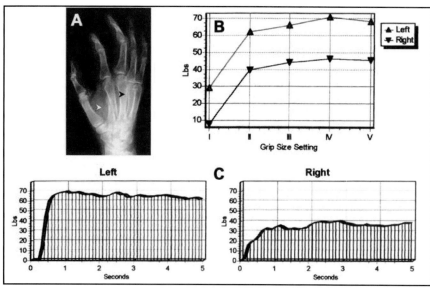

Fig. 4 A 51-year-old right-handed patient who worked on an assembly line had weakness, cramping, and loss of endurance in the right hand. **A,** Radiograph showing healed fractures of the index and ring metacarpals and a malunion of both (*arrowheads*). Digital motion was nearly normal. The patient had no pain at rest and no swelling, warmth, discoloration, or tenderness. **B,** Five-position grip-testing demonstrated a 30% loss of strength. **C,** Single sustained grip-testing revealed a similar loss. Although there is a certain amount of anatomic forgiveness in hand fracture management, disregard of the principle of a stable anatomic (or near-anatomic) reduction of a hand fracture is not always entirely innocuous.

transverse or oblique. Oblique fractures may be short (less than twice the diameter of the bone adjacent to or at the site of the fracture) or long (at least twice the adjacent bone diameter). Long oblique fractures may be uniplanar or spiral. Short oblique fractures are essentially always uniplanar. Other metacarpal shaft fractures may have comminuted patterns or bone loss.

Transverse metacarpal shaft fractures may be caused by axial loading but usually result from a dorsal impact. Undisplaced, minimally displaced, and fully reduced fractures can be successfully treated with protective splinting or functional bracing.[9,36,37] Skin necrosis overlying the fracture is a risk. If displacement recurs during the first 3 to 4 weeks of healing and before fracture callus is visualized on radiographs, closed remanipulation and percutaneous K-wire stabilization are indicated. Thereafter, open reduction

and either re-creation of the fracture or corrective osteotomy may be necessary. In such cases, some type of internal fixation, often a miniplate, is indicated.

Some closed transverse metacarpal fractures may be accompanied by such extensive swelling that reduction is impossible. Others may redisplace after reduction because of extensive periosteal disruption. In such instances, either intramedullary splinting[20] (Fig. 5) or fixation with K or composite wire[38] or with straight tubular or low-contact dynamic compression miniplates[26,27,39-48] may provide an optimal solution. The use of two plate holes on both sides of the fracture, allowing the secure purchase of four cortices (also on both sides of the fracture), provides sufficient and reliable fixation[26,27] (Fig. 6).

The treatment of short oblique fractures of the metacarpal shaft may be similar to that of transverse fractures of

the metacarpal shaft. Alternatively, sagittal short oblique fractures can be treated with a laterally inserted minilag (compression) screw. A five-hole miniplate is then centered with the middle hole over the fracture site and is secured without compression by the insertion of miniscrews into the center of the two plate holes on either end of the miniplate. The center hole is left free to accommodate the underlying laterally applied minilag screw.[26,27] A miniplate applied in this fashion is called a "neutralization miniplate." Such plates counteract the bending, rotational, and shear forces that might act on the minilag screw. Coronal short oblique fractures can be treated by application of a five-hole straight tubular or low-contact dynamic compression miniplate that drives the adjacent corner of the fracture into the miniplate. A minilag screw is then inserted through the center plate hole and across the fracture.[26,27] This is the strongest of the miniplate constructs because it compresses the fracture by both miniplate and screw application.

An unstable long oblique fracture of the metacarpal shaft can be treated with transcutaneous K-wires if closed reduction is performed and with either K-wires or two or more minilag screws if open reduction is performed.[26,27,39-46] Although K-wires can be used after open reduction, minilag screws provide more secure fixation and require no more dissection than K-wires do. The length of the fracture is divided by the width of the bone adjacent to or at the site of the fracture to determine the number of miniscrews that should be used. If the fracture is twice as long as the adjacent bone diameter, the fracture is divided into thirds and the miniscrews are inserted at the juncture of each third. If the fracture is three times as long as the adjacent bone diameter, the fracture is divided into quarters and the miniscrews are inserted at the juncture of each quarter. A minilag screw provides maximal compression

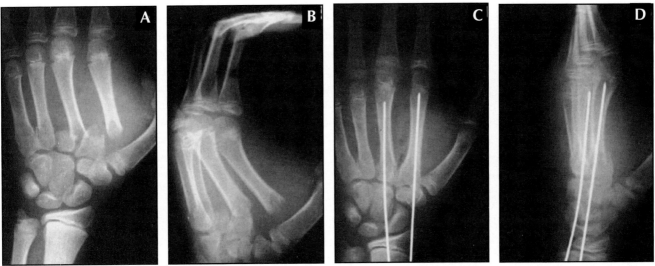

Fig. 5 An adolescent boy who had severely displaced transverse fractures of the second and third metacarpals. **A** and **B,** Preoperative AP and oblique radiographs. **C** and **D,** AP and oblique radiographs made after K-wires were inserted into the medullary canals of both metacarpals.

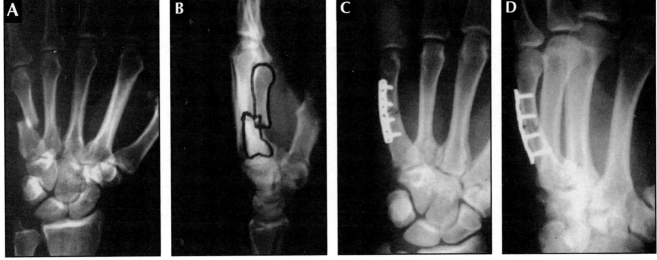

Fig. 6 An adult patient who had a transverse fracture in the middle of the fifth metacarpal shaft that was irreducible by closed manipulation. **A** and **B,** Preoperative AP and lateral radiographs. **C** and **D,** Radiographs made after ORIF with a four-hole straight low-contact miniplate applied under dynamic compression. A gradual bend of 5° was contoured over the entire length of the plate prior to its application. A small amount of prebend in the miniplate ensures that the cortex across from the plate will be under compression and that there will be uniform compression across the entire fracture. If the plate is left straight, the opposite cortex will distract as the miniplate is placed under tension. If a plate is bent at a single site rather than across the entire plate, the bend will occur at the weakest site (a plate hole), increasing the risk of fatigue fracture of the plate.

when inserted perpendicular to the fracture (in which case it is known as a compression screw) and maximal shear resistance when inserted perpendicular to the long axis of the bone (in which case it is known as a neutralization screw). Uniplanar fractures are treated with at least one neutralization screw. The remaining screw or screws can be inserted as compression screws. In long spiral oblique fractures, the intervals for division and insertion remain the same, but the spiral fracture plane is followed (Fig. 7). At one or more points, a miniscrew can be inserted both perpendicular to the fracture and perpendicular to the long axis of the bone (such a screw is known as a perfect screw). Again, once the requirement for neutralization (one miniscrew) is satisfied, the remaining miniscrews can be inserted in the com-

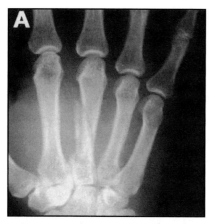
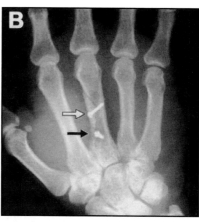

Fig. 7 A, A malrotated irreducible spiral oblique fracture of the third metacarpal. **B,** Radiograph made after the fracture was stabilized by insertion of miniscrews along the fracture plane. The proximal miniscrew (*black arrow*) is perpendicular to both the fracture (for maximal compression) and the long axis of the bone (for maximal resistance to shear displacement). The distal miniscrew (*white arrow*) is perpendicular to the fracture (for maximal compression). The miniscrews neutralize rotational and bending forces. The third metacarpal is also protected by intact metacarpal pillars on either side.

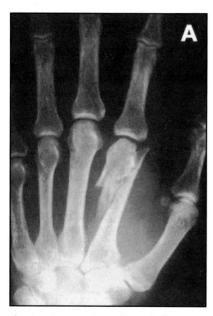
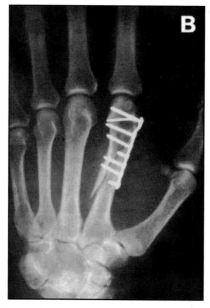

Fig. 8 A, Preoperative radiograph showing a closed, unstable comminuted subcapital fracture of the second metacarpal. **B,** Radiograph made after the fracture was reduced and stabilized by the application of a minicondylar plate applied from the lateral side.

pression mode. If they neutralize as well, so much the better.

Miniplates are almost always essential for unstable comminuted metacarpal fractures (Fig. 8) and metacarpal fractures with bone loss. Multiple displacement metacarpal fractures (Fig. 9) usually are unstable and require closed or open internal fixation.

An axial load resulting from impact against a clenched fist causes most sub-

capital or metacarpal neck fractures (boxer fractures). The fifth metacarpal is most commonly injured, followed by the fourth metacarpal. Rotational and lateral deviation deformities should be corrected. Shortening may occur as a result of impaction, angulation, or a combination of the two. There is some latitude for acceptance of dorsal angulation. As noted above, in general, dorsal angulation of as much as 10° more than the amount of motion in the respective carpometacarpal joint may be accepted. Consequently, up to 15° of dorsal angulation can be accepted in the second and third metacarpals. Subcapital fractures with as much as 50° of dorsal angulation in the fourth metacarpal and 70° in the fifth metacarpal have healed without pain or subjective functional deficit, although with varying degrees of cosmetic deformity.[49-51] A functional deficit may also be masked by low demand. The greater the dorsal angulation upon presentation, the more likely that there is an injury to an adjacent metacarpal at the carpometacarpal joint in the form of a fracture, dislocation, or a combination of the two.[27] Consequently, it is important to survey these areas for coexisting injury during physical examination and when viewing radiographs.

Although we have detailed the extremes of acceptable parameters, if a fracture approaches or exceeds these limitations and is seen early enough that reduction can be achieved, an effort to achieve anatomic or near-anatomic reduction should be undertaken. The coexistence of clawing, apparent angular deformity, malrotation, or any obstruction of digital motion makes fracture reduction even more compelling. The Jahss maneuver is an effective reduction method.[52] In this maneuver, the metacarpophalangeal joint is flexed 70° to 90°. The proximal fragment is compressed in a palmar direction by the physician's fingers while the physician's thumb applies dorsally directed axial pressure to the metacarpal head through the proximal phalanx. When a reduced fracture is unstable, any of a number of transcutaneous K-wire applications is effective for splinting the site until callus is visualized on a radiograph. In the rare case when open reduction is needed, K-wires can still be used just as with closed reduction. More secure fixation may provide the advantage of allowing earlier and more intensive rehabilitation with no additional soft-tissue dissection other than that necessary for the open reduction itself. Minicondylar plates are ideal in terms of both size and design.[47,48] They also have a lower profile than mini-T, mini-L, or angled plates, and they are more versatile in that they can be applied dorsally on any metacarpal and laterally on the metacarpals of the thumb, the index finger, and the small finger.

Fractures of the metacarpal base of a finger are generally stable, but even minor rotational malalignments at this level are greatly magnified at the fingertips and may interfere with function. These fractures are easily missed at the time of initial evaluation because of poor-quality radiographs or poor positioning. Treatment of an extra-articular fracture of the metacarpal base is similar to that of a fracture of the shaft. Minicondylar plates are more adaptive than straight plates in the region of the metaphyseal-diaphyseal junction. Displaced articular fractures are reduced and stabilized with K-wires or minilag screws.

An intra-articular fracture of the metacarpal base of a finger may be unicondylar (a reverse Bennett fracture) or comminuted. Displaced unicondylar and bicondylar fractures are reduced and stabilized with pins, screws, metaphyseal plates, or a combination of these implants. Subluxated and dislocated carpometacarpal joints must be reduced and incorporated into the fixation.

Intra-articular fractures of the metacarpal head of the fingers and thumb are treated similarly.[53] A condylar fracture of the metacarpal head may be associated

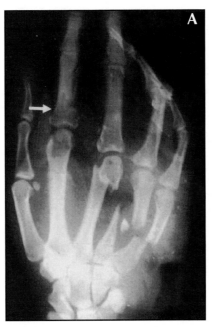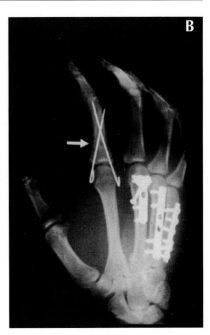

Fig. 9 A, Preoperative radiograph showing open, displaced, highly unstable fractures of the third, fourth, and fifth metacarpals and a closed extra-articular fracture of the base of the proximal phalanx of the index finger (*arrow*). **B,** Radiograph made after open reduction and stabilization of the metacarpal fractures with use of miniplates and screws and after closed reduction and fixation of the proximal phalanx of the index finger with use of crossed K-wires (*arrow*).

with a complex metacarpophalangeal joint dislocation. This fracture usually is on the ulnar side of the metacarpal head when the complex dislocation occurs in a finger. Whenever an articular fracture is treated with open reduction, great care should be taken to preserve soft-tissue attachments to the articular fragments to preserve their blood supply.

Phalangeal Fractures

Proximal phalangeal shaft fractures typically exhibit palmar angulation because of muscle imbalance. The proximal fragment is flexed by the interossei insertions. The distal fragment is extended by the central extensor slip.[30,31] Palmar angulation causes commensurate shortening of the proximal phalanx. This compromises extensor tendon function and causes an extensor lag that averages 12° at the proximal interphalangeal joint for every millimeter of bone-tendon discrepancy.[54]

Palmar angulation may also prevent full digital flexion, with commensurate weakness of pinch and grip and a loss of endurance. More than 25° of palmar angulation causes a functional deficit accompanied by a cosmetic deformity and should usually be corrected.[6]

Most simple undisplaced phalangeal fractures can be treated by static protective or dynamic functional splinting for up to 4 weeks regardless of configuration because of the integrity and stabilizing effect of the periosteum and adjacent soft-tissue structures.[7-14] When functional splinting techniques are used, the extensor mechanism acts as a tension band and exerts a progressive compression force on the phalangeal fracture site during finger flexion.[9]

Undisplaced or minimally displaced simple extra-articular fractures of any configuration usually are stable because of an intact periosteum. Some physicians

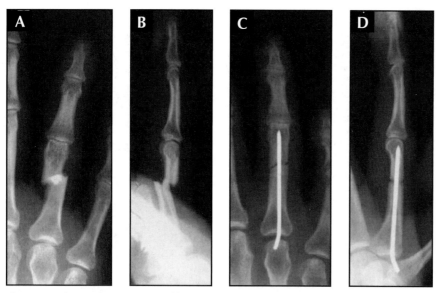

Fig. 10 A and **B**, Preoperative AP and lateral radiographs of a closed displaced transverse fracture of the shaft of the proximal phalanx of the right ring finger. **C** and **D**, Postoperative AP and lateral radiographs. A small (limited) dorsal incision was made to complete the fracture reduction, and an intramedullary K-wire was used to hold the reduction.

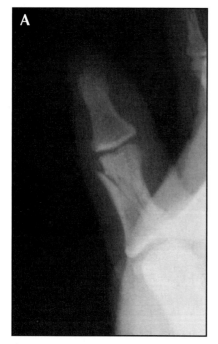
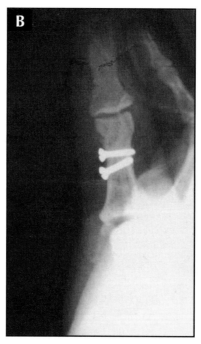

Fig. 11 A, Preoperative radiograph of a displaced uniplanar oblique fracture of the proximal phalanx of the thumb. **B,** Radiograph made after closed reduction and percutaneous fixation with miniscrews.

stabilized if they displace. Transcutaneous pinning is usually sufficient,[6,8,12,14-16] but open fixation with K- or another type of wire or application of miniscrews or a plate may be required in some instances.[12,14,17,19,39-48,55-57]

Displaced transverse and short oblique extra-articular phalangeal fractures may be stable after reduction, especially with the hand and digits functionally positioned to balance the muscles. They can then be treated similar to undisplaced fractures, with the exception that buddy-splinting alone is insufficient. No more than 25° of palmar angulation should be accepted.[6] One or more intramedullary or two crossed K-wires should be inserted by either transcutaneous or open technique to stabilize unstable fractures.[15,16] Fractures that cannot be reduced with closed manipulation should be opened and internally stabilized (Fig. 10). To avoid distraction, the K-wires should cross proximal or distal to but not at the fracture. Miniplates can be applied when the fracture is irreducible or open or when there are multiple fractures. They can also be used when there is comminution or bone loss and when a patient has multiple traumatic injuries or is noncompliant.[39-48,55,56] Minicondylar plates are designed for proximal and distal phalangeal fractures and can be applied on either the radial or the ulnar side of the proximal phalanx.[47,48] Distal application of a minicondylar plate on either the radial or the ulnar side of the proximal phalanx minimizes injury to or impingement on the central slip and the consequent risk of a boutonnière deformity at the proximal interphalangeal joint.

Displaced long oblique extra-articular phalangeal fractures are almost always unstable. Transcutaneous transverse or oblique K-wire pinning provides sufficient fixation and a good outcome in a compliant patient.[15,16] Miniscrews can be used at the surgeon's discretion, with an increase in stability and little additional soft-tissue damage[22] (Fig. 11). Such fractures rarely are treated with open re-

have successfully treated these fractures with buddy-splinting (or taping) alone,[7,13] while others have used static or dynamic functional splinting.[7-14] These fractures should be monitored during the course of treatment and should be reduced and

duction unless closed reduction or transcutaneous fixation fails. Open injury; multiple fractures in the hand, extremity, spine, or pelvis; and patient noncompliance are all indications for open treatment.[58-60]

Undisplaced unicondylar articular fractures of the base of the proximal or middle phalanx and displaced unicondylar articular fractures involving less than 25% of the articular surface that are not associated with joint subluxation or deformity can be treated with buddy-splinting (or taping) to the finger adjacent to the fracture and with early mobilization.[7,44] If more than 25% of the articular surface is involved and the fracture is displaced, closed reduction should be performed. This is best accomplished with use of C-arm fluoroscopy, digital traction, and pointed reduction forceps. Use of a cannulated reduction forceps facilitates placement of the K-wire. If closed reduction is not possible, open reduction is recommended. A midaxial incision is centered over the fracture fragment and is extended obliquely over the metacarpal head, parallel with the Langer lines. Although the incision is drawn to allow an extensive exposure of the fracture, the smallest possible portion of this incision is used to reduce the fracture. The goal is to reduce the fracture by aligning its superior border while preserving the soft-tissue attachments and blood supply to the condylar fragment. Fluoroscopy provides additional assistance with this task. Regardless of whether the fracture is reduced with a closed or open technique, fixation with two or more K-wires or with one or more minilag screws is appropriate.[44,55,56] Tension-banding can be added to smaller or less stable fragments.[61-63] Fragments of any size associated with subluxation of the metacarpophalangeal joint should be reduced and fixed.

Bicondylar fractures of the base of the proximal or middle phalanx are almost always displaced. If closed reduction (a

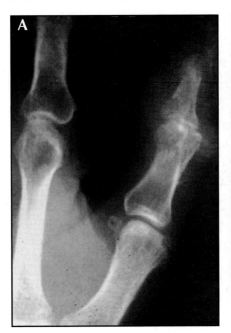
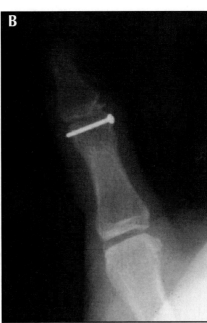

Fig. 12 A, Radiograph showing a slightly displaced unicondylar fracture of the proximal phalanx of the thumb. The fracture was treated with open reduction through a limited midaxial incision and alignment of the proximal portion of the fracture without opening the interphalangeal joint. **B,** Radiograph showing fixation of the fragment with a miniscrew.

combination of traction, manipulation, and use of transcutaneously applied pointed reduction forceps) is possible, transcutaneous K-wire fixation can be carried out. This method of fracture reduction and K-wire insertion and its governing principles can be used for any bicondylar intra-articular fracture of the hand. The major condylar fragments and their articular surfaces are reduced and stabilized with one or more transverse K-wires inserted parallel or nearly parallel to the joint surface. Smaller ("vassal") fragments either follow the major fragments during their reduction or may be ignored. This is called the "rule of the majority" or the "vassal rule."[55] The repaired metaphysis is then reduced, aligned, and secured to the diaphysis with two K-wires inserted at or near the tip of each condyle proximally. Both of these K-wires are driven past the fracture site and into the medullary canal of the distal fragment, where they continue down the canal to or near the end of the diaphysis

or engage or traverse the diaphyseal cortex. If they traverse the diaphysis, their points should go just slightly past the exterior cortex to avoid any abrasion or penetration of either the extensor mechanism or the flexor tendons. This same technique can be applied if open reduction is necessary, and it is especially useful for smaller condylar fragments. When there are larger fragments, a minicondylar plate can be applied laterally. The lateral band and oblique retinacular fibers can be excised to allow access for insertion of a minicondylar plate.[25] Excision of this single lateral band prevents the intrinsic tightness, adhesions, or rubbing over the miniplate that might occur with incision and repair. The major condylar fragments and their adjacent joint surfaces are reduced and are stabilized by the spike of the minicondylar plate. This spike is measured and cut to the proper length prior to insertion. The metaphysis and the stem of the minicondylar plate are reduced, aligned, and secured to the

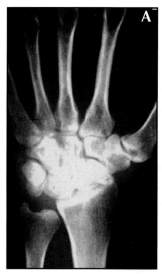 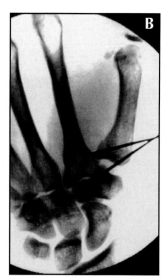 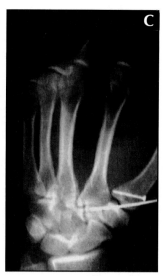 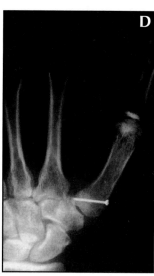

Fig. 13 A, Preoperative radiograph of a displaced Bennett fracture. **B,** Radiograph made after reduction with closed traction and manipulation and stabilization with transcutaneous K-wires. **C,** The wire across the fracture site has been replaced by a transcutaneously applied minilag screw. The buttressing K-wire remains. **D,** The buttressing K-wire was removed 3 weeks after surgery.

diaphysis. The remaining plate holes are filled with miniscrews to complete the fixation.

While early mobilization of joints adjacent to undisplaced intra-articular fractures of the base of the proximal phalanx may be safe, digits with undisplaced unicondylar fractures of the distal portion of the proximal or middle phalanx are probably more safely mobilized only after transcutaneous pin fixation or limited open miniscrew fixation through a portal-sized (1- to 2-cm) incision.[7,44,55,64] Displaced unicondylar fractures can be treated similarly following closed or open reduction (Fig. 12). A small midaxial incision is preferred. This allows fracture reduction with a minimum of soft-tissue dissection. The condyle can be reduced without opening the proximal interphalangeal joint by aligning the proximal spike of the condylar fragment with the shaft of the phalanx. Intraoperative fluoroscopy is helpful. A more extensive dorsal incision can be made, and the joint can be exposed between the lateral band and the extensor slip if more exposure is needed. Sometimes such an incision is necessary, but it is associated with a

greater risk of scarring and stiffness. Fixation with K-wires or minilag screws results in the best final motion. Tension-band wiring can be added for smaller and less stable fragments.[61-63] A bicondylar fracture of the distal portion of the proximal phalanx is treated with similar methods, principles, and implants, as is a bicondylar fracture of the base of the proximal phalanx.

Subluxation and dislocation of the proximal interphalangeal joint occurs either in a dorsal direction as a result of a volar lip fracture of the base of the middle phalanx adjacent to the insertion of the palmar plate or in a palmar direction as a result of a dorsal avulsion or marginal impact fracture at the dorsal base of the middle phalanx adjacent to the insertion of the central slip. True lateral radiographs are essential in the confirmation and evaluation of these diagnoses. Additional oblique radiographs may also be helpful. Dorsal fracture-dislocations result from axial compression and may be comminuted, often involving a substantial portion of the palmar articular surface. Reduction and extension block-splinting in moderate flexion usually maintains a reduced and

congruent joint when less than 40% of the palmar articular surface is involved.[65,66] For fractures involving more than 40% of the palmar articular surface, internal fixation should be considered if there is a single large fragment.[67] Optimal treatment requires a stable congruent joint reduction, early motion, and smooth gliding of the middle phalanx around the proximal phalangeal head. Anatomic restoration of the articular surface is desirable but of less importance. Subluxation and hinging of the joint must be prevented. When the palmar fragments can be restored, they provide a restraint to dorsal subluxation and resurface an irregular and deficient palmar articular surface. These goals are much more easily stated than achieved. Buttress extension-block pinning, traction, and a variety of static and dynamic external fixation techniques are options when there is severe comminution and a congruent reduction cannot otherwise be maintained.[67,68] Arthroplasty with a palmar plate can be used as a salvage procedure after an early or late failure for up to 2 years after injury.[69-71]

Comminuted fractures of the articular surface of the base of the middle phalanx caused by axial compression are called pilon fractures. One or more of the articular fragments may be depressed. Splinting, miniskeletal traction, mini-external fixation, open reduction, internal fixation, and bone grafting are among the treatment options.[72-75] This is a devastating injury, and stiffness is the rule rather than the exception. The goal is to recover as much of the functional midrange of motion as possible, recognizing that the extremes of flexion and extension may be lost. Patients treated with traction or dynamic mini-external fixation tend to have the best results with regard to the active range of motion, grip strength, radiographic appearance, and pain control. Immobilization produces the poorest results.

For irreparable interphalangeal joint fractures, primary or early arthroplasty or arthrodesis may provide the best and most timely outcome. Both procedures provide reliable pain relief and restore joint alignment and stability. Both constrained silicone and nonconstrained bicondylar implants are available for arthroplasty of the proximal interphalangeal joint.[76-78] The silicone implants are unstable to pinch in the index finger, but the bicondylar implants hold up quite well and provide an alternative to arthrodesis. Consequently, arthrodesis may be reserved for joint destruction that is beyond arthroplastic salvage.[79]

Thumb Fractures

Although the forces acting to displace phalangeal fractures and metacarpal shaft fractures of the thumb may differ from those acting on the fingers, fractures of the thumb can be evaluated and treated similarly. The metacarpal of the thumb has no suspensory protection from shortening after fracture but is quite tolerant of this component of deformity. When intra-articular or extra-articular fractures of the base of the thumb metacarpal are unstable, the abductor pollicis longus and the adductor pollicis shorten the thumb

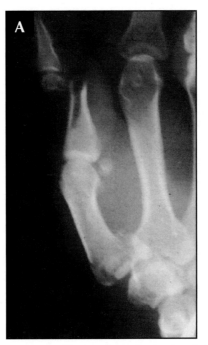
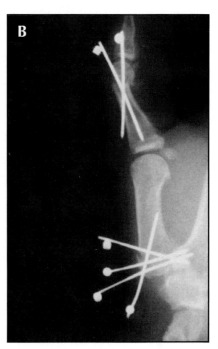

Fig. 14 A, Oblique radiograph of a closed, displaced transverse subcondylar fracture of the proximal phalanx of the thumb and a closed Rolando fracture. **B,** The Rolando fracture was reduced with traction and manipulation. The joint surface was aligned, and the major metaphyseal fragments were stabilized with two K-wires inserted parallel to the articular plane. The repaired metaphysis was then fixed to the diaphysis with crossed K-wires. The transverse subcondylar fracture of the proximal phalanx was reduced and transcutaneously pinned with crossed K-wires.

and the adductor pollicis adducts the thumb. This narrows the thumb web space and results in a decreased span of grasp with accompanying limitations of pinch and grip. This may seriously limit hand function.

With an extra-articular fracture of the thumb metacarpal base, an adduction deformity of up to 30° is acceptable because of the compensatory capacity of the trapeziometacarpal joint, but greater deformity usually should be corrected.[79,80] A reduction should be performed for deformities accompanied by compensatory hyperextension of the metacarpophalangeal joint. Successful closed reduction can be stabilized with transcutaneous K-wires. If open reduction is necessary, metaphyseal minifragment plates such as the minicondylar, mini-T, or mini-L plates are appropriate for application.

An axial force along a partially flexed thumb may produce an articular fracture of the metacarpal base. This is termed a Bennett fracture and is distinguished by a nondisplaced palmar radial fragment attached to the anterior oblique ligament and by dorsal, radial, and proximal displacement of the base of the shaft caused by the unopposed pull of the abductor pollicis longus. The distal part of the metacarpal is adducted, and the thumb web space is narrowed by the adductor pollicis. Most surgeons strive to reestablish articular congruity in a fresh Bennett fracture by closed reduction. Reliable fixation of this inherently unstable fracture is achieved with K-wires. Deformity is concurrently corrected. This fracture is especially suited for exchange of a K-wire for one or more minilag screws, thus enhancing the stability of the construct (Fig. 13). While symptomatic posttrau-

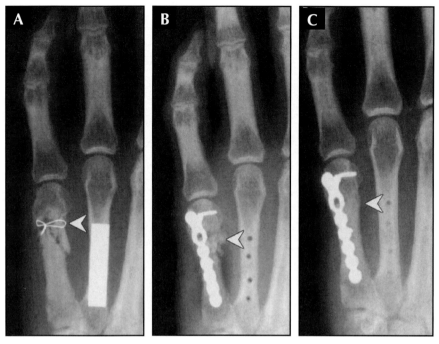

Fig. 15 A, A comminuted subcapital fracture of the fifth metacarpal was inadequately stabilized with a circumferential malleable wire, resulting in a painful nonunion (*arrowhead*). A fracture of the fourth metacarpal healed after fixation with a miniplate. Both the ring and small fingers were stiff. **B,** An extensor tenolysis and implant removal was performed on both fingers. The sclerotic bone fragments were removed from the fracture site (*arrowhead*) of the fifth metacarpal. The ununited fracture was stabilized, and bone-grafting was done with compressed cancellous bone obtained from the distal aspect of the ipsilateral radius. **C,** The fracture of the fifth metacarpal (*arrowhead*) healed. The motion of both fingers substantially improved.

matic arthritis does not always correlate with articular incongruity, minimally traumatic restitution of the joint surface and normal joint mechanics appears to be the most reliable deterrent.[3,4,81,82] Open reduction rarely is necessary or indicated. When a Bennett fracture that is detected more than 2 to 3 weeks after injury is solid or cannot be completely reduced by closed manipulation, an allowance for a small amount of joint step-off may be preferable to the surgical trauma necessary to restore joint congruity.

Comminuted fractures of the base of the metacarpal of the thumb are caused by mechanisms similar to those that cause a Bennett fracture but with higher energy. A Rolando fracture is a T- or Y-shaped intra-articular fracture of the base of the metacarpal of the thumb

that has two major articular fragments. The deformity is similar to that occurring after a Bennett fracture. Closed reduction with use of ligamentotaxis and periosteotaxis often is possible by application of distal traction to the thumb. Temporary transcutaneous K-wire fixation may adequately stabilize this fracture during healing[83] (Fig. 14). More highly comminuted fractures may require miniexternal fixation or traction to reestablish and maintain congruity of the shattered base of the metacarpal of the thumb.[84] Larger fragments can be incorporated into the construct with K-wires in most instances; occasionally, however, miniscrews are used. Compacted cancellous bone can be added if there are defects that produce instability.

Open Fractures

Infection at the site of an open fracture in the hand is uncommon, probably because of the excellent blood supply. The prevalence has been reported to range from 5% (9 of 173) to 11% (16 of 146).[5] The infection rate has been shown to substantially increase in the presence of gross wound contamination, extensive soft-tissue and skeletal crush injury, systemic illness, or a delay in treatment exceeding 24 hours.[85,86] McLain and associates[86] showed that a delay in treatment of up to 12 hours did not increase the infection rate or influence the outcome. Swanson and associates[85] found that infection rates were not increased by the presence of internal fixation, immediate wound closure, large wound size, or complex injury in well-débrided, surgically clean open fractures. They recommended delayed wound closure in fractures associated with gross contamination.

Duncan and associates[5] reported that the functional outcome of open hand fractures, evaluated on the basis of digital motion, correlated highly with the initial severity of the injury. Metacarpal fractures had substantially better results than did proximal phalangeal fractures. Fractures of the proximal phalanx had the poorest outcome, especially if they were intra-articular or were associated with a tendon injury.[5,87] In mutilating injuries involving multiple fractures in a hand, the outcome may be predicted with use of the scoring system described by Campbell and Kay.[88]

Initial treatment consists of irrigation and débridement. Simple fractures can be definitively treated as we have outlined. Simple lacerations of tendons, nerves, and vessels as well as simple wounds can be repaired primarily. When comminution or bone loss is accompanied by simple wounds that can be closed primarily, and in most cases of low-velocity gunshot wounds, the fracture can be stabilized and treated with bone-grafting initially.[88-90] When comminution or bone loss is accompanied by integumentary loss, provisional fracture fixation is achieved with spacer wires, transfixation wires, or mini-external fixators. Definitive delayed primary treatment with mini-internal fixation, bone-grafting, and coverage is best done within 3 days after injury or as soon thereafter as possible.[59,89-92]

Complications

Stiffness resulting from tendon adhesions and joint contractures is the most common complication associated with hand fractures.[2,14] Stiffness has been shown to be directly correlated with the severity of the initial fracture, the presence and severity of soft-tissue injury, excessive immobilization (more than 4 weeks), and the extent of surgical dissection necessary for miniplate application.[5,14,87] Conversely, fractures that require miniplate fixation but are treated without fixation or with inadequate fixation still lead to stiffness and are associated with an increased rate of nonunion and malunion.[21,60] Immobilization in inappropriate positions and an inadequate rehabilitation program also may contribute to stiffness.

Chronic pain rarely is a compelling long-term problem following hand fractures, even in the event of posttraumatic arthritis.[2-4] Occasionally, however, arthroplasty or arthrodesis is indicated and may improve function as well as relieve pain.[76-79]

Malunion and nonunion are more likely to occur at the site of unstable fractures that are inadequately reduced, poorly stabilized, and not treated with bone grafting than they are at the site of those that are treated with adequate reduction, stable fixation, and bone-grafting of defects.[21,60] Adjacent joint stiffness and tendon adhesions are common. If malunion or nonunion is sufficiently symptomatic, surgical reconstruction is indicated (Fig. 15). One must go back to the fundamentals of fracture

treatment and start anew. Anatomic correction of deformity, sufficient stability to allow simultaneous bone healing and digital rehabilitation, respect for soft-tissue and vascular integrity, pain control, and early intensive rehabilitation are required. Miniplate fixation usually is the most reliable method of stabilizing these reconstructed fractures while they heal. Corrective osteotomies are performed for malunions, and some of these may require bone grafting. A nonunion often requires compression, bone grafting, or both. Tenolysis, capsulotomy, or both may be done concurrently if aggressive rehabilitation can begin immediately after surgery or independently at a later time.

Botte and associates,[93] in a review in which 422 pins were used to stabilize hand and wrist fractures in 137 patients, reported 34 complications involving 45 pins (11%) in 24 patients (18%). Sixty-nine percent of the complications, which included infection, pin loosening, loss of reduction, symptomatic nonunion, and impaled extensor and flexor tendons, occurred in the phalanges. Poor initial pin placement and patient noncompliance correlated most highly with these complications. In most cases of poor pin placement, the problem was not discovered until after surgery. Therefore, pin placement should be confirmed by radiographs at the time of surgery. Care of the skin surrounding the pins and removal of the pins as soon as bone healing (radiographic evidence of callus) allows (usually 3 to 6 weeks after insertion) eliminates much of the risk of pin loosening and pin-tract infection.

The complication rate associated with miniplate fixation has been reported to be 67% (6 of 9) when phalangeal fractures were involved and 34% (10 of 29) when metacarpal shaft fractures were involved.[14,94] Stiffness was the most common complication. The soft-tissue dissection necessary for miniplate application and the interference with tendon

excursion were the main causes. Twenty-five percent of the miniplates were removed because of discomfort or stiffness. The smaller lower-profile miniplates that are currently available may provide better results.

K-wires are almost always used for temporary fixation and are removed after the early appearance of fracture callus on radiographs. Miniscrews and plates usually are only removed for cause. Reasons for removal may include prominence and irritation under the skin, loosening, pull-out, or breakage. Loosening or breakage may herald delayed union, nonunion, or malunion. Implants may also be removed at the time of tenolysis or capsulotomy.

References

1. Freeland AE, Jabaley ME, Hughes JL (eds): *Stable Fixation of the Hand and Wrist.* New York, NY, Springer-Verlag, 1986, pp 3-35.
2. O'Rourke SK, Gaur S, Barton NJ: Long-term outcome of articular fractures of the phalanges: An eleven year follow-up. *J Hand Surg Br* 1989; 14:183-193.
3. Kjaer-Petersen K, Langhoff O, Andersen K: Bennett's fracture. *J Hand Surg Br* 1990;15: 58-61.
4. Livesley PJ: The conservative management of Bennett's fracture-dislocation: A 26-year follow-up. *J Hand Surg Br* 1990;15:291-294.
5. Duncan RW, Freeland AE, Jabaley ME, Meydrech EF: Open hand fractures: An analysis of the recovery of active motion and of complications. *J Hand Surg Am* 1993;18: 387-394.
6. Coonrad RW, Pohlman MH: Impacted fractures in the proximal portion of the proximal phalanx of the finger. *J Bone Joint Surg Am* 1969;51:1291-1296.
7. Barton N: Fractures of the phalanges of the hand. *Hand* 1977;9:1-10.
8. Barton NJ: Fractures of the hand. *J Bone Joint Surg Br* 1984;66:159-167.
9. Burkhalter WE: Hand fractures. *Instr Course Lect* 1990;39:249-253.
10. Corley FG Jr, Schenck RC Jr: Fractures of the hand. *Clin Plast Surg* 1996;23:447-462.
11. Ip WY, Ng KH, Chow SP: A prospective study of 924 digital fractures of the hand. *Injury* 1996; 27:279-285.
12. Kozin SH, Thoder JJ, Lieberman G: Operative treatment of metacarpal and phalangeal shaft fractures. *J Am Acad Orthop Surg* 2000;8: 111-121.

13. Maitra A, Burdett-Smith P: The conservative management of proximal phalangeal fractures of the hand in an accident and emergency department. *J Hand Surg Br* 1992;17:332-336.

14. Stern PJ: Management of fractures of the hand over the last 25 years. *J Hand Surg Am* 2000;25: 817-823.

15. Green DP, Anderson JR: Closed reduction and percutaneous pin fixation of fractured phalanges. *J Bone Joint Surg Am* 1973;55:1651-1654.

16. Belsky MR, Eaton RG, Lane LB: Closed reduction and internal fixation of proximal phalangeal fractures. *J Hand Surg Am* 1984;9: 725-729.

17. Widgerow AD, Edinburg M, Biddulph SL: An analysis of proximal phalangeal fractures. *J Hand Surg Am* 1987;12:134-139.

18. Edwards GS Jr, O'Brien ET, Heckman MM: Retrograde cross-pinning of transverse metacarpal and phalangeal fractures. *Hand* 1982;14:141-148.

19. Gonzalez MH, Igram CM, Hall RF: Intramedullary nailing of proximal phalangeal fractures. *J Hand Surg Am* 1995;20:808-812.

20. Gonzalez MH, Hall RF: Intramedullary fixation of metacarpal and proximal phalangeal fractures of the hand. *Clin Orthop* 1996;327: 47-54.

21. Jupiter JB, Koniuch MP, Smith RJ: The management of delayed union and nonunion of the metacarpals and phalanges. *J Hand Surg Am* 1985;10:457-466.

22. Freeland AE (ed): *Hand Fractures: Repair, Reconstruction, and Rehabilitation*. Philadelphia, PA, Churchill Livingstone, 2000, pp 25-29.

23. Pratt DR: Exposing fractures of the proximal phalanx of the finger longitudinally through the dorsal extensor apparatus. *Clin Orthop* 1959; 15:22-26.

24. Littler JW: Hand, wrist, and forearm incisions, in Littler JW, Cramer LM, Smith JW (eds): *Symposium On Reconstructive Hand Surgery*. St Louis, MO, CV Mosby, 1974, pp 87-97.

25. Field LD, Freeland AE, Jabaley ME: Midaxial approach to the proximal phalanx for fracture fixation. *Contemp Orthop* 1992;25:133-137.

26. Freeland AE, Geissler WB: Plate fixation of metacarpal shaft fractures, in Blair WF, Steyers CM (eds): *Techniques in Hand Surgery*. Baltimore, MD, Williams & Wilkins, 1996, pp 255-264.

27. Freeland AE, Jabaley ME: Open reduction internal fixation: Metacarpal fractures, in Strickland JW (ed): *The Hand*. Philadelphia, PA, Lippincott-Raven, 1998, pp 3-33.

28. Freeland AE: External fixation for skeletal stabilization of severe open fractures of the hand. *Clin Orthop* 1987;214:93-100.

29. Freeland AE, Geissler WB: Distal radial fractures: Open reduction internal fixation, in Wiss DA (ed): *Fractures*. Philadelphia, PA, Lippincott-Raven, 1998, pp 185-209.

30. Smith RJ: Balance and kinetics of the fingers under normal and pathological conditions. *Clin Orthop* 1974;104:92-111.

31. Smith RJ: Intrinsic muscles of the fingers: Function, dysfunction, and surgical reconstruction. *Instr Course Lect* 1975;24:200-220.

32. Eglseder WA Jr, Juliano PJ, Roure R: Fractures of the fourth metacarpal. *J Orthop Trauma* 1997; 11:441-445.

33. Strauch RJ, Rosenwasser MP, Lunt JG: Metacarpal shaft fractures: The effect of shortening on the extensor tendon mechanism. *J Hand Surg Am* 1998;23:519-523.

34. Birndorf MS, Daley R, Greenwald DP: Metacarpal fracture angulation decreases flexor mechanical efficiency in human hands. *Plast Reconstr Surg* 1997;99:1079-1085.

35. Royle SG: Rotational deformity following metacarpal fracture. *J Hand Surg Br* 1990;15: 124-125.

36. Viegas SF, Tencer A, Woodard P, Williams CR: Functional bracing of fractures of the second through fifth metacarpals. *J Hand Surg Am* 1987;12:139-143.

37. Konradsen L, Nielsen PT, Albrecht-Beste E: Functional treatment of metacarpal fractures 100 randomized cases with or without fixation. *Acta Orthop Scand* 1990;61:531-534.

38. Greene TL, Noellert RC, Belsole RJ, Simpson LA: Composite wiring of metacarpal and phalangeal fractures. *J Hand Surg Am* 1989;14: 665-669.

39. Ford DJ, el-Hadidi S, Lunn PG, Burke FD: Fractures of the metacarpals: Treatment by A.O. screw and plate fixation. *J Hand Surg Br* 1987;12:34-37.

40. Bosscha K, Snellen JP: Internal fixation of metacarpal and phalangeal fractures with AO minifragment screws and plates: A prospective study. *Injury* 1993;24:166-168.

41. Chen SH, Wei FC, Chen HC, Chuang CC, Noordhoff S: Miniature plates and screws in acute complex hand injury. *J Trauma* 1994;37: 237-242.

42. Pun WK, Chow SP, So YC, et al: A prospective study on 284 digital fractures of the hand. *J Hand Surg Am* 1989;14:474-481.

43. Dabezies EJ, Schutte JP: Fixation of metacarpal and phalangeal fractures with miniature plates and screws. *J Hand Surg Am* 1986;11:283-288.

44. Hastings H: Unstable metacarpal and phalangeal fracture treatment with screws and plates. *Clin Orthop* 1987;214:37-52.

45. Melone CP: Rigid fixation of phalangeal and metacarpal fractures. *Orthop Clin North Am* 1986;17:421-435.

46. Diwaker HN, Stothard J: The role of internal fixation in closed fractures of the proximal phalanges and metacarpals in adults. *J Hand Surg Br* 1986;11:103-108.

47. Buchler U, Fischer T: Use of a minicondylar plate for metacarpal and phalangeal periarticular injuries. *Clin Orthop* 1987;214:53-58.

48. Ouellette EA, Freeland AE: Use of the minicondylar plate in metacarpal and phalangeal fractures. *Clin Orthop* 1996;327:38-46.

49. Ford DJ, Ali MS, Steel WM: Fractures of the fifth metacarpal neck: Is reduction or immobilisation necessary? *J Hand Surg Br* 1989;14: 165-167.

50. McKerrell J, Bowen V, Johnston G, Zondervan J: Boxer's fractures: Conservative or operative management? *J Trauma* 1987;27:486-490.

51. Ashkenaze DM, Ruby LK: Metacarpal fractures and dislocations. *Orthop Clin North Am* 1992; 23:19-33.

52. Jahss SA: Fractures of the metacarpals: A new method of reduction and immobilization. *J Bone Joint Surg Am* 1938;20:178-186.

53. Light TR, Bednar MS: Management of intra-articular fractures of the metacarpophalangeal joint. *Hand Clin* 1994;10:303-314.

54. Vahey JW, Wegner DA, Hastings H III: Effect of proximal phalangeal fracture deformity on extensor tendon function. *J Hand Surg Am* 1998;23:673-681.

55. Freeland AE, Sennett BJ: Phalangeal fractures, in Peimer CA (ed): *Surgery of the Hand and Upper Extremity*. New York, NY, McGraw-Hill, Health Professions Division, 1996, pp 921-937.

56. Baratz ME, Divelbiss B: Fixation of phalangeal fractures. *Hand Clin* 1997;13:541-555.

57. Ford DJ, el-Hadidi S, Lunn PG, Burke FD: Fractures of the phalanges: Results of internal fixation using 1.5mm and 2mm A. O. screws. *J Hand Surg Br* 1987;12:28-33.

58. Hall RF Jr: Treatment of metacarpal and phalangeal fractures in noncompliant patients. *Clin Orthop* 1987;214:31-36.

59. Freeland AE, Jabaley ME: Stabilization of fractures in the hand and wrist with traumatic soft tissue and bone loss. *Hand Clin* 1988;4:425-436.

60. Lester B, Mallik A: Impending malunions of the hand: Treatment of subacute, malaligned fractures. *Clin Orthop* 1996,327.55-62.

61. Jupiter JB, Sheppard JE: Tension wire fixation of avulsion fractures in the hand. *Clin Orthop* 1987;214:113-120.

62. Jupiter JB, Lipton HA: Open reduction and internal fixation of avulsion fractures in the hand: The tension band wiring technique. *Tech Orthop* 1991;6:10-18.

63. Bischoff R, Buechler U, De Roche R, Jupiter J: Clinical results of tension band fixation of avulsion fractures of the hand. *J Hand Surg Am* 1994;19:1019-1026.

64. Weiss AP, Hastings H: Distal unicondylar fractures of the proximal phalanx. *J Hand Surg Am* 1993;18:594-599.

65. Dobyns JH, McElfresh EC: Extension block splinting. *Hand Clin* 1994;10:229-237.

66. Inoue G, Tamura Y: Treatment of fracture-dislocaton of the proximal interphalangeal joint using extension-block Kirschner wire. *Ann Chir Main Memb Super* 1991;10:564-568.

67. Freeland AE, Benoist LA: Open reduction and internal fixation method for fractures at the proximal interphalangeal joint. *Hand Clin* 1994; 10:239-250.

68. Kiefhaber TR, Stern PJ: Fracture dislocations of the proximal interphalangeal joint. *J Hand Surg Am* 1998;23:368-380.

69. Eaton RG, Malerich MM: Volar plate arthroplasty of the proximal interphalangeal joint: A review of ten years' experience. *J Hand Surg Am* 1980;5:260-268.

70. Malerich MM, Eaton RG: The volar plate reconstruction for fracture-dislocation of the proximal interphalangeal joint. *Hand Clin* 1994; 10:251-260.

71. Durham-Smith G, McCarten GM: Volar plate arthroplasty for closed proximal interphalangeal joint injuries. *J Hand Surg Br* 1992;17:422-428.

72. Schenck RR: Advances in reconstruction of digital joints. *Clin Plast Surg* 1997;24:175-189.

73. Morgan JP, Gordon DA, Klug MS, Perry PE, Barre PS: Dynamic digital traction for unstable comminuted intra-articular fracture-dislocations of the proximal interphalangeal joint. *J Hand Surg Am* 1995;20:565-573.

74. Stern PJ, Roman RJ, Kiefhaber TR, McDonough JJ: Pilon fractures of the proximal interphalangeal joint. *J Hand Surg Am* 1991;16:844-850.

75. Weiss AP: Cerclage fixation for fracture dislocation of the proximal interphalangeal joint. *Clin Orthop* 1996;327:21-28.

76. Nagle DJ, af Ekenstam FW, Lister GD: Immediate silastic arthroplasty for non-salvageable intraarticular phalangeal fractures. *Scand J Plast Reconstr Surg Hand Surg* 1989;23:47-50.

77. Gerard F, Garbuio P, Galleze B, Obert L, Tropet Y: Value of Swanson implants in complex traumatic lesions of the proximal interphalangeal joint. *Ann Chir Main Memb Super* 1996; 15:158-166.

78. Buchler U, Aiken MA: Arthrodesis of the proximal interphalangeal joint by solid bone grafting and plate fixation in extensive injuries to the dorsal aspect of the finger. *J Hand Surg Am* 1988;13:589-594.

79. Linscheid RL, Murray PM, Vidal MA, Beckenbaugh RD: Development of a surface replacement arthroplasty for proximal interphalangeal joints. *J Hand Surg Am* 1997;22: 286-298.

80. Surzur P, Rigault M, Charissoux JL, Mabit C, Arnaud JP: Recent fractures of the base of the 1st metacarpal bone: A study of a series of 138 cases. *Ann Chir Main Memb Super* 1994;13: 122-134.

81. Kahler DM: Fractures and dislocations of the base of the thumb. *J South Orthop Assoc* 1995; 4:69-76.

82. Cannon SR, Dowd GS, Williams DH, Scott JM: A long-term study following Bennett's fracture. *J Hand Surg Br* 1986;11:426-431.

83. Timmenga EJ, Blokhuis TJ, Maas M, Raaijmakers EL: Long-term evaluation of Bennett's fracture: A comparison between open and closed reduction. *J Hand Surg Br* 1994;19: 373-377.

84. Langhoff O, Andersen K, Kjaer-Petersen K: Rolando's fracture. *J Hand Surg Br* 1991;16: 454-459.

85. Swanson TV, Szabo RM, Anderson DD: Open hand fractures: Prognosis and classification. *J Hand Surg Am* 1991;16:101-107.

86. McLain RE, Steyers C, Stoddard M: Infections in open fractures of the hand. *J Hand Surg Am* 1991;16:108-112.

87. Strickland JW, Steichen JB, Kleinman WB, Hastings H: Phalangeal fractures: Factors influencing digital performance. *Orthop Rev* 1982; 11:39-50.

88. Campbell DA, Kay SP: The Hand Injury Severity Scoring System. *J Hand Surg Br* 1996; 21:295-298.

89. Gonzalez MH, Hall M, Hall RF Jr: Low-velocity gunshot wounds of the proximal phalanx: Treatment by early stable fixation. *J Hand Surg Am* 1998;23:150-155.

90. Gonzalez MH, McKay W, Hall RF: Low-velocity gunshot wounds of the metacarpal: Treatment by early stable fixation and bone grafting. *J Hand Surg Am* 1993;18:267-270.

91. Freeland AE, Jabaley ME, Burkhalter WE, Chaves AM: Delayed primary bone grafting in the hand and wrist after traumatic bone loss. *J Hand Surg Am* 1984;9:22-28.

92. Godina M: Early microsurgical reconstruction of complex trauma of the extremities. *Plast Reconstr Surg* 1986;78:285-292.

93. Botte MJ, Davis JL, Rose BA, et al: Complications of smooth pin fixation of fractures and dislocations in the hand and wrist. *Clin Orthop* 1992;276:194-201.

94. Stern PJ, Wieser MJ, Reilly DG: Complications of plate fixation in the hand skeleton. *Clin Orthop* 1987;214:59-65.

Current Concepts in the Treatment of Distal Radial Fractures

David S. Ruch, MD
Andrew J. Weiland, MD
Scott W. Wolfe, MD
William B. Geissler, MD
Mark S. Cohen, MD
Jesse B. Jupiter, MD

Abstract

Surgical indications for the treatment of distal radial fractures are evolving. It is important to identify the various articular fragments and their significance to facilitate optimal surgical treatment of these fragments from the standpoint of both internal and external fixation. New techniques in the visualization and stabilization of the articular surface and the treatment of defects in the metaphysis, including the use of cement to buttress the articular surface, have been brought to the forefront. A treatment algorithm for associated injuries to the distal radioulnar joint is also helpful.

In 1951, Gartland and Werley[1] evaluated the treatment outcomes for fractures of the distal radius in adults and concluded that the loss of the palmar tilt of the distal end of the radius was the single most important predictor of patient outcome. In 1986, Knirk and Jupiter[2] focused attention on the significance of a 2-mm intra-articular step-off in the development of posttraumatic osteoarthritis in younger adults. In 1994, Trumble and associates[3] subsequently concluded that "the degree to which articular step-off, gap between fragments, and radial shortening are improved by surgery is strongly correlated with improved outcome."

Since that time, several studies have raised additional questions about the optimal treatment of these common fractures. Although bridging external fixation preserved radial length, studies indicated that it was difficult to restore palmar tilt.[4,5] The subsequent enthusiasm for the use of dorsal plates to maintain palmar tilt and prevent radial collapse was diminished by reports of tenosynovitis and attritional rupture.[6-8] These concerns have led to the introduction of palmar plates, fixed angle devices, and the use of small implants with and without external fixation.[9-12] The role of internal fixation with the multitude of choices available requires definition. The introduction of arthroscopy both to assist in reduction and diagnose soft-tissue injuries indicates that many complaints after treatment may be referable to either interosseous ligament injury or distal radioulnar joint (DRUJ) disruption.[13-15] Finally, Young and Rayan[16] noted that the correlation between patient outcome and radiographs may not apply in older patients. These studies and others highlight a need to (1) document surgical indications for distal radial fractures, (2) identify the significance of anatomic reduction of the characteristic fragments in an intra-articular fracture, (3) establish specific applications for each type of plate available for internal fixation, (4) examine the indications for arthroscopy and its role in treating associated DRUJ injuries, and (5) examine the role of associated bone graft to prevent loss of reduction.

Surgical Indications

There is currently no consensus regarding the treatment of unstable distal radial fractures, which are defined by the presence of metaphyseal comminution, intra-articular extensions, shearing fractures, radiocarpal fracture-dislocations, or reduction that cannot be maintained with a cast.[17] Contemporary treatment issues include identifying the relative indications, advantages, and risks of external skeletal fixation compared with open reduction and stable internal fractures; determining whether functional outcome is enhanced by early motion following stabilization; and defining the role of bone substitutes or cements.[18-20]

The literature since the early 1970s reports varying degrees of success using external fixation to treat distal radial fractures. Although some studies report excellent functional and radiologic outcomes,[21] others reflect complication rates as high as 60%,[22] failure to achieve or maintain congruous articular reduction,[18] or loss of radiocarpal mobility because of the longitudinal distraction provided by the external fixation frame.[23]

Unfortunately, the majority of the expansive literature on the treatment of distal radial fractures is flawed from a scientific perspective. Most clinical trials are too small, have methodologic shortcomings, and lack standardization and validated functional outcomes. In addition, the generalization and application of limited trial results often become widespread without sufficient foundation.

Interest in avoiding the perceived stiffness associated with external fixation resulted in the development of mobile nonbridging external fixation devices. These devices, however, failed to adequately control unstable fractures of the DRUJ,[24] and several prospective studies failed to show improved motion or function compared with the use of standard external fixation frames.[25]

Despite the lack of evidence to support improved outcomes with early range of motion, many of the complications associated with these injuries can be minimized with internal fixation. Unfortunately, the literature on open reduction and internal fixation (ORIF) has varying methods of analysis, variability in techniques and fractures, and generally includes extended case series without comparative controls.[26-28]

A recent randomized, prospective, multicenter study compared the outcomes of external fixation with percutaneous Kirschner wires (K-wires) with ORIF for intra-articular distal radial fractures (HJ Kreder, MD; DP Hanel, MD; J Agel, MD; MD McKee, MD; TE Trumble, MD, Toronto, Canada, unpublished data presented at the Orthopaedic Trauma Association 18th annual meeting, 2002). Eighty-eight patients were randomized to have external fixation and 91 to have ORIF. (Eight patients from the external fixation group had ORIF because of inadequate reduction.) The patients were observed for 24 months and evaluated using the musculoskeletal functional analysis upper extremity module and Jebsen-Taylor hand function testing and were further evaluated for pain, wrist and forearm motion, and grip strength. At 2 years, the external fixation group had significantly better upper extremity function ($P = .014$) and pinch strength ($P = .020$). No statistically significant difference between the groups was reported for all other modalities of evaluation, and complication rates were relatively equal in both groups.

When other prospective studies are examined critically, whether comparing ORIF and immobilization, bridging and nonbridging external fixation,[5] or bone cement and cast or external fixation,[29,30] the ultimate range of motion seems to be unaffected by early motion.

Despite the inconclusive data in the literature, there has been increasing enthusiasm for using ORIF to treat distal radial fractures. Several factors may account for this. Radiologic advances including CT and three-dimensional reconstructions have more accurately defined articular fracture patterns, especially those that would not fare well with closed treatment.[31,32] These imaging studies have also helped to define the functional significance of the anatomic elements of the distal end of the radius. Some investigators have independently recognized the importance of the cortical margins around the "radial column,"[27] which has led to the development of implants specifically designed to support this aspect of the radial metaphysis and accommodate various anatomic aspects of the dorsal or volar aspects of the radius.

Plate Design

Until recently, the use of and indications for plate fixation have been limited, especially in the treatment of fractures of the dorsal aspect of the distal radius. Early plate designs were bulky and did not allow for contouring to the normal osseous anatomy. Moreover, early plate designs were notorious for irritating the overlying extensor tendons, frequently necessitating plate removal. The early plate designs also had limited variability in the location of screw insertion sites as well as screw types, which confined their use to only very specific fracture patterns. Plate design eventually evolved toward a low-profile, malleable plate with numerous screw options that would theoretically obviate problems with tendon irritation and rupture.

One of the first-generation distal radial fracture plates was the AO oblique T plate (Synthes, Paoli, PA)

(Figure 1). Although this dorsally placed plate was relatively thin and somewhat malleable, the screw insertion sites were few, requiring the use of proportionately large 3.5-mm screws. The 3.5-mm screws used distally in this plate caused several problems. The bulk of the heads on the 3.5-mm screws contributed to irritation and attrition of the overlying extensor tendons. In addition, the size of the screw restricted use of the plate to the treatment of fractures with large fragments.

In an attempt to alleviate the problems encountered with the oblique T plate, the Pi plate (Synthes,) (named for its resemblance to the Greek letter Pi) was created (Figure 2). This dorsally applied plate had a low-profile contour, recessed screw heads, and improved malleability, all of which would theoretically decrease extensor tendon irritation. The distal limb of the plate was created to confine the articular fragments and had numerous holes for the placement of smaller 2.4-mm screws or 1.8-mm buttress pins. In addition, this generation of plate design introduced two new elements into the evolution of plate design: (1) titanium for plate construction and (2) screws that locked into the plate, creating a fixed-angle buttress effect for the fixation of comminuted articular fragments. Although the new design was created to reduce the risk of tendon irritation, the Pi plate was associated with a high rate of tendon irritation and attritional rupture of the overlying extensor tendons.[33,34] A second generation of Pi plate design was subsequently released with tapered skids at the distal screw insertion sites and stainless steel composition.

At the same time the second-generation Pi plate design was released, the Forte Plate (Zimmer, Warsaw, IN) was introduced. This plate

was essentially an oblique T-shaped plate. However, the design included recessed screw heads to reduce tendon irritation. A template that is pre-shaped to the contour of an uninjured dorsal distal radius is used with this system to aid in reduction and drilling of the countersunk screws.

Other dorsal plating systems have used a low-profile design and multiple fixed-angle buttress prongs to maintain a buttress support of the subchondral bone as well as the dorsal aspect of the distal radius. The SCS plate (Avanta, San Diego, CA) uses this buttressing technique to allow the plate to act as a load-sharing device when placed either on the dorsal or volar surfaces of the distal radius. The fixed-angle plate has been shown in the laboratory to be up to 2.4 times stronger and more rigid than conventional plate-screw interfaces.[35] However, the shape of the plate necessitates the use of a drill guide to predrill the distal radius before placement and may also require additional fixation methods for varying fracture patterns.

A recently developed low-profile dorsal plate, the LoCon-T (Wright Medical Technologies, Inc, Arlington, TN), combines several previously successful design features with several innovations (Figure 3). Anatomically individualized shapes and improved malleability allows the plate to conform better to the distal radius. In addition, the shape of the distal limb of the plate allows for a variety of low-profile head screw options, thereby decreasing the risk of extensor tendinitis. An optional variable angle-extending device can also be used to capture small radial-sided fragments.

Two new plate design features have recently been introduced: fragment-specific fixation and fixed-angle volar plating. Fragment-specific

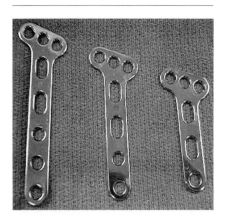

Figure 1 AO oblique T plate. (Synthes, Paoli, PA.)

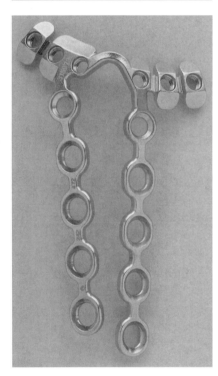

Figure 2 Pi plate. (Synthes, Paoli, PA.)

fixation uses multiple small, low-profile plates and K-wires.[36] Peine and associates[11] reported that lower-profile, less rigid implants such as the TriMed System (TriMed, Valencia, CA) when placed in an orthogonal position to the deforming forces of the wrist maximized their biomechanical stability (Figure 4). The fixed-angle volar plating system DVR (Hand Innovations, Miami, FL) is

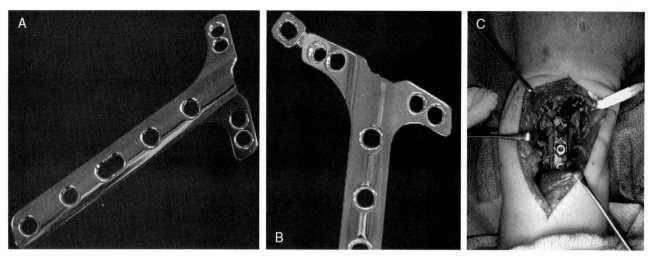

Figure 3 A through **C,** LoCon-T plate. (Wright Medical Technologies, Inc, Arlington, TN.)

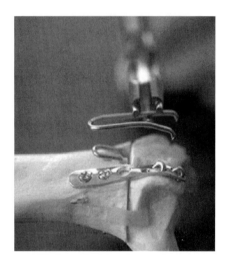

Figure 4 TriMed system. (TriMed, Valencia, CA.)

used for dorsally displaced intra-articular fractures. Like the fixed-angle plate designs before it, fixed-angle volar plating uses subchondral support pegs to support the distal fracture fragments. In addition, this plating system allows for either the use of fixed-angle or regular threaded screws to allow for increased variability in the screw placement patterns. Orbay and Fernandez[37] recently described the use of an extended flexor carpi radialis approach in conjunction with the use of this plate to achieve reduction of the dorsal pieces through a volar approach.

One problem with traditional methods of internal fixation is that surgeons are expected to mold the fracture to the particular hardware available. This may leave individual fracture fragments poorly stabilized or require extensive soft-tissue disruption on both the dorsal and palmar sides of the wrist when dual-plating systems are placed. In an effort to reduce the complications associated with traditional internal fixation devices, steady improvements in the methods of internal fixation been made and fracture outcomes have improved as a result. Critical improvements over the past decade include: (1) appreciation of the complexity of distal radial fracture patterns, (2) improved comprehension of the high mechanical forces across the wrist fracture site, (3) enhancements in hardware design, and (4) the liberal use of bone graft. In particular, the development of columnar fixation has radically changed the approach to internal fixation of complex distal radial fractures over the past 10 years.

Columnar Fixation

Peine and associates[11] and Jakob and associates[27] have been particularly instrumental in advancing the columnar approach to treat distal radial fractures. The distal forearm can be conceptualized as having three longitudinal columns: radial, intermediate, and ulnar. The radial column consists exclusively of the radial styloid. The intermediate column consists of the lunate die-punch fragments and the critical components of the sigmoid notch. The ulnar column consists of the ulna, DRUJ, and triangular fibrocartilage complex. Each column has unique characteristics that must be considered for fracture stability and restoration.

In mechanical studies, Peine and associates[11] demonstrated that strategic placement of ultra–low-profile (2.0-mm) implants provided increased stability of fixation when compared with traditional T plate and Pi plate implants for distal radial fixation. Their model used a dorsal metaphyseal defect, and loading was performed in compression using a servohydraulic testing system (MTS, Eden Prairie, MN). The authors concluded that the strategic placement of these low-profile implants at 50° to 90° angles from each other more effectively reduced external forces when compared with a dorsally applied plate. In a similar study, Dodds and associates[38] demonstrated that although internally fixed specimens were allowed to fully flex and extend under applied load, the application of thin implants along the radial and intermediate columns in an orthogonal relationship (orthogonal 90° fixation) provided increased stability when compared with traditional techniques of augmented external fixation (Figure 5).

Specific Columnar Applications

Radial Column Restoration of radial columnar height is the cornerstone of unstable distal radial fracture fixation, and it can be compared with the restoration of the lateral malleolus when reconstructing complex bimalleolar fractures of the ankle. The radial column is approached through a volar-radial incision that parallels the traditional Henry incision but lies 5 mm radial to the radial artery. The incision is 3 to 4 cm in length and begins at a prominent tubercle on the radial styloid. The brachioradialis can be split longitudinally to allow subperiosteal exposure of the entire radial column and the volar aspect of the distal radius. With traction applied through the use of a fingertrap or a traction table, the large radial styloid fragment is reduced and stabilized.

Intermediate Column Each of the individual fracture fragments that comprise the intermediate column (the dorsal cortical, volar lip, dorsal-ulnar, and volar-ulnar fragments) should be identified. Each of these individual fracture fragments can exist individually or in combination in any particular fracture. It is important to realize that the dorsal-ulnar

and volar-ulnar fragments constitute the entire sigmoid notch and thus the seat for radioulnar joint stability. The dorsal cortical and volar lip fragments are generally created by compression-type forces and often include a separate articular impaction component.

These fragments must be reduced to provide stability for the articular surface. Bone graft may be required to support the elevated articular surface. Using a variety of implants, the intermediate column can be restored and stabilized. The implants must be modular to allow customization of the implant to the particular fracture characteristics.

The intermediate column is approached through a utilitarian dorsal incision beginning at Lister's tubercle and coursing approximately 3 to 5 cm proximally. Exposure of the fracture fragments is generally performed through the third dorsal compartment in a subperiosteal fashion. An isolated approach to the dorsal-ulnar fragment can be performed through the same incision, developing an interval through the fifth dorsal compartment directly to the dorsal lip of the sigmoid notch.

An often overlooked but critical component of intermittent column fractures is the volar-ulnar component. Unless reduced anatomically and held with stable fixation, the lunate can translate palmarly and leave the entire carpus subluxated. The volar-ulnar fragment is best visualized with oblique radiographs or CT and can be approached through a limited incision on the volar-ulnar aspect of the forearm. The ulnar neurovascular bundle can be retracted to the ulnar side and the median nerve and flexor tendons to the radial side to expose the pronator quadratus and the volar aspect of the sigmoid notch. With elevation of the pronator

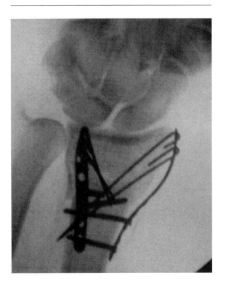

Figure 5 Fragment-specific fixation with the TriMed implant system. (Reproduced with permission from Barrie KA, Wolfe SW: Internal fixation for intraarticular distal raduis fractures. *Tech Hand Upper Extremity Surg* 2002;6;10-20.)

quadratus, the fracture fragment is readily exposed and can be fixed with a tension band, a wireform implant, or a small contoured plate.

Ulnar Column The stability of the ulnar column must be evaluated before leaving the operating room. Fractures that involve the base of the ulnar styloid can entirely disrupt the dorsal and palmar radial ulnar ligaments and may need fixation to restore stability. Similarly, ulnar neck fractures can be comminuted and unstable, requiring separate fixation of the ulnar shaft or neck. Failure to appreciate and stabilize the ulnar column can result in painful instability of the radioulnar joint and dramatic loss of forearm rotation.

Arthroscopic Treatment of Intra-Articular Distal Radial Fractures

Displaced intra-articular fractures are a unique subset of distal radial fractures. These fractures are usually the result of a high-energy injury and can be associated with soft-tissue injuries. The prognosis for these injuries has been shown to depend on radial shortening, residual extra-articular angulation, both radiocarpal and radioulnar articular congruity, and associated soft-tissue injuries. Wrist arthroscopy can be a valuable adjunct in the treatment of these difficult fractures, particularly when articular congruity and associated soft-tissue injuries are also present.

Articular Congruity

Auge and Velazquez[39] reviewed the results of arthroscopic evaluation of the articular surface after fluoroscopic reduction and pinning in 15 patients and found that with arthroscopic evaluation, 33% of the patients had an articular step-off of 1 mm that appeared anatomically reduced under fluoroscopy. The authors also noted that adjunctive arthroscopy might detect residual gapping not seen with traditional fluoroscopy.

Soft-Tissue Lesions

The fact that intracarpal soft-tissue injuries can occur with fractures of the distal radius has been well documented; however, whether intracarpal soft-tissue injuries truly affect the prognoses and treatment results is still unknown. Four separate wrist arthrography studies noted a high incidence of tears of the triangular fibrocartilage complex associated with fractures of the distal radius. Fontes and associates[40] noted a 66% incidence of tears of the triangular fibrocartilage complex in 58 patients with distal radial fractures. Similarly, Mohanti and Kar[41] found a 45% incidence of tears of the triangular fibrocartilage complex in a series of 60 patients. Additionally, in a report on 60 patients with intra-articular fractures of the distal radius who underwent arthroscopic

evaluation, Geissler and associates[15] found that 49% of the patients had a tear of the triangular fibrocartilage complex. Injuries to the scapholunate and lunotriquetral interosseous ligaments were also present but were less common. Tears of the scapholunate interosseous ligament were present in 32% of the patients and injury to the lunotriquetral interosseous ligament was present in 15%.[15] In a similar arthroscopic study of 50 patients, Lindau and associates[42] reported that 78% had a tear of the triangular fibrocartilage complex, with 54% having injury to the scapholunate interosseous ligament and 16% having a tear to the lunotriquetral interosseous ligament.

Radial styloid fractures, die-punch fractures, three-part T-fractures, and four-part fractures are all ideal fracture patterns for arthroscopically assisted reduction and internal fixation. Four-part fractures are generally treated with a combination of open arthrotomy combined with arthroscopic fixation where the joint surface is not opened. After the articular surface is stabilized, a small incision may be made between the fourth and fifth dorsal compartments and bone graft added to supplement the fixation. Additional indications for fixation may be a minimally displaced fracture of the distal radius and a suspected soft-tissue injury. Radial styloid fractures are highly associated with injury to the scapholunate interosseous ligament and may be evaluated arthroscopically and the fragments anatomically reduced. Rotation of the radial styloid is best judged by looking across the wrist through the 6-R portal. A probe or blunt trocar may be inserted in the 3-4 portal to help reduce the radial styloid fragment with the use of the K-wire joy stick. Once the fracture has been arthroscopically judged to be anatomic, the K-wire is then advanced across the fracture, and two K-wires

are placed across the fracture site through a soft-tissue protector.

Impaction Fractures

Three-part fractures are more difficult to treat than radial styloid fractures. The radial styloid may be closed, reduced, and pinned under fluoroscopy. The radial styloid fragment then may be used as a landmark to arthroscopically elevate the depressed medial fragment. After the radial styloid fragment has been closed, reduced, and pinned, the wrist is suspended in traction. The fracture debris is lavaged out, the arthroscope is placed in the 3-4 portal, and the depressed medial fragment is visualized. An 18-gauge needle may be placed percutaneously through the wrist directly over the fracture fragment and used as a landmark where a Steinmann pin will be placed (approximately 2 cm proximal to the 18-gauge needle onto the bone fragment). Under arthroscopic visualization, the fragment is then elevated percutaneously with a large Steinmann pin. A bone tenaculum can also be used to further reduce the sagittal gap. One point of the tenaculum is placed on the radial styloid and the second on the medial fragment to further close the sagittal gap, if present. Once the fracture is judged to be anatomic under fluoroscopy, it is pinned transversely. Two K-wires may be placed subchondrally into the medial fragment. If the medial fragment is a dorsal die-punch fragment, it is important to aim the pins dorsally to capture this fragment. It is also important to pronate and supinate the wrist after placement of the transverse pins to ensure that the pins have not violated the DRUJ. As in radial styloid fractures, headless cannulated screws may be used. One screw may be placed to stabilize the radial styloid and a second subchondrally and transversely to stabilize the medial fragment. This prevents protruding K-wires from causing soft-tissue irritation and allows for earlier range of motion.

Four-part fractures are treated with a combination of open arthrotomy and arthroscopically assisted fixation. The volar medial fragment often cannot be reduced by closed manipulation; it rotates with traction on the volar capsule. The radial styloid fragment is reduced under closed manipulation in fluoroscopy. Two K-wires are provisionally placed to stabilize the radial styloid fragment. A longitudinal incision is then made between the flexor tendons and the ulnar neurovascular bundle. Dissection between these structures is done down to the volar medial radius. The pronator quadratus is then elevated, exposing the fragment. A 2.7- or 3.5-mm buttress plate is then placed on the volar aspect of the distal radius to stabilize the volar medial fragment, which is important to radioulnar joint congruency and stability of the DRUJ. Screws are placed in the proximal screw holes but not in the very distal aspect of the plate because they can potentially block reduction of the dorsal fragments. The wrist is then suspended in the traction tower, and the arthroscope is placed in the 3-4 portal. To best view the dorsal fragments, the arthroscope is transferred to the 6-R portal. Although adequate visualization of the dorsal fragment is usually achieved with the arthroscope in the 6-R portal, the arthroscope may be placed in a volar portal, which is located between the radioscaphocapitate ligament and the long radiolunate ligament.

The fracture now is treated as a three-part fragment, and the volar medial fragment can be used as a ful-crum to reduce the dorsal fragment. This fragment is reduced percutaneously with a Steinmann pin elevated to both the radial styloid and the volar medial fragment, which are used as landmarks when visualized arthroscopically. Once the dorsal medial fragment is elevated, it is pinned transversely. Once the fragment has been pinned, screws in the distal portion of the plate may be placed to capture the dorsal fragment. Any associated soft-tissue injuries may then be treated.

The Role of Cement

The use of cement for distal radial fracture fixation was first reported in the 1980s and involved the use of polymethylmethacrylate bone cement.[43,44] Cement fixation is possible because most distal radial fractures are reducible. Dorsal comminution and bone loss are responsible for fracture collapse and failure of conservative treatment methods. Unfortunately, acrylate cement is neither remodeled nor incorporated and is exothermic, potentially impairing fracture healing. In the liquid state, it is cytotoxic and extravasation from the fracture site can cause soft-tissue morbidity.[45]

A variety of materials are currently available to replace compromised cancellous bone in the metaphysis following fracture. In 1995, a bioactive bone cement (Norian, Synthes), was introduced that can be injected in paste form. It rapidly cures in vivo (at body temperature and pH level) to form an osteoconductive carbonated apatite cement.[46-48] This material has chemical and physical properties similar to the mineral phase of bone. It hardens in approximately 10 minutes, at which time it reaches a compressive strength of 10 MPa. After approximately 12 hours at body temperature, it reaches its ultimate compressive strength of 55

MPa, which lies between the compressive strength of cancellous and cortical bone. The cement is weak in shear and tension to the order of 2 to 3 MPa, which is lower than that of cancellous bone.[49] It is ultimately incorporated and remodeled in a cell-mediated process without stimulating an immune response.

The largest randomized, prospective clinical trial evaluating this bone cement involved 323 patients from multiple centers.[29] Unstable distal radial fractures were randomized to be treated with either conventional methods (casting or external fixation) or bone cement. The cement-treated patients began an early range-of-motion program at approximately 2 weeks versus 6 to 8 weeks for the patients treated with conventional methods. Results showed that the cement-treated patients had a more rapid return of motion and improved outcome measures when evaluated at 6 to 8 weeks. Although differences normalized by 3 months, the use of the bone cement clearly moved the rehabilitation curve to the left allowing for a more rapid return of function following injury. Fortunately, this was not at the expense of healing and radiographic parameters. The bone cement thus permitted earlier mobilization and improved the rate of functional recovery and patient satisfaction in the early postoperative period.

The primary technical difficulty in the use of the bone cement in this study was inadequate metaphyseal filling leading to fracture settling (Figure 6). This occurred early in the series when the bone cement was administered percutaneously. It became clear that there was a zone of compromised cancellous bone around the cement that was inherently less stable than the cement itself. A technique was developed using a limited open

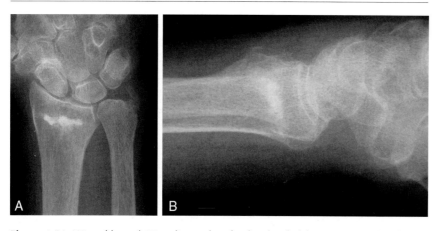

Figure 6 PA (**A**) and lateral (**B**) radiographs of a distal radial fracture treated with percutaneous placement of Norian (Synthes) bone cement. Note the poor metaphyseal fill and settling that have occurred, leading to shortening and collapse. This was the most common complication of the largest prospective study evaluating this material.

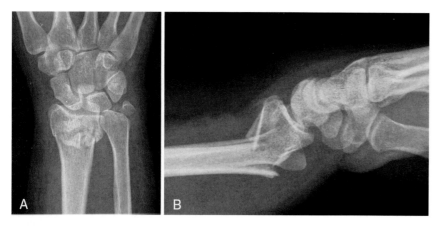

Figure 7 PA (**A**) and lateral (**B**) radiographs of a distal radial fracture with dorsal angulation and comminution. Note the associated ulnar styloid base fracture.

protocol was used to create extra-articular bending fractures of the distal radius. All fractures were reduced, and three treatment groups were studied: (1) percutaneous cementing alone, (2) open cementing through a dorsal exposure with manual creation of a metaphyseal cavity, and (3) a balloon tamp with percutaneous cementing. After curing, the specimens were cyclically loaded using linear variable transducers to measure displacement. Overall, the volume of cement injected was related to the treatment used, with more cement injected with the balloon tamp method than the other methods. Both the open and balloon tamp groups had less axial settling and angular collapse than the group with percutaneous cementing alone. Thus, percutaneous cement delivery with a minimally invasive bone tamp was equal to open methods of fracture cementing when tested in the laboratory.

Treatment of Associated DRUJ Injuries

Studies of the treatment of distal radial fractures report that possible intra-articular incongruity resulting in arthrosis and immediate loss of function are two major outcome risks. Intra-articular incongruity is secondary to residual depression of the lunate facet, resulting in step-off in the articular surface and causing arthrosis in 7 to 10 years.[2,28,52] Loss of function is perhaps more perplexing and primarily the result of dysfunction of the DRUJ.[53] Increasingly, authors are documenting the correlation between patient-related outcome scores and DRUJ instability following fracture.[54-56] These data have shifted attention to the intermediate column of the wrist with its component sigmoid notch and DRUJ.

dorsal approach in which the hematoma was evacuated and the fragmented cancellous bone manually compressed to form a stable defect. The bone cement was then injected into the prepared cavity under direct visualization. Dorsal dissection of the soft tissues added time and morbidity to the procedure.

In an effort to return to more percutaneous and minimally invasive techniques, researchers hypothesized that balloon tamp technology could be applied to the wrist. The balloon tamp (Kyphon Inc, Sunny-vale, CA) was originally developed to reduce osteoporotic spinal wedge-compression fractures.[50] When used to treat fractures of the distal radius, the inflatable tamp could be percutaneously introduced to elevate the fracture and create a compression-resistant metaphyseal defect. The carbonated apatite cement could then be injected percutaneously (Figures 7 through 10).

This treatment method has been tested using 24 paired fresh cadavers.[51] Specimens were mounted on a testing apparatus and a standardized

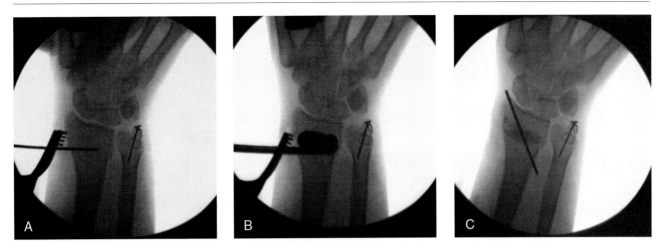

Figure 8 A, Intraoperative fluoroscopy image with the sleeve of the bone tamp in place. **B,** The tamp has been inflated, compressing the compromised cancellous bone and hematoma and creating a stable metaphyseal defect. **C,** Final intraoperative image following percutaneous bone cement injection. The patient began range-of-motion exercises 2 weeks postoperatively.

Pattern Recognition

In the treatment of acute DRUJ injuries associated with distal radial fractures, a spectrum of injury is involved consisting of either (1) bony injuries resulting from fractures of the palmar/dorsal sigmoid notch or the ulnar styloid or (2) DRUJ ligament/triangular fibrocartilage complex injuries. Successful treatment of these injuries is predicated on early recognition and maintaining the DRUJ in its reduced position. Early recognition of these injuries is critical and may be achieved with plain radiographs and examination of the patient after stabilization of the distal radius. Radiographic evidence of preoperative instability is unreliable, but a large ulnar styloid fragment that involves the hilum of the ulna may also serve as the attachment for the palmar and dorsal radioulnar ligaments. Significant displacement of the styloid implies not only an inability of these ligaments to heal but also possible tendinous interposition in the DRUJ. In the absence of a large ulnar styloid fragment, instability may be diagnosed once the radius has been anatomi-

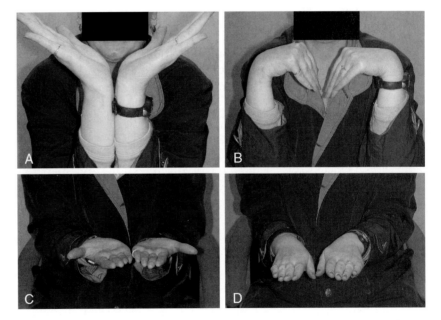

Figure 9 Clinical photographs showing wrist extension at 3 months (**A**), wrist flexion at 3 months (**B**), wrist supination at 3 months (**C**), and wrist pronation at 3 months (**D**).

cally stabilized. Although a definition of instability of this joint has not been established, more than 1 cm of palmar dorsal translational instability or gross rotational instability when compared with the contralateral radioulnar joint is a useful criterion.

Joint Stability

Several studies have examined the significance of the radioulnar ligaments in DRUJ stability, and both the palmar and dorsal radioulnar ligaments have been shown to play a significant role.[57-60] It is also significant that in cadaver models, the

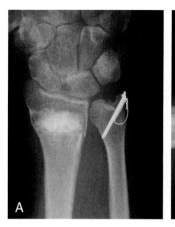
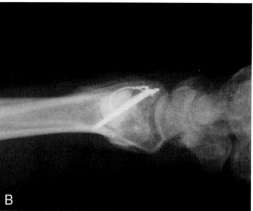

Figure 10 Final PA (**A**) and lateral (**B**) radiographs revealing maintenance of the original reduction despite early range of motion.

DRUJ subluxated or dislocated in maximum pronation, but in supination, the DRUJ was stable.[58] These data indicate that after injury to the DRUJ the position of supination will minimize residual dorsal subluxation of the ulna relative to the radius.

Osseous Injury

Osseous injury of the DRUJ may occur as either a fracture of the palmar or dorsal lunate facets (sigmoid notch) or a fracture of the ulnar styloid. Fractures of the sigmoid notch may involve either the entire lunate facet or may represent avulsion fragments of the DRUJ ligaments. Although congruity of the sigmoid notch remains a significant theoretic concern, cadaveric study data indicate that only approximately 20% of the DRUJ stability is provided by articular contact between the radius and ulna.[57] It appears, therefore, that the ligamentous attachments of these structures are primarily responsible for the stability of the DRUJ. In regard to the significance of either the palmar and dorsal lunate facet, the majority of cadaveric study data suggest that the major constraint to the dorsal translation of the distal ulna relative to the radius is the palmar ra-

dioulnar ligament.[57] Malunion of this palmar lunate facet results in residual loss of supination of the DRUJ. With regard to the dorsal lunate facet, although the cadaveric studies indicate that the dorsal ligaments are significant in maintaining the stability of the DRUJ, residual depression of this dorsal lunate facet appears to be relatively common following external fixation of distal radial fractures. Outcome studies indicate that as much as a 20° loss of palmar tilt (residual depression of the dorsal lunate facet) may still result in excellent functional outcome and a stable DRUJ.[61] Therefore, the sigmoid notch apparently provides minimal bony constraint to the DRUJ, and the palmar radioulnar ligaments that attach to the palmar lunate facet are the most important structures to restore anatomically.

Fractures of the ulnar styloid are common following fractures of the distal radius. These fractures must be identified as either fractures that extend into the hilum of the distal ulna or more distal fractures. Several authors have documented the significance of distal ulnar fractures in association with distal radial fractures.[57,62] These fractures may occur

in isolation or in association with a ligamentous disruption[63] (Figure 11).

The optimal treatment of ulnar styloid base fractures has not been completely elucidated; however, the position of the styloid relative to the shaft of the ulna on a true lateral view must be assessed. If the ulnar styloid lies palmar to the axis of the ulna on a true lateral view and the ulna is displaced relative to it, stability to the DRUJ is compromised and must be restored. As these fractures typically will reduce in supination, one option is to place the patient in full supination, document reduction, and maintain this position for 4 to 6 weeks before initiating range-of-motion exercises. If the styloid does not reduce in supination or the position of forearm rotation is unacceptable, then ORIF of the styloid should be performed using either tension-band wiring or a single screw. Regardless of the technique used, verification that stability of the DRUJ has been restored must be achieved after fixation of the styloid fragment. This is in contradistinction to tip of the ulnar styloid fractures, which represent either direct trauma to the tip of the styloid or avulsion of the dorsal capsule. Stability will not be restored by fixation of these distal fractures, and the DRUJ must be examined as if this represents a pure ligamentous injury.

Ligamentous Injury

Injury to the DRUJ ligaments at either the radial or peripheral attachments may result in significant instability and symptoms following fracture.[63] Treatment of these injuries depends on whether the joint can be maintained in a reduced position. When preoperative radiographs demonstrate significant shortening of the radius relative to the ulna and no evidence of an ulnar styloid base fracture, cadaveric studies indicate that disruption of the

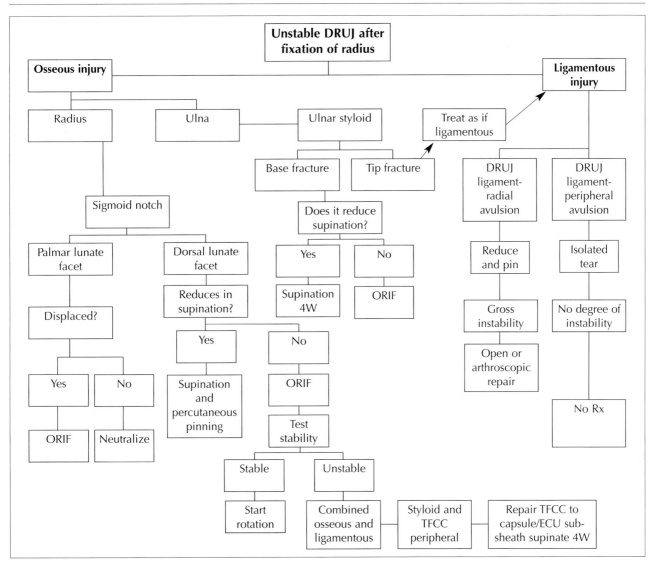

Figure 11 Algorithm for the treatment of DRUJ injuries. TFCC = Triangular fibrocartilage complex, ECU = extensor carpi ulnaris, 4W = 4 weeks.

DRUJ ligaments have occurred.[64] In the absence of an ulnar styloid base fracture, the ligaments must be stripped off the distal ulna. In the face of gross instability with this pattern following fixation of the radius, the ligamentous injury should be treated. If arthroscopy has been used as an adjunctive tool for fixation of the fracture, arthroscopic repair of the triangular fibrocartilage complex should be considered. If arthroscopic repair is not an option, then the sigmoid notch should be assessed. If there is no ev-

idence of avulsion of the sigmoid notch by these ligaments, the forearm should be placed in supination for 3.5 to 4 weeks to allow the DRUJ to heal in a reduced position before initiation of pronation and supination. This can be accomplished via either cross pins or the use of an external fixator device with an outrigger to the ulna (Orthofix, McKinney, TX).

Combined Injuries
A significant incidence of soft-tissue injuries in association with ulnar sty-

loid base fractures has been documented.[65] Fixation of the sigmoid notch and the ulnar styloid may not result in complete restoration of stability because the ligaments may be either avulsed from these fragments or ruptured along their anatomic course. Following fixation of these fragments, if DRUJ stability is not accomplished, then the patient should be placed in supination for 4 to 6 weeks, followed by gradual mobilization into pronation to avoid the instability associated with chronic ligamentous disruption.

Summary

Fractures of the distal radius may be successfully managed using a variety of techniques. The keys to a successful outcome appear to be (1) understanding the patient's needs and expectations; (2) adequate imaging to enable identification of displacement of key bony and soft-tissue components; and (3) adequate reduction and stabilization of these "critical" fragments. Although newer implant technology may make stabilization more rigid and less invasive, an understanding of the fracture fragments and their natural history if they heal in a displaced position ultimately determines whether the patient will have an acceptable outcome.

References

1. Gartland J, Werley C: Evaluation of healed Colles' fractures. *J Bone Joint Surg Am* 1951;33:895-907.

2. Knirk J, Jupiter J: Intraarticular fractures of the distal end of the radius in young adults. *J Bone Joint Surg Am* 1986;68:647-659.

3. Trumble TE, Schmitt S, Vedder NB: Factors affecting functional outcome of displaced intra-articular distal radius fractures. *J Hand Surg Am* 1994;19:325-340.

4. Bartosh RA, Saldana MJ: Intraarticular fractures of the distal radius: A cadaveric study to determine if ligamentotaxis restores radiopalmar tilt. *J Hand Surg Am* 1990;15:18-21.

5. McQueen M, Hajducka C, Court-brown C: Redisplaced unstable fractures of the distal radius. *J Bone Joint Surg Br* 1996;78:404-409.

6. Kambouroglou G, Ayres JR: Complications of the AO/ASIF titanium distal radius plate system (pi plate) in internal fixation of the distal radius: A brief report. *J Hand Surg Am* 1998;23:737-741.

7. Axelrod TS, McMurtry RY: Open reduction and internal fixation of comminuted, intraarticular fractures of the distal radius. *J Hand Surg Am* 1990;15:1-11.

8. Fitoussi F, Chow SP: Treatment of displaced intra-articular fractures of the distal end of the radius with plates. *J Bone Joint Surg Am* 1997;79:1303-1312.

9. Rikli D, Regazzoni P: Fractures of the distal end of the radius treated by internal fixation and early function. *J Bone Joint Surg Br* 1996;78:588-592.

10. Hahnloser D, Platz A, Amgwerd M, Trentz O: Internal fixation of distal radius fractures with dorsal dislocation: Pi-plate or two 1/4 tube plates? A prospective randomized study. *J Trauma* 1999;47:760-765.

11. Peine R, Rikli DA, Hoffmann R, Duda G, Regazzoni P: Comparison of three different plating techniques for the dorsum of the distal radius: A biomechanical study. *J Hand Surg Am* 2000;25:29-33.

12. Sommerkamp T, Seeman M, Silliman J, et al: Dynamic external fixation of unstable fractures of the distal part of the radius. *J Bone Joint Surg Am* 1994;76:1149-1161.

13. Zancolli EA, Ziadenberg C, Zancolli E Jr: Biomechanics of the trapeziometacarpal joint. *Clin Orthop* 1987;220:14-26.

14. Kazuteru D, Hattori Y, Otsuka K, Abe Y, Yamamoto H: Intraarticular fractures of the distal aspect of the radius: Arthroscopically assisted reduction compared with open reduction and internal fixation. *J Bone Joint Surg Am* 1999;81:1093-1110.

15. Geissler WB, Freeland AE, Savoie FH, McIntyre LW, Whipple TL: Intracarpal soft-tissue lesions associated with an intra-articular fracture of the distal end of the radius. *J Bone Joint Surg Am* 1996;78:357-365.

16. Young BT, Rayan GM: Outcome following nonoperative treatment of displaced distal radius fractures in low-demand patients older than 60 years. *J Hand Surg Am* 2000;25:19-28.

17. Fernandez DL, Jupiter JB: *Fractures of the Distal Radius*. Springer-Verlag, 2002.

18. Axelrod TS, Green J, McMurtry RY: Limited open reduction of the lunate facet in comminuted intraarticular fractures of the distal radius. *J Hand Surg Am* 1988;13:384-389.

19. Herrera M, Chapman CB, Roh M, Strauch RJ, Rosenwasser MP: Treatment of unstable distal radius fractures with cancellous allograft and external fixation. *J Hand Surg Am* 1999;24:1269-1278.

20. McQueen M, Caspers J: Colles' Fracture: Does the anatomical result affect the final function? *J Bone Joint Surg Br* 1988;70:649-651.

21. Frykman GK, Peckham RH, Willard K, Saha S: External fixators for treatment of unstable wrist fractures: A biomechanical, design feature, and cost comparison. *Hand Clin* 1993;9:555-565.

22. Weber S, Szabo R: Severely comminuted distal radial fracture as an unsolved problem: Complications associated with external fixation and pins and plaster techniques. *J Hand Surg Am* 1986;11:157-165.

23. Kaempffe FA, Wheeler DR, Peimer CA, Hvisdak KS, Senall J: Severe fractures of the distal radius: Effect of amount and duration of external fixator distraction on outcome. *J Hand Surg Am* 1993;18:33-41.

24. Sommerkamp TG, Seeman M, Silliman J, et al: Dynamic external fixation of unstable fractures of the distal part of the radius; A prospective, randomized comparison with static external fixation. *J Bone Joint Surg Am* 1994;76:1149-1161.

25. McQueen MM: Redisplaced unstable fractures of the distal radius: A randomised, prospective study of bridging versus non-bridging external fixation. *J Bone Joint Surg Br* 1998;80:665-669.

26. Carter P, Frederick H, Laseter G: Open reduction and internal fixation of unstable distal radius fractures with a low-profile plate: A multicenter study of 73 fractures. *J Hand Surg Am* 1998;23:300-307.

27. Jakob M, Rikli D, Regazzoni P: Fractures of the distal radius treated by internal fixation and early function. *J Bone Joint Surg Br* 2000,82.340-344.

28. Ring D, Jupiter JB, Brennwald J, Buchler U, Hastings H II: Prospective multicenter trial of a plate for dorsal fixation of distal radius fractures. *J Hand Surg Am* 1997;22:777-784.

29. Cassidy C, Jupiter JB, Cohen MS, et al: Norian SRS cement compared with conventional fixation in distal radial fractures: A randomized study. *J Bone Joint Surg Am* 2003;85:2127-2137.

30. Sotelo-Sanchez J, Munuera L, Madero R: Treatment of fractures of the distal radius with a remodellable bone cement. *J Bone Joint Surg Br* 2000;82:856-863.

31. Cole RJ, Bindra RR, Evanoff BA, Gilula LA, Yamaguchi K, Gelberman RH: Radiographic evaluation of osseous displacement following intra-articular fractures of the distal radius: Reliability of plain radiography versus computed tomography. *J Hand Surg Am* 1997;22:792-800.

32. Johnston GH, Friedman L, Kriegler JC: Computerized tomographic evaluation of acute distal radial fractures. *J Hand Surg Am* 1992;17:738-744.

33. Chiang PP, Roach S, Baratz ME: Failure of a retinacular flap to prevent dorsal wrist pain after titanium Pi plate fixation of distal radius fractures. *J Hand Surg Am* 2002;27:724-728.

34. Lowry KJ, Gainor BJ, Hoskins JS: Extensor tendon rupture secondary to the AO/ASIF titanium distal radius plate without associated plate failure: A case report. *Am J Orthop* 2000;29:789-791.

35. Gesensway D, Putnam MD, Mente PL, Lewis JL: Design and biomechanics of a plate for the distal radius. *J Hand Surg Am* 1995;20:1021-1027.

36. Barrie KA, Wolfe SW: Internal fixation for intraarticular distal radius fractures. *Tech Hand Upper Extrem* 2002;6:10-20.

37. Orbay JL, Fernandez DL: Volar fixation for dorsally displaced fractures of the distal radius: A preliminary report. *J Hand Surg Am* 2002;27:205-215.

38. Dodds SD, Cornelissen S, Jossan S, Wolfe SW: A biomechanical comparison of fragment-specific fixation and augmented external fixation for intra-articular distal radius fractures. *J Hand Surg Am* 2002;27:953-964.

39. Auge WK, Velazquez PA: The application of indirect reduction techniques in the distal radius: The role of adjuvant arthroscopy. *Arthroscopy* 2000;16:830-835.

40. Fontes D, Lenoble E, de Somer B, Benoit J: Lesions of the ligaments associated with distal fractures of the radius: 58 intraoperative arthrographies. *Ann Chir Main Memb Super* 1992;11:119-125.

41. Mohanti RC, Kar N: Study of triangular fibrocartilage of the wrist joint in Colles' fracture. *Injury* 1980;11:321-324.

42. Lindau T, Arner M, Hagberg L: Intraarticular lesions in distal fractures of the radius in young adults: A descriptive arthroscopic study in 50 patients. *J Hand Surg [Br]* 1997;22:638-643.

43. Kofoed H: Comminuted displaced Colles' fractures: Treatment with intramedullary methylmethacrylate stabilisation. *Acta Orthop Scand* 1983;54:307-311.

44. Schmalholz A: Bone cement for redislocated Colles' fracture: A prospective comparison with closed treatment. *Acta Orthop Scand* 1989;60:212-217.

45. Mjoberg B, Pettersson H, Rosenqvist R, Rydholm A: Bone cement, thermal injury and the radiolucent zone. *Acta Orthop Scand* 1984;55:597-600.

46. Cohen MS, Whitman K: Calcium phosphate bone cement: The Norian skeletal repair system in orthopedic surgery. *AORN J* 1997;65:958-962.

47. Constantz BR, Ison IC, Fulmer MT, et al: Skeletal repair by in situ formation of the mineral phase of bone. *Science* 1995;267:1796-1799.

48. Yetkinler DN, Ladd AL, Poser RD, Constantz BR, Carter D: Biomechanical evaluation of fixation of intra-articular fractures of the distal part of the radius in cadavera: Kirschner wires compared with calcium-phosphate bone cement. *J Bone Joint Surg Am* 1999;81:391-399.

49. Larsson S, Bauer TW: Use of injectable calcium phosphate cement for fracture fixation: A review. *Clin Orthop* 2002;395:23-32.

50. Verlaan JJ, van Helden WH, Oner FC, Verbout AJ, Dhert WJ: Balloon vertebroplasty with calcium phosphate cement augmentation for direct restoration of traumatic thoracolumbar vertebral fractures. *Spine* 2002;27:543-548.

51. Cohen MS, Ralph C, Lim TH: The use of percutaneous cement for fixation of distal radius fractures. 2 Oct; American Society for surgery of the Hand Web site. Available at: http://www.hand-surgery.org. Accessed January 12, 2004..

52. Bradway JK, Amadio PC, Cooney WP: Open reduction and internal fixation of displaced, comminuted intraarticular fractures of the distal end of the radius. *J Bone Joint Surg Am* 1989;71:839-847.

53. Geissler WB, Fernandez DL, Lamey DM: Distal radioulnar joint injuries associated with fractures of the distal radius. *Clin Orthop* 1996;327:135-146.

54. Das SK, Brown HG: In search of complications in carpal tunnel decompression. *Hand* 1976;8:243-249.

55. DePalma AF: Comminuted fractures of the distal end of the radius treated by ulnar pinning. *J Bone Joint Surg Am* 1952;34:651-662.

56. Leung K, Shen W, Leung P, Kinninmonth AWG, Chang J, Chan G: Ligamentotaxis and bone grafting for comminuted fractures of the distal radius. *J Bone Joint Surg Br* 1989;71:838-842.

57. Stuart P, Berger RA, Linscheid RL, An K: Dorsopalmar stability of the distal radioulnar joint. *J Hand Surg Am* 2000;25:689-699.

58. Kihara H, Short WH, Werner FW, Fortino MD, Palmar AK: The stabilizing mechanism of the distal radioulnar joint during pronation and supination. *J Hand Surg Am* 1995;20:930-936.

59. Sarmiento A, Zagorski JB, Sinclair W: Functional Bracing of Colles' Fracture: A prospective study of immobilization in supination vs. pronation. *Clin Orthop* 1980;146:175-183.

60. van Dijk J, Laudy F: Dynamic external fixation versus non-operative treatment of severe distal radial fractures. *Injury* 1996;27:57-61.

61. Cooney WP III, Linscheid R, Dobyns JH: External pin fixation for unstable Colles' fractures. *J Bone Joint Surg Am* 1979;61:840-845.

62. Frykman GK. Fractures of the distal radius including sequelae-shoulder-hand-finger syndrome, disturbance in the distal radio-ulnar joint and impairment of nerve function. *Acta Orthop Scand* 1967;(Suppl 108):3+.

63. Lindau T, Aldercreutz C, Aspenberg P: Peripheral tears of the triangular fibrocartilage complex cause distal radioulnar joint instability after distal radius fractures. *J Hand Surg Am* 2000;25:464-468.

64. Adams BD: Effects of radial deformity on distal radioulnar joint mechanics. *J Hand Surg Am* 1993;18:492-498.

65. Lindau T, Arner M, Hagberg L: Intraarticular lesions in distal fractures of the radius in young adults: A descriptive arthroscopic study in 50 patients. *J Hand Surg Br* 1997;22:638-643.

Complications Following Distal Radial Fractures

Jesse B. Jupiter, MD
Diego L. Fernandez, MD

Malunion of the Distal End of the Radius

Union with deformity is the most common complication following a distal radial fracture.[1-5] The deformity may be extra-articular, characterized by loss of length and metaphyseal angulation; it may be intra-articular, involving either the radio-carpal or the radioulnar joint, or both; or it may be a combination of the two.

Surgical treatment of a symptomatic malunion of the distal part of the radius has been recognized for more than 200 years. Resection of the distal aspect of the ulna for the management of pain at the distal radioulnar joint after a distal radial fracture, a procedure attributed to Darrach after his description in 1913,[6] had been suggested by Desault in 1791[7] and again by Moore in 1880.[8] In 1937, Campbell[9] described a corrective osteotomy of the distal part of the radius with use of an interpositional bone graft obtained from the distal part of the ulna. In 1945, Merle d'Aubigné and Joussement[10] described a multiple-facet curved osteotomy without the need for an interpositional bone graft. This concept is currently being revisited and is described.

A deformity following fracture of the distal part of the radius is not necessarily symptomatic. In fact, it is not uncommon for an older patient to have acceptable wrist and forearm function without pain even when there is an apparent deformity. Therefore, impairment of function rather than radiographic deformity is the reason to treat a distal radial malunion, and, consequently, the patient's wrist and forearm function must be assessed.

The most common deformity following a malunited extra-articular Colles type of fracture is the loss of the normal volar tilt of the articular surface in the sagittal plane, loss of ulnar inclination in the frontal plane, loss of length relative to the ulna, and rotational deformity of the distal fragment[11] (Fig. 1). In addition, the distal fragment may be translated in either the sagittal or the frontal plane. In a report on 27 patients undergoing a corrective osteotomy, Bilic and associates[12] noted that more than half had a translation of $\geq$ 3 mm of the distal fragment.

A patient with a dorsal deformity of the distal radial fragment, and loss of the normal volar tilt, will have loss of palmar flexion and, on occasion, an increase in wrist extension. This malalignment alters the force pattern across the wrist and can lead to posttraumatic arthrosis.[13-18] Dorsal tilt of the distal articular surface of the radius not only alters the force distribution within the radiocarpal joint but also increases the load on the distal part of the ulna.[14,19-21] In addition, radiocarpal instability can develop in a patient with a dorsally displaced carpus, even when the intercarpal ligaments are intact. This instability may produce pain at the radiocarpal articulation. The dorsal deformity can also result in problems at the midcarpal joint.[21-24] An extrinsic midcarpal dynamic instability has been noted in some patients. These patients have a painful and, at times, audible subluxation of the midcarpal joint with active ulnar deviation of the wrist while the forearm is pronated.[22] In patients with laxity of the intercarpal and radiocarpal ligaments, continued stress on the midcarpal joint results in synovitis, ligamentous stretching, and increased intercarpal deformity (Sakai K, Doi K, Ihara K, et al, Nagoya, Japan, unpublished data presented at the International Symposium on The Wrist, 1991).

A dorsal deformity of the distal radial articular surface can also produce a fixed carpal malalignment—that is, a dorsal intercalary segment instability. This instability, associated with a dorsally angulated malunion of a distal radial fracture, can be classified into two categories:[25]

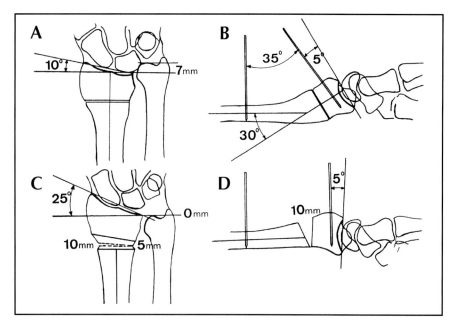

Fig. 1 Preoperative planning of the osteotomy for a Colles-type deformity. **A,** For correction in the frontal plane, the amount of shortening (7 mm in this patient) is measured between the head of the ulna and the ulnar corner of the radius on the AP radiograph. The lines for the measurement are perpendicular to the long axis of the radius. The ulnar tilt is reduced to 10° in this patient. **B,** In order to restore the ulnar tilt to normal (average, 25°), the osteotomy is opened more on the dorsoradial side than on the dorsoulnar side. **C,** For correction in the sagittal plane, the dorsal tilt (30° in this patient) is measured between the perpendicular to the joint surface and the long axis of the radius on the lateral radiograph. The K-wires are introduced so that they subtend the angle that corresponds to the dorsal tilt plus 5° of volar tilt (30° + 5° = 35° in this patient). **D,** After opening the osteotomy by the correct amount, the K-wires lie parallel to each other.

Type I: A "lax" reducible dorsal carpal malalignment that is improved, or even totally corrected, by a distal radial osteotomy. This type is more likely to be found in young individuals with lax ligaments and a good range of wrist mobility despite the deformity (Fig. 2).

Type II: A dorsal intercalary segment instability that is "fixed" and does not improve after correction of the distal radial malunion (Fig. 3).

Malunions of the distal part of the radius that are associated with loss of the normal ulnar inclination in the frontal plane may position the carpal tunnel in a radial direction, angulating the flexor tendons and decreasing their mechanical advantage. This contributes to diminished strength. Dorsal deformity has been associated with alteration of extensor tendon function[26] as well as an increase in

the intracompartmental pressure in the carpal tunnel.

Malunited Smith fractures (palmar displacement of the distal articular fragment) have an increased palmar tilt and pronation deformity of the distal fragment.[27] Disruption of the distal radioulnar joint is quite common. In contrast to the dorsally directed deformity, midcarpal instability and/or carpal malalignment is less often observed.

The distal radioulnar joint may also be impaired as a result of the distal radial deformity producing an incongruity of the sigmoid notch articulation with the ulnar head.[8,18,28-30] Radial shortening in relation to the distal part of the ulna can lead to tightening of the triangular fibrocartilage complex and impedance in the arc of forearm rotation. Long-standing radial shortening has also been shown to result in

impaction of the ulnar head onto the lunate with attrition wear in the center of the triangular fibrocartilage complex.

Several patterns of intra-articular malunion involving the radiocarpal joint have been identified.[13,31,32] Posttraumatic collapse of the lunate facet (a die-punch fracture) can affect the position of the lunate, usually in association with an intercalary segment instability. A malunited shearing Barton fracture, in addition to having intra-articular incongruity, leads to chronic volar or dorsal radiocarpal subluxation. The potential for the development of secondary arthritis is increased by these fractures, which heal with incongruity of the distal radial articular surface in the presence of intercarpal ligament injury.[33]

Preoperative Evaluation

A number of factors must enter into the decision regarding the surgical treatment of a distal radial malunion. These factors include the degree of discomfort with use of the wrist, the clinical appearance, the radiographic findings, and most importantly the patient's expectations with regard to the outcome. The physician should identify the location of the discomfort, the presence or absence of instability of the distal radioulnar joint, the range of motion of the wrist and forearm, and the grip strength compared with that on the contralateral side.

There are no fixed radiographic parameters with which to determine surgical indications for corrective osteotomy. In an analysis of 64 malunions of the distal part of the radius, Fourrier and associates[34] concluded that the lower limits of deformity at which symptoms are likely to develop include a radial deviation of the distal fragment of between 20° and 30°, a dorsal tilt in the sagittal plane of between 10° and 20°, and shortening of between 1 and 2 mm. Additional experimental evidence suggests that a dorsal tilt of between 20° and 30° should be considered as a prearthrotic condition[14,15,21] (Table 1).

The goal of a corrective osteotomy is to

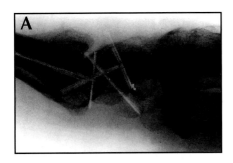

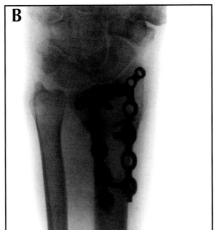

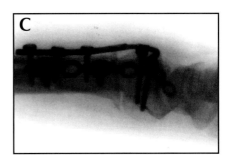

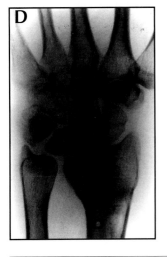

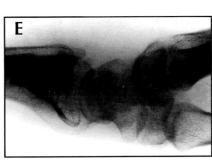

Fig. 2 A patient with a malunited distal radial fracture with dorsal intercalary segment instability (DISI) of the carpus. **A,** Preoperative radiograph. AP (**B**) and lateral (**C**) radiographs following corrective osteotomy. **D** and **E,** Radiographs made after removal of the plates show correction of the DISI.

reorient the distal articular surface of the radius in order to restore normal load distribution across the wrist joint, reestablish the normal kinematics of the midcarpal and radiocarpal joints, and restore the anatomic orientation of the distal radioulnar joint.[11] Our combined experience with nearly 200 corrective osteotomies has shown that, when these goals were accomplished, motion and function of the wrist and distal radioulnar joints as well as patient acceptance of the outcome were improved in most patients. Contraindications to surgical correction of a deformity include advanced degenerative changes in the radiocarpal and intercarpal joints, fixed carpal malalignment, limited functional disability, and advanced osteoporosis[25] (Table 1).

Timing of Osteotomy

We have performed the corrective osteotomy after a fracture as soon as it has been decided that the patient meets the criteria and the swelling has subsided. An

Table 1	
Distal Radial Osteotomy	
Relative Indications	**Contraindications**
Limitation of function	Advanced degenerative changes
Pain	Fixed carpal malalignment
Midcarpal instability	Limited functional disability
Distal radioulnar joint disruption	Extensive osteoporosis
Prearthrotic joint incongruity	

advantage of earlier intervention is that the deformity can be corrected through the immature callus of the healing fracture. This minimizes soft-tissue contracture and dysfunction of the distal radioulnar joint, which tend to develop over time. Early intervention also limits the economic and physiologic impact of the deformity.

The timing of the intervention was evaluated in a study comparing two groups of patients who had had a corrective osteotomy of a distal radial malunion.[35] One group of 10 patients had had the osteotomy at an average of 8.2 weeks after the initial injury, and a comparable group of 10 patients had had the osteotomy at an average of 39.9 weeks after the fracture. The overall functional and radiographic outcomes were similar, but earlier intervention reduced the total duration of disability. The time until the patient returned to work after the initial injury averaged 21 weeks in the early-intervention group compared with 70 weeks in the late-correction group.

Preoperative Planning

Standard biplanar radiographs of both wrists are adequate for the planning of the surgical treatment of most deformities.[11,36]

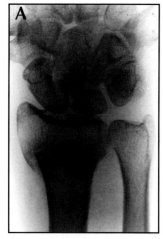

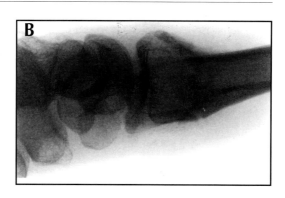

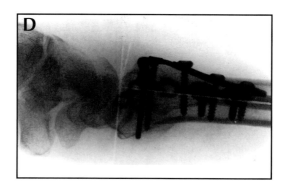

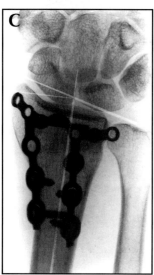

Fig. 3 A patient with a malunited distal radial fracture with fixed DISI. **A** and **B,** Preoperative radiographs. **C** and **D,** Following corrective osteotomy, the DISI persists along with limitation of palmar flexion.

Comparison with the uninjured wrist is crucial to the understanding of carpal alignment, ulnar variance, and inclination of the distal radial articular surface in the sagittal plane.[16,17,37] CT can be used to evaluate instability or incongruence of the distal radioulnar joint or rotational malalignment of the distal part of the radius.[38-40] Rotation of the distal fragment can be accurately determined by superimposition of tracings of symmetrical CT slices of both forearms obtained in neutral rotation. The proximal CT slice should include the bicipital tuberosity and the distal slice should include Lister's tubercle to serve as reference points.[38] The difference between the measurements on the uninjured and injured sides represents the amount of rotational malalignment. Three-dimensional reformatting of CT images is especially useful for patients who need both intra-articular and extra-articular corrections.[31,41-43]

Bilic and associates[12] demonstrated an effective use of computer-assisted modeling in the planning of corrective osteotomies. The use of computer-assisted design and computer-assisted manufacturing technology has facilitated the construction of three-dimensional solid models.[44]

Osteotomy Technique

The specific surgical technique depends on a number of factors: the type and direction of the deformity, the presence of intra-articular displacement, associated soft-tissue conditions, distal radioulnar dysfunction, and the surgeon's preference.[11,30,32,37,40,45-48]

Shortening of the radius in relation to the ulna is a common feature of most malunions; therefore, an opening-wedge osteotomy (transverse in the frontal plane and parallel to the articular surface in the sagittal plane) is the most frequently performed procedure.[11,30,36,45] Lengthening of the radius as much as 12 mm, restoration of the volar tilt in the sagittal plane, and rotational correction in the horizontal plane are all possible. The defect created by this approach can be filled with autogenous iliac-crest bone graft.

Dorsally Displaced Deformity

A 5- to 7-cm dorsal incision beginning 2 cm distal to Lister's tubercle and extending proximally provides excellent exposure. We open the extensor retinaculum between the second and third compartments, and we subperiosteally elevate the fourth compartment off the radius. The osteotomy is usually done 2 cm from the distal radial articular cartilage. The sagittal plane of the articular surface is determined by placing a fine Kirschner-wire (K-wire) into the radiocarpal joint parallel to the articular surface of the radius. A 2.5-mm K-wire is drilled into the radius on both sides of the intended osteotomy site. The angle between these two wires should be the planned angle of correction in the sagittal plane. After the osteotomy is made, the wire in the distal fragment can be used to help to manipulate that fragment into correct alignment and then the wires can be connected with a small external fixator frame to maintain the correction. Unless the radius needs to be lengthened >12 mm, the osteotomy should not extend completely through the volar cortex.

The osteotomy is made with a thin blade on an oscillating saw. With use of a lamina spreader, the osteotomy site is opened dorsally and radially, and the two

K-wires are connected with a small frame. Complete tenotomy or Z-lengthening of the brachioradialis tendon can be done to help gain length when a deformity is characterized by extreme radial deviation and shortening.

Use of a contoured trapezoid-shaped corticocancellous iliac-crest graft has been recommended to fill the metaphyseal defect created by the osteotomy, but we use a cancellous graft to fill the defect now that newer plates that allow screws to be placed in orthogonal directions are available (Fig. 4). Cancellous graft more readily fills the three-dimensional defect created by the osteotomy, is incorporated more rapidly, and limits donor-site morbidity because the cancellous bone can be harvested with trephine biopsy needles (Fig. 5).

Another option for the stabilization of the site of the corrective osteotomy is an external fixator with the pins placed in the distal fragment rather than in the metacarpals. This allows postoperative adjustment should the restoration of length or alignment prove to be inadequate.[47]

A number of investigators have utilized computer-generated data and/or CT scans to develop a more accurate preoperative representation of the deformity.[12,38] The better the surgeon's understanding of the deformity, the simpler the operation. Angular deformity in the frontal and sagittal planes can be determined by superimposition of orthogonal radiographs of the injured and normal wrists. Rotational deformity can be determined by the comparative CT scan technique described by Bindra and associates.[38] On the basis of these data, an osteotomy can be created by opening the dorsal and radial sides hinging on the volar and ulnar sides of the metaphysis.[25] The precise center of rotation can be determined preoperatively. The osteotomy is done so that the center of rotation lies in, on, or outside the margins of the radial cortex. When the center of rotation

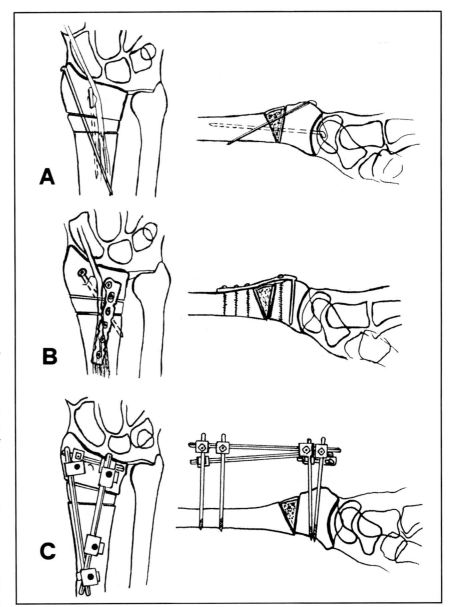

Fig. 4 Internal fixation techniques for an osteotomy of a malunited Colles fracture. **A,** Fixation with two 1.6-mm K-wires. One wire is inserted through the radial styloid process, across the graft, and into the ulnar cortex of the proximal fragment. The other wire is inserted through Lister's tubercle, across the graft, and into the volar cortex of the proximal fragment. **B,** Fixation with an AO 2.7-mm condylar plate with an optional 3.5-mm oblique lag screw. **C,** Fixation with a small external fixator (a triangular or quadrilateral frame).

needs to be within the bone margins, an incomplete opening-wedge osteotomy is necessary. When the center of rotation needs to be away from the bone, a complete osteotomy with lengthening and insertion of a corticocancellous iliac-crest bone graft is required. When the center

of rotation needs to be inside the bone and lengthening is not needed, a "rocking" type of osteotomy (opening on one side and closing on the other) is done (Fig. 6). When a rotational correction is required, the osteotomy line must be perpendicular to the axis of the distal

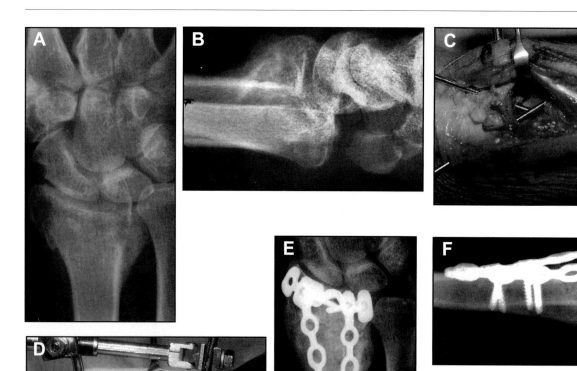

Fig. 5 A malunited Colles fracture in a 55-year-old patient. **A** and **B**, Preoperative radiographs. **C**, After an osteotomy, the reduction was maintained with two smooth Steinmann pins. **D**, Following plate placement, the defect created by the osteotomy was filled with cancellous bone graft. **E** and **F**, Excellent healing was noted at 3 months.

fragment. Two "reference" K-wires should be placed subtending the planned corrective rotational angle. Creating the osteotomy from radial dorsal to ulnar palmar allows the interposed graft to be a simple wedge rather than a more complicated trapezoidal wedge.

Palmarly Displaced Deformity

A classic volar Henry approach is used to expose the distal part of the radius for a corrective osteotomy of a palmarly angulated malunion. The malunion is exposed subperiosteally by reflecting the pronator quadratus muscle to the ulnar side. The osteotomy is done at the site of the original fracture, and the distal fragment is then extended and rotated into the correct alignment. The application of a T-shaped plate facilitates the fixation of a

rotational correction. The correction restores the alignment of both the radiocarpal and the distal radioulnar joint (Fig. 7). When the distal fragment has united in palmar flexion and is also shortened and extremely radially angulated, tenotomy or z-lengthening of shortened wrist flexors may be required to achieve the desired correction.

We reported our experience with opening-wedge osteotomy for the treatment of a malunited volarly displaced fracture of the distal part of the radius in 25 patients.[27] The average volar inclination was 24°, the average ulnar variance was 5 mm, and the average ulnar inclination of the articular surface of the distal part of the radius was 14°. At an average of 61 months after the osteotomy, the functional result was rated as very good

in 10 patients, good in 8, fair in 3, and poor in 4. The volar inclination averaged 5°, ulnar variance averaged 0 mm, and ulnar inclination averaged 22°. The grip strength improved from an average of 17 kg to an average of 30 kg. Wrist extension improved from an average of 25° to an average of 55°.

The indications for correction of an intra-articular malunion depend on the anatomy of the deformity as well as the duration since the original injury.[17,32] If the patient presents with an intra-articular malunion within 6 months after the injury, our preference is to correct the deformity. The deformities that are most suitable for correction are malunited radial styloid fractures, dorsal or volar shearing (Barton) fractures, and dorsal die-punch fractures of the lunate facet

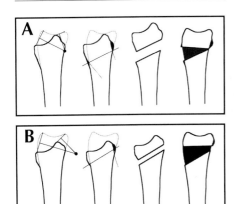

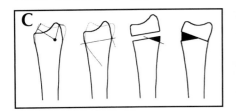

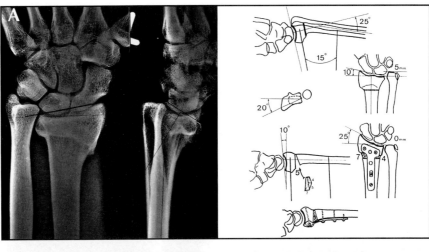

Fig. 6 Defining the center of rotation of the corrective osteotomy. **A,** Incomplete opening-wedge osteotomy. **B,** Complete full-thickness interpositional osteotomy. **C,** Rocking osteotomy. (Courtesy of Dr. Ladislav Nagy, Bern, Switzerland.)

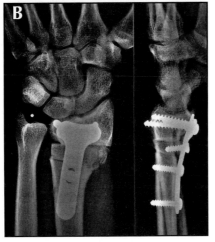

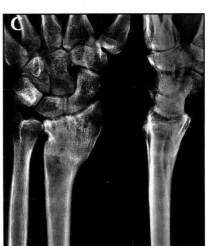

Fig. 7 A patient with a malunited Smith-Goyrand fracture with 25° of volar tilt, 5 mm of shortening, and pronational deformity of the distal fragment. **A,** Apparent dorsal subluxation of the distal part of the ulna is seen on the lateral radiograph. A 15° volar and radial opening-wedge osteotomy was performed to restore 10° of volar tilt and 25° of ulnar inclination in the frontal plane. **B,** Postoperative radiographs reveal restoration of both radiocarpal and radioulnar joint anatomy. **C,** Follow-up radiographs made at 3 years show a well-preserved joint space and good alignment of the distal radioulnar joint. Wrist function was normal.

a salvage procedure such as an arthrodesis or arthroplasty should be considered. The type of salvage procedure depends on the patient's functional requirements, hand dominance, level of pain, age, and occupation.

A proximal row carpectomy should be considered only if the degenerative changes are localized solely to the radial side of the radiocarpal joint. The articular cartilage of the lunate and capitate must be relatively normal. This is not usually the situation in a patient with degenerative arthritis of the wrist due to an intra-articular fracture.

Limited arthrodesis of the radiocarpal joint (radioscapholunate fusion) is a good alternative for a patient with localized degenerative changes in the wrist. The outcome of this procedure depends on the anatomic and functional integrity of the midcarpal joint, with a satisfactory result requiring a preserved midcarpal

joint and no carpal collapse or fixed midcarpal instability. To perform the procedure, a longitudinal incision is made from the middle metacarpal to 6 cm proximal to the wrist. The wrist is exposed between the third and fourth compartments, and a dorsal transverse capsulotomy is performed. (The posterior interosseous nerve is identified, and its distal 3 to 4 cm is resected.) The articular cartilage from the scaphoid, lunate, and distal part of the radius is removed. Wrist flexion facilitates exposure. The

(Fig. 8).

Osteonecrosis of the articular components is a risk with intra-articular osteotomy; therefore, the surgeon must be careful to minimize the soft-tissue dissection around the articular components. When choosing internal fixation, the surgeon must take into consideration the limited size of the components and the quality of the bone.

When the patient presents with a malunion associated with pain and disability 6 months or more after the injury,

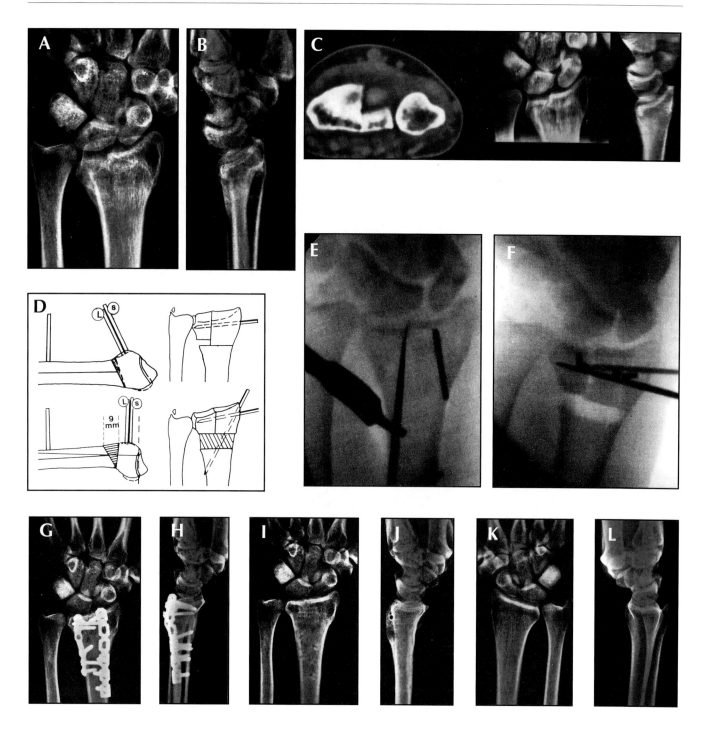

Fig. 8 A complex intra-articular malunion in a young man. (Case courtesy of Dr. Juan Gonzalez del Pino.) **A** and **B,** Anterior and lateral radiographs made 4 months postinjury. **C,** A CT scan demonstrates impaction of the dorsal lunate facet and disruption of the sigmoid notch. **D,** The preoperative plan in the sagittal and frontal planes. L = lunate facet and S = scaphoid facet. Intraoperative radiographs show placement of the guide-wires **(E)** and creation of the intra-articular and extra-articular osteotomies **(F)**. Anterior **(G)** and lateral **(H)** radiographs demonstrate stable internal fixation. One-year postoperative radiographs made following plate and screw removal **(I** and **J)** compared with radiographs of the normal, contralateral wrist **(K** and **L)**.

Table 2
Management Algorithm for Distal Radioulnar Joint Disorders Following Distal Radial Fracture

Disorder*	Management
Distal radioulnar joint incongruity	
Extra-articular	Reorientation of sigmoid notch with radial osteotomy
Intra-articular (posttraumatic arthrosis)	Depending on severity of degenerative changes, age, hand dominance, and occupation: resection arthroplasty, Sauvé-Kapandji procedure, or prosthetic replacement
Combined	Radial osteotomy and distal radioulnar joint procedure as described for intra-articular incongruity
Distal radioulnar joint instability	Reattachment of triangular fibrocartilage complex (open or arthroscopic), proximal reinsertion of ulnar styloid nonunion, capsulodesis (Herbert ulnar sling procedure), shortening osteotomy of ulna, or other ligament reconstructions
Ulnocarpal abutment (impaction)	Restoration of radioulnar index or ulnar variance to normal with ulnar shortening osteotomy, wafer procedure (Feldon), radial lengthening osteotomy, combined radioulnar osteotomies, or epiphysiodesis and/or distraction-osteogenesis techniques in growing skeleton
Symptomatic (painful) nonunion of ulnar styloid process	Simple excision
Capsular retraction, pronation contracture of distal radioulnar joint	Capsulotomy or pronator quadratus release and palmar capsulotomy
Radioulnar impingement (painful radioulnar contact following resection of distal stump or unstable stump after Sauvé-Kapandji procedure)	Ulnar head prosthesis

*If two of these conditions are present, two or more procedures may need to be combined. A classic example is a malunited Colles fracture and degenerative changes of the distal radioulnar joint.

exposed bone of the scaphoid and lunate is held against the radius. Cancellous bone, obtained from either the distal part of the radius or the iliac crest, is used to fill the intercarpal space. The fusion site is fixed with K-wires, screws, or a dorsal plate with the distal screws placed in the scaphoid and lunate.

Disorders of the Distal Radioulnar Joint Associated With Distal Radial Malunion

A malunited distal radial fracture is commonly associated with residual derangement of the distal radioulnar joint.[2] The three conditions responsible for wrist pain associated with limited forearm rotation are incongruity, impaction, and instability of the distal radioulnar joint. These may present in isolation or in combination. Other, less frequent causes of wrist pain are a painful nonunion of the ulnar styloid process not associated with instability of the distal radioulnar joint, palmar capsular contracture of the joint with loss of active supination,

radioulnar impingement after resection of the distal part of the ulna,[6] or an unstable distal ulnar stump after a Sauvé-Kapandji procedure.[49]

Incongruity of the distal radioulnar joint may be due to extra-articular deformity of the radius or ulna leading to abnormal orientation of the joint surfaces, intra-articular disruption of the joint surfaces by the fracture, or a combination of extra-articular and intra-articular factors. Incongruity produces cartilage overload with degenerative joint changes, painful limitation of forearm rotation, and loss of grip strength.

Ulnocarpal impaction (ulnocarpal abutment syndrome) is abnormal contact between the ulnar head and the carpus. This occurs as a result of radial shortening. Impaction of the ulnar head against the carpus produces attenuation and degenerative tears of the triangular fibrocartilage complex; chondromalacia of the ulnar head, lunate, or triquetrum; attenuation and tears of the triquetrolunate ligament; and, finally, ulnocarpal osteoarthritis.

Instability is due to loss of ligament support after rupture or avulsion of the triangular ligament. Damage to secondary joint stabilizers (the capsular ligaments, the sheath of the extensor carpi ulnaris, the interosseous membrane, and the pronator quadratus) or extra-articular and intra-articular osseous disruption of the joint surface may increase the degree of laxity.

Careful clinical assessment of the joint is necessary to localize the source of ulnar-sided pain. Specifically, the examiner should try to localize the tenderness, swelling, and crepitation to the joint, the ulnar styloid process, the extensor carpi ulnaris sheath, or the lunotriquetral joint. Next, the examiner should determine if pain increases with forced supination, pronation, or ulnar deviation or with transverse compression of the joint. The stability and the direction of subluxation of the ulnar head (dorsal, palmar, or combined) should be assessed, and the effect of forearm rotation on the position of the ulnar head should be determined.

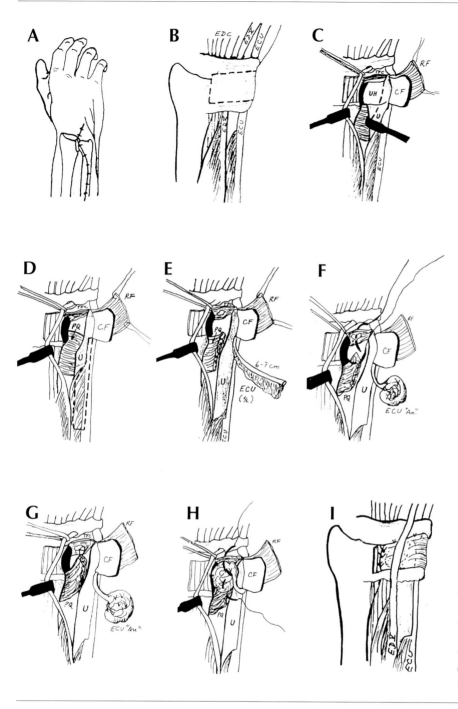

Fig. 9 Surgical treatment of intra-articular incongruity of the distal radioulnar joint. **A,** Skin incision. A dorsoulnar longitudinal incision is curved radially at the level of the distal radioulnar joint and is continued distally on the dorsum of the hand. This incision does not interfere with the course of the superficial branch of the ulnar nerve. **B,** A 2-cm-wide ulnarly based retinacular flap (RF in following illustrations) is elevated over the fourth dorsal compartment and dissected ulnarly, with care taken not to open the sheath of the extensor carpi ulnaris (ECU) tendon. EDC = extensor digitorum communis, and EDV = extensor digiti quinti minimi. **C,** The extensor digiti quinti tendon is separated radially, and the dorsal aspect of the distal radioulnar joint capsule (CF) is elevated from the sigmoid notch and dissected ulnarly to expose the ulnar head (UH) and the triangular fibrocartilage complex (TFC). The ulnar metaphysis is exposed subperiosteally, and the ulnar head is resected obliquely from the base of the ulnar styloid process to the radial aspect of the ulnar neck (dotted line), while care is taken to preserve the attachments and integrity of the TFC. U = ulna. **D,** A 6- to 7-cm-long distally based tendon-muscle strip from the radial half of the ECU tendon is dissected (dotted line). **E,** The pronator quadratus (PQ) is released and elevated from its volar attachment to the distal part of the ulna. **F,** The extensor carpi ulnaris tendon-muscle strip is rolled to form an "anchovy" (ECU "An") with use of reabsorbable sutures. **G,** With use of 2-0 sutures, the ulnar border of the PQ is brought up into the distal radioulnar joint space and tied to the TFC. **H,** Next, the rolled ECU anchovy is placed in the defect that was left after the ulnar head was resected and is fixed both to the PQ and to the dorsal edge of the triangular fibrocartilage. **I,** For closure, both the retinacular and the capsular flaps are sutured with transosseous stitches to the dorsal lip of the sigmoid notch.

Finally, active and passive forearm rotation, wrist motion, and grip strength should be measured. Injection of a local anesthetic may help to localize the specific site of pain.

Radiographic Evaluation

Standardized AP and lateral radiographs of both wrists are helpful in the evaluation of radial deformity, subluxation, ulnar variance, and cartilage width in the frontal plane. Ulnar variance increases with pronation and grip and decreases with supination and no grip. Dynamic radioulnar impingement after total or partial resection of the ulnar head can be clearly demonstrated on a lateral radiograph of the distal part of the forearm and the wrist made while the patient holds a weight of 2.5 lb (1.1 kg). Abnormal contact between the radius and the ulna can be seen on these radiographs. Superimposing transverse slices of a CT scan at the level of Lister's tubercle and the bicipital tuberosity allows assessment of rotational deformity of the distal part of the radius. Furthermore, the CT scan is useful for the detection of step-offs, degenerative changes, and subluxation of the distal radioulnar joint. CT arthrography and/or MRI may be indicated occasionally for suspected soft-tissue and cartilage damage of the triangular fibrocartilage complex, damage to the intercarpal ligaments, synovitis, ganglions, and tendon lesions. Arthroscopy of the wrist remains, however, the ideal method for evaluation and treatment of lesions of the triangular fibrocartilage complex.

Management

Our preferred treatment options for disorders of the distal radioulnar joint after a radial fracture are summarized in Table 2. Extra-articular incongruity of the distal radioulnar joint is managed by restoration of radial anatomy and reorientation of the sigmoid notch to the ulnar head with a radial osteotomy. After the osteotomy, if the distal radioulnar joint is stable, full passive pronation and supination are possible, and the normal anatomic relationship between the sigmoid notch and the ulnar head has been restored, no additional surgery is necessary. When intra-articular incongruity of the distal radioulnar joint is seen on plain radiographs or CT scans, a resection arthroplasty, a Sauvé-Kapandji procedure, or a prosthetic replacement is indicated depending on the severity of the degenerative changes and the patient's age, hand dominance, and occupation. Currently, we reserve partial resection of the ulnar head (a Bowers hemiresection interpositional technique[1]) for patients who make low demands on the wrist. To prevent ulnar convergence or radioulnar impingement, both the pronator quadratus and a "rolled anchovy" consisting of a distally based strip of the extensor carpi ulnaris tendon are used as interpositional material (Fig. 9). Both interposed structures are sutured to the proximal edges of the triangular fibrocartilage complex. Partial ulnar resection does not alter the ulnar variance, and therefore an addition-

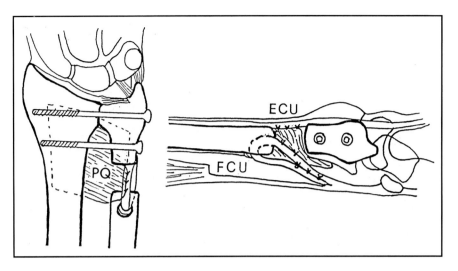

Fig. 10 Modified Sauvé-Kapandji technique. Two screws are used to ensure rotational stability. Note the tenodesis of the ulnar stump with a distally based strip of the flexor carpi ulnaris (FCU) tendon. The pronator quadratus (PQ) is used as interpositional material and is sutured to the sheath of the extensor carpi ulnaris (ECU) tendon.

al ulnar shortening either at the styloid level or at the ulnar shaft should be done with this procedure to prevent impingement of the ulnar styloid process on the carpus.

We have had very satisfactory results with the Bowers hemiresection interpositional technique combined with radial osteotomy in patients with posttraumatic deformity associated with degenerative changes at the distal radioulnar joint.[1] We reviewed our experience with this procedure in 15 patients who had radiographically evident degenerative changes, predominantly ulnar-sided pain, and limited rotation of the forearm.[30] At an average of 3 years, 13 patients were free of pain but two had some pain at the extremes of forearm rotation. All 15 distal radioulnar joints were stable, the average grip strength had increased by 30%, and the outcome was very good in four patients, good in eight, and fair in three.

In elderly patients, total resection of the ulnar head (the Darrach procedure)[6,50] still has a place in the treatment of derangement or osteoarthritis of the distal radioulnar joint. In this age group, the disadvantages of this operation

(reduction of grip strength and potential instability of the ulnar stump) are remarkably well tolerated. The most important technical details are (1) the resection is not extended higher than the level of the ulnar neck, and (2) the sheath of the extensor carpi ulnaris tendon is closed carefully to prevent dorsal subluxation. Breen and Jupiter[51] suggested that, when the ulnar head is subluxated before the operation, a primary tenodesis of the ulnar stump after head resection should be done with distally based tendon strips of the flexor carpi ulnaris and extensor carpi ulnaris.

The Sauvé-Kapandji procedure (fusion of the distal radioulnar joint with creation of a proximal ulnar pseudarthrosis)[49] is recommended for younger patients who make high functional demands on the wrist and forearm. Specific clinical and radiographic indications for a Sauvé-Kapandji procedure are posttraumatic osteoarthritis of the joint, chronic irreducible dislocation of the ulnar head with extensive limitation of forearm rotation, posttraumatic synostosis of the distal part of the forearm, simultaneous arthritic or posttraumatic

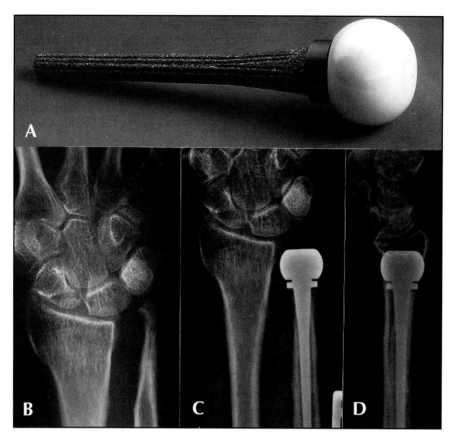

Fig. 11 A, The Herbert ulnar head prosthesis with a titanium stem for noncemented fixation and a ceramic modular head. **B** through **D,** Radiographic appearances of the prosthesis used in a patient with a failed partial resection of the distal part of the ulna with stylocarpal impingement.

destruction of the sigmoid notch and lunate fossa, and the need for salvage after a failed hemiresection arthroplasty.[52]

The two most difficult complications of the Sauvé-Kapandji procedure are reossification of the pseudarthrosis site in the ulna and instability of the proximal ulnar stump. To prevent the latter complication, we use an additional palmar tenodesis with a distally based tendon strip of the flexor carpi ulnaris to stabilize the proximal stump.[30] We do this because of the difficulty of obtaining adequate stability with pronator quadratus interposition alone. In addition, two screws are used for fixation (Fig. 10). We believe that ectopic bone formation is reduced by careful periosteal resection, the elimination of "sawdust," and soft-tissue interposition of the flexor carpi ulnaris and pronator quadratus. This operation preserves the triangular fibrocartilage complex, the ulnocarpal ligaments, and the osseous support of the ulnar side of the carpus, which perhaps explains why there frequently is, together with the pain relief offered by the arthrodesis, a satisfactory increase in grip strength. A stable and painless nonunion of the distal part of the ulna reliably restores forearm rotation. Although some degree of passive instability of the distal stump may be detected on clinical examination, it usually disappears during forceful grip. We believe that active contraction of both the extensor and the flexor carpi ulnaris muscles may be responsible for additional dynamic stabilization of the distal ulnar stump during active use of the hand.

Our modification of the Sauvé-Kapandji procedure with a flexor carpi ulnaris tenodesis was evaluated in 18 patients who had posttraumatic derangement of the distal radioulnar joint after a distal radial fracture.[52] All patients had painful limitation of forearm rotation. After an average duration of follow-up of 5 years, the average forearm supination improved from 16° preoperatively to 77° postoperatively and the average forearm pronation improved from 42° to 81°. Pain relief was satisfactory, and the average grip strength improved from 36% of the strength on the unaffected side preoperatively to 72% of the strength on the unaffected side postoperatively.

A more recent option that obviates the disadvantages of distal ulnar resection is prosthetic replacement of the ulnar head, as proposed by van Schoonhoven and associates[53] (Fig. 11). After a distal radial fracture, the aim of ulnar head replacement is to restore pain-free forearm rotation while maintaining ulnar support to the carpus. The prerequisites for ulnar head replacement after a fracture with incongruity of the distal radioulnar joint are a normally oriented sigmoid notch and adequate soft-tissue coverage. Therefore, if there is a metaphyseal deformity, a radial osteotomy should be done to reorient the sigmoid notch in the frontal and sagittal planes so that the radius can rotate freely around the prosthetic head (Fig. 12).

Through a dorsal approach, an ulna-based capsuloretinacular flap is made. This allows access to the distal part of the ulna and the triangular fibrocartilage complex and will be used to accomplish a stable soft-tissue repair. The apex of the flap lies in the bed of the extensor digiti minimi tendon, where the joint capsule attaches to the rim of the sigmoid fossa. The extensor retinaculum (containing the extensor carpi ulnaris tendon) is raised in a single layer with the joint capsule and is freed from the dorsal surface of the triangular fibrocartilage complex and from its osseous attachments to the ulna. The triangular fibrocartilage com-

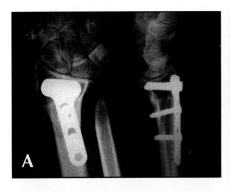

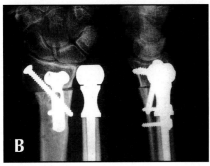

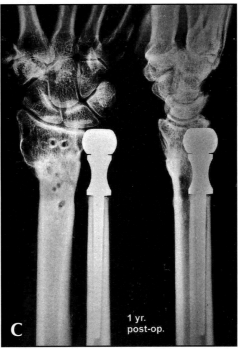

Fig. 12 A patient with a painful and unstable distal part of the ulna after resection, associated with a malunited distal aspect of the radius (20° of volar tilt and 30° of ulnar inclination). **A,** Radiograph made before the arthroplasty. **B,** Ulnar head replacement was combined with radial osteotomy to guarantee proper orientation of the sigmoid notch, a prerequisite for restoration of stability of the distal radioulnar joint. **C,** Follow-up radiographs made at 1 year reveal improved overall wrist alignment and a stable prosthesis. The patient was free of pain and had a 160° arc of forearm rotation.

plex is inspected and is repaired if necessary. Templates are used preoperatively to determine the level of the osteotomy. After the osteotomy and reaming of the ulnar shaft, a trial prosthesis is used to establish the correct size of the head and stem. Fluoroscopy can be used to make a final selection of the prosthesis. The flap is then sutured back onto the triangular fibrocartilage complex and is advanced over the prosthesis and reattached to the dorsal rim of the sigmoid fossa. Transosseous nonabsorbable sutures are placed, under sufficient tension to ensure adequate stability.

A removable above-the-elbow splint is used to prevent forearm rotation for the first 2 weeks. Active motion and physiotherapy are started 10 days to 2 weeks after the surgery. A removable ulnar gutter or sugar-tong splint, allowing 30° of pronation and supination, is used to protect the repair from undue stress during the healing period. The splint is discarded 6 weeks after the surgery, and the patient is allowed to gradually return to normal activities. The

head of the prosthesis maintains transverse radioulnar load transmission. This prevents radioulnar convergence and restores the interosseous space between the radius and ulna.

The prosthesis has gained popularity for the treatment of patients with painful radioulnar impingement after a partial or total resection of the ulnar head. This condition is often seen in association with an unstable distal ulnar stump after a distal ulnar resection (a Darrach procedure) or a Sauvé-Kapandji procedure. The patient complains of a painful "click" or "catching" sensation during forceful forearm rotation or when lifting objects. Removal of the ulnar head (the keystone of the distal radioulnar joint) allows the radius to fall toward the ulna when objects are lifted with the forearm in neutral rotation (Fig. 13). The insertion of a prosthesis that will remain stable is more difficult in these patients than it is in patients who have not been operated on previously. Soft-tissue stabilization of the prosthesis is critical. Creation of an "annular" ligament with a free tendon

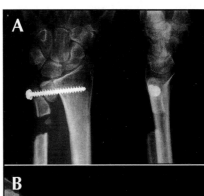

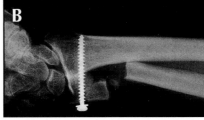

Fig. 13 A, A failed Bowers arthroplasty was converted into a Sauvé-Kapandji procedure. The patient had painful radioulnar impingement due to substantial instability of the ulnar stump. **B,** Horizontal lateral radiograph of the wrist, demonstrating abnormal contact of the ulna and radius while the patient held a 2.5-lb (1.1-kg) weight with the forearm in neutral rotation.

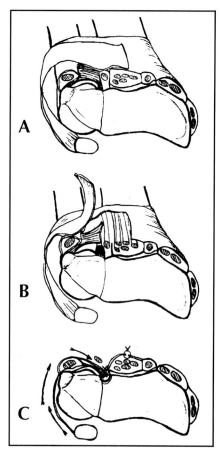

Fig. 14 The ulnar sling distal radioulnar joint capsulodesis. **A,** A 2-cm-wide dorsal retinacular flap is incised at the level of the fourth extensor compartment. **B,** The flap is carefully dissected ulnarly to the base of the sixth compartment. Care is taken not to open the sheath of the extensor carpi ulnaris tendon. The dorsal aspect of the distal radioulnar joint capsule is detached from the dorsal lip of the sigmoid notch. **C,** Both the retinacular flap and the dorsal aspect of the capsule are radially advanced and are fixed to the dorsal lip of the sigmoid notch with transosseous nonabsorbable 2-0 U-shaped sutures.

graft passed around the neck of the prosthesis and fixed palmarly and dorsally to the sigmoid notch is recommended.

Since 1995, this prosthesis has been used in an international multicenter prospective trial.[53] Twenty-three patients (11 men and 12 women) with chronic painful instability after a previous ulnar head resection have been operated on.

The average age was 45 years (range, 22 to 65 years). Previous operations included 10 Darrach-type resections, 11 Bowers-type hemiresections, and 2 failed silicone ulnar head replacements; each patient had an average of three procedures (range, 1 to 12 procedures). At 27 months, stability and a marked decrease in symptoms had been achieved in 22 patients. One prosthesis was removed because of a low-grade infection. Use of a prosthesis is contraindicated when the distal part of the ulna is severely unstable and the quality of the soft tissues is poor. With this scenario, the two possible solutions are the use of a constrained total distal radioulnar joint prosthesis or a radioulnar arthrodesis (a one-bone-forearm operation). Fusion of the distal part of the ulna to the radius in a midpronation position controls pain and instability at the cost of loss of forearm rotation.

Malposition of the sigmoid notch in the sagittal plane aggravates the condition because it creates incongruity of the joint surfaces (relative subluxation of the ulnar head). Rotational deformity of the radius plays an additional role in the etiology of instability of the distal radioulnar joint and should be kept in mind during surgical reconstruction. This is especially important for fractures that are malunited with volar and pronational displacement of the distal fragment (Smith deformity).

The most important preoperative symptom in 25 patients treated with osteotomy for a malunited Smith fracture was limitation of supination associated with dorsal subluxation of the distal part of the ulna and pain in the distal radioulnar joint.[27] Radial osteotomy alone was sufficient in 18 patients, whereas seven required an additional partial resection of the ulnar head to treat degenerative changes of the joint. At an average of 5 years after surgery, the average supination had improved from 44° preoperatively to 69° postoperatively and the average extension had improved from 25° preoperative-

ly to 55° postoperatively. The functional outcome was rated as very good in 10 patients, good in 8, fair in 3, and poor in 4.

A combined procedure is usually required when there is both an osseous deformity and deficiency of the triangular fibrocartilage complex. Arthroscopy is used to assess the triangular fibrocartilage complex. A peripheral or radial transosseous reattachment of the triangular fibrocartilage complex is performed depending on the site of the old tear. If deficiency of the triangular fibrocartilage complex is associated with a nonunion of the ulnar styloid process, proximal osseous reattachment is preferred. In most instances, we add an extra-articular capsulodesis after reconstruction of the triangular fibrocartilage complex. An ulna-based dorsal retinacular flap is made to the level of the sixth compartment. The sheath of the extensor carpi ulnaris tendon is not opened. Traction is applied to the flap, which is securely fixed with transosseous sutures to the dorsal edge of the sigmoid notch together with the dorsal aspect of the distal radioulnar joint capsule. The extensor digiti quinti tendon is left on top of the flap. This retinacular flap, modified from that described by Stanley and Herbert,[54] relocates the commonly ulnarly subluxated extensor carpi ulnaris tendon on top of the ulnar head and provides additional fibrous augmentation to the lax dorsal aspect of the capsule (Fig. 14).

Finally, if instability is associated with an ulnar-plus variance, a shortening osteotomy should be added to the procedure. Radial deformity, when present, is first corrected to provide an appropriate position of the sigmoid notch and the ulnar head.

Ulnocarpal abutment is managed by restoring the radioulnar length discrepancy to a physiologic ulnar variance, as dictated by the study of the radiographs of the patient's unaffected wrist. Prerequisites for a shortening osteotomy of the ulna are a well-oriented sigmoid notch in

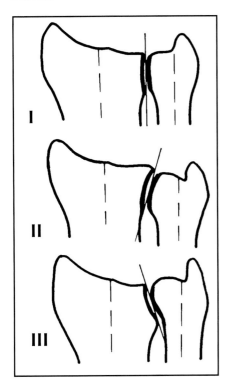

Fig. 15 Classification of distal radioulnar joint morphology described by Tolat and associates.[55]

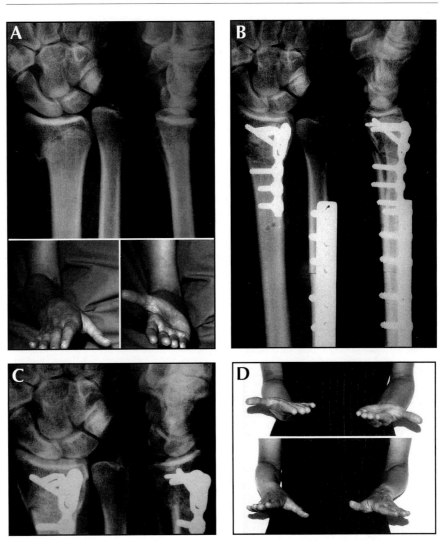

Fig. 16 A patient with a malunited distal radial fracture with painful limitation of forearm rotation. **A,** Note the distal radioulnar joint incongruity due to shortening as well as radial and dorsal deviation of the distal fragment resulting in a type III inclination of the sigmoid notch. **B,** Restoration of the distal radioulnar joint congruity with combined ulnar shortening and radial osteotomy to reorient the sigmoid notch. **C** and **D,** At 2.5 years after the operation, radiographs showed a congruent distal radioulnar joint, a healed ulnar styloid process, and no degenerative changes. Clinically the joint was stable, and pronation and supination had been fully restored.

both the frontal and the sagittal plane and no intra-articular step-offs or degenerative changes as demonstrated by CT scans.

The morphology of the sigmoid notch should be carefully assessed and classified according the system described by Tolat and associates[55] (Fig. 15). A type I distal radioulnar joint has a sigmoid notch and ulnar seat angle roughly parallel to each other and to the long axis of the ulna, type II has a joint surface that is oblique and pointing toward the distal part of the ulna, and type III has a reverse oblique orientation. If a type III sigmoid notch is present, ulnar shortening will produce joint incongruity with impingement of the ulnar head on the proximal edge of the notch. In this situation, reorientation of the sigmoid notch with a radial osteotomy is recommended (Fig. 16).

Ulnar shortening decompresses the ulnar compartment of the wrist, reestablishes distal radioulnar joint congruency, and tightens both the ulnocarpal ligaments and the triangular fibrocartilage complex, helping to stabilize the distal part of the ulna.[56] For ulnocarpal abutment with ≤ 3 mm of ulnar-plus variance and no instability, a wafer arthroscopic resection of the distal end of the ulnar head is an alternative, minimally invasive procedure.[57] In cases in which radial shortening exceeds 10 mm, ulnar short-

ening combined with radial lengthening and angular correction may become necessary. Bone distraction techniques combined with epiphysiodesis of the distal part of the ulna is an option in children.[25]

Symptomatic or painful nonunion of the ulnar styloid process without instability of the distal radioulnar joint is an infrequent problem. Usually fibrous unions of the tip of the ulnar styloid process are extracapsular and do not produce symptoms. When a patient with pain on the ulnar side of the wrist has an ununited ulnar styloid process, instability and incongruity of the joint should be suspected. If a local anesthetic block over the tender area relieves all symptoms, a surgical excision of the styloid process without damaging the triangular fibrocartilage complex is recommended.[58]

After a fracture of the distal part of the radius, contracture of the distal radioulnar joint capsule may be responsible for limitation of forearm rotation, especially supination. Passive stretching of the joint is recommended after joint incongruity, subluxation, radioulnar synchondrosis, contracture of the interosseous membrane, and derangement of the proximal radioulnar joint have been excluded. Surgical release of the distal radioulnar joint capsule may be necessary if nonsurgical treatment fails. The volar aspect of the joint is exposed through a longitudinal incision just ulnar to the flexor carpi ulnaris tendon. The dorsal cutaneous branch of the ulnar nerve is protected and the flexor carpi ulnaris tendon and the ulnar neurovascular bundle are retracted radially. The pronator quadratus is sectioned longitudinally 5 mm radial to its ulnar insertion. A longitudinal capsulotomy proximal to the volar edge of the triangular fibrocartilage complex, close to the sigmoid notch, is performed and is continued proximal to the neck of the ulna. Passive supination is then tested. If capsular section does not restore full supination, a total palmar capsulectomy is performed.[59] After surgery, the wrist is held in full supination for 2 weeks in a splint; then passive and active supination can be begun. Dynamic supination splinting may be necessary.

References

1. Bowers WH: Distal radioulnar joint arthroplasty: The hemiresection-interposition technique. *J Hand Surg Am* 1985;10:169-178.

2. Cooney WP III, Dobyns JH, Linscheid RL: Complications of Colles' fractures. *J Bone Joint Surg Am* 1980;62:613-619.

3. McQueen M, Caspers J: Colles' fracture: Does the anatomical result affect the final function? *J Bone Joint Surg Br* 1988;70:649-651.

4. Meine J: Early and late complications of radius fractures in the classical location. *Z Unfallchir Versicherungsmed Berufskr* 1989;82:25-32.

5. Speed JS, Knight RA: The treatment of malunited Colles's fractures. *J Bone Joint Surg* 1945;27:361-367.

6. Darrach W: Abstract: Partial excision of lower shaft of ulna for deformity following Colles's fracture. *Ann Surg* 1913;57:764-765.

7. Desault M: Extrait d'un mémoire de M. Desault sur la luxation de l'extrémité inférieure du cubitus. *J Chir (Paris)* 1791;1:78.

8. Moore EM: Three cases illustrating luxation of the ulna in connection with Colles' fracture. *Med Rec* 1880;17:305-308.

9. Campbell WC: Malunited Colles' fractures. *JAMA* 1937;109:1105-1108.

10. Merle d'Aubigné R, Joussemet L: A propos du traitement des cals vicieux de l'extrémité inférieure du radius. *Bull Mém Acad Chir* 1945;71:153-157.

11. Fernandez DL: Correction of post-traumatic wrist deformity in adults by osteotomy, bone-grafting, and internal fixation. *J Bone Joint Surg Am* 1982;64:1164-1178.

12. Bilic R, Zdravkovic V, Boljevic Z: Osteotomy for deformity of the radius: Computer-assisted three-dimensional modelling. *J Bone Joint Surg Br* 1994;76:150-154.

13. Martini AK: Secondary arthrosis of the wrist joint in malposition of healed and un-corrected fracture of the distal radius. *Aktuelle Traumatol* 1986;16:143-148.

14. Miyake T, Hashizume H, Inoue H, Shi Q, Nagayama N: Malunited Colles' fracture: Analysis of stress distribution. *J Hand Surg Br* 1994;19:737-742.

15. Pogue DJ, Viegas SF, Patterson RM, et al: Effects of distal radius fracture malunion on wrist joint mechanics. *J Hand Surg Am* 1990;15:721-727.

16. Rodriguez-Megthiaz AM, Chamay A: Traitement des cals vicieux extra-articulaires du radius distal par ostéotomie d'ouverture avec interposition d'une greffe. *Med Hyg (Genève)* 1988;46:2757-2765.

17. Saffar P: Treatment of distal radial intraarticular malunions, in Saffar P, Cooney WP (eds): *Carpal Instability: Diagnosis and Practice-Oriented Treatment.* London, England, Martin Dunitz, 1999, pp 249-258.

18. Villar RN, Marsh D, Rushton N, Greatorex RA: Three years after Colles' fracture: A prospective review. *J Bone Joint Surg Br* 1987;69:635-638.

19. Kazuki K, Kusunoki M, Shimazu A: Pressure distribution in the radiocarpal joint measured with a densitometer designed for pressure-sensitive film. *J Hand Surg Am* 1991;16:401-408.

20. Palmer AK, Werner FW: Biomechanics of the distal radioulnar joint. *Clin Orthop* 1984;187:26-35.

21. Short WH, Palmer AK, Werner FW, Murphy DJ: A biomechanical study of distal radial fractures. *J Hand Surg Am* 1987;12:529-534.

22. Lichtman DM, Schneider JR, Swafford AR, Mack GR: Ulnar midcarpal instability: Clinical and laboratory analysis. *J Hand Surg Am* 1981;6:515-523.

23. Linscheid RL, Dobyns JH, Beabout JW, Bryan RS: Traumatic instability of the wrist: Diagnosis, classification, and pathomechanics. *J Bone Joint Surg Am* 1972;54:1612-1632.

24. Taleisnik J, Watson HK: Midcarpal instability caused by malunited fractures of the distal radius. *J Hand Surg Am* 1984;9:350-357.

25. Fernandez DL, Jupiter JB (eds): *Fractures of the Distal Radius: A Practical Approach to Management.* New York, NY, Springer-Verlag, 1996.

26. Hove LM: Delayed rupture of the thumb extensor tendon: A 5-year study of 18 consecutive cases. *Acta Orthop Scand* 1994;65:199-203.

27. Shea K, Fernandez DL, Jupiter JB, Martin C: Corrective osteotomy for malunited, volarly displaced fractures of the distal end of the radius. *J Bone Joint Surg Am* 1997;79:1816-1826.

28. Boyd HB, Stone MM: Resection of the distal end of the ulna. *J Bone Joint Surg* 1944;26:313-321.

29. Castaing J: Les fractures récentes de l'extrémité inférieure du radius chez l'adulte. *Rev Chir Orthop* 1964;50:581-696.

30. Fernandez DL: Radial osteotomy and Bowers arthroplasty for malunited fractures of the distal end of the radius. *J Bone Joint Surg Am* 1988;70:1538-1551.

31. Marsh JL, Vannier MW: Surface imaging from computerized tomographic scans. *Surgery* 1983;94:159-165.

32. Marx RG, Axelrod TS: Intraarticular osteotomy of distal radial malunions. *Clin Orthop* 1996;327:152-157.

33. Knirk JL, Jupiter JB: Intra-articular fractures of the distal end of the radius in young adults. *J Bone Joint Surg Am* 1986;68:647-659.

34. Fourrier P, Bardy A, Roche G, Cisterne JP, Chambon A: Approach to a definition of malunion callus after Pouteau-Colles fractures. *Int Orthop* 1981;4:299-305.

35. Jupiter JB, Ring D: A comparison of early and late reconstruction of malunited fractures of the distal end of the radius. *J Bone Joint Surg Am* 1996;78:739-748.

36. Fernandez DL, Albrecht HU, Saxer U: Corrective osteotomy for malalignment of fractures of the distal radius. *Arch Orthop Unfallchir* 1977;90:199-211.

37. Oskam J, Kingma J, Klasen HJ: Ulnar-shortening osteotomy after fracture of the distal radius. *Arch Orthop Trauma Surg* 1993;112:198-200.

38. Bindra RR, Cole RJ, Yamaguchi K, et al: Quantification of the radial torsion angle with computerized tomography in cadaver specimens. *J Bone Joint Surg Am* 1997;79:833-837.

39. King GJ, McMurtry RY, Rubenstein JD, Ogston NG: Computerized tomography of the distal radioulnar joint: Correlation with ligamentous pathology in a cadaveric model. *J Hand Surg Am*

1986;11:711-717.

40. Mino DE, Palmer AK, Levinsohn EM: The role of radiography and computerized tomography in the diagnosis of subluxation and dislocation of the distal radioulnar joint. *J Hand Surg Am* 1983;8:23-31.

41. Sangeorzan BJ, Sangeorzan BP, Hansen ST, Judd RP: Mathematically directed single-cut osteotomy for correction of tibial malunion. *J Orthop Trauma* 1989;3:267-275.

42. Vannier MW, Totty WG, Stevens WG, et al: Musculoskeletal applications of three-dimensional surface reconstructions. *Orthop Clin North Am* 1985;16:543-555.

43. Weeks PM, Vannier MW, Stevens WG, Gayou D, Gilula LA: Three-dimensional imaging of the wrist. *J Hand Surg Am* 1985;10:32-39.

44. Jupiter JB, Ruder J, Roth DA: Computer-generated bone models in the planning of osteotomy of multidirectional distal radius malunions. *J Hand Surg Am* 1992;17:406-415.

45. Bora FW Jr, Osterman AL, Zielinski CJ: Osteotomy of the distal radius with a biplanar iliac bone graft for malunion. *Bull Hosp Jt Dis Orthop Inst* 1984;44:122-131.

46. Brown JN, Bell MJ: Distal radial osteotomy for malunion of wrist fractures in young patients.

J Hand Surg Br 1994;19:589-593.

47. Pennig D, Gausepohl T: Extraarticular and transarticular external fixation with early motion in distal radius fractures. *J Orthop Surg Tech* 1995;9:2.

48. Roesgen M, Hierholzer G: Corrective osteotomy of the distal radius after fracture to restore the function of wrist joint, forearm, and hand. *Arch Orthop Trauma Surg* 1988;107:301-308.

49. Sauvé L, Kapandji M: Nouvelle technique de traitement chirurgical des luxations récidivantes isolées de l'extrémité inférieure du cubitus. *J Chir* 1936;47:589-594.

50. Dingman PVC: Resection of the distal end of the ulna (Darrach operation): An end-result study of twenty-four cases. *J Bone Joint Surg Am* 1952;34:893-900.

51. Breen TF, Jupiter JB: Extensor carpi ulnaris and flexor carpi ulnaris tenodesis of the unstable distal ulna. *J Hand Surg Am* 1989;14:612-617.

52. Lamey DM, Fernandez DL: Results of the modified Sauvé-Kapandji procedure in the treatment of chronic posttraumatic derangement of the distal radioulnar joint. *J Bone Joint Surg Am* 1998;80:1758-1769.

53. van Schoonhoven J, Fernandez DL, Bowers WH, Herbert TJ: Salvage of failed resection arthroplasties of the distal radioulnar joint using a new

ulnar head prosthesis. *J Hand Surg Am* 2000;25:438-446.

54. Stanley D, Herbert TJ: The Swanson ulnar head prosthesis for post-traumatic disorders of the distal radio-ulnar joint. *J Hand Surg Br* 1992;17:682-688.

55. Tolat AR, Stanley JK, Trail IA: A cadaveric study of the anatomy and stability of the distal radioulnar joint in the coronal and transverse planes. *J Hand Surg Br* 1996;21:587-594.

56. Chun S, Palmer AK: The ulnar impaction syndrome: Follow-up of ulnar shortening osteotomy. *J Hand Surg Am* 1993;18:46-53.

57. Feldon P, Terrono AL, Belsky MR: Wafer distal ulna resection for triangular fibrocartilage tears and/or ulna impaction syndrome. *J Hand Surg Am* 1992;17:731-737.

58. Hauck RM, Skahen J, Palmer AK: Classification and treatment of ulnar styloid nonunion. *J Hand Surg Am* 1996;21:418-422.

59. Kleinman WB, Graham TJ The distal radioulnar joint capsule: Clinical anatomy and role in posttraumatic limitation of forearm rotation. *J Hand Surg Am* 1998;23:588-599.

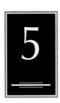

5

Acute Injuries of the Distal Radioulnar Joint and Triangular Fibrocartilage Complex

David M. Lichtman, MD
Atul Joshi, MD, MCH (Orth), FRCS

Abstract

Distal radioulnar joint disorders have become increasingly recognized. Over the past decade, advances in functional anatomy, kinematics, advanced imaging, and arthroscopy have improved understanding of distal radioulnar joint disorders and their management. In the past, injuries to the triangular fibrocartilage complex and distal radioulnar joint have been regarded as related but separate entities. The authors' classification and treatment algorithm perceives these injuries as a single entity, differing only in their progressively severe anatomic pathology and subsequent clinical manifestations. A discussion of pertinent anatomy, clinical characteristics, ancillary studies, and a new classification system help establish recommended management options of this disorder.

Distal radioulnar joint (DRUJ) dislocations were first described in 1777[1] and since then have been appearing with increasing frequency. Along with a discussion of the pertinent anatomy, clinical characteristics, and ancillary studies, a new classification system and the authors' recommended management of this disorder are presented.

Functional Anatomy

In the past, injuries to the triangular fibrocartilage complex (TFCC) and DRUJ have been regarded as related but separate entities. Our classification and treatment algorithm categorizes these injuries as a single entity, differing only in their progressively severe anatomic pathology and subsequent clinical manifestations.

The DRUJ is but one component in the integrated system called the forearm axis. Proper function requires coordination of the proximal and distal radioulnar joints coupled with appropriate geometric alignment of the ulnar and radius shafts and correct arrangement of interposing and stabilizing soft-tissue structures.

The DRUJ, like other joints, depends on its bony and ligamentous structure for stability. The sigmoid notch is designated as the point of articulation of the distal ulna with the distal radius (Fig. 1). Four types of sigmoid notches have been identified in the transverse plane: flat (42%), ski-slope (14%), hemicyclic (30%), and S-shaped (14%). The flat and ski-slope types tend to be unstable in pronation.[2] The orientation and congruity of the articular surface play important roles in DRUJ stability.

Ulnar positive variance increases the load on the TFCC and makes it more susceptible to acute or degenerative injuries.[3] In addition, ulnar abatement syndrome is common with ulnar positive variance and can exacerbate symptoms of TFCC tears. Ulnar positive variance must always be addressed when treating TFCC/DRUJ injuries.

Soft-tissue structures that play important roles in the function and stabilization of the DRUJ include triangular fibrocartilage (TFC), dorsal and palmar distal radioulnar ligaments, ulnocarpal ligaments, extensor carpi ulnaris (ECU) sheath, pronator quadratus, and interosseous membrane (Fig. 2).

Triangular Fibrocartilage Complex

The TFCC is made up of the triangular fibrocartilage or disk proper and adjacent supporting structures. The TFCC has many roles. It provides primary stabilization of the wrist, functions as a shock absorber, increases joint range of motion while increasing surface area, and helps transfer 20% of the load from the hand to the forearm.[4]

The TFC is the articular disk or disk proper (discus articularis). The disk is a semicircular fibrocartilaginous structure of variable thickness with a central and peripheral zone (Fig. 3). The central zone is avascular with sporadically organized collagen fibers, whereas the peripheral

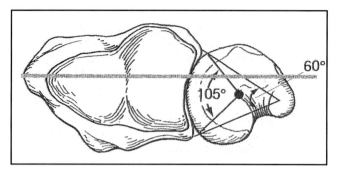

Fig. 1 The radius of curvature of the seat of the ulna is 10 mm, with the arcs subtending an angle of 105°. The radius of curvature of the sigmoid notch is approximately 60°. Thus, the distal radioulnar joint is not purely congruent. This anatomic feature allows for the translational motion of the ulna within the signoid notch during prosupination. (Reproduced with permission from Loftus J, Palmer A: Disorders of the distal radioulnar joint and triangular fibrocartilage complex: An overview, in Lichtman D, Alexander H (eds): *The Wrist and Its Disorders.* Philadelphia, PA, WB Saunders, 1997, pp 387-403.)

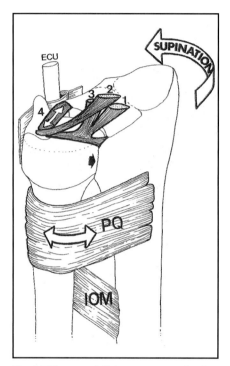

Fig. 2 Different stabilizing structures of radio-ulnocarpal joint during supination. The ulnocarpal ligaments, formed by the ulnolunate (1), ulnocapitate (2), and ulnotriquetrum (3) ligaments, pull the ulnar head palmarly as the wrist supinates. Such palmar translation tendency is counteracted by the tightness of the dorsal radioulnar ligament (4), thus increasing coaptation of the ulnar head against the palmar rim of the joint (black arrow). The constraining effects on such palmar translation vector of the dorsally located ECU and pronator quadratus (PQ) muscles also are important. Finally, the interosseous membrane (IOM), which in supination becomes extremely taut, is also to be considered. (Reproduced with permission from Garcia-Elias M: Soft-tissue anatomy and relationships about the distal ulna. *Hand Clin* 1998;14:165-176.)

zone has well-defined collagen fibers arranged in a semicircular orientation. It is important to note that the disk proper plays a role in shock absorption and load transfer but does not add significantly to DRUJ stability.

The peripheral fibers of the triangular disk consist of the dorsal and palmar radioulnar ligaments, both of which stabilize the distal ulna during pronation and supination through their origin in the radius and insertion at the base of the ulnar styloid. Exact contributions of each ligament during rotation is a topic of debate. Recent biomechanical studies have confirmed that the palmar radioulnar ligaments restrain dorsal subluxation of the ulna in the position of supination, whereas the dorsal radioulnar ligament restrains palmar subluxation of the distal ulna in pronation[5] (Fig. 4). The radius is the mobile segment; therefore, a dorsal DRUJ subluxation or dislocation is really a volar distal radius subluxation and vice versa. In keeping with tradition, however, this dislocation will be referred to as in the direction of the distal ulna. Because the central avascular zone and the peripheral zone are well vascularized at the dorsal, palmar, and ulnar attachments, healing of these fibers is possible in acute injuries.

Ulnocarpal Ligament

The ulnocarpal ligament is actually a group of ligaments that can be broadly divided into ulnotriquetral, ulnolunate, and ulnocapitate ligaments.[6] The ulnotriquetral and ulnolunate ligaments arise

from the palmar distal radioulnar ligament (Figs. 2 and 3). The ulnocapitate ligament arises from the base of the ulnar styloid. This ligament complex resists excessive rotation, usually supination, of the hand on the forearm. Failure of these ligaments is commonly seen in patients with inflammatory arthropathy, but the exact role of these ligaments is unclear in acute injury.

Extensor Carpi Ulnaris

The ECU tendon sheath has a close relationship with the ulna (sixth compartment). The fibrous subsheath is firmly attached to the dorsal TFCC at the ulnar styloid. Injury to the subsheath can result in ECU subluxation over the styloid and can decrease resistance to dorsal DRUJ subluxations.[7]

Pronator Quadratus Muscle

The pronator quadratus muscle adds stability during supination and becomes lax without a stabilizing effect in pronation.

Radioulnar Interosseous Membrane

The interosseous membrane tightens with supination and provides some DRUJ stability by preventing palmar translation of the distal ulna. The central third of the membrane is the major load-bearing portion.[8,9] Its primary focus is to transfer appropriately 80% of the forearm load from the distal radius to the proximal ulna. Damage to the central fibers along with a radial head injury can lead to proximal migration of the radial shaft

(Essex-Lopresti lesion).[6] Axial instability of the DRUJ also accompanies this injury.

Clinical Presentation

Ulnar-sided wrist pain and "clicking" are the most common presenting symptoms of DRUJ/TFCC injuries. A pertinent detailed patient history will help achieve the correct diagnosis. Salient points include duration of symptoms, painful activities or maneuvers, history of trauma, occupational activity, and recreational activity. Patients may describe various sounds, including snaps, clicks, and grinding or crepitus associated with the pain-producing activity. A high-pitched snap is often produced by a subluxating tendon or plica. Grinding or crepitus may be generated by synovitis. A medium-pitched click is indicative of the rubbing of two bones as in triquetrolunate dislocation. A low-pitched clunk represents a joint subluxation or relocation and could be diagnostic of midcarpal instability or DRUJ dislocation.

Ulnar-sided wrist pain has an extensive list of differential diagnoses (Table 1). Physical examination should be thorough and systematic, beginning with the proximal aspect of the dorsum of the wrist and proceeding distally in a stepwise fashion. The process should be repeated on the volar surface of the wrist. The presence of pain with acute ulnar deviation and compression and tender points dorsally and palmarly should be noted. Localization of pain at various stages of motion (dorsiflexion, palmar flexion, ulnar deviation, radial deviation, pronation, and supination) should also be noted. The degree of prominence of the ulnar head in comparison with the contralateral wrist should also be assessed. Pain-provoking movements should be compared with the opposite side. Stressing the DRUJ and comparing pain or laxity with the opposite side is very helpful. The piano key test involves depressing the distal ulna from dorsal to

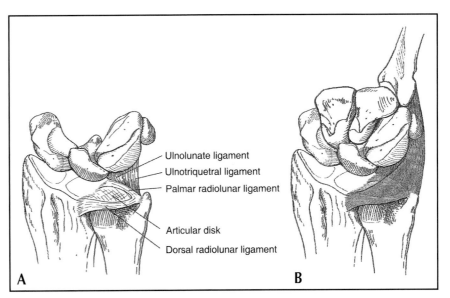

Fig. 3 A, Diagrammatic drawing of the triangular fibrocartilage complex, depicting the triangular fibrocartilage iteself with its dorsal and palmar radioulnar ligaments. The ulnolunate and ulnotriquetral ligaments run from the fovea of the ulna to the carpus. **B,** Same view as in A with the addition of the meniscal reflection. (Reproduced with permission from Loftus J, Palmer A: Disorders of the distal radioulnar joint and triangular fibrocartilage complex: An overview, in Lichtman D, Alexander H (eds): *The Wrist and Its Disorders*. Philadelphia, PA, WB Saunders, 1997, pp 385-414.)

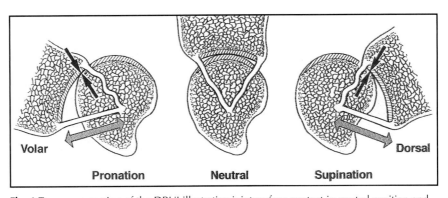

Fig. 4 Transverse section of the DRUJ illustrating joint surface contact in neutral position and minimal joint surface contact (*arrows*) in supination and pronation. (Reproduced with permission from Ekenstam F: Osseous anatomy and articular relationships about the distal ulna. *Hand Clin* 1998;14;161-164.)

volar with the forearm pronated. The test is positive if increased laxity or lack of resistance is present in comparison with the contralateral side. In inflammatory conditions, the test will elicit an expression of pain.[10] The ulnar compression test can be performed by compressing the ulnar head against the sigmoid notch while rotating the wrist. Pain or crepitus indicates a positive test, suggesting arthritis or instability.[10] Other stress tests including triquetrolunate ballottement or midcarpal shift tests aid in the differential diagnosis. An attempt to elicit ECU subluxation should be made by asking the patient to actively move the wrist from pronation to supination along with palmar flexion and ulnar deviation of the

Table 1
Differential Diagnoses in the Dorsal and Volar Zones of the Wrist

Dorsal Zone	Volar Zone
ECU	Flexor carpi ulnaris tendinitis
Subluxation	Ulnar head
Stenosing tenosynovitis	Subluxation
Inflammatory arthritis	Dislocation
DRUJ	TFCC
Arthritis (degenerative or inflammatory)	Volar tear
Incongruity	Pisiform
Intra-articular pathology (synovial,	Subluxation
rheumatoid arthritis, chondroma)	Fracture
Instability	Pisotriquetral disease
TFCC	Degenerative
Traumatic lesions	Ganglion
Degenerative tears (ulnar abutments)	Guyon's canal
Ulnar abutment	Ganglion
Degenerative lesions of TFCC	Ulnar artery thrombosis
Ulnar impaction syndrome (chondromalacia	Tunnel syndrome
of ulnar head and lunate, lunotriquetral	Hamate (hook fracture)
instability)	Fifth flexor tendon
Ulnar styloid	(synovitis/rupture)
Fracture	
Nonunion	
Lunate/triquetrum	
Kienböck disease	
Chondromalacia	
Cyst/interosseous ganglion (lunate/capitate)	
Intraosseous pathology (enchondroma,	
osteoid osteoma)	
Lunotriquetral instability (trauma or impaction)	
Midcarpal instability	
Capitate/hamate	
Osteonecrosis	
Capitolunate arthrosis	
Triquetrohamate arthrosis	
Body fracture (hamate/capitate)	
Hook fracture (hamate)	
Carpometacarpal fourth, fifth joint arthritis	
Carpal bosse third	

hand. Examination of the DRUJ is not complete without examination of the forearm and elbow.

Diagnostic Studies

Most often, a reasonably accurate diagnosis can be made from the history and physical examination. Specific diagnostic studies can then be chosen that are complementary to the clinical examination or are confirmatory prior to choosing a definitive treatment option.

Plain Radiographs

Basic radiographs should include PA and lateral views of the wrist. The PA view should be taken in neutral rotation with the patient seated, the elbow in 90° of flexion, and the shoulder in 90° of abduction.[11] Comparison films of the opposite wrist will help to delineate any minor discrepancies. This provides a reproducible method of determining ulnar variance. The lateral view is taken with the forearm in neutral and the ulnar side of the wrist

placed flat against the cassette. In a true lateral view, the lunate, proximal pole of the scaphoid, and the triquetrum are all superimposed upon one another, and the pisiform is superimposed on the volar, distal pole of the scaphoid[12] (Fig. 5). Plain radiographs are useful in the diagnosis of fractures, ulnar subluxation/dislocation, triquetrolunate subluxation, triquetral or lunate cysts, degenerative changes in radioulnar or triquetroulnar joints, Kienböck disease, and ulnar variance measurements.

Arthrography

Once commonly used, this test is performed less frequently because of the advent of MRI and arthroscopy. Arthrography usually consists of a three-compartment injection. Normally, the midcarpal joint, the radiocarpal joint, and the DRUJ are separately contained components; visualized dye flow between the compartments indicates perforation. Because of the high number of asymptomatic, degenerative, or traumatic perforations, the test has a high false-positive rate.[13,14] There are also many false-negative results because many small perforations are not seen arthrographically.

Fluoroscopy

This study is infrequently ordered but can be diagnostic for midcarpal instability or subtle proximal row (dissociative) instabilities. The wrist should be examined in both planes through an entire range of motion. Abnormal movements between carpal bones can be seen in stress and motion views. Provocative maneuvers can also be performed under fluoroscopy to aid in visualization of the various instabilities.

Radionuclide Scan

The role of nuclear bone scan is limited in ulnar-sided wrist pain but can be used if the clinical signs and symptoms are not well localized and the plain radiographs are negative. A bone scan may help to narrow the focus to a specific area of the wrist. Other modalities are then used to arrive at a more definitive diagnosis.

Computed Tomography

CT is useful in delineating osseous architecture and in identification of occult fractures. DRUJ incongruity is best studied by axial imaging in several positions from full pronation to full supination.[12] Comparison to the contralateral extremity is helpful in assessing subtle changes (Figs. 6 and 7). Objective methods have been described to assess the congruity of the DRUJ.[15]

Magnetic Resonance Imaging

MRI allows detailed structural assessment of the TFCC, intercarpal ligaments, tendons, and tendon sheaths.[16] Various signal changes can indicate soft-tissue inflammation and alteration of bone physiology. The utility of MRI in wrist pathology is dependent on good communication between the clinician and the radiologist. Improvements in three-dimensional gradient-recalled echo and use of custom-made coils will continue to improve the accuracy of MRI.

Arthroscopy

Arthroscopy allows direct visualization of carpal pathology while allowing minimally invasive surgical treatment of many conditions. Currently, arthroscopic procedures include trimming torn TFCC and triquetrolunate cartilage, removing loose bodies and inflamed synovium, TFCC repair, and capsule shrinkage.[17] As technical advances continue, arthroscopy will play an increasingly important role in the management of TFCC/DRUJ injuries.[18]

Classification of DRUJ/TFCC Disorders

TFCC and DRUJ disorders have traditionally been classified separately. TFCC tears have been classified by Palmer,[19] divided into traumatic and degenerative

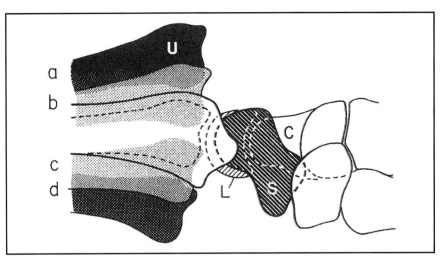

Fig. 5 Schematic representation of a true lateral radiograph of the wrist in neutral position. In a true lateral view, the radial styloid is centered over the lunate (L), and scaphoid (S). If the x-ray beam is even slightly oblique to this position, one may incorrectly diagnose DRUJ dislocation. If in position a, the ulna (u) is dorsally dislocated; if in position b, the ulna is dorsally subluxated; if in position c, the ulna is volarly subluxated; and if in position d, the ulna is volarly dislocated. (Reproduced with permission from Mino DE, Palmer AK, Levinsohn EM: The role of radiography and computerized tomography in the diagnosis of subluxation and dislocation of the distal radioulnar joint. *J Hand Surg Am* 1983;8:23-31.)

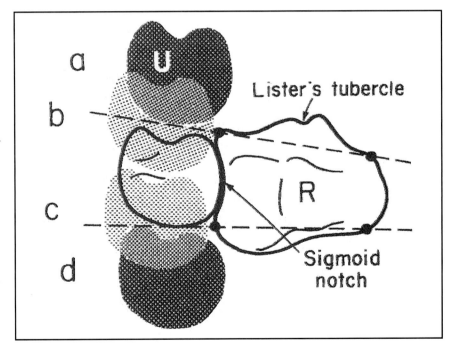

Fig. 6 Schematic representation of CT scan transverse section through the DRUJ. The distal ulna should fit snugly in the sigmoid notch of the radius (R). If in position a, the ulna is dorsally dislocated; in position b, the ulna is dorsally subluxated; in position (c) the ulna is volarly subluxated; and, in position d, the ulna is volarly dislocated. (Reproduced with permission from Mino DE, Palmer AK, Levinsohn EM: The role of radiography and computerized tomography in the diagnosis of subluxation and dislocation of the distal radioulnar joint. *J Hand Surg Am* 1983;8:23-31.)

Table 2
Palmer's Classification of TFCC Tears

Class 1 Traumatic

A   Central perforation

B   Medical avulsion (ulnar attachment)
      with distal ulnar fracture
      without distal ulnar fracture

C   Distal avulsion (carpal attachment)
      Lateral avulsion (radial attachment)
      with sigmoid notch fracture
      without sigmoid notch fracture

Class 2 Degenerative

A   Thinning of the articular disk

B   Thinning of the articular disk and
      chondromalacia

C   Tear of the articular disk and
      chondromalacia

D   Tear of the articular disk,
      chondromalacia, and partial tearing
      of the lunotriquetral ligament

E   Tear of the articular disk,
      chondromalacia, partial tearing
      of the lunotriquetral ligament, and
      arthritis of the radioulnar joint

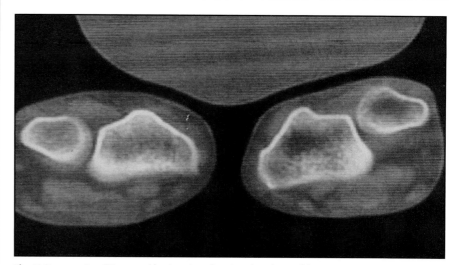

Fig. 7 Comparative CT scan of both wrists showing the ulnar subluxations.

categories. The two classes are further subdivided by location and severity as shown in Table 2. DRUJ injuries are traditionally classified as either palmar or dorsal. However, we believe that the function and pathology of the DRUJ and TFCC are integrated. Therefore, we have divided DRUJ injuries into three contiguous categories based on DRUJ stability, which in turn depends on the extent and type of TFCC injury. These categories are: stable, partially unstable, and unstable. The last category is further divided as simple or complex depending on the reducibility of the joint.

Authors' Classification

Stable Stable injuries involve isolated pathology of the nonstabilizing TFC. In a stable injury, a traumatic central (Palmer class 1A) or radial (Palmer class 1D) tear of the TFC is present (Table 2). Ulnar abutment may also cause a stable central tear of the TFCC, usually of a degenerative nature (Palmer class 2). The diagnosis is based on the clinical examination of ulnar-sided wrist pain

elicited by ulnar deviation and compression of the TFCC. Tenderness may be present over the palmar or dorsal aspect of the TFCC. There may be a history of clicking, or the click may be elicited with forearm rotation and ulnar deviation. Plain radiographs may show a positive variance of the ulna. Diagnostic confirmation can be done by MRI or arthroscopy, but most often the diagnosis is clearly elucidated by history, physical examination, and plain radiographs.

Partially Unstable Patients with partially unstable injury have a hypermobile distal ulna elicited by manual stress testing. As in stable injuries, there will be pain on ulnar deviation and TFCC compression with tenderness over the palmar or dorsal aspect of the TFCC. The pathology is usually the Palmer class 1B (peripheral TFCC tear) or class 1C (volar, peripheral TFCC tear). Ulnar abutment or ECU subluxation may coexist. Ancillary studies such as MRI and arthroscopy will confirm the pathology. Comparable axial CT imaging can be diagnostic of instability when it shows joint incongruity. In subtle cases, an axial CT stress test has been described. Plain radiographs should always be obtained to look for ulnar abutment or DRUJ degeneration (Fig. 8).

Unstable Unstable injuries, without bony pathology, are associated with massive disruption of the TFCC. The ulna is usually displaced dorsally. The plain film will identify the deformity on the true lateral view of the wrist. An axial CT revealing the dislocation is pathognomonic. MRI may also show an associated ECU or ligamentous injury. Dorsal dislocation occurs with hyperpronation. The ulnar head will be dorsally dislocated, and patients will be unable to perform supination. Palmar dislocation occurs with hypersupination. Acutely, the wrist may appear narrow, a mass (ulnar head) may be palpable palmarly, and the patient will be unable to perform pronation. Unstable injuries can be isolated to the soft tissues but more frequently are associated with concurrent fractures such as ulnar styloid fracture, distal radius fracture, radial head fracture/dislocation, and both-bone forearm fractures. The DRUJ dislocation may have interposing soft tissue, bone, or tendons that can block reduction. When reduction is difficult, the physician must be aware that open treatment of the joint is required.

The most common reported cause of an irreducible DRUJ is the Galeazzi fracture. In 1981, an interposed ECU tendon at the DRUJ that was blocking reduction

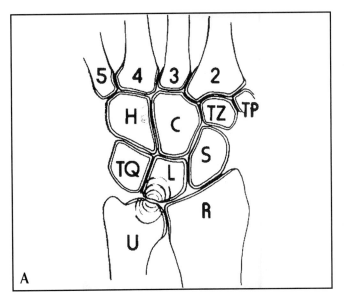
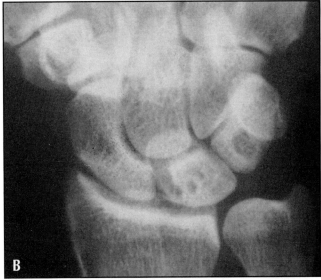

Fig. 8 A, Schematic representation of ulnar abutment. Numbers denote fifth, fourth, third, and second metacarpals. H = hamate, C = capitate, TZ = trapezoid, TP = trapezium, TQ = triquetrum, L = lunate, S = scaphoid, U = ulna, and R = radius. **B,** Radiograph showing the changes in the lunate because of ulnar abutment.

of the DRUJ was reported.[20] This condition was subsequently noted in other studies of Galeazzi fractures.[21-24] These injuries are termed "complex" DRUJ dislocations as opposed to the more common "simple" DRUJ dislocations.[25]

Treatment
Stable
Stable injuries of the TFCC, if diagnosed early, should be treated with immobilization for a period of 4 weeks. If symptoms persist, various conservative and surgical options are considered. Nonsteroidal anti-inflammatory drugs, avoidance of the inciting activity, and splinting should be tried initially. If local tenderness and inflammation persist, steroid and anesthetic injections can be used for treatment as well as to localize pathology. For the unresponsive individual, débridment of the central TFCC tear can be done arthroscopically.[26,27]

The decision to treat associated ulnar abutment is based on symptoms and the degree of ulnar variance. Appropriate radiographic studies, including studies of the opposite wrist, should be obtained. If positive variance is caused by an associated injury such as distal radius fracture, treatment should be directed toward correction of the deformity of the distal radius. For symptomatic positive or neutral ulnar variance, two treatment options are available: the open or arthroscopic wafer procedure, or ulnar shortening osteotomy. The wafer procedure, described by Feldon and associates[28] in 1992, involves excising the distal 2 to 4 mm of the ulnar head, with preservation of the TFCC. Formal shortening of the ulna is unnecessary. Some studies have reported good results but have been occasionally associated with ECU tendinitis. Wafer excision of the ulnar head can also be performed arthroscopically.[29,30] Formal ulnar shortening has withstood the test of time since first being reported in 1941.[1] Various techniques have been described to perform the osteotomy, such as the use of a dynamic compression plating with an interfragmentary lag screw at the oblique osteotomy site. Regardless of the technique, the reported outcomes have been uniformly good to excellent.

Partially Unstable
Acute injuries are generally treated by immobilization of the wrist in neutral or slight supination to promote healing of the peripheral tear. Later symptomatic partially unstable injuries can be treated arthroscopically. When examined arthroscopically, a Palmer class 1B lesion may show the "trampoline effect," a subtle yet exaggerated giving way of the articular disk when tested with a probe. Several arthroscopic techniques have been described to repair this lesion.[31-35] The goal of treatment is to débride the synovitis and to reattach the peripheral tear to the base of the ulnar styloid (fovea). Special instruments have been devised to perform the repair. When the tear and instability are pronounced, we prefer to repair the lesion using an open technique. Once again, abutment should be appropriately treated if present. In the presence of both a peripheral TFCC tear and abutment, we often perform a formal shortening of the distal ulna. This tightens the ligamentous supporting structures (TFCC) while relieving pressure on the torn TFCC. This technique has

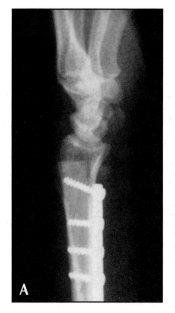 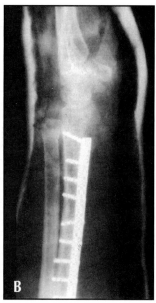 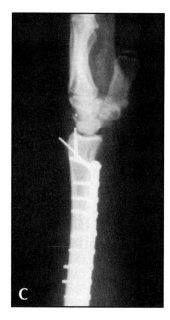

Fig. 9 A, Apparent reduction of the DRUJ after a Galeazzi fracture. **B,** Loss of DRUJ reduction in cast within 1 week after fixation. **C,** Open reduction was performed and DRUJ was stabilized with transfixing Kirschner wire and stable reduction was achieved.

been used frequently without formal débridment, and the outcome has been good.

Unstable

Unstable injuries are often associated with other significant forearm injuries or fractures, including distal radius fracture, both-bone forearm fracture, isolated radius (Galeazzi) fracture, and radial head fracture (Essex-Lopresti fracture). A basic principle of treating this injury is to treat the associated injury first and then address the TFCC. After accurate and stable fracture fixation, careful assessment of the DRUJ stability should be done. This not only includes reduction of the DRUJ but assessment as to whether the reduction is stable (Fig. 9). DRUJ stability is tested with the forearm in neutral to slight supination. If the reduction can be done easily but stability is doubtful, then two Kirschner wires are inserted from the distal ulna to the radius, avoiding the sigmoid notch. If the DRUJ cannot be relocated or the reduction has a "mushy" or "springy" feel, then there may be an anatomic block to reduction (a complex dislocation). These cases require open reduction of the DRUJ. According

to our studies and a review of the literature, the most common cause of a complex dislocation is entrapment of the ECU tendon volar to the ulnar head, often with an attached large fragment of the ulnar styloid.

Ulnar styloid fractures (with or without associated radius fractures) deserve special mention. Nondisplaced fractures can be treated by cast immobilization. Displaced fractures need assessment for DRUJ stability. If the joint is stable and the fracture is distal to the TFCC insertion at base of the styloid, then it also can be treated conservatively. If the DRUJ is unstable or the fracture is proximal to the TFCC insertion, then the fracture requires reduction with open or closed internal fixation. Open reduction and Kirschner wire fixation using a tension band technique is preferred.

Summary

Injuries of the TFCC/DRUJ represent a spectrum of instability that correlates well with the degree of the TFCC injury and associated pathology. Accurate diagnosis can be made by careful history, physical examination, and appropriate studies. By using a simple classification

system based on stability, abutment, and associated fractures, a logical treatment plan can be devised.

References

1. Alexander AH, Lichtman DM: Treatment of acute injuries of the distal radioulnar joint, in Lichtman DM, Alexander AH (eds): *The Wrist and Its Disorders,* ed 2. Philadelphia, PA, WB Saunders, 1997, pp 420-428.

2. Tolat AR, Stanley JK, Trail IA: A cadaveric study of the anatomy and stability of the distal radioulnar joint in the coronal and transverse planes. *J Hand Surg Br* 1996;21:587-594.

3. Palmer AK: The distal radioulnar joint: Anatomy, biomechanics, and triangular fibrocartilage complex abnormalities. *Hand Clin* 1987;3:31-40.

4. Viegas SF, Patterson RM: Load mechanics of the wrist. *Hand Clin* 1997;13:109-128.

5. Stuart PR, Berger RA, Linscheid RL, An KN: The dorsalpalmar stability of the distal radiolunar joint. *J Hand Surg Am* 2000;25:689-699.

6. Garcia-Elias M: Soft-tissue anatomy and relationships about the distal ulna. *Hand Clin* 1998;14:165-176.

7. Spinner M, Kaplan EB: Extensor carpi ulnaris: Its relationship to the stability of the distal radio-ulnar joint. *Clin Orthop* 1970;68:124-129.

8. Skahen JR III, Palmer AK, Werner FW, Fortino MD: The interosseous membrane of the forearm: Anatomy and function. *J Hand Surg Am* 1997;22:981-985.

9. Hotchkiss RN, An KN, Sowa DT, Basta S, Weiland AJ: An anatomic and mechanical study of the interosseous membrane of the forearm: Pathomechanics of proximal migration of the radius. *J Hand Surg Am* 1989;14:256-261.

10. Loftus J, Palmer A: Disorders of the distal radioulnar joint and triangular fibrocartilage complex: An overview, in Lichtman DM, Alexander AH (eds): *The Wrist and Its Disorders,* ed 2. Philadelphia, PA, WB Saunders Company, 1997, pp 385-414.

11. Palmer AK, Glisson RR, Werner FW: Ulnar variance determination. *J Hand Surg Am* 1982;7:376-379.

12. Mino DE, Palmer AK, Levinsohn EM: The role of radiography and computerized tomography in the diagnosis of subluxation and dislocation of the distal radioulnar joint. *J Hand Surg Am* 1983;8:23-31.

13. Hardy DC, Totty WG, Carnes KM, et al: Arthrographic surface anatomy of the carpal triangular fibrocartilage complex. *J Hand Surg Am* 1988;13:823-829.

14. Reinus WR, Hardy DC, Totty WG, Gilula A: Arthrographic evaluation of the carpal triangular fibrocartilage complex. *J Hand Surg Am* 1987;12:495-503.

15. Burk DL Jr, Karasick D, Wechsler RJ: Imaging of the distal radioulnar joint. *Hand Clin* 1991;7:263-275.

16. Rettig ME, Raskin KB, Melone CP Jr: Clinical applications of MR imaging in hand and wrist surgery. *Magn Reson Imaging Clin North Am* 1995;3:361-368.

17. Zelouf DS, Bowers WH: Arthroscopy of the distal radioulnar joint. *Hand Clin* 1999;15:475-477.

18. Johnstone DJ, Thorogood S, Smith WH, Scott TD: A comparison of magnetic resonance imaging and arthroscopy in the investigation of chronic wrist pain. *J Hand Surg Br* 1997;22:714-718.

19. Palmer AK: Triangular fibrocartilage complex lesions: A classification. *J Hand Surg Am* 1989;14:594-606.

20. Alexander AH, Lichtman DM: Irreducible distal radioulnar joint occurring in a Galeazzi fracture: Case report. *J Hand Surg Am* 1981;6:258-261.

21. Dyer CR, Kuschner SH, Brien WW: The distal radioulnar joint following Galeazzi's fracture. *Orthop Rev* 1994;23:587-592.

22. Hanel DP, Scheid DK: Irreducible fracture-dislocation of the distal radioulnar joint secondary to entrapment of the extensor carpi ulnaris tendon. *Clin Orthop* 1988;234:56-60.

23. Biyani A, Bhan S: Dual extensor tendon entrapment in Galeazzi fracture-dislocation: A case report. *J Trauma* 1989;29:1295-1297.

24. Cetti NE: An unusual cause of blocked reduction of the Galeazzi injury. *Injury* 1977;9:59-61.

25. Bruckner J, et al: Complex dislocations of the distal radioulnar joint: Recognition and management. *Clin Orthop* 1992;275:90-103.

26. Gan BS, Richards RS, Roth JH: Arthroscopic treatment of triangular fibrocartilage tears. *Orthop Clin North Am* 1995;26:721-729.

27. Dailey SW, Palmer AK: The role of arthroscopy in the evaluation and treatment of triangular fibrocartilage complex injuries in athletes. *Hand Clin* 2000;16:461-476.

28. Feldon P, Terrono AL, Belsky MR: The "wafer" procedure: Partial distal ulnar resection. *Clin Orthop* 1992;275:124-129.

29. Wnorowski DC, Palmer AK, Werner FW, Fortino MD: Anatomic and biomechanical analysis of the arthroscopic wafer procedure. *Arthroscopy* 1992;8:204-212.

30. De Smet L, De Ferm A, Steenwerck A, Dauwe D, Zachee B, Fabry G: Arthroscopic treatment of triangular fibrocartilage complex lesions of the wrist. *Acta Orthop Belg* 1996;62:8-13.

31. Osterman AL, Terrill RG: Arthroscopic treatment of TFCC lesions. *Hand Clin* 1991;7:277-281.

32. Trumble TE, Gilbert M, Vedder N: Arthroscopic repair of the triangular fibrocartilage complex. *Arthroscopy* 1996;12:588-597.

33. Hermansdorfer JD, Kleinman WB: Management of chronic peripheral tears of the triangular fibrocartilage complex. *J Hand Surg Am* 1991;16:340-346.

34. Haugstvedt JR, Husby T: Results of repair of peripheral tears in the triangular fibrocartilage complex using an arthroscopic suture technique. *Scand J Plast Reconstr Surg Hand Surg* 1999;33:439-447.

35. Bednar JM: Arthroscopic treatment of triangular fibrocartilage tears. *Hand Clin* 1999;15:479-488.

6

Scaphoid Fractures: Current Treatments and Techniques

William P. Cooney III, MD

Abstract

Scaphoid fractures are among the most common fractures of the bones of the wrist and usually result from a forceful extension of the wrist. If the diagnosis cannot be established by clinical and radiographic examination, bone scans are recommended and are preferred over tomography or MRI, which are more expensive diagnostic procedures. Scaphoid fractures should be classified as either undisplaced, stable or displaced, unstable. Nonsurgical treatment with cast immobilization (short arm–thumb spica cast) is recommended for stable fractures; however, there is increased interest in percutaneous screw (or pin) fixation. The recommended treatment for unstable scaphoid fractures is open reduction and screw fixation. Closed reduction and percutaneous screw or pin fixation can be considered in minimally displaced or reducible fractures, whereas open reduction is recommended for all other displaced fractures. The following treatment protocols are recommended: (1) bone scan or, if necessary, tomography for early diagnosis; (2) percutaneous screw fixation of nondisplaced or minimally displaced scaphoid fractures as an alternative to treatment with a thumb spica cast; (3) open reduction of displaced scaphoid fractures; (4) early mobilization of stable fractures after internal fixation; and (5) the possible use of a playing splint after athletic injuries when secure internal fixation is achieved.

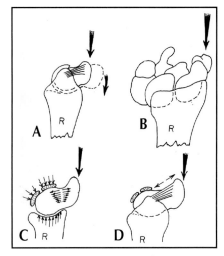

Fig. 1 Mechanism of scaphoid fractures. **A**, Lateral diagram of the wrist. Large arrow shows an axial load that produces extension of the scaphoid; with hyperextension, a tensile force occurs across the palmar waist of the scaphoid. **B**, AP diagram of the wrist showing load (*large arrow*) applied to the volar distal aspect of the carpus. **C** and **D**, Palmar radiocarpal ligaments (*small downward arrows*) hold the proximal scaphoid when load (*large arrows*) is applied, increasing the tensile force across the scaphoid waist; the scaphoid fails in tension palmarly and compression dorsally. R = radius. (Reproduced with permission from the Mayo Foundation, Rochester, MN.)

Scaphoid fractures are the most common fractures of the wrist with the exception of fractures of the distal radius. These fractures result from a significant force applied to the wrist (Fig. 1). Studies of the mechanism of specific fractures and research studies indicate that extension or hyperextension of the wrist, usually combined with radial deviation, produce fractures of the scaphoid.[1] This fracture is often the result of sports-related injuries, motor vehicle or motorcycle crashes, or a fall from a height;[2-4] with significant injuries, the scaphoid fracture fragments are displaced. In one view of perilunate dislocation of the wrist, a transcaphoid fracture represents the first step of a hyperextension injury through the greater arc that sequences across the wrist[3] (Fig. 2). Depending on the degree

of force from the injury mechanism, the scaphoid fracture may be minimally to moderately displaced as an isolated injury.[2,5,6] When there is a perilunate dislocation that involves the scaphoid, significant displacement is always present.[2,3]

A second mechanism of injury involving a pure axial load injury that produces an impaction fracture of the scaphoid that is always nondisplaced has been suggested in several studies.[6-8]

Diagnosis

A significant injury to the wrist (ie, from a fall or motor vehicle crash) and the existence of positive physical and radiographic findings are important factors that would contribute to the suspicion of a scaphoid fracture.[9,10] The history of a forceful injury is important. Some

patients have wrist pain and radiographs that show a scaphoid fracture; however, the mechanism of injury is trivial and of insufficient force to produce a scaphoid fracture. In such patients, the recent injury exacerbates a previous scaphoid nonunion, which now becomes symptomatic.[5,10,11] It is essential that these two

Table 1
Classification Systems for Scaphoid Fractures

Mayo Classification by Fracture Location
1 Tuberosity
2 Distal articular surface
3 Distal third
4 Wrist, middle third
5 Proximal pole

Russe Classification by Obliquity
HO Horizontal oblique
VO Vertical oblique
T Transverse

Herbert Classification
Type A Stable acute fractures
    A1 Fracture of tubercle
    A2 Incomplete fracture of the wrist
Type B Unstable acute fracture
    B1 Distal oblique
    B2 Complete wrist fracture
    B3 Proximal pole fracture
    B4 Transscaphoid perilunate
        dislocation fracture
Type C Delayed union
Type D Established nonunion
    D1 Fibrous nonunion (stable)
    D2 Displaced nonunion (unstable)

(Adapted with permission from Herbert TJ: *The Fractured Scaphoid.* St Louis, MO, Quality Medical Publishing, 1990.)

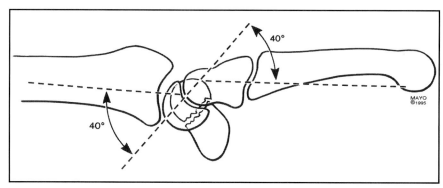

Fig. 2 Scaphoid fracture with perilunate instability. The scaphoid fracture represents the bone equivalent of scapholunate dissociation. The displacement of the proximal scaphoid and lunate from the distal scaphoid (and distal carpal row) results in a dorsal intercalated segment instability. (Reproduced with permission from the Mayo Foundation, Rochester, MN.)

diagnoses remain separate, as the treatment of an acute scaphoid fracture is considerably different than the treatment of an established scaphoid nonunion.

Physical findings of a scaphoid fracture include painful wrist motion, swelling, and loss of grip strength.[11,12] Examination of the patient's wrist may show swelling and occasional deformity; often the swelling is mild and unrelated to the degree of fracture unless the scaphoid fracture is associated with a perilunate dislocation. Direct clinical examination will reveal tenderness in the radial snuffbox, pain with radial deviation, and pain with guarding on flexion and extension of the wrist (Fig. 3). Grip strength will average 50% of that shown by the uninjured wrist. Physical examination of the distal radioulnar joint and the elbow should also be performed, but findings are usually normal.

Recommended radiographic views include a straight PA, a true lateral, and 30° supinated views from the fully pronated forearm with ulnar deviation of the wrist[5,9,13,14] (Fig. 4). If a fracture of the scaphoid is evident, the degree of displacement (minimal, moderate, or severe) or nondisplacement should be determined.[14] If more definite imaging is needed to determine displacement, polytomography or axial CT is recommended[13,15-17] (Fig. 5).

Recommendations for the Evaluation of Potential Scaphoid Fractures

If a patient has a painful wrist (wrist sprain) with negative radiographs, options for evaluating the wrist include ultrasound, bone scan, tomography, and MRI.[5,10,13,16-22] Recent studies show that a bone scan, while not specific, is the best imaging study based on its cost and diagnostic ability[10,18,23,24] (Fig. 6). Bone scans have good sensitivity but lack specificity. Ultrasound is neither specific nor as sensitive as a bone scan, but its use is advocated by some physicians.[5,25-27]

Classification of scaphoid fractures is important because it can help to direct treatment[14] (Fig. 7) (Table 1). One classification system is based on the concept of displacement or nondisplacement and on the presence or absence of osteonecrosis

(Table 2). Other classification systems, such as that of Herbert and associates,[28] have multiple components for clinical assessment and indirectly address treatment. By definition, a displaced scaphoid fracture has more than 1.0 mm of offset and an increased intrascaphoid angulation (lateral view) of greater than 30°.[15,20,29] Fracture pattern and location are also important criteria in determining treatment. For example, a transverse fracture is more suitable for percutaneous screw fixation than a comminuted or oblique fracture. CT and MRI should be reserved for assessment of displacement or avascular changes.[13,30] Tomography (axial or three-dimensional CT) is used to measure the degree of displacement and the intrascaphoid angulation of the fracture[16,17] (Fig. 5). MRI shows the fracture well and the status of the blood supply to the proximal scaphoid, although it lacks the clarity of CT in determining displacement.[21,30-32] Wrist arthroscopy can show both scaphoid displacement and associated carpal ligament injuries at the midcarpal joint.[33]

Treatment

Nondisplaced and minimally displaced fractures of the scaphoid can be treated by cast immobilization.[15,22,26,34] Differences in the healing rates between a long-

Table 2
Author's Preferred Classification of Scaphoid Fracture Stability

Acute stable
  Displacement less than 1 mm
  Normal intercarpal alignment
    C-L angle 0° to 15°*
    S-L angle 30° to 60°*
  Distal pole fractures

Acute unstable
  Displacement greater than 1 mm
  Lateral intrascaphoid angulation
    greater than 35°†
  Significant bone loss or comminution
  Perilunate fracture
  DISI alignment
    C-L angle greater than 15°*
    S-L angle greater than 60°*

± Proximal pole fractures (osteonecrosis)

---

*Normal C-L angulation is 0° to 15°, and 30° is the uppermost limit of normal; normal S-L angulation is 30° to 60°, and an angle of 61° to 80° is abnormal

†Lateral intrascaphoid angulation is most accurately determined with lateral tomography or CT. Normal lateral intrascaphoid angulation is 24° ± 5°; greater than 45° is associated with an increased risk of functional impairment

C = capitate; L = lunate; S = scaphoid; and DISI = dorsal intercalated segmental instability

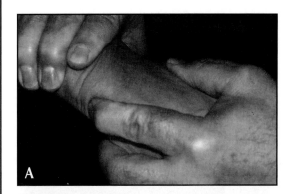

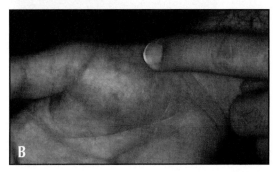

Fig. 3 Clinical examination. **A,** The finding of tenderness in the radial aspect of the wrist in the scaphoid "snuffbox" indicates a scaphoid fracture unless imaging studies prove negative. **B,** Volar distal scaphoid tenderness (with stress) also suggest a scaphoid fracture.

arm cast and short arm cast (usually thumb spica) are not of sufficient statistical significance to warrant the use of one type of cast over the other. The physician's perception of the patient's reliability may help in the choice of a long arm cast over a short arm cast.[9,26,35] For a reliable patient who would refrain from forceful use of the extremity, a short arm-thumb spica cast is usually sufficient.

It is recommended that treatment with a cast or splint immobilization should not be delayed for 2 to 3 weeks to reassess the patient because the period for proper cast treatment will have passed and further displacement can occur. Healing of the scaphoid is delayed, and malunion and nonunion rates are higher when there is a delay in treatment.[36,37] When diagnosis is delayed, limited, per-

cutaneous surgical procedures appear less reasonable.

A displaced scaphoid fracture has several treatment options. Although surgeons previously have considered cast immobilization, the rate of nonunion is statistically higher with cast immobilization of displaced fractures in comparison with nondisplaced fractures.[15] The trend has shifted to internal fixation techniques for immediate fixation of the scaphoid to avoid both nonunion and malunion.[20,29,38-40] The choices for fixation depend on the surgeon's experience and ability to realign and internally fix the scaphoid. It is important to obtain an anatomic alignment of the fracture components. Percutaneous pins placed by biplanar guidance are a reasonable, time-tested method of fixation, especially for minimally displaced fractures. Percutaneous screw fixation with limited incision of the scaphoid has recently become both popular and practical.[41-43] For surgeons experienced in wrist arthroscopy, arthroscopic fixation with guided pins or screws may be suitable.[33] Most, if not all,

of these techniques require the use of biplanar imaging with a C-arm. Clear imaging aids in the correct placement of a Kirschner wire (K-wire) within the scaphoid and in the choice of a percutaneous screw (cannulated screw over a K-wire) of a predetermined length for the final internal fixation.

If direct visualization is preferred, or in patients with comminuted, significantly displaced fractures of the scaphoid, open reduction and internal fixation is recommended.[20,39,44] This is particularly true for the transscaphoid perilunate fracture-dislocations of the wrist.[3] Usually, a volar approach is recommended for the middle to distal third fractures of the scaphoid and a dorsal approach for fractures of the proximal third.[20,45-47]

The Author's Preferences for Surgical Treatment of Acute Scaphoid Fractures
Percutaneous insertion of cannulated screws to treat nondisplaced or minimally displaced fractures and open reduction (or arthroscopic-guided reduction) is

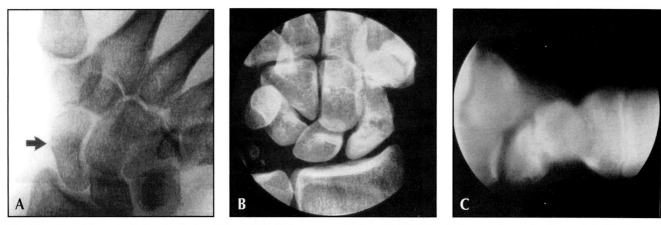

Fig. 4 Imaging of the wrist. **A,** Scaphoid view (30° supinated) shows an undisplaced scaphoid waist fracture (impaction fracture). **B,** PA view shows a comminuted delayed union of a scaphoid waist fracture. **C,** Lateral trispiral tomogram shows a scaphoid waist fracture with mild dorsal intercalated segment instability deformity.

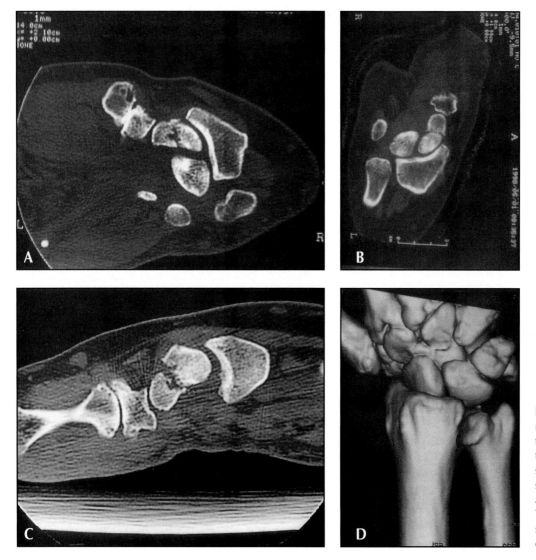

Fig. 5 A, PA view of comminuted scaphoid waist fracture using CT. **B,** CT cut at the waist of the scaphoid showing fracture of the scaphoid with reasonable alignment. **C,** Lateral CT. **D,** Three-dimensional reconstruction of the wrist based on CT.

preferred for the treatment of displaced fractures. A limited number of incisions, either dorsal or volar, is needed for the screw insertions; temporary stabilization of the fracture with K-wires is usually needed.

Surgical Techniques for Acute Fractures of the Scaphoid
Percutaneous Screw Fixation

Percutaneous screw fixation is recommended as a reasonable alternative to cast immobilization for patients with non-displaced or minimally displaced scaphoid fractures, with the exception of pediatric and elderly patients.[41] Both dorsal and volar surgical approaches are used, although the volar technique is preferred for all scaphoid fractures except the most proximal third scaphoid fractures[40] (Fig. 8). The technique of percutaneous screw fixation uses traction applied to the thumb to stabilize the hand and wrist and biplanar imaging of the scaphoid. The patient is placed in a supine position on the operating room table with overhead traction. Some surgeons prefer a standard hand table approach without traction[48] (Fig. 8, B). Two rolled towels are used to assist in hyperextension of the wrist.[41] Axillary block or general anesthesia is required and biplanar imaging is necessary to confirm anatomic reduction of the scaphoid. An incision, down to the bone, is made distally at the base of the thumb between the trapezium and the scaphoid. Through this small longitudinal incision the thumb tendons (the thumb abductor pollicis longus dorsally and thenar muscles volarly) are retracted. The radial capsule is divided, and the distal scaphoid and scaphoid tubercle identified. A K-wire is introduced within the central portion of the scaphoid (assuming that the fracture is reduced) and its position confirmed with biplanar imaging. If alignment is correct, the depth of the K-wire within the full length of the scaphoid is measured, and the K-wire is advanced into the radius so that it will not move

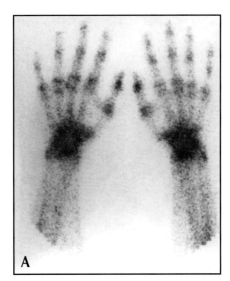
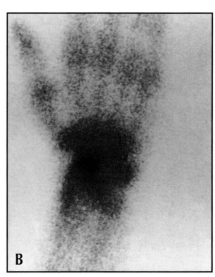

Fig. 6 Bone scan of the wrist. **A,** The increased uptake in the right wrist with uptake greater on the radial side than the ulnar side is nondiagnostic but suggestive of wrist fracture. **B,** A definitive bone scan showing acute scaphoid fracture.

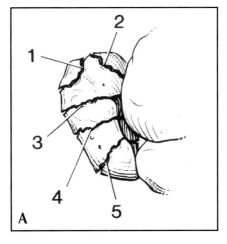

Fig. 7 A, Classification of scaphoid fractures: Distal tubercle of scaphoid (1). Distal intra-articular (2). Distal third (3). Waist (4). Proximal pole (5). **B,** The Mayo classification system for scaphoid fractures. The scaphoid union rate associated with (top) location of the fracture and (bottom) displacement (stable = undisplaced; unstable = displaced) is shown. (Reproduced with permission from the Mayo Foundation, Rochester, MN.)

Location	Number of Fractures	% Union
Distal 1/3	2	100
Middle 1/3	56	80
Proximal 1/3	32	64

Displacement	Number of Fractures	% Union
Stable	48	85
Unstable	42	65

with screw insertion. If there is concern about rotational displacement of the scaphoid, a second K-wire or guide pin should be inserted. The percutaneous screw drill is then placed over the lead K-wire followed by the tap and screw, unless the screw is self-tapping (Fig. 8, C). With the Herbert screw (noncannulated) (Zimmer, Warsaw, IN) the K-wire track is followed with a handheld drill and the tap and the screw inserted along the same path (Fig. 8, C and D). The screw length is judged by measuring the original length of the K-wire using a guide or by measuring the length of the K-wire within the scaphoid with a second K-wire of equal size.

When using a cannulated scaphoid screw, it is important to use a screw 2 to 4 mm shorter in length than that measured with the K-wire[40] (Fig. 9). A screw length of 20 mm is usually correct with a range of 18 to 22 mm. For example, the measurement of a 20-mm length would indicate the selection of an 18-mm screw. The use of a screw that is shorter than measured is necessary to avoid overcompression and a situation in which a screw crosses the joint surface and extends within the wrist. Biplanar imaging is recommended throughout the procedure to assist in proper screw alignment, placement, and determination of proper screw length.

The technique of screw insertion will vary with the type of screw chosen. When the Herbert or Herbert-Whipple screw (Zimmer, Warsaw, IN) is used, tapping of the screw track is necessary.[49] The Acutrak screw system (Acumed, Inc, Hillsboro, OR) uses a self-tapping screw that can be inserted directly after hand drilling. Biplanar imaging is recommended during screw insertion to judge fracture reduction and to ensure that no rotational displacement of the scaphoid occurs (Fig. 9).

Open Reduction and Internal Fixation

Open reduction and internal fixation is recommended for fractures displaced

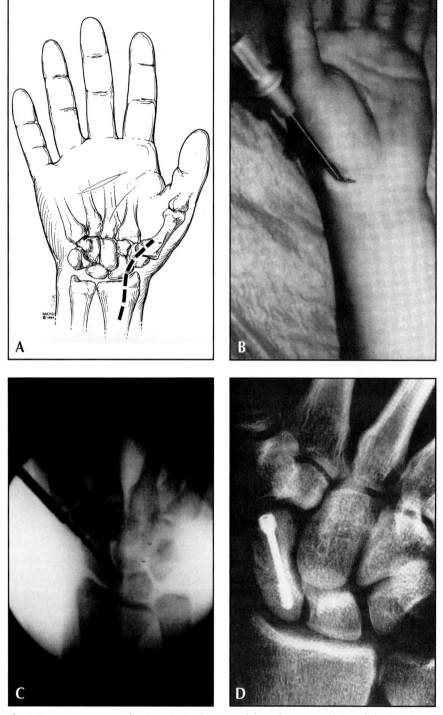

Fig. 8 Percutaneous screw fixation. **A,** A schematic of the volar approach. Distal third of this incision is advised for percutaneous screw insertion. (Reproduced with permission from the Mayo Foundation, Rochester, MN.) **B,** Incision and screw placement shown on a left wrist. **C,** After a lead K-wire determines the track within the scaphoid, the scaphoid drill and then scaphoid tap are inserted (Herbert system). **D,** Herbert screw insertion across acute, undisplaced waist fracture of the scaphoid is shown. (Figures B, C, and D are reproduced with permission from Bond CD, Shin AY, McBride MT, Dao KD: Percutaneous screw fixation or cast immobilization for nondisplaced scaphoid fractures. *J Bone Joint Surg Am* 2001;83:483-488.).

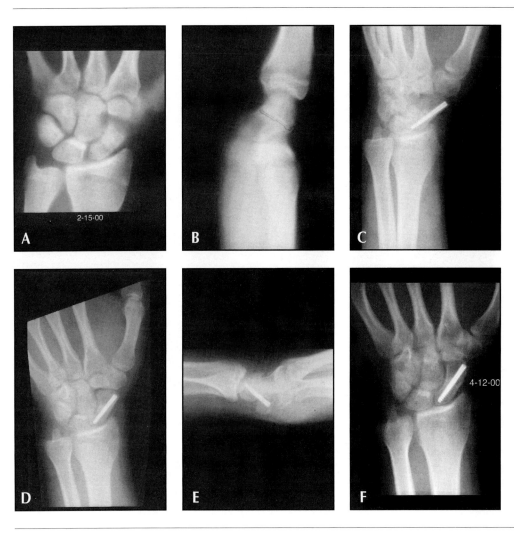

Fig. 9 Delayed union of an acute scaphoid fracture is shown. **A** and **B,** PA and lateral views of the scaphoid showing delayed healing of a scaphoid waist fracture. **C,** Scaphoid view of inserted Acutrak screw. **D** and **E,** PA and lateral views immediately after screw insertion showing anatomic alignment. **F,** PA view of healed fracture showing Acutrak screw insertion across the scaphoid waist fracture.

more than 2 mm or those with significant carpal instability (scapholunate angle greater than 70°).[15,34,39,49] The choice of surgical approach for open reduction is related to the location of the fracture with distal and middle third fractures of the scaphoid generally requiring a volar approach (Figs. 8, *A* and 10, *A*). An extended Russe incision often is needed, particularly if a compression jig is used with an internal fixation screw (Fig. 10, *B*). The volar approach involves a capsular incision between the radioscaphocapitate ligament and the long radiolunate ligament. The fracture site is identified and reduced. K-wire fixation for temporary fixation is recommended. Distal release of the scaphoid trapezial joint may be needed to insert the compression jigs[49]

(Herbert-Huene or Herbert-Whipple jigs [Zimmer, Warsaw, IN]) (Fig. 10, *C*). Biplanar radiographs are necessary to confirm jig placement and fracture reduction (Fig. 10, *D* and *E*). The proximal end of the jig must be carefully placed about the proximal pole of the scaphoid. After the compression jig is accurately placed and firm compression applied, the scaphoid is drilled, tapped, and the appropriate size screw is then inserted (Fig. 10, *F* and *G*). A second parallel K-wire is suggested to assist in maintaining reduction and preventing scaphoid fragment rotation during the screw insertion. Screw length must be predetermined and is usually reduced in length by 2 to 3 mm. The AO and Acutrak screw systems do not use a compression jig but

require careful K-wire placement that is best confirmed by radiographs.

A dorsal approach is suggested for fractures of the proximal third of the scaphoid[40,47,50,51] (Fig. 11, *A*). Because the wrist must be flexed for the dorsal approach, imaging is necessary but is more difficult. A dorsal approach to the wrist is done just radial to Lister's tubercle. The extensor retinaculum is divided in line with the incision and the dorsal capsule incised down to the scaphoid (Fig. 11, *B*). A K-wire is placed longitudinally down the waist of the scaphoid (Fig. 11, *C*). Alignment is checked with imaging and direct inspection of the direction of the K-wire. If the scaphoid is reduced and aligned, a compression screw is inserted and buried beneath the articular surface

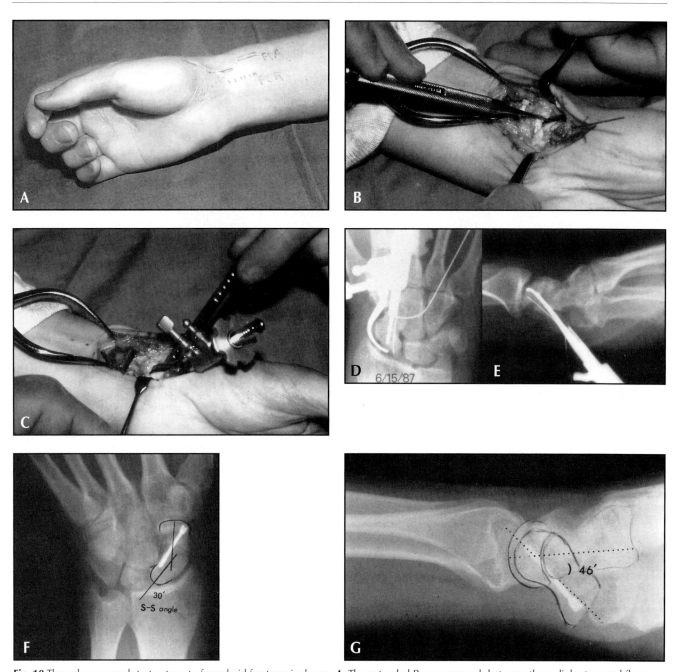

Fig. 10 The volar approach to treatment of scaphoid fractures is shown. **A,** The extended Russe approach between the radial artery and flexor carpi radialis from thumb metacarpal trapezial joint distal to the distal radius, proximal is shown. **B,** Volar Russe approach with thumb and fingers to the right is shown; a K-wire transverses the fracture site, and a Lorenz elevator supports the proximal scaphoid. **C,** A Heune jig is applied across the scaphoid prior to insertion of the Herbert screw. **D** and **E,** PA and lateral radiographs show the compression jig in place and the initial stage of drill placement across the fracture site. **F** and **G,** PA and lateral views of Herbert screw fixation of the scaphoid. PA view shows an intrascaphoid (S-S angle) of 30°, and the lateral view shows a scapholunate angle of 46°.

(Fig. 11, *D* through *F*). The Herbert screw also may be used (Fig. 12). A guiding 0.035 K-wire through the center of the scaphoid is used and the track is enlarged to a 0.065 K-wire and then hand

drilled and tapped using the Herbert instruments. A Herbert screw of the correct length is then inserted along the same track prepared by the K-wires and drill. For the small proximal pole scaphoid frac-

ture, the smaller-sized Herbert screw or the Herbert-Whipple screws are preferred. A mini-Acutrak screw is an option, but the small guide wire (0.028) can be difficult to direct into the scaphoid and is

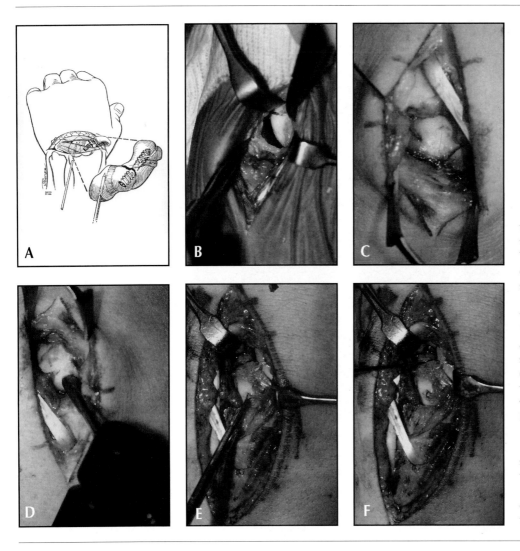

Fig. 11, A Schematic representation of the dorsal approach to treatment of scaphoid fractures. The incision and reflection of dorsal carpal ligaments with schematic of retrograde screw insertion is shown. A single K-wire stabilizes the lunate. **B,** Using the dorsal radial approach the capsule is retracted showing the scaphoid fracture (right wrist). **C,** The scaphoid fracture is reduced and pinned with 0.045 K-wire (right wrist). **D,** The scaphoid alignment guide is placed over the K-wire, which is then removed, and the scaphoid drill is inserted along the K-wire track. **E** and **F,** A Herbert screw is inserted and countersunk after drilling and tapping.

susceptible to bending and breaking; also, the head of the Acutrak screw may be proud within the proximal articular surface of the scaphoid.

Complications

Complications have occurred with both compression screws inserted by either open or percutaneous techniques and with K-wires. Displacement of the fracture during screw insertion is a risk; however, correct screw length measurements and scaphoid reduction held with a K-wire help to prevent displacement (Fig. 13, A). Inaccurate placement of both the K-wire guide or the screws has been reported. If screw placement is not accurate or fails during the procedure, K-wires

should then be used for the internal fixation. Overlength screws (ie, screws that are too long) are also a concern, especially with comminuted fractures or delayed scaphoid unions with bone resorption. The Acutrak screw requires proper drilling depth as overdrilling can lead to screw loosening (Fig. 13, A). Burying the screw head has been difficult, and stripping of the Acutrak screw head can result in a prominent screw.

Sepsis, although rare, is often catastrophic. It is essential that great care be taken during the surgical exposure, K-wire placement, and imaging to prevent intraoperative sepsis.

Nonunion after internal fixation presents a challenge if screw fixation is used

and fails, especially after a proximal pole scaphoid fracture[51,52] (Fig. 13, B). The use of screws, K-wires, or a combination of internal fixation methods, including bone grafting, must be carefully considered.

Postoperative Care and Rehabilitation

The need for cast immobilization after most scaphoid fractures, including those with internal fixation, remains an important treatment principle. The use of a cast is preferred because there is little evidence that the wrist can be left free without cast or splint support. A short arm-thumb spica cast is recommended for 6 to 8 weeks for most scaphoid fractures, including those with internal fixation. A

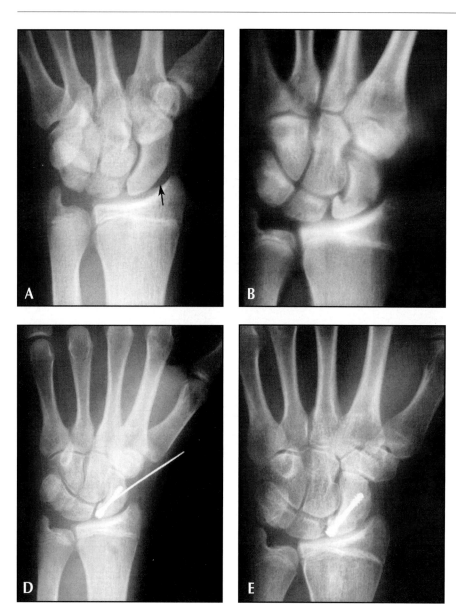

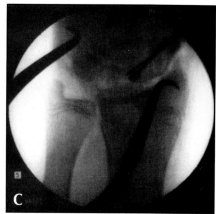

Fig. 12 Radiographs of a proximal pole (third) fracture of the scaphoid show various stages of treatment and follow-up. **A,** The acute fracture (*arrow*) appears undisplaced and is treated in a short arm-thumb spica cast. **B,** Two months later, PA tomograms show displacement of the proximal scaphoid. **C,** Treatment is done with open reduction with K-wire (rotation control) and retrograde Herbert screw fixation. **D,** Two months after surgery, early union is seen, and the K-wire is removed. Protective splinting is done. **E,** The healed scaphoid fracture proximal third is shown 4 months after surgery.

shift from a thumb spica cast to a splint after 3 weeks for undisplaced acute fractures with solid internal fixation is considered for the cooperative patient. Gentle active wrist motion may be done during this period. Radiographic union should be seen by 7 to 8 weeks (confirmed by tomography) except for proximal pole fractures, which may not show union until 10 to 12 weeks after initial treatment.

For the athlete, continued immobilization after internal fixation is recommended.[3] The use of a playing splint is controversial and the decision is best left to the surgeon in discussion with the patient and family[38,53] (Fig. 14). Rettig and associates[53] have suggested that the scaphoid can be adequately protected with a well-fitted custom-made playing splint.[38] Allowing the athlete to compete without a splint or cast may result in nonunion or delayed union.

The Author's Recommendation for Postoperative Patient Care

Patients with a scaphoid fracture should use either a cast or splint postoperatively until union is determined, usually by tomography. Participation in contact sports after internal fixation of acute scaphoid fractures is not recommended until union is evident. Comparative studies are needed to determine if participation in competitive sports for patients with an unhealed scaphoid fracture is appropriate or may contribute to screw loosening, fracture displacement, or nonunion.

Summary

Scaphoid fracture is the most common fracture of the wrist. Diagnosis is usually

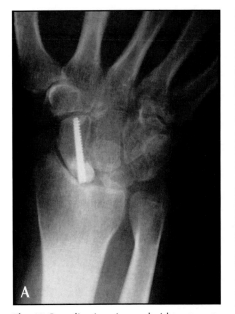
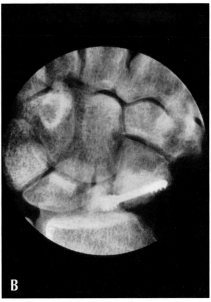

Fig. 13 Complications in scaphoid treatment are seen in these radiographs. **A,** The migration and collapse of the proximal scaphoid with osteonecrosis, nonunion, and screw penetration through the scaphoid proximal pole results when an overlength screw is used for internal fixation. **B,** A failed Herbert screw fixation of the proximal scaphoid with clear nonunion and proximal screw failure within the proximal pole of the scaphoid is shown.

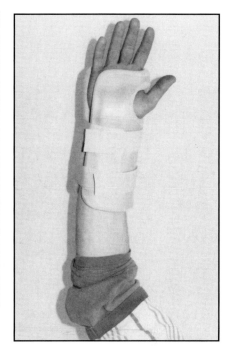

Fig. 14 A thermoplastic resin, hemisolid wrist playing splint is allowed in most state high school and college athletic competitons.

evident based on patient history, physical examination, and radiographic images. If the diagnosis is in doubt, a bone scan, which is reasonably specific and cost-effective, is recommended. CT scans or MRI can also be used to resolve uncertainty in the diagnosis of scaphoid fracture and displacement.

The type of treatment chosen is based on classification of the displacement. Undisplaced scaphoid fractures can be treated with a thumb spica cast, but fixation with percutaneous screws or K-wires currently is preferred, as such fixation allows an early return to activity and use. Open or arthroscopic-guided percutaneous scaphoid reduction and screw fixation is recommended for displaced fractures. A volar approach is recommended, except for the most proximal scaphoid fractures. Early mobilization of the wrist and hand in patients with stable fractures is suggested to decrease fracture casting morbidity and to allow earlier return to activities.

References

1. Weber ER: Biomechanical implications of scaphoid waist fractures. *Clin Orthop* 1980;149:83-89.

2. Engel AF, Keeman JN: Transscaphoid perilunate fracture dislocation and pseudarthrosis of the scaphoid. *Neth J Surg* 1990;42:128-130.

3. Moneim MS: Management of greater arc carpal fractures. *Hand Clin* 1988;4:457-467.

4. Riester JN, Baker BE, Mosher JF, Lowe D: A review of scaphoid fracture healing in competitive athletes. *Am J Sports Med* 1985;13:159-161.

5. Dias JJ, Thompson J, Barton NJ, Gregg PT: Suspected scaphoid fractures: The value of radiographs. *J Bone Joint Surg Br* 1990;72:98-101.

6. Giddins GE, Wilson-MacDonald J: Acute compression fracture of the scaphoid. *J Hand Surg Br* 1994;19:757-758.

7. Horii E, Nakamura R, Watanabe K, Tsunoda K: Scaphoid fracture as a "puncher's fracture." *J Orthop Trauma* 1994;8:107-110.

8. Hanks GA, Kalenak A, Bowman LS, Sebastianelli WJ: Stress fractures of the carpal scaphoid: A report of four cases. *J Bone Joint Surg Am* 1989;71:938-941.

9. Krasin E, Goldwirth M, Gold A, Goodwin DR: Review of the current methods in the diagnosis and treatment of scaphoid fractures. *Postgrad Med J* 2001;77:235-237.

10. Tiel-van Buul MM, Roolker W, Broekhuizen AH, Van Beek EJ: The diagnostic management of suspected scaphoid fracture. *Injury* 1997; 28:1-8.

11. Connolly JF, Smith SE, Ferlic TP: Recurrent wrist "sprain" from an unrecognized scaphoid fracture. *Nebr Med J* 1987;72:198-200.

12. Parvizi J, Wayman J, Kelly P, Moran CG: Combining the clinical signs improves diagnosis of scaphoid fractures: A prospective study with follow-up. *J Hand Surg Br* 1998;23:324-327.

13. Roolker W, Tiel-van Buul MM, Ritt MJ, Verbeeten B Jr, Griffioen FM, Broekhuizen AH: Experimental evaluation of scaphoid X-series, carpal box radiographs, planar tomography, computed tomography, and magnetic resonance imaging in the diagnosis of scaphoid fracture. *J Trauma* 1997;42:247-253.

14. Roolker W, Tiel-van Buul MM, Bossuyt PM, et al: Carpal Box radiography in suspected scaphoid fracture. *J Bone Joint Surg Br* 1996;78:535-539.

15. Cooney WP, Dobyns JH, Linscheid RL: Fractures of the scaphoid: A rational approach to management. *Clin Orthop* 1980;149:90-97.

16. Bain GI, Bennett JD, Richards RS, Slethaug GP, Roth JH: Longitudinal computed tomography of the scaphoid: A new technique. *Skeletal Radiol* 1995;24:271-273.

17. Nakamura R, Imaeda T, Horii E, Miura T, Hayakawa N: Analysis of scaphoid fracture displacement by three-dimensional computed tomography. *J Hand Surg Am* 1991;16:485-492.

18. Brown JN: The suspected scaphoid fracture and isotope bone imaging. *Injury* 1995;26:479-482.

19. Finkenberg JG, Hoffer E, Kelly C, Zinar DM: Diagnosis of occult scaphoid fractures by intrasound vibration. *J Hand Surg Am* 1993;18:4-7.

20. Kozin SH: Internal fixation of scaphoid fractures. *Hand Clin* 1997;13:573-586.

21. Raby N: Magnetic resonance imaging of suspected scaphoid fractures using a low field dedicated extremity MR system. *Clin Radiol* 2001;56:316-320.

22. Terkelsen CJ, Jepsen JM: Treatment of scaphoid fractures with a removable cast. *Acta Orthop Scand* 1988;59:452-453.

23. Fowler C, Sullivan B, Williams LA, McCarthy G, Savage R, Palmer A: A comparison of bone scintigraphy and MRI in the early diagnosis of the occult scaphoid waist fracture. *Skeletal Radiol* 1998;27:683-687.

24. Thorpe AP, Murray AD, Smith FW, Ferguson J: Clinically suspected scaphoid fracture: A comparison of magnetic resonance imaging and bone scintigraphy. *Br J Radiol* 1996;69:109-113.

25. Herneth AM, Siegmeth A, Bader TR, et al: Scaphoid fractures: Evaluation with high-spatial-resolution US initial results. *Radiology* 2001;220:231-235.

26. Kaneshiro SA, Failla JM, Tashman S: Scaphoid fracture displacement with forearm rotation in a short-arm thumb spica cast. *J Hand Surg Am* 1999;24:984-991.

27. Knight P, Rothwell AG: Intrasound vibration in the early diagnosis of scaphoid fracture. *J Hand Surg Am* 1998;23:233-235.

28. Herbert TJ, Fisher WE: Management of the fractured scaphoid using a new bone screw. *J Bone Joint Surg Br* 1984;66:114-123.

29. Szabo RM, Manske D: Displaced fractures of the scaphoid. *Clin Orthop* 1988;230:30-38.

30. Cook PA, Yu JS, Wiand W, Cook AJ II, Coleman CR, Cook AJ: Suspected scaphoid fractures in skeletally immature patients. Application of MRI. *J Comput Assist Tomogr* 1997;21:511-515.

31. Tiel-van Buul MM, van Beek EJ, Broekhuizen AH, Nooitgedacht EA, Davids PH, Bakker AJ: Diagnosing scaphoid fractures: Radiographs cannot be used as a gold standard! *Injury* 1992;23:77-79.

32. Trumble TE: Avascular necrosis after scaphoid fracture: A correlation of magnetic resonance imaging and histology. *J Hand Surg Am* 1990;15:557-564.

33. Toh S, Nagao A, Harata S: Severely displaced scaphoid fracture treated by arthroscopic assisted reduction and osteosynthesis. *J Orthop Trauma* 2000;14:299-302.

34. Smith DK, Cooney WP III, An KN, Linscheid RL, Chao EY: The effects of simulated unstable scaphoid fractures on carpal motion. *J Hand Surg Am* 1989;14:283-291.

35. Gellman H, Caputo RJ, Carter V, Aboulafia A, McKay M: Comparison of short and long thumb-spica casts for non-displaced fractures of the carpal scaphoid. *J Bone Joint Surg Am* 1989;71:354-357.

36. Amadio PC, Berquist TH, Smith DK, Ilstrup DM, Cooney WP III, Linscheid RL: Scaphoid malunion. *J Hand Surg Am* 1989;14:679-687.

37. Nakamura R, Imaeda T, Miura T: Scaphoid malunion. *J Bone Joint Surg Br* 1991;73:134-137.

38. Rettig AC, Kollias SC: Internal fixation of acute stable scaphoid fractures in the athlete. *Am J Sports Med* 1996;24:182-186.

39. Rettig ME, Kozin SH, Cooney WP: Open reduction and internal fixation of acute displaced scaphoid waist fractures. *J Hand Surg Am* 2001;26:271-276.

40. Rettig ME, Raskin KB: Retrograde compression screw fixation of acute proximal pole scaphoid fractures. *J Hand Surg Am* 1999;24:1206-1210.

41. Bond CD, Shin AY: Percutaneous cannulated screw fixation of acute scaphoid fractures. *Tech Hand Upper Ext Surg* 2000;4:81-87.

42. Inoue G, Shionoya K: Herbert screw fixation by limited access for acute fractures of the scaphoid. *J Bone Joint Surg Br* 1997;79:418-421.

43. Wozasek GE, Moser KD: Percutaneous screw fixation for fractures of the scaphoid. *J Bone Joint Surg Br* 1991;73:138-142.

44. O'Brien L, Herbert T: Internal fixation of acute scaphoid fractures: A new approach to treatment. *Aust NZ J Surg* 1985;55:387-389.

45. Adams BD, Blair WF, Reagan DS, Grundberg AB: Technical factors related to Herbert screw fixation. *J Hand Surg Am* 1988;13:893-899.

46. Botte MJ, Gelberman RH: Modified technique for Herbert screw insertion in fractures of the scaphoid. *J Hand Surg Am* 1987;12:149-150.

47. DeMaagd RL, Engber WD: Retrograde Herbert screw fixation for treatment of proximal pole scaphoid nonunions. *J Hand Surg Am* 1989;14:996-1003.

48. Bayer LR, Widding A, Diemer H: Fifteen minutes bone scintigraphy in patients with clinically suspected scaphoid fracture and normal x-rays. *Injury* 2000;31:243-248.

49. Sommerkamp TG: Scaphoid arthroscopically assisted reduction and internal fixation of scaphoid fractures. *J Am Soc Surg Hand* 2001;1:192-210.

50. Herbert TJ, Filan SL: Proximal scaphoid nonunion-osteosynthesis. *Handchir Mikrochir Plast Chir* 1999;31:169-173.

51. Trumble TE, Duc Vo: Proximal pole scaphoid fractures and nonunions. *J Am Soc Surg Hand* 2001;1:155-171.

52. Nakamura R, Horii E, Watanabe K, Tsunoda K, Miura T: Scaphoid nonunion: Factors affecting the functional outcome of open reduction and wedge grafting with a Herbert screw fixation. *J Hand Surg Br* 1993;18:219-224.

53. Rettig AC, Weidenbener EJ, Gloyeske R: Alternative management of midthird scaphoid fractures in the athlete. *Am J Sports Med* 1994;22:711-714.

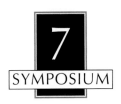

Difficult Elbow Fractures: Pearls and Pitfalls

Shawn W. O'Driscoll, PhD, MD

Jesse B. Jupiter, MD

Mark S. Cohen, MD

David Ring, MD

Michael D. McKee, MD, FRCSC

Abstract

Complex elbow fractures are exceedingly challenging to treat. Treatment of severe distal humeral fractures fails because of either displacement or nonunion at the supracondylar level or stiffness resulting from prolonged immobilization. Coronal shear fractures of the capitellum and trochlea are difficult to repair and may require extensile exposure. Olecranon fracture-dislocations are complex fractures of the olecranon associated with subluxation or dislocation of the radial head and/or the coronoid process. The radioulnar relationship usually is preserved in anterior but disrupted in posterior fracture-dislocations. A skeletal distractor can be useful in facilitating reduction. Coronoid fractures can be classified according to whether the fracture involves the tip, the anteromedial facet, or the base (body) of the coronoid. Anteromedial coronoid fractures are actually varus posteromedial rotatory fracture subluxations and are often serious injuries. These patterns of injury predict associated injuries and instability as well as surgical approach and treatment. The radial head is the bone most commonly fractured in the adult elbow. If the coronoid is fractured, the radial head becomes a critical factor in elbow stability. Its role becomes increasingly important as other soft-tissue and bony constraints are compromised. Articular injury to the radial head is commonly more severe than noted on plain radiographs. Fracture fragments are often anterior. Implants applied to the surface of the radial head must be placed in a safe zone.

Complications such as stiffness, malunion, nonunion, instability, posttraumatic osteoarthritis, and ulnar neuropathy are common following complex elbow fractures. Restoration of stability takes priority over motion because mobility usually can be improved with capsular excision, but instability may damage the articular surface irreversibly.

One or more of the authors or the departments with which they are affiliated have received something of value from a commercial or other party related directly or indirectly to the subject of this chapter.

Comminuted Distal Humeral Fractures

Despite advances in surgical techniques and implants, comminuted fractures of the distal humerus are difficult to treat.[1-4] Because of the complex anatomy of the distal humerus, obtaining and maintaining an anatomic reduction is inherently more challenging than for many other fractures. Factors that increase the complexity of these difficult injuries include open soft-tissue wounds, neurovascular injuries, intra-articular comminution, anterior osteochondral shearing fractures in the coronal plane, metaphyseal comminution, and associated injuries.[5-7]

Furthermore, many of these fractures occur in osteoporotic bone, which makes fracture fixation difficult. Although it may not be possible to restore the elbow to normal function, several techniques and methods can be used to optimize outcome. On occasion, especially in severely osteoporotic bone, rigid fixation is not feasible, and elbow arthroplasty may be indicated in the elderly individual.[8] If the fracture involves only the articular bone, a prosthetic hemiarthroplasty can be used to replace the distal humerus only. Otherwise, a linked elbow replacement is required.

Treatment

Surgical Exposure Exposure is critical in the successful treatment of these injuries.[9] It generally is accepted that a posterior surgical approach is optimal for comminuted intra-articular fractures of the distal humerus that require surgical fixation.[1,4,6,10] Typically, exposure is through either an olecranon osteotomy or reflection or splitting of the triceps muscle and tendon. The triceps can be reflected either from side to side[11] or elevated in continuity with the anconeus and reflected proximally as in the triceps-anconeus pedicle (TRAP) approach.[12] Objective muscle strength testing following surgical repair of distal humeral fractures has shown no difference in elbow extension strength after osteotomy or triceps splitting.[10,13] In patients with open intra-articular distal humeral fractures, the shaft of the humerus typically ruptures through the triceps muscle, producing a posterior skin lesion. This defect in the triceps can be easily incorporated into a triceps-splitting approach. These approaches are complementary rather than mutually exclusive; with them the surgeon can be prepared to take advantage of whatever injury is present to facilitate the exposure, be it a large rent in the triceps or an associated olecranon fracture.

An apex-distal chevron-shaped osteotomy is initiated with an oscillating saw and completed by levering it open with a small osteotome. This procedure will create an interdigitating surface to facilitate later repair. The olecranon fragment and triceps are then mobilized proximally. The osteotomy will be repaired with two parallel 0.045-in Kirschner wires (K-wires) drilled obliquely to engage the anterior ulnar cortex distal to the coronoid process and two 22-gauge stainless steel figure-of-8 tension band wires or a precontoured congruent olecranon plate.

Before performing an olecranon osteotomy, it is wise to consider the possibility of having to do a total elbow arthroplasty. In such cases, the olecranon should be preserved. When performing a semiconstrained total elbow arthroplasty for a comminuted distal humeral fracture, it often is possible to preserve the entire extensor mechanism by releasing the triceps muscle from the distal aspect of the humeral shaft and working on either side of it. Excision of the fractured condyles creates a distal working space that facilitates component insertion.[8] This procedure decreases time in surgery and triceps-related complications, and it enhances rapid restoration of elbow strength and motion. However, it may be more difficult to instrument the ulna with the triceps intact.

Surgical Techniques The most technically challenging aspect of the surgical repair of a comminuted distal humeral fracture is severe intra-articular comminution.[1,5,7] (**DVD-10.1**) Although conventional teaching is to reassemble the articular fragments first and then reattach this construct to the metaphysis, alternate methods may be useful in some situations. If one large fragment of the joint surface can be anatomically reduced to either medial or lateral columns, it can be used to the surgeon's advantage in the setting of severe articular comminution. Once this stable construct has been reestablished, the other articular fragments can be assembled to it. This technique requires the surgeon either to use precontoured plates or to contour them. Fortunately, precontoured anatomically congruent plates are available in a range of sizes for the medial, lateral, and posterolateral aspects of the distal humerus. It is important to maintain the dimensions of the trochlea so that the proximal ulna articulates normally. If there is comminution of the trochlea and lag screw compression is applied, the groove may be narrowed, and the ulna will not seat properly. This problem can be avoided by inserting the 3.5-mm screws typically used for this fixation in a nonlag fashion or by adding an intercalary bone graft to the trochlear defect to maintain its width. One advantage of using the triceps-splitting or TRAP approach is that the proximal ulna remains intact and can be used as a bony template against which the trochlear reduction can be judged.[10]

Although small osteochondral fragments may not have nonarticular areas to which conventional plates and screws can be applied, they are important structurally. The use of Herbert screws countersunk through the articular surface perpendicular to the fracture line has been successful in stabilizing these fragments. The head of the screw is inserted flush with the level of the subchondral bone to maximize purchase and avoid prominence in case of cartilage loss. These screws also can be used to repair anterior fragments fractured in the coronal plane. It is important to remember that the screw itself provides relatively little compres-

sion; instead it maintains compressive force obtained through use of fracture-reduction forceps.[5] Alternative fixation options include minifragment 2.0- or 2.7-mm screws countersunk through the articular surface or small diameter threaded wires that can be cut off and then burred down flush with the subchondral bone surface. Disadvantages of these options include a greater amount of cartilage surface area lost and the potential for wire prominence if there is loss of cartilage.

Plate fixation of both the medial and lateral columns is necessary to reestablish stability of the distal humerus in bicondylar fractures (Fig. 1). Despite the many biomechanical and clinical studies on the ideal shape and orientation of the plates, some controversy exists.[1,2,9,14,15] What is clear is that two plates placed directly posteriorly on the medial and lateral columns (in the plane of motion of the joint) are biomechanically suboptimal. However, two parallel plates (one on each side) approximately in the sagittal plane are just as strong as two plates perpendicular to each other (ie, one medial and one posterolateral). Stronger 3.5-mm compression plates or plates designed specifically for the distal humerus are preferable. One-third tubular plates are too weak for most distal humerus fractures; they have a higher failure rate, especially when there is metaphyseal comminution in the supracondylar area. Precontoured commercially available plates have proved to be advantageous because they cradle the distal fragments or enable fracture reduction to the plate.[5,9,10] This is useful when severe comminution makes reestablishing the columns difficult. Longer (45 to 70 mm) screws passed through the plates across to the opposite column will also improve fracture construct stability by creating a closed box or triangle effect.

Treatment of severe distal humerus fractures fails either because of nonunion at the supracondylar level (Fig. 2) or stiffness resulting from prolonged immobilization that has been used in an attempt to avoid failure of inadequate fixation. Either way, the limiting factor is fixation of the distal fragments to the shaft. To obtain union and maintain elbow mobility after a severe fracture of the distal humerus, two principles must be satisfied: fixation in the distal fragment must be maximized, and all fixation in the major distal fragments should contribute to stability between the distal fragments and the shaft.[16] There are seven technical objectives by which these principles are met. Every screw in the major distal fragments should: (1) pass through a plate, (2) engage a fragment on the opposite side that also is fixed to a plate, (3) be as long as possible, and (4) engage as many articular fragments as possible. In addition, (5) as many screws as possible should be placed in the distal fragments, and the plates should be applied such that compression (6) is achieved at the supracondylar level for both columns and (7) is strong enough to resist failure before union occurs at the supracondylar level. Severe metaphyseal comminution and/or bone loss can be managed by a supracondylar shortening osteotomy[17] (Fig. 3), which allows restoration of bony contact and functional motion provided the following three guidelines are followed. First, shortening should be limited to 2 cm or less (preferably 1 cm). Second, the distal fragments can be translated laterally or medially with respect to the center of the humeral canal to improve bone contact at the metaphyseal level, but the rotational and varus-valgus alignments of the distal articular surface are carefully restored. Third, the coronoid and olecranon are prevented from impinging on the distal humerus in the functional arc of motion (30° to 130°). A convenient method to provide room for the coronoid and olecranon is to translate the epiphyseal segment anteriorly (to avoid losing flexion) and to sculpt the olecranon fossa with a burr once the fix-

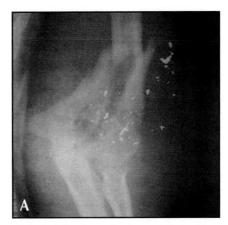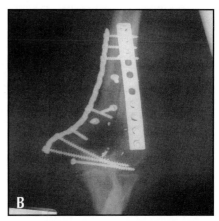

Fig. 1 A, AP radiograph of a comminuted, intra-articular distal humeral fracture caused by a gunshot wound. Fragments of the bullet can be seen in the soft tissues, and by their appearance and the anterior entry and posterior exit wounds a significant defect in the triceps muscle could reasonably be expected. The patient had a complete radial nerve palsy. **B,** This triceps defect was incorporated in the approach, and a triceps split was performed. Rigid fixation with two plates allowed early postoperative motion and enhanced the functional result. The radial nerve was explored and found to be contused but intact. At 1-year follow-up, the fracture had healed, the patient had a 115° arc of flexion-extension, and the radial nerve had recovered fully.

ation is complete (to avoid losing extension). The tip of the olecranon also can be resected to allow extension to at least 20° or 10°. For anatomic repairs, it is important to leave these fossae free of any fixation devices that may impede motion. Intraoperative radiographs will help confirm this is the case.

In certain fractures, the combination of articular comminution and osteoporosis may make stable fixation unattainable. In such circumstances, a linked total elbow arthroplasty is indicated if the patient is elderly. This option is reserved for older patients because prosthesis longevity is a concern, and the decision to proceed will depend on the surgeon's experience with both fracture fixation and arthroplasty.[8] If an arthroplasty is contemplated, it is usually necessary to use a linked device, and to preserve the olecranon (important for ulnar component stability) by using a triceps splitting or reflecting approach.

Postoperative Management
Ideally, when repairing comminuted intra-articular distal humeral fractures,

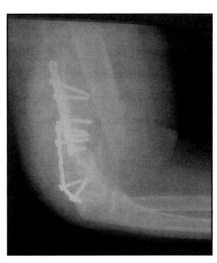

Fig. 2 Fixation failure following surgical repair of a distal humeral fracture. The posterior placement of both plates and lack of screw purchase distal to the fracture contributed to the displacement at the fracture site.

sufficient stability is gained surgically to allow early motion of the injured elbow. Prolonged immobilization in an attempt to protect tenuous fixation typically results in stiffness. In a retrospective review, Waddell and associates[9] showed that immobilization for longer than 3

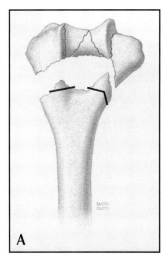 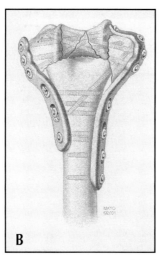 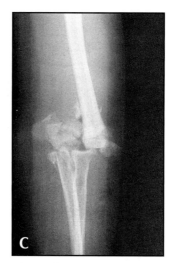 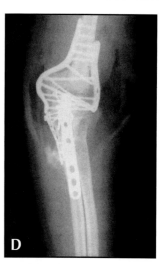

Fig. 3 Supracondylar shortening osteotomy. In cases of supracondylar bone loss and severe comminution, supracondylar shortening osteotomy is a viable option when an anatomic reconstruction is not believed to be possible. **A,** A small amount of bone from the distal end of the shaft is resected (dark lines) (never the articular segments) to enhance and permit compression contact between the distal articular segment and the shaft. **B,** Medial and lateral precontoured plates are placed slightly oblique to the sagittal plane. The distal screws should be as long as possible, passing through as many fragments as possible, and engaging the condyle or epicondyle of the opposite column. The coronoid fossae and radial fossa are best preserved by offsetting the distal segment anteriorly. To preserve terminal extension, the olecranon fossa can be recreated by burring the distal end of the shaft and removing the tip of the olecranon. **C,** Radiographic example of a distal humerus fracture with extensive bone loss and comminution, as well as fractures of the olecranon and coronoid. **D,** A supracondylar shortening osteotomy of 1.5 cm was performed and the fractures rigidly fixed using the Mayo Clinic Congruent Elbow plates (Acumed, Beaverton, OR) that are specially designed for these fractures. All of this patient's fractures healed and final range of motion was 25° to 120°. (Reproduced with permission from the Mayo Foundation, Rochester, MN.)

weeks caused disabling stiffness. Even with optimal surgery and early motion, normal flexion-extension has rarely been reported following this injury. McKee and associates[10] reported a mean flexion-extension arc of 108° (range, 55° to 140°) with a mean flexion contracture of 25° in a recent review of 25 elbows that were splinted for a week after surgical repair of an intra-articular distal humeral fracture and then treated with active range-of-motion (ROM) exercises. To decrease postoperative swelling, the arm should be elevated with the elbow held extended in a well-padded splint. The splint usually is removed 48 hours after surgery in isolated injuries, and active physiotherapy is initiated. The patients are carefully counseled regarding a home exercise program and given an instruction booklet. Some surgeons prefer the patient to use a continuous passive motion device at home for the first 4 weeks. Resisted extension is

avoided for the first 6 weeks to protect the extensor mechanism.

The patient is expected to show steady improvement in terms of ROM. Recalcitrant patients are managed with turnbuckle and nighttime extension splinting and flexion strapping. Although prophylactic measures against heterotopic bone may not be used routinely, indomethacin is used in patients with concomitant head injuries (25 mg three times a day orally for 3 weeks).

Although there is a wide range of reported results following this severe injury, the average patient can expect a relatively pain-free, functional,[18] 105° arc of motion, with approximately 75% normal strength if current standards of rigid anatomic fixation and early motion are followed.

Pearls
The surgeon should take advantage of any disruption of the extensor mecha-

nism in the approach (ie, if there is an open fracture and triceps defect, a triceps splitting approach should be considered; if there is an olecranon fracture, it can be used instead of an osteotomy). In addition, the surgeon should make sure that all screws in the major articular fragments also contribute to stability at the supracondylar level. In elderly patients with severe comminution, alternatives to olecranon osteotomy should be considered in case an elbow replacement is required. If a truly unfixable fracture is limited to the articular segment with no supracondylar involvement, replacement can be performed with a distal humeral hemiarthroplasty rather than a total elbow arthroplasty.

Pitfalls
Common complications following surgical intervention for displaced intra-articular fractures of the distal humerus

include fixation failure, nonunion, stiffness, elbow weakness, ulnar neuropathy, and infection.[2-4] Fixation failure usually is attributable to inadequate techniques, implants such as thin plates (Fig. 2), or K-wire fixation alone. A common pitfall is prolonged immobilization in an attempt to compensate for such inadequate fixation; severe stiffness is the inevitable result. Another common pitfall is placement of screws in the major articular fragments before plate application, only to find that fixation of those fragments to the shaft is then limited by the number of screws that can be placed into the distal fragments through the plates.

Yet another common pitfall is the placement of hardware adjacent to the ulnar nerve, which then becomes painful and/or impaired as a result of scarring and fibrosis. Ulnar neurolysis and transposition during elbow reconstruction are usually helpful, but nerve recovery may take up to 2 years.[4]

Elbow flexion and extension strength are significantly decreased to about 75% of contralateral strength despite apparently successful fracture treatment.[10,13] This degree of weakness may not be functionally disabling for sedentary individuals, but it may explain the sense of weakness and loss of endurance that more active patients have when they attempt to return to rigorous tasks following this injury.[10]

Coronal Shear Fractures of the Capitellum and Trochlea

A constellation of articular fractures primarily involving the articular surface of the distal humerus has been identified; some of these fractures have little or no supporting metaphyseal subchondral bone.[19] A precise morphologic definition of these different fracture patterns is useful in surgical decision making and choice of surgical techniques and should help in the assessment of outcome in comparisons with alternative techniques such as total elbow arthroplasty.[8]

Table 1	
Classification of Articular Shearing Fractures of the Distal Humerus	
Type	**Description**
Type I	A single articular fragment, including the capitellum and a portion of the trochlea; previously described as a coronal shear fracture.
Type II	A shearing fracture of the articular surface, including the lateral epicondyle.
Type III	The shearing articular fragmentation anteriorly, including impaction of the most distal metaphyseal bone of the lateral column.
Type IV	The articular fractures include the anterior and posterior trochlea as separate fragments.
Type V	Involvement of the medial and lateral epicondyles.

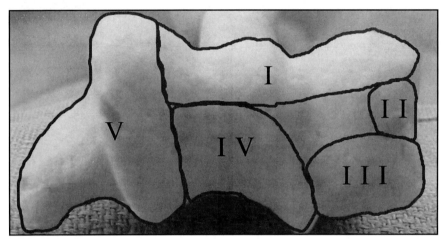

Fig. 4 Patterns of articular shearing fractures of the distal humerus. See Table 1 for descriptions of each pattern.

Patterns of Injury

These fractures have been classified based on involvement of articular surfaces extending from lateral to medial (Fig. 4, Table 1). Although established fracture classifications such as the AO/ASIF include some components of these injuries either in the frontal plane alone or as part of complex multifragmented intercondylar fractures, none depict the variety of patterns that exist with these primarily articular injuries.[20-23] Recognition of the morphology of these complex chondral fractures is critical for preoperative planning and deciding on the most appropriate surgical exposure. Three-dimensional CT has added immeasurably to defining these lesions and, when available, should be considered (Fig. 5).

Chondral articular fractures are difficult to repair because they require extensile surgical exposure, realignment of small and at times impacted articular fragments, and the precise placement of implants that must be countersunk beneath the joint surface. The specific fracture types represent a progression of injury severity extending from an isolated articular component displaced in the frontal plane to combinations of shearing and impaction injury to the capitellum and trochlea with a limited zone of metaphyseal bone support.[1,24-28]

Despite separation from the underlying metaphyseal bone and the complete lack of any soft-tissue attachments, osteonecrosis of these small articular fragments is uncommon, which may be because the stability has been adequate to

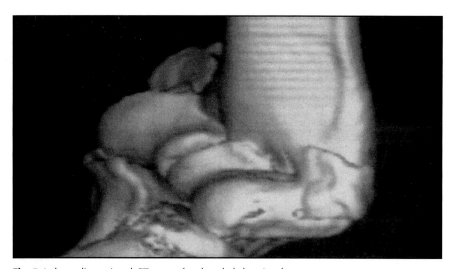

Fig. 5 A three-dimensional CT scan of a chondral shearing fracture.

permit rapid revascularization from the underlying metaphyseal bone support. When osteonecrosis does occur, it can be treated by hemiarthroplasty if the ulna and radial head remain normal.

Treatment

Surgical Exposure Patients whose fractures do not involve the medial epicondyle can be treated using an extensile lateral Kocher exposure. Those fractures extending to involve the medial epicondyle can be treated through an olecranon osteotomy or TRAP approach.[12] For treatment of a fracture of the lateral epicondyle, the lateral exposure is facilitated by elevating and retracting the epicondyle distally along with the attached origins of the wrist and digital extensor muscles and lateral collateral ligament (LCL) complex. The more proximal origins of the radial wrist extensor muscles are elevated from the lateral supracondylar ridge to improve the access to the anterior articular fragments. The exposure is completed by elevating the lateral triceps from the distal humerus and lateral aspect of the proximal olecranon, which permits the elbow joint to be hinged open, providing exposure to the anterior and posterior articular surfaces of the distal humerus.

Surgical Techniques The fracture frag-ments should be individually identified, repositioned, and provisionally secured with smooth 0.045- or 0.062-in K-wires. Inability to anatomically realign some of the anterior articular fragments may be the result of impaction of the posterior aspect of the lateral bony column or impaction of part or all of the posterior trochlea. Definitive internal fixation of the isolated articular fracture fragments is facilitated using Herbert screws alone or in combination with small threaded K-wires. Alternatively, if an olecranon osteotomy or TRAP approach is used, a lateral precontoured plate in addition to screws from the medial side can be used (Fig. 6).

If it is of sufficient size, the lateral epicondylar fragment is best reattached with a plate and screws. The epicondylar plate and screw fixation can be reinforced with a 22-gauge stainless steel wire placed distally through the soft-tissue insertions and proximally through a drill hole in the distal humerus. A figure-of-8 wire alone will be sufficient when the epicondylar fragment is too small to support screw fixation (Fig. 7).

Patients with a type I single articular fragment require varus distraction but not actual subluxation of the ulnotrochlear articulation for exposure, and the fragment can be reduced and secure-ly stabilized by elevation of the anterior capsule through this lateral approach. If the articular fragment is so comminuted or osteoporotic as to render fixation impossible, prosthetic replacement of the distal humerus is an option.

Postoperative Management

The extremity is splinted in extension overnight, and then active motion is initiated on the first or second postoperative day using gravity to assist flexion.

Pearls

Inability to reduce a coronal shear fracture anatomically usually implies metaphyseal impaction (shortening at the supracondylar level) or impaction of the posterior trochlea. Medial extension to involve the medial epicondyle requires the same exposure as a distal humeral fracture.

Pitfalls

There is a tendency to malreduce the capitellum, leaving it displaced proximally. Ulnohumeral subluxation can impede reduction of a fracture involving the medial trochlea. This subluxation occurs as a result of impingement of the coronoid against the medial trochlear fragment. Such fractures should be reduced through an olecranon osteotomy or a TRAP approach.

Olecranon Fracture-Dislocations

Olecranon fracture-dislocations are complex fractures of the olecranon associated with subluxation or dislocation of the radial head and or the coronoid process (Fig. 8). The fracture of the proximal ulna in an olecranon fracture-dislocation is usually multifragmented.[29,30]

Patterns of Injury

It is useful to distinguish anterior and posterior displacement patterns of olecranon fracture-dislocation. Anterior fracture-dislocations of the olecranon have been described as transolecranon frac-

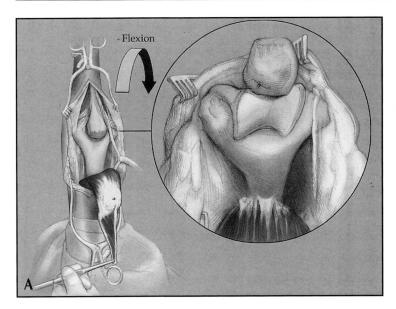

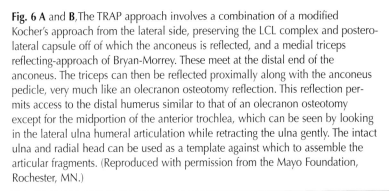

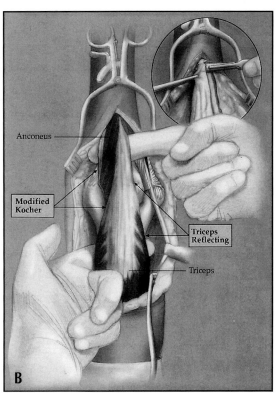

Fig. 6 A and **B**, The TRAP approach involves a combination of a modified Kocher's approach from the lateral side, preserving the LCL complex and posterolateral capsule off of which the anconeus is reflected, and a medial triceps reflecting-approach of Bryan-Morrey. These meet at the distal end of the anconeus. The triceps can then be reflected proximally along with the anconeus pedicle, very much like an olecranon osteotomy reflection. This reflection permits access to the distal humerus similar to that of an olecranon osteotomy except for the midportion of the anterior trochlea, which can be seen by looking in the lateral ulna humeral articulation while retracting the ulna gently. The intact ulna and radial head can be used as a template against which to assemble the articular fragments. (Reproduced with permission from the Mayo Foundation, Rochester, MN.)

ture-dislocations of the elbow[29,31] because the trochlea of the distal humerus appears to have fractured through the olecranon process as the forearm displaced anteriorly (Fig. 8, *A*). Distinction of anterior from posterior fracture-dislocations is straightforward because the radial head is displaced anteriorly rather than posteriorly relative to the capitellum; however, anterior radiocapitellar dislocation often leads to misidentification of this injury as an anterior (Bado type 1[32]) Monteggia fracture-dislocation.[29,30,33] Anterior fracture-dislocations of the olecranon destabilize the ulnohumeral joint, but the radioulnar relationship usually is preserved[29,31,34] (Fig, 8 *B*). In contrast, anterior Monteggia fractures are fracture-dislocations of the forearm in which the ulnohumeral joint is not involved.[33]

Posterior fracture-dislocations of the olecranon can be considered the most proximal injury type among the spectrum of posterior (Bado type 2)[32] Monteggia fractures because the principles and pitfalls of treatment are similar.[30,35] Posterior Monteggia injuries are characterized by an apex posterior fracture of the ulna, posterior dislocation of the radial head with respect to the capitellum, and in about two thirds of injuries, fracture of the radial head[30,32,35-37] (Fig. 8, *B*). These injuries, like more distal posterior Monteggia fractures, threaten both elbow and forearm function.

Fractures of the coronoid process of the ulna are common among both anterior and posterior fracture-dislocations of the olecranon.[29,33] The fracture of the coronoid is usually a basal fracture (see section

on coronoid fractures) involving between 50% and 100% of the height of the coronoid process. There can be a single large fragment or comminution (Fig. 9). In some patients, the fracture may be oblique so that it involves the anteromedial facet of the coronoid, particularly in posterior fracture-dislocations of the olecranon.

In some patients with complex fractures of the proximal ulna, the relationship between the radius and ulna and the trochlea may have been restored either spontaneously or by manipulative reduction. The displacement was probably posterior if the radial head is fractured, particularly if some of the fragments remain posterior. The distinction is important because anterior olecranon fracture-dislocations are stable once the alignment of the olecranon and coronoid

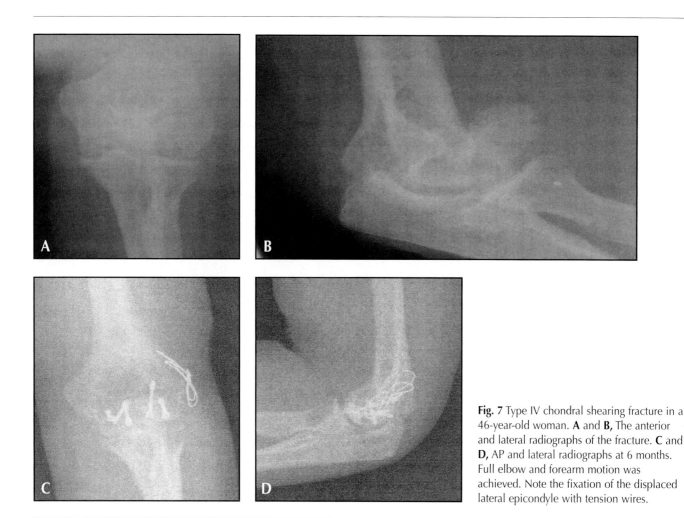

Fig. 7 Type IV chondral shearing fracture in a 46-year-old woman. **A** and **B,** The anterior and lateral radiographs of the fracture. **C** and **D,** AP and lateral radiographs at 6 months. Full elbow and forearm motion was achieved. Note the fixation of the displaced lateral epicondyle with tension wires.

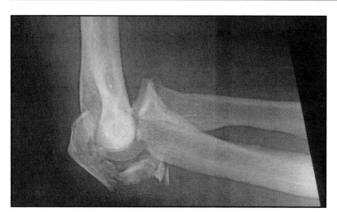
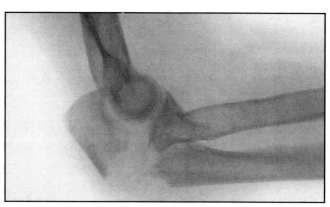

Fig. 8 A, Anterior fracture-dislocations of the olecranon. **B,** Posterior fracture-dislocations of the olecranon.

are restored, and forearm function is rarely in jeopardy.[29] In contrast, ulnohumeral instability is common after posterior olecranon fracture-dislocations, and forearm function often is compromised.[30,33]

Treatment

Surgical Exposure A posterior midline incision is used for exposure.[38,39] The treatment of posterior olecranon fracture-dislocations often requires the creation of a broad lateral skin flap to access the radi-

al head. A medial skin flap can be created if access to the coronoid process from the medial side is required. **(DVD-10.2)**

Exposure of the ulna should preserve periosteal and muscle attachments. A contoured dorsal plate can be applied

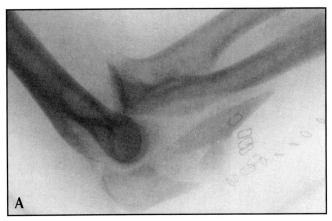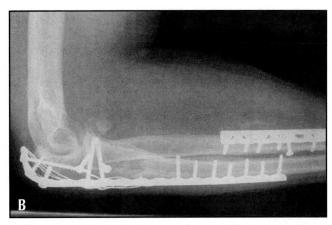

Fig 9 Anterior fracture-dislocations of the olecranon can be so complex that they are not identified as olecranon fracture-dislocations. **A,** Lateral radiograph demonstrates extensive fragmentation extending into the diaphysis. **B,** Six months later the fracture is solidly healed, the elbow is stable, and good elbow function has been restored.

directly over a portion of the triceps insertion at the olecranon and on the apex of the ulnar diaphysis distally without elevating muscle attachments (Fig. 9). This procedure preserves blood supply and optimizes healing. If olecranon comminution is extensive, the plate can be extended proximally through a triceps split to the tip of the olecranon. Despite extensive fragmentation, bone grafts[40] are rarely necessary if the soft-tissue attachments are preserved.

The fractures of the radial head and coronoid process can be evaluated and sometimes definitively treated through the exposure provided by the fracture of the olecranon process.[41-43] With little additional dissection, the olecranon fragment can be mobilized proximally, providing exposure of the coronoid through the ulnohumeral joint (Fig. 9, *B*). If the radial head is fragmented and will be replaced with a prosthesis, replacement can be done through this traumatic exposure in most cases. Doing so, however, makes alignment of the radial head more challenging. If surgical fixation of the radial head with a plate is considered, the use of a separate muscle interval (eg, Kocher's or Kaplan's intervals)[44] rather than further mobilization of the musculature separating the proximal radius and

ulna may help limit the potential for synostosis formation.

Posterior olecranon fracture-dislocations often require a lateral exposure to address a fracture of the radial head or coronoid, or to repair the LCL. When the LCL is injured, it may be avulsed at its ulnar insertion or from the lateral epicondyle. This avulsion facilitates both exposure and repair. The LCL origin and common extensor musculature can be mobilized distally. Improved exposure of the coronoid can be obtained by releasing the origins of the radial wrist extensors from the lateral supracondylar ridge and elevating the brachialis from the anterior humerus and by excising the fractured radial head.[43]

A medial exposure (as described in the section on coronoid fractures) may be needed to address a complex fracture of the coronoid, particularly if it involves the anteromedial facet of the coronoid process.

Surgical Techniques The fracture of the coronoid often can be reduced directly through the elbow joint using the limited access provided by the olecranon fracture. However, failure to fix an anteromedial coronoid fragment can seriously jeopardize the result. Provisional fixation can be obtained using K-wires to

attach the fragments either to the metaphyseal or diaphyseal fragments of the ulna or to the trochlea of the distal humerus when there is extensive fragmentation of the proximal ulna.[42] An alternative when there is extensive fragmentation of the proximal ulna is the use of a skeletal distractor (a temporary external fixator).[29,45] External fixation applied between a wire driven through the olecranon and up into the trochlea and a second wire in the distal ulnar diaphysis often can obtain reduction indirectly when distraction is applied between the pins. Definitive fixation usually can be obtained with screws applied under image intensifier guidance. The screws are placed through the plate when there is extensive fragmentation of the proximal ulna. The proximal olecranon fragment is grasped with a tenaculum forceps through the triceps insertion and provisionally secured to the trochlea of the distal humerus using a stout, smooth K-wire (usually 5/64 in). **(DVD-10.3)**

A precontoured plate is used, or a long plate is contoured to wrap around the proximal olecranon.[46] The plate can lie directly on a portion of the triceps insertion, or the insertion can be split longitudinally and mobilized slightly so that the plate is in direct contact with the

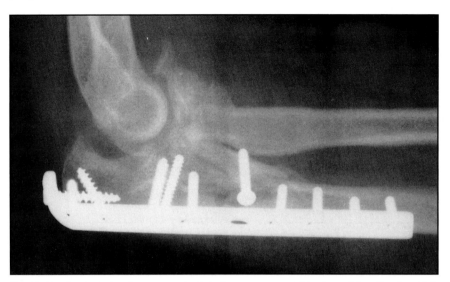

Fig. 10 A radiograph showing a comminuted olecranon coronoid fracture-dislocation in which the anteromedial coronoid fragment remains displaced despite attempts to lag the coronoid fragments in place. This resulted in joint incongruity and early posttraumatic arthritis, requiring a total elbow arthroplasty later.

bone. This proximal contour of the plate makes it possible to insert a greater number of screws in the olecranon fragment and to have those screws interdigitate. In addition, the orthogonal orientation of the most proximal screws to the more distal screws may provide a stronger hold on the fragment. When the olecranon is fragmented, a plate and screws alone may not provide reliable fixation. In this situation, it has proved useful to use ancillary tension-wire fixation through the triceps insertion to control the olecranon fragments.[29]

Direct dorsal placement of the plate is straightforward, requires no soft-tissue stripping, allows more strategic screw placement, and allows the plate to function as a tension band under the influence of the brachialis and triceps muscles. Proximally, a dorsally applied plate rests on the relatively flat surface of the olecranon, but distally it lies directly over the apex of the ulna. In muscular patients, the interval between the flexor carpi ulnaris and the extensor carpi ulnaris must be split to expose the ulna. A very long plate may be needed (between 12 and 16 holes), particularly when there is extensive fragmentation or the bone quality is poor (Fig. 9).

Postoperative Management

In young patients with good bone quality, it is usually possible to obtain fixation secure enough to initiate active gravity-assisted elbow ROM exercises 1 or 2 days after surgery. Patients are also encouraged to use the injured arm for light functional activities.

Posterior olecranon fracture-dislocations are common among older women, and osteoporosis may influence the quality of the fixation. In addition, the coronoid fixation may be somewhat tenuous. In these circumstances, it may prove wise to rest the elbow at 90° of flexion in a removable posterior plastic splint for 4 weeks prior to initiating elbow mobilization. Exercises to prevent digit swelling and stiffness are important during this rest period.

Pearls

Transolecranon fracture-dislocations tend to be intrinsically stable after fracture fix-

ation because the injury is mostly through bone and less through soft tissues. Two key predictors of stability after treatment of a transolecranon fracture-dislocation are the integrity of the LCL complex and that of the anteromedial coronoid. A precontoured plate (commercially available or contoured by the surgeon) that is placed on the posterior surface of the ulna and wraps around the tip of the olecranon should be used. A skeletal distractor can be useful in facilitating reduction.

Pitfalls

Perhaps the most common pitfall is failure to obtain or maintain reduction of the coronoid (Fig. 10). If the coronoid fixation loosens, but the ulnohumeral joint remains stable and concentrically aligned, healing in an adequate position often can be obtained by protecting the elbow in a removable posterior elbow splint for 4 weeks. Stability takes priority over motion because mobility usually can be improved with capsular excision,[29,47,48] but instability may damage the articular surface irreversibly.[49] If the ulnohumeral joint is malaligned, then another attempt to improve coronoid alignment and fixation may be warranted.

Another pitfall to be avoided is placement of the plate on the medial or lateral aspect of the proximal ulna, which provides less fixation than a contoured posterior plate.[30] Failure occurs in these instances by loosening of the screws in the proximal fragment. In contrast, a dorsally applied plate rarely fails by loosening proximally but can loosen from the ulnar diaphysis if the plate is too short or the bone quality is poor. Application of a long plate will ensure correct contouring to prevent malunion. The surgeon should be certain that long plates are available because many commonly used plate and screw sets do not routinely include these longer plates.

Another subtle pitfall is failure to recognize ulnohumeral instability with a posterior olecranon fracture-dislocation.[49] The surgeon should anticipate this problem and ensure that all of the following have been achieved: (1) the radial head has either been repaired or replaced with a prosthesis so that radiocapitellar contact is restored, (2) the ulna has been realigned so that the radial head is aligned with the capitellum, (3) the coronoid has been realigned and secured, and (4) LCL injury has been identified and repaired. If ulnohumeral instability persists even though all of these have been achieved, hinged external fixation of the elbow may be necessary.[49]

Coronoid Fractures

Coronoid fractures are most commonly encountered in association with radial head fractures as part of the terrible triad (coronoid fracture, radial head fracture, and elbow dislocation).[50] Less commonly, they are seen either as isolated fractures or as part of complex olecranon fracture-dislocations. Until recently, understanding of these fractures has been lacking; thus, little has been written regarding their management.[51-56]

Patterns of Injury

Regan and Morrey[57] classified these fractures into three types according to the height of the coronoid involved. However, experience has dictated the need for a new classification system. For example, fractures of the anteromedial coronoid may not involve the tip and thus are not classifiable. The patterns of injury that take into account the anatomic location, amount of coronoid fractured, comminution, elbow stability, and associated injuries should be considered (Fig. 11, Table 2). Fortunately, these injury patterns provide a guide to surgical approach and treatment.

Coronoid Tip Fractures The fracture line is in the coronal plane, rarely involves more than about one third of the height of the coronoid, and does not extend medially past the sublime tubercle

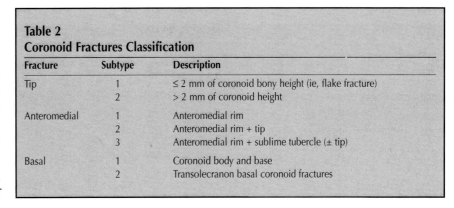

Table 2
Coronoid Fractures Classification

Fracture	Subtype	Description
Tip	1	≤ 2 mm of coronoid bony height (ie, flake fracture)
	2	> 2 mm of coronoid height
Anteromedial	1	Anteromedial rim
	2	Anteromedial rim + tip
	3	Anteromedial rim + sublime tubercle (± tip)
Basal	1	Coronoid body and base
	2	Transolecranon basal coronoid fractures

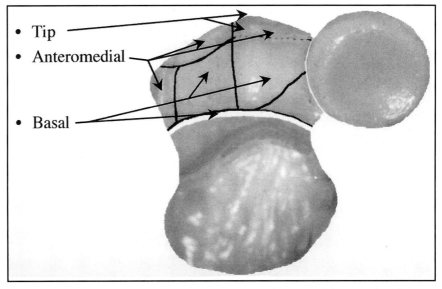

Fig. 11 Schematic showing proposed classification system for coronoid fractures, based on anatomic location with subtypes according to the severity of coronoid involvement, considers the mechanism of injury along with the associated fractures and soft-tissue injuries and dictates surgical approach and treatment (see Table 2 for details).

or into the body of the coronoid. A tip subtype 1 fracture is a small flake off the tip (≤ 2 mm). It may be seen in isolation or as part of a fracture-dislocation. A tip subtype 2 fracture involves a larger segment of the tip (> 2 mm), but does not extend more than about a third of the way into the body of the coronoid or past the sublime tubercle medially. It almost always is seen in association with a radial head fracture in a dislocated elbow, a combination of injuries that has been termed the terrible triad.[50]

Coronoid tip fractures occur as a result of an elbow subluxation or disloca-

tion via a posterolateral rotatory displacement of the ulna under the trochlea.[56,58] The mechanism is a fall onto the outstretched hand, with valgus and supination moments applied to the ulna as it flexes on the humerus during axial loading.[59] The implication of these fractures is that the elbow had subluxated or dislocated, just as a bony Bankart lesion of the glenoid does for anterior shoulder instability.[59,60] Their effect on elbow stability is proportionate to the amount of coronoid lost or fractured. The LCL is disrupted in virtually all instances in which a dislocation has occurred (all of those resulting

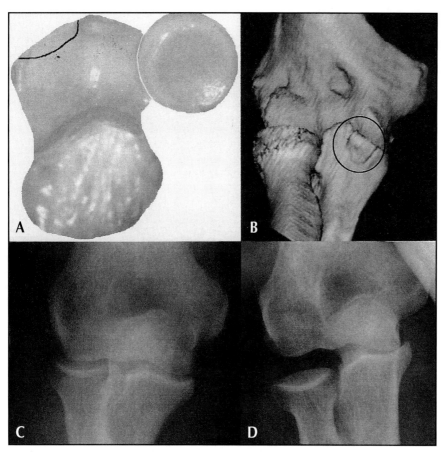

Fig. 12 A and **B,** Location of the anteromedial coronoid fracture fragment shown in a schematic and a three-dimensional CT reconstruction. (Fracture fragment indicated by black outlines.) **C** and **D,** AP radiographs with and without a varus/posteromedial rotatory stress applied contrast show what initially appears to be an almost normal radiograph with one revealing significant varus instability and apparent narrowing of the medial ulnohumeral joint.

from falls), although the medial collateral ligament (MCL) can remain at least partially or functionally intact in these fracture-dislocations.

Anteromedial Coronoid Fractures
Anteromedial fractures have not been addressed in the literature. The initial fracture (subtype 1) is located anteromedially, between the tip of the coronoid and the sublime tubercle in an oblique plane between the coronal and sagittal planes (Fig. 12). Medially, the fracture line usually exits the cortex in the anterior half of the sublime tubercle, ie, in the anterior portion of the anterior bundle of the MCL. Laterally, the fracture exits just medial to the tip of the coronoid.

Comminution can extend to involve the tip (subtype 2), the sublime tubercle (the attachment site of the anterior bundle of the MCL) (subtype 3), and the body of the coronoid (see section on basal fractures), depending on the energy of the injury.

The mechanism is a varus/posteromedial rotation injury with axial loading. Flexion and abduction torque at the shoulder, while the elbow is flexing under axial load, cause the elbow to go into varus (disrupting the LCL) and the medial trochlea to ride up onto the anteromedial coronoid, which is fractured off by a shearing mechanism (Figs. 12 and 13).

Associated injuries include disruptions of the LCL and posterior band of the MCL. The radial head may be fractured, but usually only in the more severe types (eg, subtype 3). It is safe to assume that in the presence of an anteromedial coronoid fracture the LCL has been disrupted. The LCL usually is avulsed beneath the common extensor tendon origin.

The significance of this injury is that the elbow has a tendency to articulate incongruently under axial load or gravitational varus stress (Fig. 14). On lateral tomograms or sagittal CT reconstructions, the medial trochlea can be seen to articulate with the small coronoid fragment, but not with most of the ulna (Fig. 14, *C*). Instead, there is point loading at the fracture site on the ulna, which causes high stresses on the cartilage of the medial trochlea. This pattern of fracture-subluxation is somewhat analogous to that of a Bennett's fracture-dislocation of the thumb. Joint incongruity such as this naturally can (and does appear to) lead to rapid onset arthritis (Fig. 15). Confirming the incongruity may require lateral tomograms or CT reconstruction. To demonstrate this incongruity, the elbow should be imaged while under normal gravitational force. Patients often present with painful contracture several weeks after a minor coronoid fracture. The ulnar nerve is prone to compressive neuritis because of swelling of the torn posterior band of the MCL.

Closkey and associates[53] may have derived a misleading conclusion concerning the effect of coronoid fractures on elbow stability in a recent biomechanical study. They found that a loss of up to 40% of the coronoid did not change the elbow's resistance to direct posterior subluxation. However, they did not evaluate stability with coupled motions in posterolateral or varus-posteromedial rotation. It has been verified (S O'Driscoll, MD, Rochester, MN, unpublished data, 2002) that simulation of an anteromedial subtype 1 coronoid fracture in a cadaver, in association with LCL detachment, permits varus-posteromedial rotatory instability as seen clinically. The key to considering this diagnosis is to recognize the isolated coronoid fracture, ie, a coronoid fracture without a radial head fracture (especially in the absence of apparent dislocation). This injury may appear benign, but it has a predisposition to rapid posttraumatic arthritis as a result of the persistent slight incongruity of the medial ulnohumeral joint. Thus, these fractures generally should be treated surgically.

Basal Coronoid Fractures Basal fractures involve the body of the coronoid, indicated by at least 50% of the height of the coronoid being fractured. These fractures are usually quite comminuted, but they may result in a single fragment if part of an olecranon fracture-dislocation (see section on olecranon fracture-dislocations). Although elbow congruity and stability may have been severely disrupted, the extent of soft-tissue disruption is often less than that seen with tip fractures; therefore, the prognosis may be good once the fracture has been fixed. The principle distinction between basal subtype 1 and 2 fracture is that the latter involves a fracture of the olecranon.

A basal subtype 1 fracture is comminuted and usually has fragments corresponding to those seen in the anteromedial subtype 3 fractures in addition to a die-punch fragment just dorsal to the anteromedial subtype 1 fracture fragment. Fracture lines extend into the proximal radioulnar articulation as well. The radial head often is fractured with these basal subtype 1 fractures, and the ulnohumeral joint is usually unstable.

A basal subtype 2 fracture through the body or base of the coronoid also involves a fracture of the olecranon. These fractures sometimes have a single large coronoid fragment, and much of the soft tissue still may be preserved, which means that once fracture reduc-

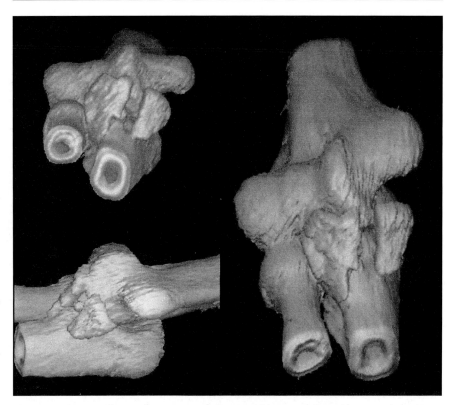

Fig. 13 Mechanism of injury for anteromedial coronoid fractures. Three-dimensional CT reconstruction of an anteromedial subtype 3 coronoid fracture shows involvement of not just the anteromedial fragment but the tip and the sublime tubercle as well. Under varus and axial loads, while the elbow is flexing, flexion and abduction torques at the shoulder cause the medial trochlea to ride up onto the anteromedial coronoid, which is fractured off by a shearing mechanism.

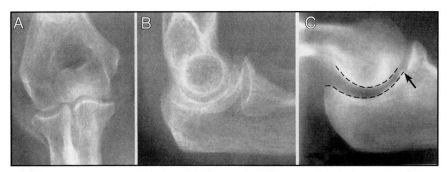

Fig. 14 A and **B,** AP and lateral radiographs of an anteromedial subtype 2 coronoid fracture, showing what appears to be no significant displacement and anatomic joint alignment. **C,** Lateral trispiral tomogram (taken with slight gravitational varus stress on the elbow) through the medial portion of the ulnaohumeral articulation shows an anteromedial subtype 2 fracture (involving the anteromedial coronoid and the tip) with joint incongruity caused by varus posteromedial rotatory subluxation. In this case, the medial trochlea has displaced anteriorly and distally along with the anteromedial coronoid fragment that it displaced and with which it remains congruent. This results in point contact between the medial trochlea and the coronoid at the fracture site (*arrow*), which over the course of a few months leads to medial trochlear erosion. The incongruity is indicated by the ulnohumeral joint being widened posteriorly and converging anteriorly (indicated by converging dotted lines).

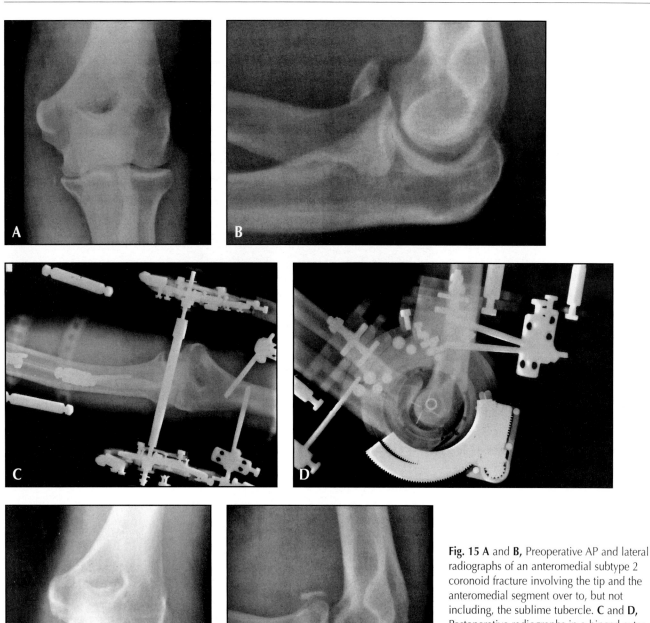

Fig. 15 A and **B,** Preoperative AP and lateral radiographs of an anteromedial subtype 2 coronoid fracture involving the tip and the anteromedial segment over to, but not including, the sublime tubercle. **C** and **D,** Postoperative radiographs in a hinged external fixator after arthroscopic reduction and suture fixation of the fragments, revealing concentric joint alignment and slightly nonanatomic reduction of the fragments. **E** and **F,** AP and lateral radiographs taken 1 year after surgery showing medial ulnohumeral collapse and early arthritis.

tion and stability have been achieved, the prognosis can be quite good.

Treatment

As part of the preoperative evaluation, the presence of a coronoid fracture should be suspected following an elbow dislocation or a fracture of the radial head or olecranon. Clinical examination should include evaluation for tenderness and/or bruising at the origin of the collateral ligament complexes and common flexor and extensor origins, especially on the lateral side where avulsion may not be obvious without an index of suspicion.

Plain AP and lateral radiographs are sometimes adequate, but oblique views can be helpful. CT scans with sagittal and/or three-dimensional reconstruction are also quite helpful in determining the fracture pattern and severity of comminution. Stress radiographs may be necessary to rule out unsuspected instability, especially with anteromedial fractures (Fig. 12).

As is the case for all articular fractures, obtaining and maintaining fracture reduction and joint stability so that early motion can be commenced is the treatment that most predictably assures preservation of function of the joint and limb. Thus, except for stable undisplaced fractures, the treatment of coronoid fractures is usually surgical.

The goal of treatment is to prevent displacement caused by either of the two primary deforming forces: (1) a varus gravitational force with placement of the hand in space and (2) the valgus/posterolateral rotatory stress experienced with axial load across the elbow.

Surgical Exposures The surgical approach depends on the fracture type and the need for other surgery such as ligament repair. A posterior skin incision, just off the midline, permits deep access laterally and medially. Tip fractures can be reduced and fixed through a lateral arthrotomy by retracting the fractured radial head. Anteromedial fractures usually require a medial exposure, which can be obtained either by reflecting a portion of the common flexor-pronator origin or by elevating the flexor carpi ulnaris muscle and tendon origin from the proximal ulna and MCL after transposing the ulnar nerve. If more exposure is required, the entire common flexor-pronator origin can be reflected. The optimum approach remains to be confirmed. An alternative treatment for some of these fractures is to perform an arthroscopic reduction with the fracture under image intensification. Basal subtype 1 coronoid fractures require a medial exposure as just described. However, basal subtype 2 fractures are transolecranon fracture-dislocations; therefore, the coronoid sometimes can be

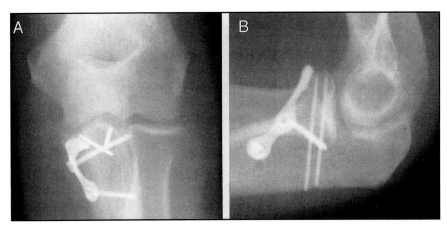

Fig. 16 AP **(A)** and lateral **(B)** radiographs of an anteromedial coronoid fracture fixed with a congruent plate and two fine threaded K-wires.

adequately accessed through the olecranon fracture before placing a precontoured posterior plate.

Surgical Techniques Several options exist for the fixation of coronoid fractures. These include, in various possible combinations, (1) transosseous sutures (or wires) through the ulna, (2) fine threaded K-wires, (3) lag screws, and (4) plate fixation. Neutralization can be achieved either by plate fixation or with a hinged external fixator. The choice of fixation depends on the fracture type, the integrity of the soft tissues, and the presence of associated injuries.

Tip Fractures Tip fractures may not require treatment because they sometimes are very small (≤ 2 mm). Larger tip fractures can be fixed adequately with transosseous sutures and/or fine threaded K-wires. Perfect anatomic reduction of these smaller fragments is not as important as restoration of the anterior buttress, including the capsular insertion of the ulna. Rigid fixation does not seem to be as important with this fracture as it is with an anteromedial or basal coronoid fracture. Two strong sutures or wires are placed through the ulna from the subcutaneous border, emerging at the proximal (articular) edge of the fracture. These are then passed over the coronoid fragment, through the attached capsule, and back

down through two separate holes in the ulna just proximal to the distal edge of the fracture and tied tightly. The use of a threaded K-wire pin to position the fracture fragment anatomically, in addition to the two sutures over the top to hold the fragment down, is quite useful. The capsule inserts 4 to 6 mm distal to the tip of the coronoid so it may not be attached to very small fragments.[52] The technique is based on principles similar to those for a volar plate advancement arthroplasty for proximal interphalangeal fracture-dislocations. It is done through the lateral exposure used for treating the radial head fracture. The fractured radial head is simply retracted while working on the coronoid.

Although the optimal treatment of anteromedial coronoid fractures has yet to be determined, these fractures appear to demand surgical treatment, which might include anatomic reduction and either rigid internal fixation or protection with a hinged external fixator. In addition, the LCL must be repaired if a hinged fixator is not being used. One option is anatomic reduction held with threaded 0.062-in K-wires placed through the ulna into the anteromedial fracture fragments and a precontoured buttress plate (Acumed, Beaverton, OR) that has sharp prongs proximally to grasp the fragments (Fig. 16).

Anteromedial Subtype 1 Fractures Anteromedial subtype 1 fractures are deceitfully benign in their presentation, yet appear to have a guarded prognosis. They usually are seen in isolation, without prior dislocation or radial head fracture. Displacement is not great and may be only about 2 mm. Because of their propensity for permitting ulnohumeral incongruity, they may be reduced and fixed and the LCL complex repaired.

Anteromedial Subtype 2 Fractures In anteromedial subtype 2 fractures, the primary fracture is still in an oblique plane from the sublime tubercle but extends laterally in the coronal plane to involve the tip of the coronoid, which also is fractured off (Fig. 11). This fracture must be distinguished from what could mistakenly be thought of as a comminuted fracture of the coronoid tip. These fractures are treated identically to the anteromedial subtype 1 fractures, except that additional threaded 0.062-in Steinmann pins and sometimes sutures are used to hold the tip reduced (Fig. 16). The buttressing of the primary anteromedial fragment or neutralization with a hinged external fixator is still necessary as described above. The LCL is repaired as well.

Anteromedial Subtype 3 Fractures Anteromedial subtype 3 fractures represent a more comminuted version of anteromedial subtypes 1 and 2. In subtype 3 fractures, medial extension occurs in the sagittal plane, fracturing off the sublime tubercle, which represents the insertion of the anterior bundle of the MCL (Fig. 11). These fractures are treated identically to the anteromedial subtype 2 fractures, but they require additional fixation with screws, threaded wires, a second plate, or suture anchors to fix the sublime tubercle. The buttressing of the primary anteromedial fragment is still necessary as described above. The LCL is repaired as well.

Basal Fractures Basal subtype 1 fractures are treated somewhat similarly to anteromedial fractures: the fragments are reduced and held with fine wires or screws and neutralized with a plate placed on the anteromedial surface of the ulna. A key distinction, however, is the need to elevate a depressed medial/central fragment of the coronoid. The elbow also can be neutralized with a hinged external fixator, which is necessary if stable anatomic reduction is not attainable. Any ligamentous disruption (usually the LCL complex or annular ligament) is repaired.

Transolecranon fracture-dislocations (basal subtype 2 fractures) are treated by first attempting a reduction of the coronoid fragment through the olecranon fracture. Special techniques for this reduction are discussed in the section on olecranon fracture-dislocations. A critical factor is to obtain adequate reduction and stability of the anteromedial coronoid fragment. Failure to do so will likely result in joint incongruity and early posttraumatic arthritis (Fig. 10). A posterior contoured plate is used for these fractures.

Postoperative Management

Postoperative management in all cases consists of brief splinting of the elbow in extension for about 36 hours, followed by early motion. A hinged brace offers some protection, but only when the elbow is relatively extended. When the security of fixation is in question, motion is limited to an arc from 30° to 110° for the first 3 to 6 weeks. Stiffness is likely to result if the elbow is immobilized after surgical repair of these fractures, so motion should be started in almost all cases. A hinged external fixator is used to protect the elbow in those cases in which fracture displacement or joint subluxation would be a concern. If for any reason the surgeon is forced to choose between stability and mobility, it is important to realize that a stiff but congruent elbow is less of a problem to correct than an elbow that has been chronically incongruent, as a result of the cartilage erosion that occurs in the latter.

Pearls

An isolated coronoid fracture (ie, no apparent radial head fracture or elbow dislocation) appears benign but is usually a fracture-subluxation with avulsion of the LCL. The LCL injury will be missed unless stress radiographs are taken or the injury explored (including exposing the ligament beneath the common extensor tendon). The anteromedial facet of the coronoid (between the tip and sublime tubercle) is the critical fragment to be buttressed. A dislocated elbow with a radial head fracture usually has an associated coronoid fracture. A coronoid fragment is bigger than it appears on the radiograph because of its cartilage cap.

Pitfalls

Several pitfalls commonly are seen in the treatment of coronoid fractures. Excision of the coronoid fragment, which is mistaken as part of the radial head, can be avoided if the surgeon realizes that any bone fragment sitting in the coronoid fossa on the radiograph is almost always from the coronoid. Another pitfall is the conclusion that small pieces of coronoid are unimportant. However, in patients with terrible triad injury, even small tip fractures are important and should be repaired if the capsule is still attached to them (as it usually is).

A pitfall experienced by most surgeons is misidentification of an anteromedial fracture as a tip fracture. The latter can be treated by near-anatomic reduction and nonrigid fixation if the radial head is replaced or fixed. However, the former must be reduced anatomically and held rigidly (or the elbow neutralized with an external fixator).

The most common complications following coronoid fractures are elbow instability or stiffness. The joint resultant force vector, which is posterior and superior, requires the coronoid to resist posterior displacement of the ulna under the humerus. Thus, the likelihood and severity of such instability is directly related to how much coronoid is lost or displaced. Gravitational varus stress in the postoperative period is probably the major culprit causing displacement of the coronoid. This stress can be avoided by neutralizing the elbow with a hinged external fixator.

Radial Head and Neck Fractures

Fractures of the radial head are the most common skeletal injury in the adult elbow. Most occur in middle-aged individuals between 20 and 60 years of age, with a 2:1 ratio of women to men.[61,62] The most common injury mechanism involves a fall on the outstretched hand with the forearm pronated and the elbow partially extended. Experimentally, axial load applied from 35° to 80° of elbow flexion leads to isolated radial head failure.[51]

The radiocapitellar joint functions in load bearing. The radial head acts as a secondary stabilizer of the MCL to valgus load,[63-65] and together with the coronoid it bears axial load and provides an anterior buttress resisting posterolateral rotatory subluxation of the elbow joint in a secondary capacity.[59,62,66] During strenuous activities, axial force of up to 90% body weight can be transmitted to the radiocapitellar articulation from the hand-forearm unit.[67] Contact forces at this joint are greatest in pronation, which also results in slight anterior translation of the radial head on the capitellum.

The radial head is slightly elliptical in shape with an offset concavity that articulates with the capitellum. The radial head and neck are angulated and offset with respect to the shaft and the neck. The anterolateral third of the head surface lacks thick articular cartilage and strong subchondral support, making this region more susceptible to fracture.

Treatment

Radiographs of the radial head must be centered on and perpendicular to its surface. This is made difficult following fracture because full elbow extension typically cannot be obtained. Studies have shown a high degree of interobserver and intraobserver variability in classifying radial head fractures based on plain radiographs.[68] Oblique views and specialized projections can be helpful.[69] Plain radiographs commonly underestimate the degree of articular involvement and surface depression, and CT scans may be indicated.

Radial head fractures can be complex either as a result of adjacent fractures or of disruption of the ligaments of the elbow and forearm. Joint dislocation is seen in approximately 3% to 10% of radial head fractures.[70] Failure of the interosseous ligament of the forearm with radial head fracture is more rare.[71-74] It is in these settings that all attempts should be made to reconstruct and preserve the radial head or replace it.

Surgical Exposure Internal fixation of comminuted radial head fractures is technically demanding and is predicated on adequate exposure. For most fracture patterns, regardless of the skin incision, deep dissection is centered over the radiocapitellar joint. The white, shiny extensor aponeurosis fascia is split longitudinally in line with its fibers. The midline of the radiocapitellar articulation marks the deep interval between the extensor carpi radialis brevis anteriorly and the extensor digitorum communis posteriorly.[75] Full-thickness flaps are developed in a single plane through the annular ligament and capsule, which are not identifiable as separate structures surgically. Fracture fragments are often anterior; in such cases, it is useful to expose the radial head between the extensor carpi radialis longus and brevis.

For more complex fractures involving the head and neck of the radius, a larger distal exposure is required. One option is simply to split the extensor fascia and tendon origin distally with elevation of the underlying supinator muscle from posterior to anterior exposing the radial neck. The supinator will help protect the posterior interosseous nerve, which is not in direct jeopardy when using a standard 4.0-cm long plate if dissection is not carried distal to the tuberosity.[76,77] However, to avoid a traction neuropathy, care must be taken not to vigorously retract the soft-tissue envelope anteriorly.

If a longer plate is required at and distal to the tuberosity, the posterior interosseous nerve branches must be identified and protected (Fig. 17). Following fracture fixation, a meticulous repair is required, facilitated by large running, locking sutures placed through drill holes in the humerus (or less commonly with suture anchors). These sutures are tied with the forearm in pronation, which reduces the posterolateral joint subluxation.

Surgical Techniques Often the impacted segments of the radial head are covered with an intact periosteal hinge at the radial neck. Central articular depression is not uncommon and can be elevated with fine instruments. The fracture line must be opened gently to remove any interposed osteochondral fragments, which may block reduction. These occasionally include shear fragments off the capitellum[78] (Fig. 18). Once the fracture is reduced, provisional K-wire fixation is helpful.

When the fracture involves only a segment of the radial head, the wires are replaced with small screws for definitive fixation. Two-millimeter and occasionally 1.5-mm implants are used most commonly and are countersunk beneath the articular surface. Alternatively, headless screws can be used. Maximum screw lengths are typically less than 20 to 24 mm in the average adult radial head. Care must be taken to ensure that the screws do not protrude through the opposite cortex. Full rotation of the forearm is documented prior to a careful closure. If the tendon or ligament origins had been torn or avulsed, they must be repaired as well.

It is important to understand that implants applied to the surface of the radi-

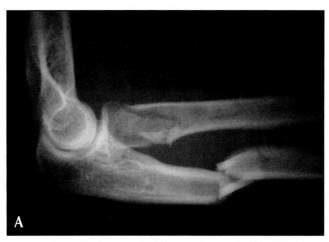
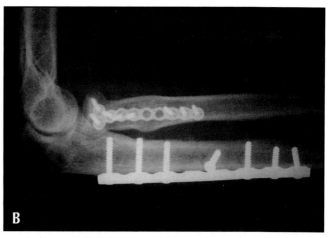

Fig. 17 A, Lateral radiograph depicting comminuted ulnar shaft fracture with associated displaced fracture of the radial neck (Monteggia variant). Note that the radius fracture line extends to nearly the midpoint of the tuberosity. The supinator was retracted anteriorly, protecting the posterior interosseous nerve, and a 2.4-mm plate was applied. Nerve identification is required if dissection is carried out distal to the radial tuberosity. **B,** Final lateral radiograph following internal fixation.

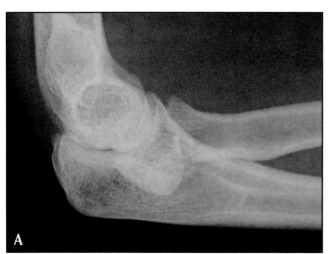
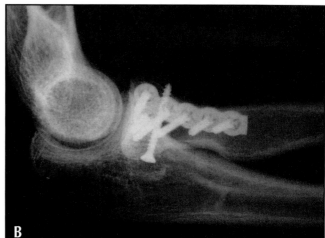
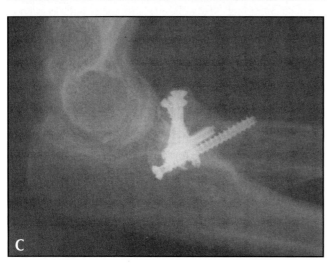

Fig. 18 A, Lateral radiograph of a radial neck fracture with complete displacement. The fracture pattern is oblique in nature, allowing placement of an interfragmentary compression screw. However, it runs from anterior to posterior. (Courtesy of Dr. Graham King, University of Western Ontario, London, Ontario, Canada.) **B,** The plate must still be placed in the safe zone, now functioning in a neutralization mode. A lag screw was applied perpendicular to the main fracture line. **C,** An alternative method of fixing radial head and neck fractures uses crossed cannulated screws.

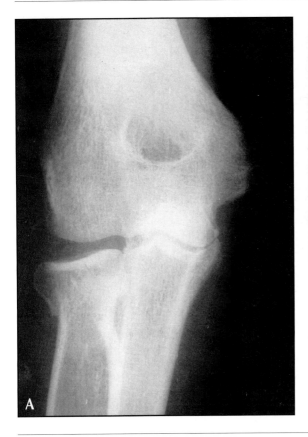

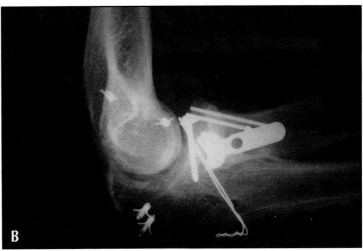

Fig. 19 A, Lateral radiograph depicting malunion of a radial head and neck fracture. In extension, the joint subluxates. **B,** Radial neck and coronoid osteotomies were performed with corticocancellous autograft placed into the radial defect. Note that the plate is not placed in a biomechanically optimal position, sitting approximately 90° to the osteotomy. It must still be applied to the safe zone of the radial head. It was therefore augmented with two threaded K-wires.

al head and neck must be placed in a safe zone so they do not limit forearm rotation. This zone refers to a 110° arc of the head circumference that does not articulate with the radial notch of the ulna.[79,80] The safe zone is perhaps most easily defined as follows: with the forearm in neutral rotation the safe zone is a 90° arc centered on the lateral side of the radial head, with 20° extra added anteriorly (total 110° arc). For fractures involving the radial neck, an interfragmentary compression screw occasionally will be required perpendicular to the fracture line, with a plate then applied as a neutralization device in the safe zone (Fig. 19).

Most commonly, 2.0- and 2.4-mm plates are used to secure and buttress the radial head. Low-profile implants are required because of the close approximation of the annular ligament and overlying soft tissues. These lie in a potential space, and, even if properly placed, implants may impinge on the overlying soft tissues, limiting full forearm rotation. Following fixation, autogenous bone graft often is required to support depressed articular fragments or replace comminuted defects of the radial neck. Graft can be obtained from the distal humerus or the ipsilateral olecranon or distal radial metaphysis.

When radial head fractures are too comminuted to allow for internal fixation with screws, three options are available: (1) fixation with multiple fine threaded K-wires, (2) excision, or (3) replacement. Severely comminuted radial head fractures can sometimes be fixed with good results using five to eight fine threaded K-wires that are cut off and burred down to the cartilage-bone junction. Additional stability can be provided to the radial neck by crisscrossing longitudinal threaded K-wires passed through the rim of the head and down the shaft.

In complex fracture-dislocations, MCL disruption, or forearm interosseous ligament failure, metallic implants are indicated when internal fixation is not possible.[81,82] Silicone arthroplasty is no longer recommended because newer metallic radial head implants are now available.[83-85] The indications and techniques for replacement of the severely fractured head are rapidly evolving. Use of a metal radial head prosthesis restores valgus and axial loading functions of the radius and allows proper healing of the soft tissues. Resection will not result in motion loss but will lead to weakness in grip, rotation, and axial forearm loading.[86-88] If resection is being considered, however, it is important to examine the elbow intraoperatively to rule out occult valgus or axial instability following radial head resection.

Postoperative Management
After surgery, patients are immobilized for 1 or 2 days in a compressive dressing with the elbow extended and elevated.

ROM exercises of the elbow and forearm are then begun with interval protective splinting for comfort and support. Prolonged immobilization is avoided because it is associated with increased stiffness and functional loss.[68,89] A nighttime elbow extension splint may be helpful to decrease the development of a flexion contracture. Terminal elbow extension and full forearm supination are hardest to recover, and therapy should concentrate on these functions. Progressive loading and strengthening are typically not permitted for approximately 6 weeks and often longer depending on the injury and the fixation obtained.

In more severe trauma with extensive soft-tissue injury, some surgeons consider using short-term nonsteroidal anti-inflammatory medication as prophylaxis against heterotopic ossification. This condition is poorly understood but is related, in part, to the severity of the original injury.[90] It also may be associated with a larger surgical dissection, repeated surgical insults to the traumatized elbow, and possibly a delay in surgical intervention.[91]

Pearls

Articular injury to the radial head is commonly more severe than noted on plain radiographs of the elbow. Even simple fractures often involve chondral injury to the capitellum and some degree of collateral ligament trauma. Late symptoms may be attributable to these unrecognized injuries. If the coronoid is fractured, the radial head becomes a critical factor in elbow stability. The role of the radial head becomes increasingly important as other soft-tissue and bony constraints are compromised. Loss of the radial head results in weakness of grip and strength of the forearm both in rotation and axial loading. Implants applied to the surface of the radial head must be placed in a safe zone, which involves a 110° arc of the articular circumference, that is almost directly lateral when the forearm is in neutral rota-

tion. Following radial head injury, loss of terminal elbow extension is more common than loss of forearm rotation. Forearm supination is typically more difficult to recover than pronation. Prolonged immobilization leads to a greater likelihood of joint stiffness.

Pitfalls

Open reduction and internal fixation of radial head fractures is technically difficult and can be fraught with pitfalls and complications. One pitfall is the failure to recognize the need for bone grafting of defects caused by fracture impaction. A low threshold should exist to bone graft areas of comminution, especially in the radial neck, and care must be taken to place internal fixation without excessive stripping of the periosteal sleeve. Another common pitfall is the placement of hardware in positions permitting impingement against the ulna. Provisional fixation of the fracture with K-wires is very helpful to stabilize reduced fragments and allow planning for subsequent definitive fixation in the safe zone.

The complication that occurs most often is loss of motion, especially when plates are used for internal fixation. A common pitfall in attempting to prevent this problem is to provide inadequate protection for patients with nonrigid fixation. The use of a long-arm orthosis between exercises during the early postoperative period may help protect the construct from excessive loads. Occasionally, it is necessary to remove the hardware once union has matured. When problematic, early implant removal is recommended at 4 to 6 months, especially for cancellous injuries. However, this does not always lead to return of full forearm rotation.

Summary

Difficult elbow fractures are defined as those posing challenges in diagnosis, exposure, and treatment or causing serious uncertainty regarding prognosis.

These include comminuted fractures of the distal humerus, often with bone loss; complex fracture patterns of the articular surfaces, such as shearing injuries; and certain fractures of the coronoid and the radial head. Improved techniques for achieving adequate stability in complex distal humerus fractures have contributed significantly to advances in treatment. The recent understanding of complex instability patterns, including varus posteromedial rotatory instability, have provided important information on the relevance of the pattern and location of fractures of the coronoid. Anteromedial coronoid fractures can present a benign appearance but pose a serious threat of incongruity and early posttraumatic arthritis. An understanding of the relevant biomechanics (such as the interdependent contributions of the coronoid and radial head) and specific principles of maintaining elbow stability allow the surgeon to treat and appropriately rehabilitate the patient with a difficult elbow fracture while avoiding some of the common pitfalls in the process.

References

1. Jupiter JB, Neff U, Holzach P, Allgower M: Intercondylar fractures of the humerus: An operative approach. *J Bone Joint Surg Am* 1985;67:226-239.

2. Jupiter JB: Complex fractures of the distal part of the humerus and associated complications. *Instr Course Lect* 1995;44:187-198.

3. McKee M, Jupiter J, Toh CL, Wilson L, Colton C, Karras KK: Reconstruction after malunion and nonunion of intra-articular fractures of the distal humerus. *J Bone Joint Surg Br* 1994;76:614-621.

4. McKee MD, Jupiter JB, Bosse G, Goodman L: Outcome of ulnar neurolysis during post-traumatic reconstruction of the elbow. *J Bone Joint Surg Br* 1998;80:100-105.

5. McKee MD, Jupiter JB: Trauma to the adult elbow and fractures of the distal humerus, in Browner B (ed): *Skeletal Trauma*. Philadelphia, PA, WB Saunders, 1998, vol 2, pp 1455-1522.

6. McKee MD, Kim J, Kebaish K, Stephen DJ, Kreder HJ, Schemitsch EH: Functional outcome after open supracondylar fractures of the humerus. *J Bone Joint Surg Br* 2000;82:646-651.

7. Zagorski JB, Jennings JJ, Burkhalter WE, Uribe JW: Comminuted intraarticular fractures of the distal humeral condyles: Surgical vs nonsurgical treatment. *Clin Orthop* 1986;202:197-204.

8. Cobb TK, Morrey BF: Total elbow arthroplasty as primary treatment for distal humeral fractures in elderly patients. *J Bone Joint Surg Am* 1997;79:826-832.

9. Waddell JP, Hatch J, Richards R: Supracondylar fractures of the humerus: Results of surgical treatment. *J Trauma* 1988;28:1615-1621.

10. McKee MD, Wilson TL, Winston L, Schemitsch EH, Richards RR: Functional outcome following surgical treatment of intra-articular distal humeral fractures through a posterior approach. *J Bone Joint Surg Am* 2000;82:1701-1707.

11. Bryan RS, Morrey BF: Extensive posterior exposure of the elbow: A triceps-sparing approach. *Clin Orthop* 1982;166:188-192.

12. O'Driscoll SW: The triceps-reflecting anconeus pedicle (TRAP) approach for distal humeral fractures and nonunions. *Orthop Clin North Am* 2000;31:91-101.

13. Kasser JR, Richards K, Millis M: The triceps-dividing approach to open reduction of complex distal humeral fractures in adolescents: A Cybex evaluation of triceps function and motion. *J Pediatr Orthop* 1990;10:93-96.

14. Helfet DL, Hotchkiss RN: Internal fixation of the distal humerus: A biomechanical comparison of methods. *J Orthop Trauma* 1990;4:260-264.

15. Schemitsch EH, Tencer AF, Henley MB: Biomechanical evaluation of methods of internal fixation of the distal humerus. *J Orthop Trauma* 1994;8:468-475.

16. Sanchez-Sotelo J, Torchia ME, O'Driscoll SW: Principle-based internal fixation of distal humerus fractures: *Tech Hand Upper Extrem Surg* 2001;5:179-187.

17. O'Driscoll S, Sanchez-Sotelo J, Torchia ME: Management of the smashed distal humerus. *Orthop Clin North Am* 2002;33:19-33.

18. Morrey BF, Askew LJ, Chao EY: A biomechanical study of normal functional elbow motion. *J Bone Joint Surg Am* 1981;63:872-877.

19. McKee MD, Jupiter JB, Bamberger HB: Coronal shear fractures of the distal end of the humerus. *J Bone Joint Surg Am* 1996;78:49-54.

20. Muller M, Nazarian S, Koch P, Schatzker J (eds): *Comprehensive Classification of Fratures of Long Bones.* New York, NY, Springer, 1990, pp 75-85.

21. Robertson R, Bogart F: Fracture of the capitellum and trochlea combined with fracture of the external humeral condyl. *J Bone Joint Surg Am* 1933;15:206-213.

22. Inoue G, Horii E: Combined shear fractures of the trochlea and capitellum associated with anterior fracture-dislocation of the elbow. *J Orthop Trauma* 1992;6:373-375.

23. Lansinger O, Mare K: Fracture of the capitulum humeri. *Acta Orthop Scand* 1981;52:39-44.

24. Milch L: Fractures and fracture dislocations of the humeral condyles. *J Trauma* 1964;4:592-607.

25. McKee MD, Jupiter JB: A contemporary approach to the management of complex fractures of the distal humerus and their sequelae. *Hand Clin* 1994;10:479-494.

26. Jupiter JB, Neff U, Regazzoni P, Allgower M: Unicondylar fractures of the distal humerus: An operative approach. *J Orthop Trauma* 1988;2:102-109.

27. Simpson LA, Richards RR: Internal fixation of a capitellar fracture using Herbert screws: A case report. *Clin Orthop* 1986;209:166-168.

28. Grantham SA, Norris TR, Bush DC: Isolated fracture of the humeral capitellum. *Clin Orthop* 1981;161:262-269.

29. Ring D, Jupiter JB, Sanders RW, Mast J, Simpson NS: Transolecranon fracture: Dislocation of the elbow. *J Orthop Trauma* 1997;11:545-550.

30. Ring D, Jupiter JB, Simpson NS: Monteggia fractures in adults. *J Bone Joint Surg Am* 1998;80:1733-1744.

31. Biga N, Thomine JM: Trans-olecranal dislocations of the elbow. *Rev Chir Orthop Reparatrice Appar Mot* 1974;60:557-567.

32. Bado JL: The Monteggia lesion. *Clin Orthop* 1967;50:71-86.

33. Ring D, Jupiter JB, Waters PM: Monteggia fractures in children and adults. *J Am Acad Orthop Surg* 1998;6:215-224.

34. Balakim G, Wippula E: Fractures of the olecranon complicated by forward dislocation of the forearm. *Ann Chir Gyn Fenn* 1971;60:105-108.

35. Jupiter JB, Leibovic SJ, Ribbans W, Wilk RM: The posterior Monteggia lesion. *J Orthop Trauma* 1991;5:395-402.

36. Penrose J: The Monteggia fracture with posterior dislocation of the radial head. *J Bone Joint Surg Br* 1951;33:65-73.

37. Pavel A, Pittman J, Lance E, Wade P: The posterior Monteggia fracture: A clinical study. *J Trauma* 1965;5:185-199.

38. Dowdy PA, Bain GI, King GJ, Patterson SD: The midline posterior elbow incision: An anatomical appraisal. *J Bone Joint Surg Br* 1995;77:696-699.

39. Patterson SD, Bain GI, Mehta JA: Surgical approaches to the elbow. *Clin Orthop* 2000;370:19-33.

40. Ikeda M, Fukushima Y, Kobayashi Y, Oka Y: Comminuted fractures of the olecranon: Management by bone graft from the iliac crest and multiple tension-band wiring. *J Bone Joint Surg Br* 2001;83:805-808.

41. Heim U: Kombinierte verletzungen von radius und ulna im proximalen unterarmsegment. *Hefte Unfallchir* 1994;241:61-79.

42. Hastings H II, Engles DR: Fixation of complex elbow fractures: Part II. Proximal ulna and radius fractures. *Hand Clin* 1997;13:721-735.

43. Ring D, Jupiter JB: Operative fixation and reconstruction of the coronoid. *Tech Orthop* 2000;15.

44. Morrey BF: Surgical exposures of the elbow, in Morrey BF (ed): *The Elbow and Its Disorders*, ed 2. Philadelphia, PA, WB Saunders, 1993, pp 139-166.

45. Mast J, Jokob R, Ganz R: *Planning and Reduction Technique in Fracture Surgery.* New York, NY, Springer-Verlag, 1989, pp 1-254.

46. O'Driscoll SW: Technique for unstable olecranon fracture-subluxations. *Op Tech Orthop* 1994;4:49-53.

47. Mansat P, Morrey BF: The column procedure: A limited lateral approach for extrinsic contracture of the elbow. *J Bone Joint Surg Am* 1998;80:1603-1615.

48. Cohen MS, Hastings H II: Post-traumatic contracture of the elbow: Operative release using a lateral collateral ligament sparing approach. *J Bone Joint Surg Br* 1998;80:805-812.

49. Ring D, Jupiter JB: Reconstruction of posttraumatic elbow instability. *Clin Orthop* 2000;10:44-56.

50. Hotchkiss RN: Fractures and dislocations of the elbow, in Rockwood CA, Green DP, Bucholz RW, Heckman JD (eds): *Fractures in Adults*, ed 4. Philadelphia, PA, Lippincott Raven, 1996, pp 980-981.

51. Amis AA, Miller JH: The mechanisms of elbow fractures: An investigation using impact tests in vitro. *Injury* 1995;26:163-168.

52. Cage DJ, Abrams RA, Callahan JJ, Botte MJ: Soft tissue attachments of the ulnar coronoid process: An anatomic study with radiographis correlation. *Clin Orthop* 1995;320:154-158.

53. Closkey RF, Goode JR, Kirschenbaum D, Cody RP: The role of the coronoid process in elbow stability: A biomechanical analysis of axial loading. *J Bone Joint Surg Am* 2000;82:1749-1753.

54. Norris TR (ed): *Orthopaedic Knowledge Update: Shoulder and Elbow.* Rosemont, IL, American Academy of Orthopaedic Surgeons, 1997, pp 405-413.

55. Regan W, Morrey B: Fractures of the coronoid process of the ulna. *J Bone Joint Surg Am* 1989;71:1348-1354.

56. O'Driscoll SW: Elbow instability. *Hand Clin* 1994;10:405-415.

57. Regan W, Morrey BF: Classification and treatment of coronoid process fractures. *Orthopaedics* 1992;15:845-848.

58. Frymoyer JW (ed): *Orthopaedic Knowledge Update 4.* Rosemont, IL, American Academy of Orthopaedic Surgeons, 1993, pp 335-352.

59. O'Driscoll SW, Bell DF, Morrey BF: Posterolateral rotatory instability of the elbow. *J Bone Joint Surg Am* 1991;73:440-446.

60. O'Driscoll SW: Classification and spectrum of elbow instability: Recurrent instability, in Morrey BF (ed): *The Elbow and Its Disorders.* Philadelphia, PA, WB Saunders, 1993, pp 453-463.

61. Mason M: Some observations on fractures of the radial head with a review of one hundred cases. *Br J Surg* 1954;42:123-132.

62. Morrey BF: Radial head fracture, in Morrey BF (ed): *The Elbow*, ed 3. Philadelphia, PA, WB Saunders, 2000, pp 341-364.

63. Hotchkiss RN, Weiland AJ: Valgus stability of the elbow. *J Orthop Res* 1987;5:372-377.

64. Morrey BF, An KN: Articular and ligamentous contributions to the stability of the elbow joint. *Am J Sports Med* 1983;11:315-319.

65. Morrey BF, Tanaka S, An KN: Valgus stability of the elbow: A definition of primary and secondary constraints. *Clin Orthop* 1991;265:187-195.

66. Cohen M, Hastings HS: Rotatory instability of the elbow: The anatomy and role of the lateral stabilizers. *J Bone Joint Surg Am* 1997;79:225-233.

67. Morrey BF, An KN, Stormont TJ: Force transmission through the radial head. *J Bone Joint Surg Am* 1988;70:250-256.

68. Morgan SJ, Groshen SL, Itamura JM, Shankwiler J, Brien WW, Kuschner SH: Reliability evaluation of classifying radial head fractures by the system of Mason. *Bull Hosp Jt Dis* 1997;56:95-98.

69. Greenspan A, Norman A, Rosen H: Radial head: Capitellum view in elbow traima: Clinical application and radiographic anatomic correlation. *AJR Am J Roentgenol* 1984;143:355-359.

70. Bakalim G: Fractures of radial head and their treatment. *Acta Orthop Scand* 1970;41:320-331.

71. Bock GW, Cohen MS, Resnick D: Fracture-dislocation of the elbow with inferior radioulnar dislocation: A variant of the Essex-Lopresti injury. *Skeletal Radiol* 1992;21:315-317.

72. Essex-Lopresti P: Fractures of the radial head with distal radio-ulnar dislocation. *J Bone Joint Surg Br* 1951;33:244-247.

73. Hotchkiss RN, An KN, Sowa DT, Basta S, Weiland AJ: An anatomic and mechanical study of the interosseous membrane of the forearm: Pathomechanics of proximal migration of the radius. *J Hand Surg Am* 1989;14:256-261.

74. Trousdale RT, Amadio PC, Cooney WP, Morrey BF: Radio-ulnar dissociation: A review of twenty cases. *J Bone Joint Surg Am* 1992;74:1486-1497.

75. Cohen M, Romeo A: Lateral epicondylitis: Open and arthroscopic treatment. *J Amer Soc Surg Hand* 2001;3:172-176.

76. Strauch RJ, Rosenwasser MP, Glazer PA: Surgical exposure of the dorsal proximal third of the radius: How vulnerable is the posterior interosseous nerve? *J Shoulder Elbow Surg* 1996;5:342-346.

77. Tornetta P III, Hochwald N, Bono C, Grossman M: Anatomy of the posterior interosseous nerve in relation to fixation of the radial head. *Clin Orthop* 1997;345:215-218.

78. Geel CW, Palmer AK, Ruedi T, Leutenegger AF: Internal fixation of proximal radial head fractures. *J Orthop Trauma* 1990;4:270-274.

79. Hotchkiss RN: Displaced fractures of the radial head: Internal fixation or excision? *J Am Acad Orthop Surg* 1997;5:1-10.

80. Smith GR, Hotchkiss RN: Radial head and neck fractures: Anatomic guidelines for proper placement of internal fixation. *J Shoulder Elbow Surg* 1996;5:113-117.

81. King GJ, Zarzour ZD, Rath DA, Dunning CE, Patterson SD, Johnson JA: Metallic radial head arthroplasty improves valgus stability of the elbow. *Clin Orthop* 1999;368:114-125.

82. Popovic N, Gillet P, Rodriguez A, Lemaire R: Fracture of the radial head with associated elbow dislocation: Results of treatment using a floating radial head prosthesis. *J Orthop Trauma* 2000;14:171-177.

83. Judet T, Garreau de Loubresse C, Piriou P, Charnley G: A floating prosthesis for radial-head fractures. *J Bone Joint Surg Br* 1996;78:244-249.

84. Knight DJ, Rymaszewski LA, Amis AA, Miller JH: Primary replacement of the fractured radial head with a metal prosthesis. *J Bone Joint Surg Br* 1993;75:572-576.

85. Moro JK, Werier J, MacDermid JC, Patterson SD, King GJ: Arthroplasty with a metal radial head for unreconstructible fractures of the radial head. *J Bone Joint Surg Am* 2001;83:1201-1211.

86. Ikeda M, Oka Y: Function after early radial head resection for fracture: A retrospective evaluation of 15 patients followed for 3-18 years. *Acta Orthop Scand* 2000;71:191-194.

87. Jensen SL, Olsen BS, Sojbjerg JO: Elbow joint kinematics after excision of the radial head. *J Shoulder Elbow Surg* 1999;8:238-241.

88. Morrey BF, Chao EY, Hui FC: Biomechanical study of the elbow following excision of the radial head. *J Bone Joint Surg Am* 1979;61:63-68.

89. Broberg MA, Morrey BF: Results of treatment of fracture-dislocations of the elbow. *Clin Orthop* 1987;216:109-119.

90. Thompson HC III, Garcia A: Myositis ossificans: Aftermath of elbow injuries. *Clin Orthop* 1967;50:129-134.

91. Morrey BF: Ectopic ossification about the elbow, in Morrey BF (ed): *The Elbow,* ed 3. Philadelphia, PA, WB Saunders, 2000, pp 437-446.

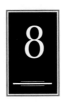

Diaphyseal Humeral Fractures: Treatment Options

Augusto Sarmiento, MD
James P. Waddell, MD, FRCSC
Loren L. Latta, PE, PhD

Several modalities of treatment are currently available for the management of diaphyseal humeral fractures. A long arm cast, a functional brace, an external fixator, a compression plate, and an intramedullary rod are different devices used to achieve the same ultimate results, but the biologic mechanisms through which they accomplish this vary. Each one of these devices has a place in the management of humeral shaft fractures, and no one treatment is superior under all circumstances.

Understanding how the fracture heals with each form of treatment is essential for selection of the most appropriate choice for any specific fracture. It is the responsibility of the treating physician to understand the appropriate indications for each treatment modality, to recognize the biologic and technical aspects that underlie its usage, to appreciate the importance of any residual deviation from normal as well as harmful sequelae, and to be familiar with all possible complications and their management. This chapter describes the four most commonly used treatments: a functional brace, an external fixator, a plate and screws, and an intramedullary rod. An outline of the biologic mechanisms of fracture repair with each of the four methods of treatment is included.

Biomechanics of Fracture Healing and Fracture Stability
Fracture Motion
Two types of motion occur at the fracture site: elastic motion and plastic motion. Elastic motion is a displacement of the bone fragments that is completely reversed after the load is relaxed. This motion is acceptable and allows healing with satisfactory alignment. Plastic motion is a displacement of the bone fragments that is not reversed after the load is relaxed, resulting in a change in the position of the fracture fragment. This motion is not acceptable. It may lead to nonunion and, even if union occurs, malalignment is present.

Elastic motion with rigid fixation (plate-and-screw fixation) allows motion on the order of micrometers at the fracture site under normal loading conditions.[1] With this degree of motion, the medullary circulation is reestablished rapidly. In areas of contact, cutting cones of bone remodeling may cross the fracture site directly, and the fracture heals with direct formation of new bone on the original bone with little or no external callus.[2] The strength of the healing bone reaches a peak within a few months (about 8 weeks in dogs), and the strength of the bone with a plate is approximately the same as that of the intact bone during the early stage

of healing; but the underlying bone does not reach its original strength and even loses strength over the next few months due to cancellization of the cortical bone beneath the plate.[3-5] This change from dense cortical bone to cancellous-like bone may be due to stress protection provided by the plate, to a change in the blood supply caused by the surgical procedure, or to a combination of the two. New procedures and devices have been designed to reduce the compromise to the blood supply, to minimize the stress protection, and to improve the long-term effects on the healing bone. The full strength of the bone with the plate in place is not reestablished for approximately 2 years.[6]

With the less rigid forms of fixation (intramedullary rods without locking, external fixators, casts, and braces), the elastic motion at the fracture site is at least 1 mm and can be as much as 1 cm with normal activities. When there is displacement between the fracture fragments or motion of more than a few micrometers at the fracture site, the medullary blood vessels cannot cross the fracture site until the fragments have been connected and immobilized by callus.[7]

With rigid fixation, the neovascularity necessary for fracture healing comes principally from the medullary circula-

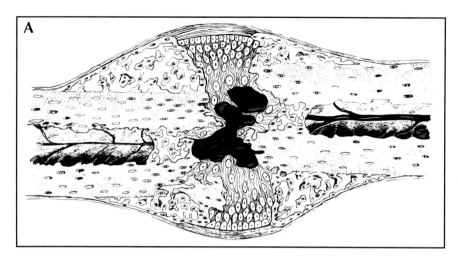

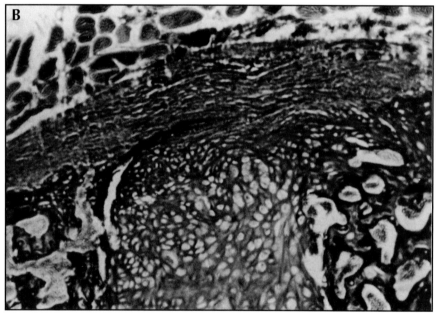

Fig. 1 Soft callus forms under the influence of early function and creates a compliant but strong, tough connection between the bone ends. The soft callus is made up of dense, well-oriented collagen fiber bundles in the periphery (**A**) covering a wedge of cartilage and loose fibrous tissue with a hematoma at the center (**B**). This is the stage of healing when use of casts or external fixators can be discontinued, braces can be applied, and comfortable function can progress rapidly.

the mechanical properties of the plate-and-screw fixation. This is why the strength of the bone at the fracture site for the first few months after plate removal is only about one half the strength of the original bone.[3,4] The new bone remodels and normal strength returns only after the plate is removed and normal stresses are applied. With less rigid fixation, new bone is formed on the surface of the bone adjacent to the fracture and, until this periosteal callus bridges the fracture site to immobilize the fracture, it is in a stage of instability.[7] Initially, a soft callus is formed.

Radiographically, the callus shows no evidence of bridging bone because the tissues bridging the fracture site are composed of hematoma, cartilage, and fibrous tissue and are not yet mineralized. A dense fibrous layer forms in the most peripheral portion of the bridging callus with well-oriented collagen fibers guided by early stresses. Beneath this layer is a wedge of cartilage (Fig. 1). This construct of callus bridging the fracture fragments acts mechanically much like the intervertebral disk, allowing a strong yet compliant connection between the bone segments. The dense, well-oriented collagen-fiber layer acts like the anulus fibrosus, providing tensile resistance to bending and torsion. The centrally confined cartilage acts like the nucleus pulposus, providing a hydraulic-like compression resistance for load transfer. Although this soft callus is relatively strong, it is vulnerable to painless creep with deformation under static loading, such as that which occurs when leaning on the arm.[9]

Within a few weeks, the peripheral callus begins to mature. The peripheral portion of the bridging callus just beneath the soft tissues surrounding the bone begins to mineralize[7] (Fig. 2). Thus, the first portion of the bridging callus to ossify is the farthest from the neutral axis. Bone in this location has a mechanical advantage compared with bone near the

tion.[8] With less rigid fixation systems, the surrounding soft tissue provides almost all of the neovascularity to the callus bridging the fracture site. With less rigid fixation, early muscle activity and the resulting localized inflammatory response are important for early bone formation. It is important to understand how these types of callus form and how they can provide adequate

strength to resist plastic deformation while allowing elastic motion during normal functional activities.

With rigid fixation, the early bone forms primarily in the microscopic gaps between the bone ends, with occasional direct osteon-to-osteon new bone formation at the contact points. This new bone is mostly shielded from the normal stress of functional activities because of

neutral axis because its resistance to bending and torsion is proportional to the fourth power of the diameter of the callus. This means that a callus twice as wide as another callus is 16 times more effective at resisting bending and torsion. A wide bridging callus can make the site of the healing fracture quite strong, and yet the fracture gap may be visible on the radiograph even when the bone has regained its strength (Fig. 2). In a rat model of femoral fracture healing, this occurred at about 5 weeks.[7] As the fracture consolidates and the callus remodels, the callus does not become stronger but the fracture line fills with bone, the peripheral callus shrinks, and the medullary canal is reconstituted.

Fracture Stability

Fracture stability is reflected by the degree of plastic motion or progressive deformity that can occur at the fracture site. It relates to the strength of fixation of the fracture. The basic parameters that determine fracture stability are coaptation, compression, neutralization, and a tension band with a buttress. Each of these factors must be addressed with each fracture-fixation method.

Accurate coaptation of the fracture fragments is important with rigid internal fixation because good bone contact is required for both strength and rigidity. With less rigid fixation, accuracy of coaptation is important only for cosmetic appearance and function. Coaptation is achieved at surgery by direct repositioning of the fragments. With functional bracing, gravity alignment and early function provide coaptation.

Compression of the fracture surfaces helps to provide stability as well as to apply strains to the healing tissues to guide their alignment. With rigid internal fixation, compression can be applied passively with the hardware at the time of surgery. With less rigid fixation and especially with functional bracing, muscle activity pro-

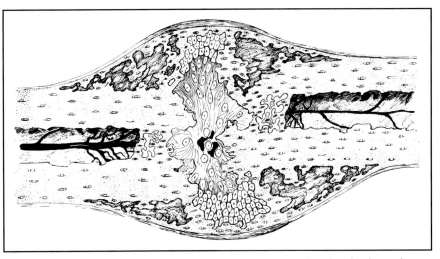

Fig. 2 Hard callus creates a rigid connection between the bone ends with a thin layer of new bone at the periphery. This bone is vascularized from the surrounding tissues and covers the cartilage and soft tissue in the center of the callus. Because of the large mechanical advantage (moment of inertia) of the thin layer of bone, the callus is rigid and strong while the radiographic image continues to have a radiolucency in the center. The fracture is mechanically healed at this stage, and all external supports and, if indicated, intramedullary nails may be removed.

vides active compression at the fracture site.

Neutralization refers to the forces applied to the fracture that balance the forces displacing it. Without adequate neutralization, the fracture deforms plastically and fixation is lost. Neutralization with rigid plate-and-screw fixation requires at least eight cortices of screw fixation through the plate on each side of a fracture of the humerus. Less fixation may lead to screw pull-out and separation of the plate from the bone. Neutralization with intramedullary nails is provided by one of two mechanisms. If a length of the medullary canal that is 2.5 times or more the diameter of the humerus can be reamed for a tight fit of the nail in one of the fragments, and there is cortical contact at the fracture site, the neutralization for that fragment is generally adequate to resist angulation and rotation. If the fragment is short and the length of the tight fit is less than 2.5 times the diameter, neutralization must be achieved by additional fixation. With most systems, transcortical

screws are used through the proximal or distal end of the nail. Other devices deploy some sort of intramedullary cancellous fixation mechanism, such as blades and pins. When there is a gap at the fracture site, these same mechanisms are necessary to maintain length and rotational alignment.

Although the most rigid, strong, and visible components in a typical external fixator construct are the connectors joining the pins between the bone fragments, the parameters that control neutralization of the fracture are related more to the pins. The pin parameters over which the surgeon has control include diameter, material, separation, and span. Plastic and elastic bending of the pins is responsible for most of the fracture site movement. Plastic bending resistance is proportional to the area moment of inertia of the pin's cross section (the fourth power of the diameter). Elastic deformation of the pins contributes to pin loosening, and pin loosening is the most common mode of loss of neutralization associated with external fixation of humeral fractures. The elastic bending resistance of a 5-mm pin is 2.5 times greater than that of a 4-mm pin of the same material. The strength of the pin in bending is related to the third power of the diameter; thus, the ability of a 5-mm pin to transmit bending without plastic deformation is twice that of a 4-mm pin of the same material. Pin strength also is affected by pin material. The stiffness of a stainless steel pin is almost twice that of a titanium pin of the same diameter. Pin span is the distance between the pin-bone interface and the pin-clamp interface, or the "free span" of the pin between its connections. The neutralization of any construct is inversely proportional to the square of the pin spans in the construct. The closer the pin clamps can be placed to the skin, the stronger and more rigid the fixation. Pin separation is the distance between any two pins within the same bone fragment. This distance provides the leverage by the pin cluster to resist angulation of that fragment in the plane of those pins. Thus, pins that are widely separated and are not all in the same plane improve the neutralization, or strength and rigidity of hold, for the construct on that fragment. Placing a third pin (or more) out of the plane of the first two pins substantially reduces the bending of all of the pins and thus their tendency to loosen.

Neutralization with a functional brace is accomplished primarily by soft-tissue compression. Circumferential wrapping of the soft tissue with any material that can be closely fit to the shape of the arm and can be adjusted to maintain compression of the tissue throughout the period of treatment provides the neutralization required for early functional activities. The hardness and rigidity of the material is not important mechanically;[7,9] only the ability of the device to be adjusted to maintain soft-tissue compression and suspension of the system is important. Thus, many

soft, compliant, and comfortable materials can be used successfully. Soft cast materials or thermoplastics applied directly to the patient's arm with custom-fit or compliant prefabricated braces are more comfortable than rigid, hard, or thick thermoplastic sheets or plaster. Comfort is important for the early introduction of functional activities.

Tension band systems resist bending by having a buttress, or compression-resistant area, on the concave side of the bend. The distance of the buttress from the line of action of the tension band provides the leverage. This distance and the strength and rigidity of the tension band determine the strength and rigidity of the fixation.

With plate-and-screw fixation, the tension band is the plate. Thus, the tension is both rigid and strong. The buttress is the contact of the bone fragments beneath the plate, with the maximal leverage related to the diameter of the bone. Because there is a tension band on only one side of the bone, the plate should be placed on the convex (tension) side of the bone. For the humerus, this is lateral because the most common tendency is for varus angulation of the fracture.[9] Bending in any other plane is resisted mostly by the bending resistance of the plate only.

With intramedullary fixation, the tension band is the nail. The buttress is the fracture-surface contact on the concave side of the bend, with a lever arm of about one cortical thickness from the nail. Thus, in a noncomminuted fracture, a buttress is available on all sides to resist bending in all planes.

An external fixator acts as a tension band only when there is bone contact to provide a buttress. The fixator provides excellent leverage only in the direction of its placement. If placed laterally, it resists varus angulation; if placed anteriorly, it resists anterior bowing. In all other planes, the resistance is related to the bending resistance of the frame only.

With functional bracing, the tension bands are compliant and are provided by the soft tissues.[9] The buttress is provided by bone contact or callus. Both the buttress and the tension bands in the upper arm are symmetric and provide resistance in all planes of angulation with compliant but strong resistance to bending.

Indications for Surgery

The role of open treatment of fractures of the humerus remains controversial. Routine surgical management of humeral shaft fractures probably is not appropriate because the results of nonsurgical treatment are generally satisfactory; acceptable alignment and healing occur in at least 90% of patients managed nonsurgically.[10-12]

The generally accepted indications for surgical treatment are a type III open fracture, polytrauma with substantial chest and/or head injury, an ipsilateral fracture of both bones of the forearm (floating elbow), and extensive local associated injury involving the joint, brachial plexus, muscle, or tendon.

If open treatment is required, the choice of implants includes plates and screws, intramedullary nails (with or without reaming and with or without locking), or external fixators.[13] External fixation is indicated only for open fractures with extensive bone loss or when extensive comminution precludes the use of internal fixation.[14]

Plate Fixation

Most surgeons favor an extensile anterolateral approach for exposure of the humerus. This exposure has the advantage of allowing the radial nerve to be visualized and protected.[15] An alternative approach is through the posterior aspect of the arm with splitting of the triceps. Fractures of the distal aspect of the humeral diaphysis can be exposed through a posterior approach.[16,17]

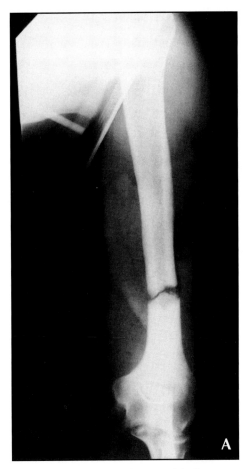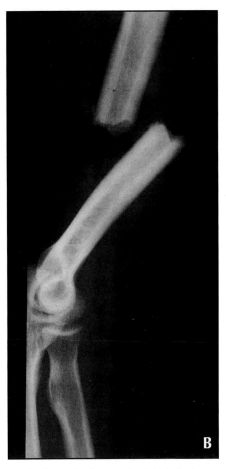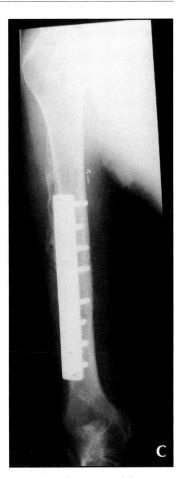

Fig. 3 A distal, transverse fracture of the humerus. **A** and **B,** Radiographs show major initial displacement through the soft tissues and thus extensive soft-tissue damage. **C,** Stability was achieved with the use of an anterior plate with eight cortices of fixation in both the proximal and the distal fragment, sufficient to maintain excellent alignment throughout healing.

Plate fixation requires accurate reduction of the major fracture fragments.[18] For comminuted fractures that cannot be reduced anatomically, bridge-plating techniques may be used.[18] Fractures that have large comminuted fragments or oblique spiral fractures should be reduced anatomically with lag-screw fixation, followed by plate fixation.[4,18,19] A broad plate with staggered holes is recommended. With the staggered holes, there is no possibility of crack propagation from the fracture site into adjacent screw holes.[18] It is essential that adequate purchase of the screws be achieved on both sides of the fracture.[20] A minimum of six and preferably eight cortices on both sides of the fracture should be engaged by the screws

(Fig. 3). The radial nerve must be protected throughout the entire surgical procedure.

Plate fixation of open fractures of the humerus require the same general principles of treatment as those applied to open fractures elsewhere in the skeleton. These include meticulous wound débridement, fracture stabilization, appropriate soft-tissue management, and the use of prophylactic antibiotics.[21,22] Once the wound has been appropriately débrided, routine plate fixation is done with particular attention paid to obtaining rigid fixation. Unless the wound is anterolateral, it is best not to apply the plate through the traumatic wound. Instead, after wound débride-

ment, a formal anterolateral approach to the humerus should be used.

There are a number of arguments for primary surgical fixation of humeral fractures in a patient with polytrauma.[22,23] Most closed methods of treatment depend on the patient's being upright, allowing the weight of the arm to contribute to fracture stabilization. In a patient in the recumbent position, it is difficult to control the fracture with closed treatment. In addition, patients with concomitant chest injury are poor candidates for the use of a sling and swath. In such circumstances, plate fixation is an option for stabilization of the fracture without interfering with the general treatment of the patient. Rigid internal fixation should be obtained so that the extremity does not require protection from movement and the patient can be mobilized early.

Concomitant fractures of the humerus and both bones of the forearm occur in a small percentage of patients, and most are associated with extensive soft-tissue injury.[24] Early mobilization of the elbow helps to maintain elbow function, and the forearm fractures accompanying such extensive skeletal injury usually are treated with internal fixation. Therefore, in most situations, primary internal stabilization of the humerus is indicated. Internal fixation of the humerus should be performed at the same time as internal fixation of the radius and ulna.

Fractures of the humerus associated with dislocation of the glenohumeral joint or dislocation of the elbow pose a difficult treatment problem. Early mobilization of the injured joint after reduction is important for optimal rehabilitation of the joint and a maximum useful range of motion. Mobilization usually requires the humerus to be stable. Rigid plate fixation provides stability to the humerus so that the injured joint can be properly treated.

A radial nerve palsy sustained concomitantly with a humeral fracture is not an indication for exploration of the nerve or for internal fixation of the fracture. Conversely, when a radial nerve palsy develops while the fracture is being reduced, the radial nerve should be explored. Whenever the nerve is explored and the humerus is not healed, internal fixation of the humerus is recommended. In addition, patients with associated brachial plexus injury should have internal fixation.[25] Stabilization of the humerus in this case permits earlier rehabilitation of the injured extremity and shortens the hospital stay.

A patient with a humeral shaft fracture and a lower limb injury who requires crutches or a walker to walk usually is mobilized more quickly after surgical stabilization of the upper limb injury. An axially stable fixation with supplementary fixation with a plaster cast or a brace permits some weight to be taken through the volar surface of the forearm and the medial aspect of the arm. Transverse fractures or spiral fractures with anatomic reduction and good lag-screw fixation are best suited for plate fixation and for shared weight bearing. Internal fixation of one or both humeral fractures with a plate and screws is recommended for a patient who has sustained a bilateral humeral fracture.[26] Self-care is improved, and the patient can be independent.

Impending or established pathologic fracture due to metastatic cancer is a well-recognized indication for surgical treatment.[27] The use of plate fixation in these circumstances permits active use of the limb as well as direct treatment of the metastatic lesion by curettage. Supplemental methylmethacrylate may be needed to improve the fixation of the screws to the bone. Intramedullary fixators can be used, but they do not allow removal of the metastatic deposits. Removal of the metastatic deposits is not always recommended, but occasionally it is necessary. If intramedullary fixators are used for a pathologic fracture due to metastatic cancer, the fixation should be rigid.

Segmental fractures occasionally are best treated with internal fixation. The location of the segmental fractures is an important factor in the selection of the most appropriate type of fixation. Intramedullary fixation is not effective for fractures in the proximal or distal quarter of the humerus; when associated with a diaphyseal fracture, these segmental injuries are best treated by plate fixation. Fractures occurring in the proximal and distal quarters without an intervening diaphyseal fracture should be treated separately. They are exposed through separate incisions and fixed with separate plates.[28]

Segmental fractures confined to the middle half of the humerus are ideal for intramedullary nail fixation.[21,29-31] The ability to achieve a satisfactory closed reduction of both fractures is a prerequisite for the use of intramedullary fixators and, if such a reduction cannot be obtained, plate fixation is a better option.[32]

The final indication for internal fixation is failure of closed treatment, which includes the inability to obtain or maintain a satisfactory closed reduction, the inability of the patient to tolerate external splinting, and a delayed union or nonunion.[33] Closed treatment of a transverse fracture with a gap often fails because the gap increases as a result of the distraction of the fracture fragments by the weight of the arm.[11,12] Closed treatment also often fails in obese patients[22] or in women with large breasts because the arm cannot be brought to the side without angulating the fracture. Furthermore, in obese patients, the plaster irritates the skin in the axilla. Under these circumstances, early recognition of the failure of the closed treatment and subsequent surgical treatment are recommended. Plate fixation is preferred for these patients.

A full discussion of delayed union and nonunion of the humerus is beyond the scope of this article;[5,11,21,34,35] however, for patients in whom union has not been obtained by 12 to 16 weeks after good closed treatment, surgical intervention should be considered. Direct exposure of the fracture site with careful protection of the radial nerve, rigid fixation, and onlay circumferential cancellous bone-grafting will result in satisfactory healing in the majority of these patients.[36]

The best reason to use a plate is that it allows control of the fracture. With the use of a plate and screws, the rotation, length, and angulation of the humeral diaphysis are controlled. The quality of reduction is better with a plate and screws than with other methods of surgical treatment. The use of a plate allows injury to the adjacent joints to be avoided, and it minimizes morbidity, particularly that related to the shoulder. Plate fixation does require a wide surgical exposure. Exposing the fracture, obtaining the reduction, and securing the fixation require more time than that needed for intramedullary fixation. There is an increased prevalence of nerve injury and a relatively high prevalence of failure of fixation in patients in whom the quality of the bone is not ideal, particularly in those with extensive comminution or osteopenia.

Randomized, controlled trials comparing plate fixation with intramedullary fixators have produced contradictory results.[19,30,37-40] Both techniques, if performed properly, provide satisfactory outcomes for most patients.[39] The question for the surgeon is which technique is the most effective in his or her hands for the management of a particular fracture pattern. Another consideration is that a nonunion after treatment with intramedullary nailing poses a more difficult problem than does nonunion after plate fixation.[41,42] Therefore, plate fixation often remains the primary choice for patients in whom surgical fixation is thought to be appropriate.

Intramedullary Nailing

Flexible or semirigid pins, usually several of them, can be used for intramedullary fixation. The operation can be done with the patient in the supine, lateral decubitus, or beach chair position. A closed reduction is done and confirmed with the use of image intensification. For antegrade insertion, an incision is made over the greater tuberosity of the humerus with splitting of the proximal portion of the deltoid muscle. The greater tuberosity is palpated, and a drill hole of appropriate diameter is made at the insertion of the rotator cuff on the greater tuberosity. A flexible nail, such as an Ender nail, of appropriate length

and diameter is then introduced through this drill hole into the proximal fragment and is directed distally, under image intensification, to the fracture site.[43] With the fracture reduced, the nail is advanced across the fracture site into the distal fragment. A stiffer, straight, or slightly bent nail such as a Rush rod also may be used. Rush rods have a tendency to displace the distal fragment into varus alignment as the rod is inserted across the fracture site. This should be avoided. It is possible to insert two or more small-diameter rods across the fracture. Rotational stability is improved by using different insertion points in the proximal portion of the humerus and by spreading the rods in the distal fragment. These types of intramedullary fixation are usually supplemented by some form of external immobilization to control rotation at the fracture site.

Problems associated with this technique include limited rotational stability, inability to control shortening of the humerus, and interference with shoulder function as a result of rotator cuff impingement or subacromial impingement of proximally migrated pins. Although the lack of rotational stability may be compensated for by the use of external immobilization, shortening cannot be addressed by external immobilization. With shortening, proximal pin migration may occur with a subsequent increase in shoulder problems.

Fixation by means of retrograde pin insertion has been used to avoid problems around the shoulder that occur as a result of antegrade pin insertion.[26,44] Small-diameter flexible pins are recommended for this technique.[45,46] The patient is positioned in the supine or lateral decubitus position. With the arm prepared and draped free, a midline incision is made over the posterior aspect of the distal part of the humerus. The muscle fibers of the triceps are split longitudinally, exposing the humerus just proximal to the olecranon fossa. A

window approximately 1 cm wide and 3 cm long is made in the posterior cortex of the humerus, beginning just proximal to the olecranon fossa, and the nails are inserted in a retrograde fashion, crossing the fracture site and continuing into the proximal portion of the humerus. The use of an image intensifier is essential for this technique to be carried out safely and expeditiously.[47] Problems with retrograde nail insertion include difficult access to the narrow medullary canal in the distal part of the humerus, irritation of the triceps by pin prominence, a decreased range of motion of the elbow, and fracture at the level of the nail insertion site.[48]

Intramedullary fixation with a larger device allowing proximal and distal locking has been developed. This concept is attractive because the problems of maintaining length and control of rotation can be overcome. However, initial efforts have met with a number of problems.[49,50] The nails were straight, necessitating a relatively medial insertion point for antegrade nailing. This medial insertion point interfered both with the rotator cuff and with the articular surface of the humerus. The increased diameter of the nail, which was necessary to obtain locking, led to a considerably larger entry portal in the proximal portion of the humerus, contributing to the postoperative problems associated with shoulder function.[33] Distal locking was also a problem with early versions of these intramedullary nails. The use of an expansion bolt to deploy fins on the distal end of the nail proved to be inadequate to control rotation in many patients;[32] side-to-side locking is impractical by virtue of the shape of the distal part of the humerus[21] (which also precludes effective intramedullary reaming into the metaphysis of the distal fragment). This necessitated AP locking with an attendant risk to the neurovascular structures in the front of the arm as well as interference with the biceps and brachialis muscles.[51]

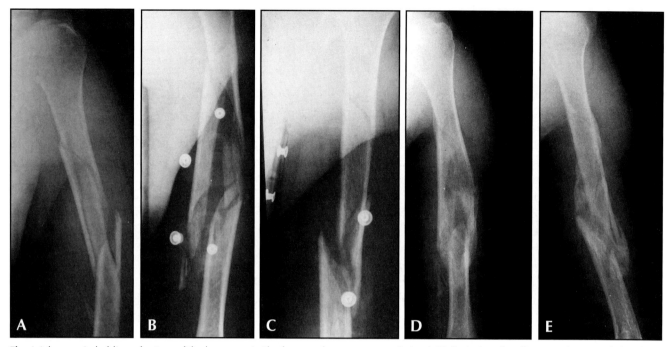

Fig. 4 A long, spiral oblique fracture of the humerus. **A,** The fracture shows varus angulation initially, before the elbow can be extended and gravity and function can align the fragments. **B** and **C,** With early function and adequate alignment afforded by gravity while the fracture is still mobile, the angulation is corrected. **D** and **E,** Final healing occurred with good alignment in both the frontal and the sagittal planes.

In later designs, the nails have had a smaller diameter with smaller locking screws and have permitted the use of multidirectional locking screws in the proximal fragment to avoid the possibility of iatrogenic injury to the axillary nerve.[52]

The success of intramedullary nailing of the humerus should be measured by both fracture union and functional outcome. However, reports in the literature have been contradictory, and few have directly compared intramedullary nail fixation with other forms of fracture treatment. In reports in which plate fixation has been directly compared with intramedullary fixation, the rate of complications associated with locked intramedullary nails appears to be higher than that associated with plate fixation.[19] The increase in complications after intramedullary nailing appears to be related primarily to the rates of union, which are somewhat lower than those after plate fixation, and to a substantial increase in functional symptoms, such as shoulder pain and stiffness.[52,53] Complications such as radial nerve palsy, infection, delayed union, and failure of fixation appear to occur at a similar rate after both types of fixation.

The indications for nailing are limited. Intramedullary nail fixation has a place in the management of pathologic fractures of the humerus, particularly when there is more than one metastatic deposit within the bone.[38,54,55] It is also useful in the management of comminuted and segmental humeral shaft fractures that require surgical treatment.

Functional Bracing of Humeral Fractures

The principles behind functional bracing of humeral fractures are that, in most patients, gravity results in adequate alignment of the fractured bone, and physiologically induced motion at the fracture site promotes osteogenesis.[56-62] Functional braces do not immobilize the fracture; they simply stiffen the upper arm through soft-tissue compression. The orthopaedic community has long recognized that stabilization of humeral diaphyseal fractures in a cast results in union in the vast majority of patients. The hanging cast and coaptation splint, which have been popular for several decades, are the methods of choice of most orthopaedists. Functional bracing often fails to restore anatomic alignment of fracture fragments, and varus angulation after healing is common. However, the angulation is, in almost all instances, cosmetically and functionally acceptable.[7,58-63] The high prevalence of union[57,60,63-66] and the avoidance of infection, which can occur after surgery, imply an earlier return to the activities of daily living and a lower overall cost of care.

The fact that functional bracing does not immobilize the joints adjacent to the fracture makes early restoration of motion possible. Rotatory deformities are also rarely encountered, perhaps because of the corrective effect of muscular forces associated with the early introduction of function.[60] As is true with all methods of treatment, functional bracing is not applicable to all diaphyseal humeral fractures. The method has its appropriate indications, and the management protocol requires a clear understanding by the treating physician as well as the cooperation of the patient.

Functional bracing requires that the patient be able to stand or sit erect. In the absence of gravity acting on the injured extremity, correction of angular deformities usually is not possible. Conversely, most isolated closed diaphyseal fractures, regardless of their geometry, can be treated with functional bracing. However, transverse fractures, particularly if they are nondisplaced, are the ones most likely to develop angular deformity. In the case of comminuted or oblique fractures, the muscle contractions produce desirable positioning at the fracture site without creating permanent deformity (Fig. 4).

The level of the fracture does not influence the ultimate result. Fractures at various levels heal at the same speed and with similar degrees of angulation. The fact that the brace does not fully cover every proximal or distal fragment is irrelevant. As long as the soft tissues of the extremity are compressed by the adjustable brace and the arm hangs freely at the side of the body, the desirable environment for healing is present. The presence of a radial nerve palsy in association with a closed fracture is not a contraindication to the use of functional bracing if the palsy appeared concomitantly with the injury. The probability of spontaneous recovery is very high.[57,59,61-63,65] Because the arm is allowed to hang at the side of the body in a normal fashion, there is no need to hold the wrist in a cock-up splint. Gravity brings the wrist into a neutral position and prevents a flexion contracture of the joint. Active use of the wrist and fingers is recommended.

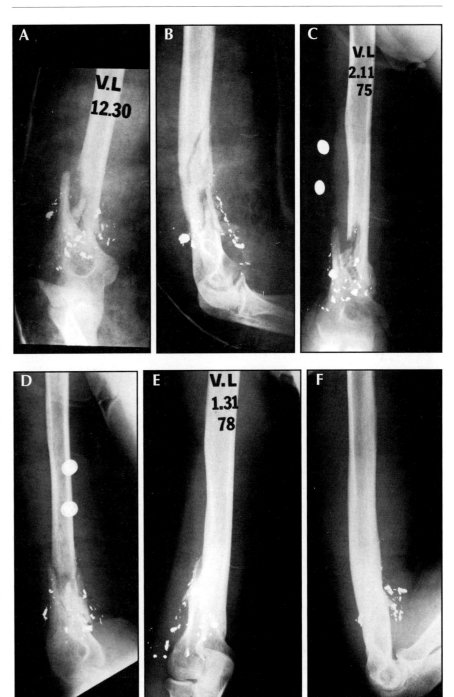

Fig. 5 A patient with a low-velocity gunshot wound in the distal part of the humerus. **A** and **B,** The wound was cleaned, and the arm was immobilized in a cast for 3 weeks. **C** and **D,** Early function in the brace improved the alignment. **E** and **F,** Final healing was uneventful.

Open fractures produced by low-velocity projectiles and associated with a minimal or moderate degree of soft-tissue damage are usually good candidates for functional bracing (Fig. 5). Local cleaning of the wound and antibiotic prophylaxis are recommended.

Obesity in itself is not a contraindication. Angular deformities are more severe in obese patients. However, the larger

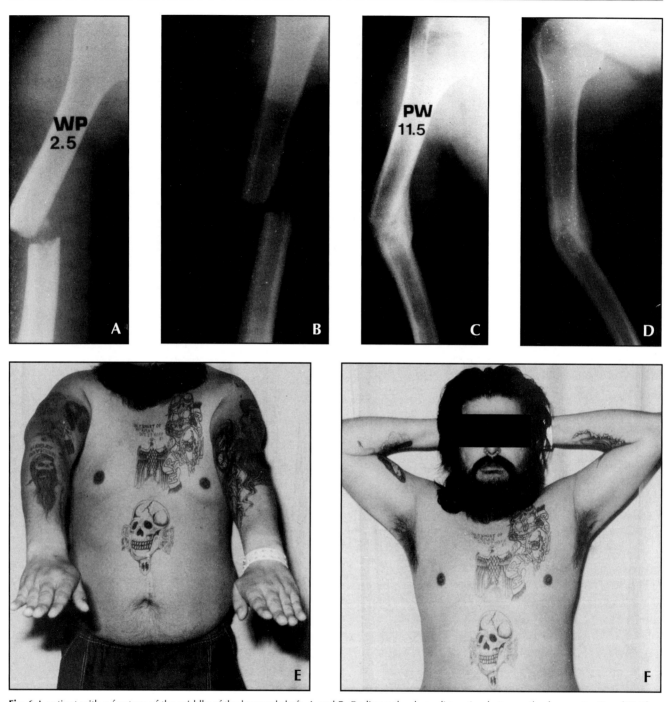

Fig. 6 A patient with a fracture of the middle of the humeral shaft. **A** and **B,** Radiographs show distraction between the fragments. **C** and **D,** The patient was lost to follow-up for several months, and the fracture healed with an unacceptable degree of angulation radiographically. **E** and **F,** The functional and cosmetic results were acceptable, demonstrating the wide tolerance for imperfect alignment in the humerus.

amount of adipose tissue usually camouflages the deformities effectively (Fig. 6).

Functional bracing is contraindicated in certain circumstances. Fractures with axial distraction between the fragments suggest a high degree of soft-tissue damage. These fractures are more likely to have a delayed union or nonunion. Surgical stabilization is usually the treatment of choice. Open fractures with major soft-tissue damage preclude successful management with functional bracing, particularly when there is an associated peripheral nerve injury. Other treatment modalities are more appropriate. Patients with bilateral humeral fractures are usually better managed with surgical stabilization if the treating surgeon has the necessary expertise. Patients with polytrauma who are unable to walk are best treated by surgical stabilization. Functional bracing is likely to result in unacceptable angular deformities in such patients. Fractures associated with vascular injuries that require surgical repair usually should be internally stabilized. However, if surgical stabilization is not done at the time that the injured vessels are surgically repaired, delayed bracing can be used.

Diaphyseal humeral fractures managed with functional bracing are initially stabilized in a hanging cast or coaptation splint. As soon as possible after the application of the stabilizing device, pendulum exercises should be initiated to prevent or lessen long-lasting limitation of motion of the shoulder. The use of a collar and cuff is essential to provide comfort and to prevent AP deformity.

The initial cast is removed when the symptoms allow. This may be as early as a few days or as late as 2 weeks after application of the cast. The brace must be adjustable to ensure that the soft tissues of the arm can be compressed as swelling decreases and atrophy ensues (Fig. 7). Frequent tightening of the Velcro straps is necessary during the first 2 weeks. Cylindrical sleeves have a tendency to slide distally and irritate the antecubital space as the circumference of the arm decreases. The brace should begin approximately 1 in (2.5 cm) distal to the axilla and should terminate distally 1 in proximal to the humeral condyles. Supra-acromial and supracondylar humeral extensions are not necessary. Patients should be able to put the brace on and take it off easily by themselves.

With the collar and cuff in place, pendulum exercises are continued. The patient should remove the arm from the sling several times a day to passively flex and extend the elbow, emphasizing

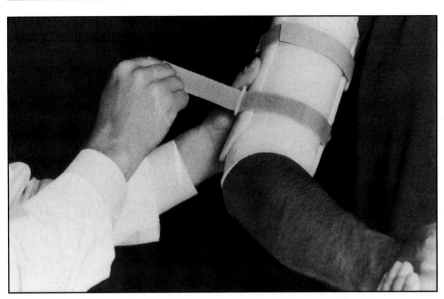

Fig. 7 The functional brace must be adjustable to maintain soft-tissue compression (which encourages function of the extremity and provides protection to the soft tissues) and to maintain fit and suspension to the limb.

extension of the joint. Active exercises are started as soon as symptoms allow. Active abduction and elevation of the shoulder must be avoided because they may produce angular deformities. Such exercises may be conducted only after the fracture has become clinically stable. Leaning on the elbow should be avoided because it is likely to cause varus angulation, especially of transverse, non-displaced fractures. Active contraction of the biceps and triceps assists in correcting the inferior subluxation of the shoulder that is occasionally seen in patients with a fracture of the proximal third of the humerus. Most patients fully extend the elbow 1 week after the application of the brace. At this time, the pendulum exercises are continued without the collar and cuff. Use of the collar and cuff may be discontinued if the patient wishes. However, use of the collar and cuff during recumbency is recommended until clinical union of the fracture has taken place. Use of the brace is permanently discontinued when union of the fracture has been confirmed on clinical and radiographic examination.

The rate of nonunion reported in the literature in recent years has ranged from 1% to 5.8%.[59,62-66] In one study,[61] the rate of nonunion was 1.5% for closed fractures, with the brace removed between 10 and 13 weeks, and 5.8% for open fractures.

Summary

All of the current modalities have a place in the treatment of diaphyseal humeral fractures. Functional bracing renders a high rate of union and seems to be a safe method of treatment for most closed fractures. Type II and III open fractures seem to respond best to plate fixation or external fixation, particularly when there are associated neural or vascular pathologic findings. Patients with polytrauma who are unable to walk are also best treated with plate fixation. Plate fixation is also the best method of treatment when adequate alignment cannot be obtained with nonsurgical methods. Intramedullary nailing remains controversial because its complication rate is higher than that associated with either plate fixation or functional bracing.

None of the treatments described is a panacea, and complications may occur with each one of them. An appropriate appreciation of the biologic response to the three modalities; an understanding of the indications, contraindications, and possible complications of the treatments; and a mastery of the techniques of application are essential for the attainment of satisfactory clinical results.

References

1. Perren SM: Physical and biological aspects of fracture healing with special reference to internal fixation. *Clin Orthop* 1979;138:175-196.

2. Rahn BA, Gallinaro P, Baltensperger A, Perren SM: Primary bone healing: An experimental study in the rabbit. *J Bone Joint Surg Am* 1971; 53:783-786.

3. Uhthoff HK, Dubuc FL: Bone structure changes in the dog under rigid internal fixation. *Clin Orthop* 1971;81:165-170.

4. Kato S, Latta LL, Malinin T: The weakest link in the bone-plate-fracture system: Changes with time, in Harvey JP, Games RF (eds): *Bone Plates*. Philadelphia, PA, ASTM, 1994, vol STP 1200.

5. Otsuka NY, McKee MD, Liew A, et al: The effect of comorbidity and duration of nonunion on outcome after surgical treatment for nonunion of the humerus. *J Shoulder Elbow Surg* 1998;7:127-133.

6. Perren SM, Rahn BA: Biomechanics of fracture healing: I. Historical review and mechanical aspects of internal fixation. *Orthop Survey* 1978;2:108-143.

7. Sarmiento A, Latta LL, Tarr RR: Principles of fracture healing: Part II. The effects of function in fracture healing and stability. *Instr Course Lect* 1984;33:83-106.

8. Milner JC, Rhinelander FW: Compression fixation and primary bone healing. *Surg Forum* 1968;19:453-456.

9. Sarmiento A, Latta LL (eds): *Functional Fracture Bracing: Tibia, Humerus, and Ulna*. Berlin, Germany, Springer-Verlag, 1995.

10. Balfour GW, Marrero CE: Fracture brace for the treatment of humerus shaft fractures caused by gunshot wounds. *Orthop Clin North Am* 1995;26:55-63.

11. Foulk DA, Szabo RM: Diaphyseal humerus fractures: Natural history and occurrence of nonunion. *Orthopedics* 1995;18:333-335.

12. Tytherleigh-Strong G, Walls N, McQueen MM: The epidemiology of humeral shaft fractures. *J Bone Joint Surg Br* 1998;80:249-253.

13. Mulier T, Seligson D, Sioen W, van den Bergh J, Reynaert P: Operative treatment of humeral shaft fractures. *Acta Orthop Belg* 1997;63: 170-177.

14. Wisniewski TF, Radziejowski MJ: Gunshot fractures of the humeral shaft treated with external fixation. *J Orthop Trauma* 1996;10: 273-278.

15. Mills WJ, Hanel DP, Smith DG: Lateral approach to the humeral shaft: An alternative approach for fracture treatment. *J Orthop Trauma* 1996;10:81-86.

16. Blum J, Rommens PM: Surgical approaches to the humeral shaft. *Acta Chir Belg* 1997;97: 237-243.

17. Moran MC: Modified lateral approach to the distal humerus for internal fixation. *Clin Orthop* 1997;340:190-197.

18. Müller ME, Perren SM, Allgöwer M (eds): *Manual of Internal Fixation: Techniques Recommended by the AO-ASIF Group*, ed 3. Berlin, Germany, Springer-Verlag, 1991.

19. Modabber MR, Jupiter JB: Operative management of diaphyseal fractures of the humerus: Plate versus nail. *Clin Orthop* 1998;347:93-104.

20. Simon JA, Dennis MG, Kummer FJ, Koval KJ: Schuhli augmentation of plate and screw fixation for humeral shaft fractures: A laboratory study. *J Orthop Trauma* 1999;13:196-199.

21. Heim D, Herkert F, Hess P Regazzoni P: Surgical treatment of humeral shaft fractures: The Basel experience. *J Trauma* 1993;35: 226-232.

22. Jensen AT, Rasmussen S: Being overweight and multiple fractures are indications for operative treatment of humeral shaft fractures. *Injury* 1995;26:263-264.

23. Bleeker WA, Nijsten MW, ten Duis HJ: Treatment of humeral shaft fractures related to associated injuries: A retrospective study of 237 patients. *Acta Orthop Scand* 1991;62:148-153.

24. Ward EF, Savoie FH, Hughes JL: Fractures of the diaphyseal humerus, in Browner BD, Jupiter JB, Levine AM, Trafton PG (eds): *Skeletal Trauma: Fractures, Dislocations, Ligamentous Injuries*. Philadelphia, PA, WB Saunders, 1992, vol 2, pp 1177-1200.

25. Brien WW, Gellman H, Becker V, Garland DE, Waters DL, Wiss DA: Management of fractures of the humerus in patients who have an injury of the ipsilateral brachial plexus. *J Bone Joint Surg Am* 1990;72:1208-1210.

26. Lin J, Inoue N, Valdevit A, Hang YS, Hou SM, Chao EY: Biomechanical comparison of antegrade and retrograde nailing of humeral shaft fracture. *Clin Orthop* 1998;351:203-213.

27. Dabezies EJ, Banta CJ II, Murphy CP, d'Ambrosia RD: Plate fixation of the humeral shaft for acute fractures, with and without radial nerve injuries. *J Orthop Trauma* 1992;6:10-13.

28. Gill DR, Torchia ME: The spiral compression plate for proximal humeral shaft nonunion: A case report and description of a new technique. *J Orthop Trauma* 1999;13:141-144.

29. Karas EH, Strauss E, Sohail S: Surgical stabilization of humeral shaft fractures due to gunshot wounds. *Orthop Clin North Am* 1995; 26:65-73.

30. Lin J: Treatment of humeral shaft fractures with humeral locked nail and comparison with plate fixation. *J Trauma* 1998;44:859-864.

31. Rodriguez-Merchan EC: Compression plating versus Hackethal nailing in closed humeral shaft fractures failing nonoperative reduction. *J Orthop Trauma* 1995;9:194-197.

32. Riemer BL, Foglesong ME, Burke CJ III, Butterfield SL: Complications of Seidel intramedullary nailing of narrow diameter humeral diaphyseal fractures. *Orthopedics* 1994; 17:19-29.

33. Thomsen NO, Mikkelsen JB, Svendsen RN, Skovgaard N, Jensen CH, Jorgensen U: Interlocking nailing of humeral shaft fractures. *J Orthop Sci* 1998;3:199-203.

34. Jupiter JB, von Deck M: Ununited humeral diaphyses. *J Shoulder Elbow Surg* 1998;7: 644-653.

35. Wu CC, Shih CH: Treatment for nonunion of the shaft of the humerus: Comparison of plates and Seidel interlocking nails. *Can J Surg* 1992; 35:661-665.

36. Ring D, Perey BH, Jupiter JB: The functional outcome of operative treatment of ununited fractures of the humeral diaphysis in older patients. *J Bone Joint Surg Am* 1999;81: 177-190.

37. Chiu FY, Chen CM, Lin CF, Lo WH, Huang YL, Chen TH: Closed humeral shaft fractures: A prospective evaluation of surgical treatment. *J Trauma* 1997;43:947-951.

38. Dijkstra S, Stapert J, Boxma H, Wiggers T: Treatment of pathological fractures of the humeral shaft due to bone metastases: A comparison of intramedullary locking nail and plate osteosynthesis with adjunctive bone cement. *Eur J Surg Oncol* 1996;22:621-626.

39. Hee HT, Low BY, See HF: Surgical results of open reduction and plating of humeral shaft fractures. *Ann Acad Med Singapore* 1998;27: 772-775.

40. Wade RH: Letter: Closed humeral shaft fractures: A prospective evaluation of surgical treatment. *J Trauma* 1998;44:1115.

41. Emmerson KP, Sher JL: A method of treatment of non-union of humeral shaft fractures following treatment by locked intramedullary nail: A report of three cases. *Injury* 1998;29: 550-552.

42. McKee MD, Miranda MA, Riemer BL, et al: Management of humeral nonunion after the failure of locking intramedullary nails. *J Orthop Trauma* 1996;10:492-499.

43. Liebergall M, Jaber S, Laster M, Abu-Snieneh K, Mattan Y, Segal D: Ender nailing of acute humeral shaft fractures in multiple injuries. *Injury* 1997;28:577-580.

44. Crates J, Whittle AP: Antegrade interlocking nailing of acute humeral shaft fractures. *Clin Orthop* 1998;350:40-50.

45. Rodriguez-Merchan EC: Hackethal nailing in closed transverse humeral shaft fractures after failed manipulation. *Int Orthop* 1996;20: 134-136.

46. Zatti G, Teli M, Ferrario A, Cherubino P: Treatment of closed humeral shaft fractures with intramedullary elastic nails. *J Trauma* 1998;45:1046-1050.

47. Shazar N, Brumback RJ, Vanco B: Treatment of humeral fractures by closed reduction and retrograde intramedullary Ender nails. *Orthopedics* 1998;21:641-646.

48. Rommens PM, Blum J, Runkel M: Retrograde nailing of humeral shaft fractures. *Clin Orthop* 1998;350:26-39.

49. Hems TE, Bhullar TP: Interlocking nailing of humeral shaft fractures: The Oxford experience 1991 to 1994. *Injury* 1996;27:485-489.

50. Svend-Hansen H, Skettrup M, Rathcke MW: Complications using the Seidel intramedullary humeral nail: Outcome in 31 patients. *Acta Orthop Belg* 1998;64:291-295.

51. Rupp RE, Chrissos MG, Ebraheim NA: The risk of neurovascular injury with distal locking screws of humeral intramedullary nails. *Orthopedics* 1996;19:593-595.

52. Lin J, Hou SM, Inoue N, Chao EY, Hang YS: Anatomic considerations of locked humeral nailing. *Clin Orthop* 1999;368:247-254.

53. Flinkkila T, Hyvonen P, Lakovaara M, Linden T, Ristiniemi J, Hamalainen M: Intramedullary nailing of humeral shaft fractures: A retrospective study of 126 cases. *Acta Orthop Scand* 1999;70:133-136.

54. Damron TA, Rock MG, Choudhury SN, Grabowski JJ, An KN: Biomechanical analysis of prophylactic fixation for middle third humeral impending pathologic fractures. *Clin Orthop* 1999;363:240-248.

55. Flinkkila T, Hyvonen P, Leppilahti J, Hamalainen M: Pathological fractures of the humeral shaft. *Ann Chir Gynaecol* 1998;87:321-324.

56. Latta LL, Sarmiento A, Tarr RR: The rationale of functional bracing of fractures. *Clin Orthop* 1980;146:28-36.

57. Sarmiento A, Kinman PB, Galvin EG, Schmitt RH, Phillips JG: Functional bracing of fractures of the shaft of the humerus. *J Bone Joint Surg Am* 1977;59:596-601.

58. Sarmiento A, Mullis DL, Latta LL, Tarr RR, Alvarez R: A quantitative comparative analysis of fracture healing under the influence of compression plating vs. closed weight-bearing treatment. *Clin Orthop* 1980;149:232-239.

59. Sarmiento A, Horowitch A, Aboulafia A, Vangsness CT: Functional bracing for comminuted extra-articular fractures of the distal third of the humerus. *J Bone Joint Surg Br* 1990;72:283-287.

60. Sarmiento A, Latta LL: Functional fracture bracing. *J Am Acad Orthop Surg* 1999;7:66-75.

61. Sarmiento A, Zagorski JB, Zych GA, Latta LL, Capps CA: Functional bracing for the treatment of fractures of the humeral diaphysis. *J Bone Joint Surg Am* 2000;82:478-486.

62. Sharma VK, Jain AK, Gupta RK, Tyagi AK, Sethi PK: Non-operative treatment of fractures of the humeral shaft: A comparative study. *J Indian Med Assoc* 1991;89:157-160.

63. Zagorski JB, Latta LL, Zych GA, Finnieston AR: Diaphyseal fractures of the humerus: Treatment with prefabricated braces. *J Bone Joint Surg Am* 1988;70:607-610.

64. Klestil T, Rangger C, Kathrein A, Brenner E, Beck E: The conservative and surgical therapy of traumatic humeral shaft fractures [German]. *Chirurg* 1997;68:1132-1136.

65. Ostermann PAW, Ekkernkamp A, Muhr G: Abstract: Functional bracing of shaft fractures of the humerus: An analysis of 195 cases. *60th Annual Meeting Proceedings*, Rosemont, IL, American Academy of Orthopaedic Surgeons, 1993, p 69.

66. Zych GA, Zagorski JB, Latta LL: Current concepts in fracture bracing: Part I. Upper extremity. *Orthop Surg Update* 1986;18:4.

Nonprosthetic Management of Proximal Humeral Fractures

Joseph P. Iannotti, MD, PhD
Matthew L. Ramsey, MD
Gerald R. Williams, Jr, MD
Jon J.P. Warner, MD

Abstract

Many proximal humeral fractures can be treated without the need for hemiarthroplasty. Treatment choice is affected by fracture location and pattern, as well as by patient factors including age, activity level, quality of bone, and ability to comply with a regimen of therapy. Successful diagnosis and treatment of proximal humeral fractures is dependent on good-quality radiographs, but in some cases, intraoperative assessment of the fracture pattern is required for a complete and accurate diagnosis of the fracture pattern and severity. A discussion of nonsurgical and surgical treatment options and techniques needed to achieve anatomic reduction and stable fixation is important.

Indications and Diagnosis

Most proximal humeral fractures are not sufficiently displaced or angulated to require surgical management. It is estimated that 20% of all proximal humeral fractures should be treated surgically,[1] and humeral head replacement is the preferred method of treatment of many of those fractures. An indication for hemiarthroplasty is the classic four-part fracture or four-part fracture-

One or more of the authors or the departments with which they are affiliated have received something of value from a commercial or other party related directly or indirectly to the subject of this chapter.

dislocation, particularly when the articular segment of the humeral head is separated from the tuberosities and the humeral shaft, because of the expected high risk of osteonecrosis. Other indications for hemiarthroplasty are fragmentation of the articular surface and severe osteoporosis. On the other hand, reduction and internal fixation can be accomplished for displaced fractures associated with an intact humeral head with good quality bone. The indications for open or closed reduction and internal fixation are related to the fracture pattern, the quality of the bone, the status of the rotator cuff, and the age and activity level of the patient. The goal of reduction and fixation of

a proximal humeral fracture is to obtain nearly anatomic reduction and stable fixation to allow an early range of motion.[2] Recently, there has been an emphasis on the use of less invasive open procedures for reduction and fixation, thereby minimizing periarticular scarring and decreasing the risk of vascular insult to the articular humeral head segment from the surgical exposure.[3-5]

Accurate diagnosis and effective management of proximal humeral fractures require good quality radiographs in at least two orthogonal planes. In general, basic radiographs include an AP view, an axillary view, and a scapular lateral (Y) view. Sometimes, in an emergency department setting, it is not easy to obtain all three of these views with sufficient quality to make a clear diagnosis and define the best treatment options. A CT scan can be of value when the plain radiographs do not clearly define the size of the fragments or the degree of displacement. Although MRI is rarely needed, it is indicated when the patient has symptoms suggestive of a preinjury shoulder disorder such as a rotator cuff tear. It can

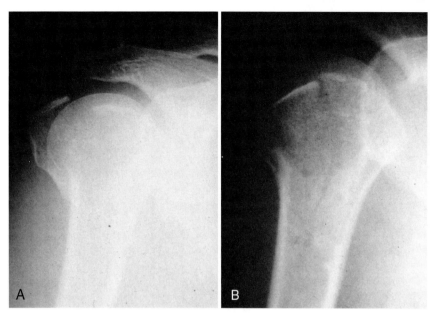

Figure 1 A small fragment of the greater tuberosity treated with a figure-of-8 suture technique through a deltoid-splitting incision. Sutures are passed through the tendon-bone insertion of the rotator cuff and then into the diaphyseal cortical bone. **A,** Preoperative radiograph. **B,** Postoperative radiograph.

also be useful in the evaluation of the rotator cuff when the patient has persistent pain after the fracture has healed.

Isolated Fracture of the Greater Tuberosity

Fractures of the greater tuberosity can be associated with an acute glenohumeral dislocation or a tear of the rotator cuff. When associated with a glenohumeral dislocation, the greater tuberosity fracture fragment is usually small and lies in a satisfactory position after reduction of the dislocation of the humeral head. In these cases, the size of the fragment, the amount of residual displacement, and the presence of a full-thickness rotator cuff tear determine the need for surgical management. In Neer's review of displaced proximal humeral fractures, 1 cm or more of displacement was considered an indication for surgical management.[1,6] This general guideline may not apply to all cases of greater tuberosity fracture. Nonsurgical treatment is usually recommended for such fractures that have less than 0.5 cm of superior displacement or less than 1 cm of posterior displacement. The difference between the amount of allowable superior displacement and the amount of allowable posterior displacement is because of the greater likelihood of symptoms associated with subacromial impingement when there is superior displacement. Patient age and activity level influence the decision to reduce and internally fix a displaced fracture of the greater tuberosity as nonsurgically treated fractures are likely to cause more pain in active individuals.

Results of Surgery

Flatow and asssociates[7] evaluated the results in 12 patients in whom an isolated acute fracture of the greater tuberosity had been treated with open reduction and internal fixation with use of a deltoid-splitting approach and suture fixation. The results were uniformly good or excellent. In that study, 0.5 cm of superior displacement was considered to be a sufficient indication for open reduction and internal fixation.

Surgical Technique

The superior surgical approach, such as splitting of the deltoid, is ideal for smaller fracture fragments and for fractures associated with a rotator cuff tear. This approach allows direct exposure and repair of both the rotator cuff and the greater tuberosity (Figure 1). The innervation of the deltoid by the axillary nerve limits the distal extent of the superior approach to approximately 5 cm from the lateral aspect of the acromion. A large fracture fragment with diaphyseal extension is difficult to mobilize, reduce, and fix through the superior approach without undue risk to the axillary nerve and should be managed surgically through a deltopectoral approach. The deltopectoral approach enables distal placement of sutures, a plate, or screws into the fragment with less risk of injury to the axillary nerve. When a large fragment of the greater tuberosity is displaced posteriorly and is behind the humeral head, a bone hook can be used to pull the fragment into the surgical field. Then, placement of a traction suture into the rotator cuff to control and manipulate the fragment allows the fragment to be anatomically reduced to the proximal part of the humerus.

A fragment of the greater tuberosity is excised only when it is less than 1 cm in size. If the fragment is larger, excision makes rotator cuff repair very difficult, if not impossible. Therefore, most displaced fragments of the greater tuberosity should be saved and treated with open reduction and internal fixation. The method of fixation depends on several factors, including the size of the fragment, the quality of the bone, the degree of comminution, and the presence of an associated rotator cuff tear. Suture fixation with use of the rotator cuff for proximal fixation is preferable, particularly for smaller and comminuted fragments or for osteoporotic bone. Most fractures of the greater tuberosity are secured with a figure-of-8 suture as well as an intraosseous suture with No. 5 or larger nonabsorbable suture material. Cancellous bone screws can be used for large noncomminuted fragments when the bone is of good quality. Bone screw fixation is often supplemented with a figure-of-8 suture (Figure 2).

Malunions

Persistent pain as a result of malunion of the greater tuberosity can occur with as little as 0.5 cm of superior displacement. The symptoms result from subacromial impingement. Such subacromial pain can be treated with subacromial decompression if the displacement is less than 1 cm. If the displacement is minimal and the fragment is 1 cm or smaller in size, excision of the osseous prominence that is causing impingement followed by rotator cuff repair can yield a satisfactory result. When the greater tuberosity is displaced more than 1 cm, an osteotomy of the fragment is the preferred treatment (Figure 3). The fragment is then mobilized by dissection and release of scar tissue and the underlying capsule associated with the torn and scarred rotator cuff. Mobilization of the retracted rotator cuff tissue is required to reduce the greater tuberosity fragment to an anatomic position. Mobilization of the rotator cuff requires release of the rotator in-

terval and the underlying capsule at the site of the fracture.

Beredjiklian and associates[8] evaluated the results at an average of 44 months after surgical management of a proximal humeral malunion in 39 patients, 11 of whom had an isolated malunion of a fracture of the greater tuberosity. These 11 malunions were treated with a combination of osteotomy and fixation of the tuberosity or subacromial decompression and excision of a portion of the impinging fracture fragment. When the tuberosity was osteotomized, capsular release was required to obtain a full passive arc of motion and to achieve cuff repair. Nine patients had a satisfactory result. The results of the surgical management of malunions of the greater tuberosity have been reported to be less favorable than the results of reduction and fixation of acute fractures.[9] However, the results of surgical management of an isolated greater tuberosity malunion are generally more favorable than the results of surgical management of malunions that also involve the surgical neck or both tuberosities (three- and four-part malunions).

Surgical Neck Fractures

Surgical neck fractures are often undertreated and are associated with a relatively high risk of malunion or nonunion. Malunion can be fairly well tolerated if the relationship of the articular surface and the tuberosities is not distorted. Fracture classifications, although very good, tend to underestimate or overestimate the severity of the fractures because the quality of the bone or the health and understanding of the patient are not always considered.[1,10,11] With this in mind, one can define two distinct patient groups who should be treated with different approaches, even when the fracture is the same.[12]

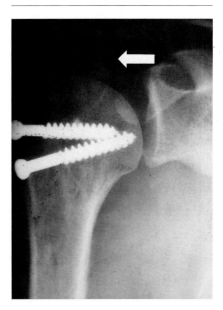

Figure 2 A fracture of the greater tuberosity associated with anterior dislocation of the humerus was treated with two screws with good fixation and an anatomic reduction. Three weeks after the surgery, the patient had a minor fall and sustained a fracture of the greater tuberosity proximal to the superior screw (*arrow*). Supplemental figure-of-8 fixation through the tendon-bone insertion reduces this complication with isolated screw fixation.

One group consists of young patients, more often male, who sustain high-energy trauma. This sometimes causes fragments to be impacted, but more often than not there is comminution. Typically, the bone quality is good with thick cortices and dense cancellous structure. The patient is usually able to comply with postoperative therapy. This group can be treated with a variety of surgical methods, including open reduction and internal fixation.

The second group consists of elderly patients, more often female. Minor trauma, such as a fall, causes impaction or comminution of thin cortices and porous cancellous bone. An unstable configuration of thin bone fragments is the rule. Elderly

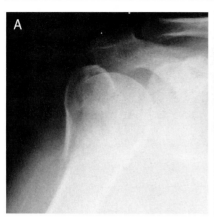
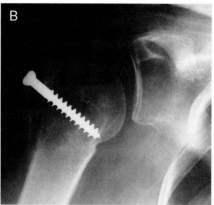

Figure 3 A, A radiograph of a malunion of the greater tuberosity. **B,** The malunion was treated with an osteotomy, reduction, and internal fixation.

patients sometimes have a poor understanding of the nature of the surgery or their role in postoperative rehabilitation, may have comorbid medical conditions that adversely affect the outcome, and often are frail and have a limited social support system to aid in postoperative recovery. Rigid internal fixation devices often fail when applied to thin porous bone, so fixation options may be more limited in these patients. In some cases, it is better to perform a hemiarthroplasty because of poor-quality bone.

Indications for stabilization of a surgical neck fracture include a displaced unstable fracture, multiple trauma, association with other upper extremity fractures, vascular injury, and a patient who will comply with a postoperative regimen.

Percutaneous internal fixation is an excellent option for a displaced two-part fracture that can be reduced with closed manipulation. While this technique can be difficult and tedious, it offers several advantages. There is almost no dissection of the soft tissues, which minimizes the risk of the articular segment becoming avascular.

Surgical Technique

The technique of closed reduction and percutaneous fixation of proximal humeral fractures was originally described by Bohler[13] for the treatment of fractures in children, but it has become a standard treatment method for displaced two-part fractures when the patient has good-quality bone and minimal comminution.

There are several pitfalls with this treatment. The first is improper patient selection. The ideal indication is a displaced two-part fracture of the surgical neck that can be reduced by closed manipulation with the patient under anesthesia. Marked comminution or the inability to reduce the fracture are contraindications to this technique. Another pitfall is related to patient positioning, draping, and fluoroscope placement in the operating room. The patient should be positioned on the operating table so that the arm is free to be manipulated and biplanar fluoroscopic image intensification is possible. While use of a fluoroscopic operating table is preferred by some, we prefer to place the patient supine onto a long bean bag that can be contoured around the

scapula, allowing the patient to be moved sufficiently laterally for C-arm visualization. The C-arm is brought in from a cranial direction, and a closed reduction, confirmed in two planes, is performed before preparation and draping of the shoulder for surgery (Figure 4).

A third pitfall is related to the reduction maneuver. Usually, two-part fractures have an apex anterior angulation. In such cases, some longitudinal traction is applied while posteriorly directed pressure on the humerus is used to correct the anterior angulation. It is helpful to have a sterile arm-positioner to hold the arm in place of an assistant. Once the reduction is confirmed, the arm is prepared in a sterile fashion and fixation pins are placed under image-intensification control. Two and a half-millimeter terminally threaded pins (AO; Synthes, Paoli, PA) are preferred for the internal fixation. The terminal threads of these pins help to prevent migration. In some patients, cannulated 4.0-mm screws can be used to fix the fracture.

The pinning technique has been described in detail previously.[14] After the fracture has been reduced, a pin is held in front of the shoulder and an image in the AP plane confirms proper orientation. A small stab incision is then made, and a straight clamp is used to spread the soft tissue down to the lateral humeral cortex. Two pins are then inserted, from inferior and lateral up into the articular fragment, and biplanar confirmation of proper pin placement is performed. Next, a third pin is placed from a more anterior and distal orientation. In the case of a three-part fracture with an unstable greater tuberosity fragment, one or two additional pins can be placed through this fragment and down into the humeral shaft (Figure 5). The pins are

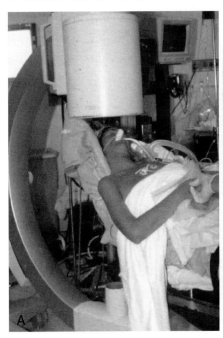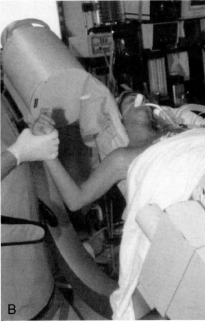

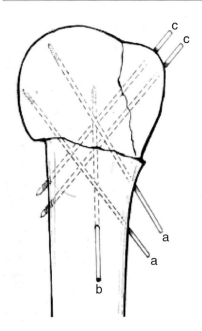

Figure 4 A, A patient positioned in the beach-chair position, with the body held in place with a large bean bag. The image intensifier is placed at the head of the table. **B,** The image intensifier can be positioned for both AP and axillary views of the proximal part of the humerus.

Figure 5 Two pins (a) are inserted from inferior and lateral up into the articular segment, and biplanar confirmation of proper placement is performed. A third pin (b) is placed from a more anterior and distal orientation. Two additional pins (c) can be used to stabilize a greater tuberosity fragment. (Reproduced with permission from Jaberg H, Warner JJ, Jakob RP: Percutaneous stabilization of unstable fractures of the humerus. *J Bone Joint Surg Am* 1992;74;508-515.)

trimmed so that they lie underneath the skin, and then all incisions are closed with sutures. The shoulder is placed in an immobilizer, which the patient wears for 4 to 6 weeks. Pendulum exercises are instituted immediately after treatment of two-part fractures. When a proximal pin was used to secure a greater tuberosity fragment, no motion is begun until 3 weeks after the surgery, at which time the proximal pins are removed and pendulum exercises are begun. The patient should be evaluated weekly in the physician's office for the first 2 postoperative weeks to ensure that the pins do not become prominent as the soft-tissue swelling around the pins subsides. Serial radiographs are made at each visit to monitor for movement of the pins. If the pins do become prominent, they should be trimmed back to a subcutaneous position. The pins are usually removed between 4 and 6 weeks

after surgery, either in the physician's office or in an operating room. After the pins have been removed, active motion is commenced. In general, stiffness is not a problem as the joint was not violated by surgical dissection.

Intramedullary fixation with use of combinations of rods, wires, and sutures to treat two-part fractures of the surgical neck has also been described.[15] Although this method has been successful when it has been performed properly by some surgeons, there are concerns about torsional rigidity and the risk of displacement. Furthermore, impingement by a prominent rod can be a problem (Figure 6).

An elderly patient with a two-part fracture of the surgical neck may have osteoporotic bone, precluding rigid fixation. To address this, Banco and associates[16] described a method of fixation termed the "parachute

technique." With this method, heavy sutures of 5-mm Dacron are placed through the rotator cuff tendons and then through drill holes in the humeral shaft distal to the fracture so that stability is achieved through impaction and compression of the fracture (Figure 7).

A displaced comminuted surgical neck fracture associated with good-quality bone can be treated successfully with a special blade-plate (Figure 8). Preoperative planning is essential, especially when there is extensive comminution, so that length can be restored. Long arm radiographs of both humeri allow the surgeon to determine the proper length and to restore the fractured humerus

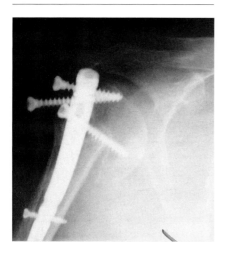

Figure 6 Nonunion of the surgical neck treated with a locking intramedullary rod. Failure of fixation and reduction lead to healing in varus malunion and prominent hardware in the subacromial space.

to match the humerus on the contralateral side. An AO distractor can be used to restore length, and then the blade-plate can be applied. Because no dissection is required in the region of the medial soft tissues adjacent to the bicipital groove, the risk of devascularizing the humeral head fragment is reduced.

Three-Part Fractures

The muscles that are attached to the fracture fragments create deforming forces. Awareness of the common patterns of three-part proximal humeral fractures and an understanding of the muscle forces that act on the fracture fragments allow one to adjust the treatment of each patient.

Deforming Forces

In three-part fractures, fracture lines occur through the surgical neck and the greater or lesser tuberosity. Involvement of the greater tuberosity is much more common than involvement of the lesser tuberosity. The greater tuberosity is displaced superiorly and posteriorly by the pull of the attached supraspinatus, infraspina-

tus, and teres minor. The degree of displacement depends largely on the location of the fracture line with respect to the rotator cuff insertion. The humeral head fragment is pulled into internal rotation by the attached subscapularis, and the shaft is displaced anteriorly and medially by the pull of the pectoralis major. These forces, combined with the proximal pull of the deltoid, produce retroversion of the humeral head.

With a three-part fracture with a lesser tuberosity fragment, the lesser tuberosity is displaced medially by the attached subscapularis. The humeral head and the greater tuberosity fragment are pulled into adduction and external rotation. The shaft is pulled anteriorly and medially by the pectoralis major and proximally by the deltoid.

An understanding of the deforming forces is critical because these forces must be neutralized to achieve a satisfactory reduction of the fracture and the fixation devices must be capable of withstanding the continuous muscle forces. The options for internal fixation include interfragmentary fixation with sutures or wire, percutaneous pinning, plate-and-screw fixation, and intramedullary fixation with and without suture supplementation.

Surgical Technique

Regardless of the method of fixation, adequate surgical exposure is critical. For most three-part fractures, an extended deltopectoral approach provides the exposure necessary to mobilize and fix the surgical neck and tuberosity components of the fracture. The fracture of the greater tuberosity is more easily managed through a superior deltoid-splitting approach, but fixation of the surgical neck portion of a three-part fracture through this approach is possible

only with an intramedullary rod.

There are two goals in the surgical management of three-part proximal humeral fractures. The first is to obtain an anatomic reduction of the fracture fragments, and the second is to neutralize the deforming forces to prevent displacement of the fragments following fixation. Often these two goals can be achieved simultaneously within the fixation construct. However, several techniques achieve these goals independently.

Interfragmentary Fixation Interfragmentary fixation with suture or wires is an established method for fixing three-part fractures of the proximal part of the humerus.[17,18] Neutralization of the forces about the humerus requires achievement of both horizontal and vertical stability across the fracture. To obtain adequate suture fixation in osteopenic bone or comminuted tuberosity fragments, the sutures must be passed at the tendon-bone junction of the tuberosity. Accurate placement of the sutures into the humeral head in the anterior-to-posterior and superior-to-inferior directions is imperative. When the sutures that have been passed through the tuberosity are then passed into the humeral head fragment, they must be placed at the margin of the fracture bed because, when they are placed in the fracture site, the tuberosity fragment tends to be displaced as the sutures are tied. The same is true for the sutures directed in the superior-to-inferior direction. Superior displacement of the tuberosity fragment should be avoided because it can cause subacromial impingement.

The sutures form a figure-of-8 tension-band configuration. Heavy nonabsorbable suture is recommended. We currently use No. 2 fiberwire suture (Arthrex, Naples, FL). Drill holes are made in the shaft

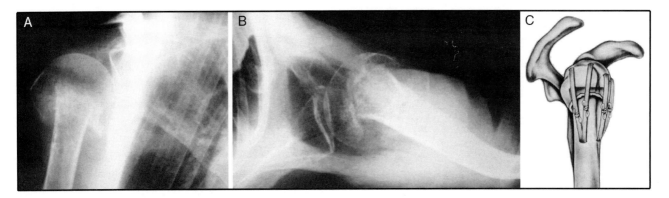

Figure 7 AP (**A**) and axillary (**B**) radiographs of a surgical neck fracture treated with the "parachute technique" of fixation described by Banco and associates.[16] **C,** Heavy sutures have been placed through the rotator cuff tendons and then through drill holes in the humeral shaft distal to the fracture.

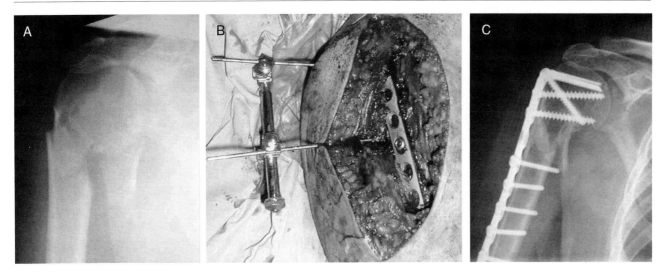

Figure 8 A, Preoperative AP radiograph of a comminuted surgical neck fracture with loss of humeral length. **B,** Intraoperative exposure with use of an AO distractor to restore length. A blade-plate is then applied. **C,** Postoperative AP radiograph showing restoration of humeral length, anatomic reduction, and excellent fixation of both major fragments.

fragment about 1 to 2 cm distal to the fracture site along the medial and lateral ridges of the bicipital groove. Horizontal sutures are then passed through the fractured tuberosity fragment at the bone-tendon junction and through the intact tuberosity of the humeral head fragment. Finally the sutures are crossed and passed through the drill holes in the shaft fragment, forming a figure-of-8. As these sutures are tied, the major deforming forces across the fracture are neutralized (Figure 9).

A potential complication associated with use of the figure-of-8 tension-band technique as the only means of fixation is overlap of the fracture fragments as the sutures are tied. To maintain the fracture reduction as the sutures are tied, interfragmentary sutures can be placed through the fracture site.[12] Drill holes are placed at the fracture margins, on corresponding sides of the fracture fragments, and a figure-of-8 suture is passed with the suture crossing at the fracture site. This pre-

vents the fracture fragments from overlapping when the tension-band neutralization suture is tightened.

Hawkins and associates[17] reported satisfactory results in 12 of 14 patients treated with a wire tension-band construct. However, forward elevation was limited to approximately 120°, and osteonecrosis of the humeral head developed in two patients.

Percutaneous Pinning Percutaneous pinning of three-part proximal humeral fractures requires advanced

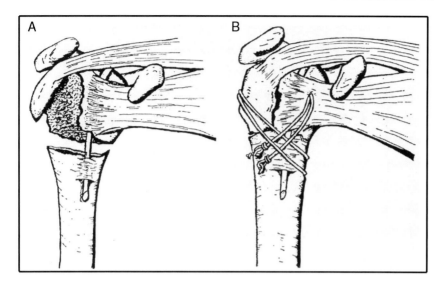

Figure 9 Displaced three-part proximal humeral fracture (**A**) treated with a figure-of-8 fixation suture (**B**) as described by Hawkins and associates.[17] (Reproduced with permission from Hawkins RJ, Bell RH, Gurr K: The three-part fracture of the proximal part of the humerus: Surgical treatment. *J Bone Joint Surg Am* 1986;68;1410-1414.)

skills; good bone stock; minimal comminution, particularly of the tuberosity fragment; and a patient who is able and willing to cooperate with treatment. A retrograde lateral pin, a retrograde anterior pin, or a retrograde anterolateral pin can be used. The retrograde anterolateral pin is most commonly used to achieve percutaneous fixation of the shaft to the humeral head. A fourth option, an antegrade superolateral pin, can supplement the retrograde pin if instability is a problem, but it will slow rehabilitation because it will impinge on the acromion.

Necessary equipment includes a C-arm and image intensifier, 2.5-mm terminally threaded pins, a pin cutter, a small cannulated-screw system, a small- to medium-sized periosteal elevator, and a reduction pick or hook. A knowledgeable assistant is always helpful, and a skillful radiology technician to operate the C-arm and image intensifier is mandatory.

The patient is placed in the beach-chair position with the back of the operating table elevated approximately 30°. The C-arm is positioned so that AP and axillary images can be made. Through a stab incision at the level of the surgical neck, the humeral head is elevated with a reduction tool, reestablishing the neck-shaft angle. The retrograde pins are placed to obtain fixation of the humeral head to the humeral shaft. The greater tuberosity fragment is reduced to the head-shaft composite with use of a reduction pick and is provisionally fixed with a guide-wire for the 4.0-mm cannulated screw set. When the tuberosity has been reduced satisfactorily, a screw of appropriate length is placed.

Percutaneous pinning of three-part fractures of the proximal part of the humerus is technically demanding. A transitional step before performing the fully percutaneous technique is performing open reduction and internal fixation of the greater tuberosity fragment through a superior deltoid-splitting approach fol-lowed by percutaneous pinning of the surgical neck component of the fracture. The deltoid split is performed between the anterior and middle thirds of the deltoid, with the anterior third of the deltoid released in continuity with its periosteal sleeve from the acromion. The tuberosity fragment is then fixed to the head fragment with an interfragmentary suture technique. The surgical neck component can be anatomically reduced through the superior deltoid split. Under fluoroscopic guidance, the surgical neck component can then be fixed percutaneously. Once the surgeon has become comfortable with this technique, he or she can transition to a fully percutaneous technique.

Resch and associates[5] reported good to very good functional results with percutaneous pinning of three-part proximal humeral fractures. At 24 months, no patient in their study showed radiographic evidence of necrosis of the humeral head. The expertise required to obtain such outstanding results of the treatment of these difficult fractures cannot be overstated.

Plate-and-Screw Fixation The results of plate-and-screw fixation of three-part proximal humeral fractures have been mixed. Although some authors have reported excellent results,[19,20] this approach has typically been associated with a high complication rate, particularly in elderly patients.[21-25] Earlier implants were poorly designed, and placement of those implants required extensive soft-tissue stripping, which placed the vascular supply to the humeral head at risk. Currently, there is a renewed interest in plate-and-screw fixation with the development of better implants, including the fixed-angle blade-plate and the locking anatomic proximal humeral plates.

The indication for plate-and-screw fixation is a comminuted fracture, particularly one involving the tuberosity and the surgical neck and requiring rigid fixation. An extended deltopectoral incision is used to approach the fracture, and the tuberosity fragment is first reduced to the humeral head with interfragmentary sutures. If a blade-plate is used, a guide-wire is advanced into the humeral head under fluoroscopic guidance and a plate of appropriate length is selected. If an anatomic proximal humeral locking plate is chosen, it is placed along the greater tuberosity and diverging, locked screws are placed into the humeral head. Then, the head is anatomically reduced to the shaft, and bicortical shaft fixation is performed.

If bone quality is a concern, neutralization sutures can be placed at the bone-tendon junction and passed through one of the holes of the plate to counteract the pull of the rotator cuff on the head and tuberosity fragments.

Intramedullary Fixation There are two types of intramedullary fixation of three-part proximal humeral fractures: (1) intramedullary fixation as the sole means of fixation,[2] and (2) intramedullary fixation with Ender rods supplementing a tension band. The second type is the preferred method of intramedullary fixation because it provides longitudinal and rotational stability to the fracture.

These methods are technically demanding. Because the fracture line in the greater tuberosity fragment is at the articular margin, insertion of an intramedullary rod at the articular margin may displace the fragment. When there is a fracture of the lesser tuberosity, the entry point for the medullary canal is unaffected. Therefore, intramedullary fixation is probably better for three-part fractures with a fracture of the lesser tuberosity than it is for those with a fracture of the greater tuberosity.

Management of the Ender rods and sutures can be cumbersome, even in two-part fractures of the proximal part of the humerus. The application of this technique to three-part proximal humeral fractures requires, in addition, management of the tuberosity fragment.

The peril associated with Ender rod fixation of three-part fractures involving the greater tuberosity is the need for a bone bridge between the margin of the tuberosity fracture and the articular margin to place the rods into the medullary canal. It has been recommended that the Ender rods be modified by creation of an additional hole above the manufactured hole through which to place sutures and keep the rod distal to the level of the greater tuberosity[15] (Figure 10). The superior hole is used to form a tension-band construct that neutralizes the deforming forces across the surgical neck. Two additional sutures are placed through the lower hole, with one limb of each suture coming out of drill holes placed in the shaft fragment. These sutures counteract the tension band suture that is trying to pull the Ender rod out of the medullary canal.

Valgus Impacted Four-Part Fractures

The valgus impacted four-part fracture is characterized by impaction of the lateral aspect of the humeral articular surface through a fracture of the anatomic neck.[3-5,26,27] This lateral impaction results in a valgus deformity of the humeral head such that the articular surface faces superiorly, toward the acromion, rather than medially, toward the glenoid. As the articular surface is imploded into the proximal humeral metaphysis, the greater and lesser tuberosities typically displace from each other as well as from the humeral shaft through intertubercular and surgical neck fractures lines.

Although this displacement pattern may fit Neer's criteria for four-part fractures,[1] the fracture does not behave as such because of at least two important factors. First, true valgus impacted four-part fractures are characterized by little or no displacement (ie, translation) of the medial aspect of the humeral articular surface with respect to the medial aspect of the shaft. Second, the shaft, periosteum, displaced tuberosities, glenohumeral joint capsule, and rotator cuff form a single continuous sleeve of tissue.[3-5,26,27] The lack of displacement between the medial aspect of the humeral articular surface and the shaft preserves the inferomedial part of the periosteum and its associated vessels. Therefore, the prevalence of necrosis of the humeral head (5% to 10%) is much lower than that associated with standard four-part fractures.[3-5,26,27] Moreover, the continuous sleeve of tissue connecting the shaft, tuberosities, glenohumeral joint capsule, and rotator cuff imparts substantial stability and encourages anatomic or nearly anatomic reduction of the tuberosities when the head is reduced.[3-5,26,27]

Radiographic Features

Initial radiographs should include an AP view in the scapular plane, a transscapular lateral view (the Y view), and an axillary view.[1] At first glance, the severity of valgus impacted four-part fractures may be underestimated. Closer inspection reveals the humeral articular surface to be facing superiorly. The displacement of the greater and lesser tuberosities (especially the greater tuberosity) may seem severe,

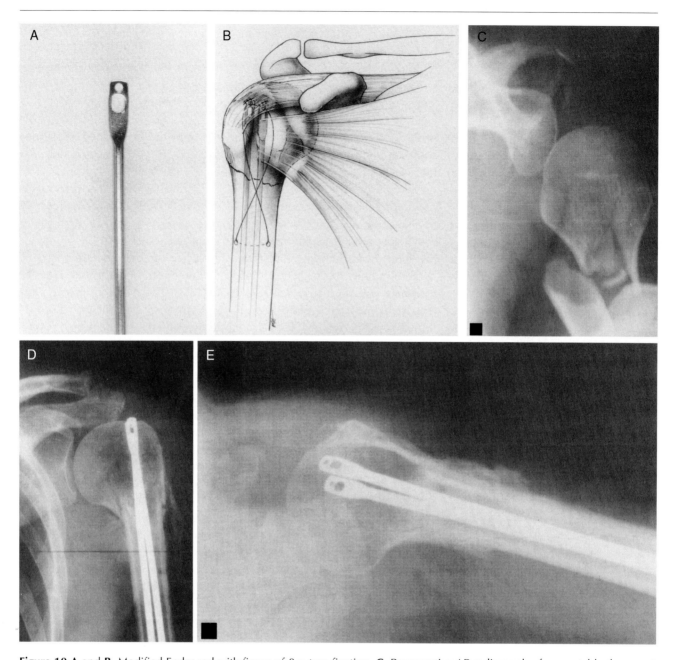

Figure 10 A and **B,** Modified Ender rod with figure-of-8 suture fixation. **C,** Preoperative AP radiograph of an unstable three-part fracture. **D** and **E,** Postoperative radiographs. (Reproduced with permission from Cuomo F, Flatow EL, Maday MG, Miller SR, McIlveen SJ, Bigliani LU: Open reduction and internal fixation of two- and three-part displaced surgical neck fractures of the proximal humerus. *J Shoulder Elbow Surg* 1992;1;287-295.)

but the relative tuberosity displacement is primarily the result of the valgus impaction of the humeral head (Figure 11). The intertubercular fracture line is typically posterior to the bicipital groove. This is an important consideration when surgical reduction is being contemplated.

Treatment Options

Potential treatment options include early mobilization, percutaneous reduction and internal fixation, open reduction and internal fixation, and hemiarthroplasty. The vast majority of valgus impacted four-part fractures are amenable to percutaneous reduc-

tion and internal fixation. Nonsurgical treatment often results in painful malunion and therefore is indicated only for elderly, sedentary patients with medical comorbidities that preclude surgical treatment. Percutaneous reduction and internal fixation is an excellent option for patients who

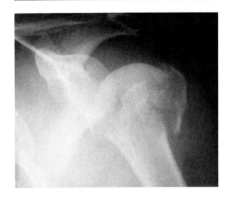

Figure 11 AP radiograph of a classic valgus impacted four-part fracture. The displacement of the tuberosities is secondary to the valgus impaction of the articular segment. There is unimportant displacement of the humeral shaft in relation to the humeral head consistent with an intact medial periosteal soft-tissue sleeve and an intact blood supply in this area.

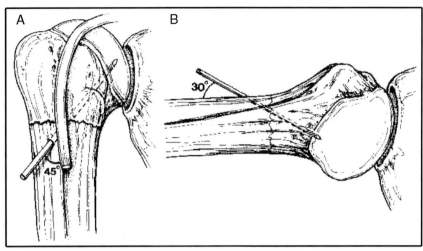

Figure 12 Percutaneous fixation of the head fragment with two pins. First, the pin is placed on the anterolateral surface of the humerus and advanced to within 1 cm of the subchondral surface of the head under fluoroscopic guidance. Accurate placement typically requires the pin to be angled 45° medially **(A)** and 30° posteriorly **(B)**. A second pin is then placed parallel and slightly superior or inferior to the first.

have an acute injury (7 to 10 days old), good bone quality, and minimal comminution and can be relied on to cooperate with treatment. Open reduction and internal fixation is primarily indicated for acute fractures that are not reducible by closed means, for severe osteopenic bone, for extensive comminution, or for fractures that are between 10 days and 4 months old. Hemiarthroplasty is reserved for fractures that are more than 4 months old or the rare acute fracture in an elderly, sedentary patient with severe osteopenia.

Percutaneous Reduction and Internal Fixation The patient is positioned so that radiographs can be made in two orthogonal planes. This should be verified before sterile preparation and draping. The optimal patient position is semirecumbent in a beach-chair configuration, with the back of the table elevated 30° to 45°. The affected extremity should be positioned off the edge of the table to allow adequate C-arm access. The anesthesia equipment is

moved to the opposite side of the table to allow the C-arm to enter the surgical field from superior with the plane of the C-arm parallel to the table's edge (Figure 4). The arm and shoulder are then prepared and draped.

Successful percutaneous reduction and internal fixation may be accomplished by following a series of individual steps: percutaneous reduction of the articular segment, fixation of the head, reduction and fixation of the greater tuberosity, and reduction and fixation of the lesser tuberosity.[1] Reduction and fixation is not always required for both tuberosities. This decision is made after reduction and fixation of the head.

A small Cobb periosteal elevator is used to reduce the humeral head on the shaft through a small incision in the skin. With the arm held in 20° to 30° of abduction and neutral rotation, the level of the intertubercular fracture is identified with fluoroscopy. A 1.5- to 2.0-cm incision is made on the anterolateral surface of the

arm over the fracture. The elevator is placed through this incision, through the deltoid, and into the fracture under fluoroscopic guidance. It is then placed under the lateral portion of the humeral head. This position is again verified radiographically. A superiorly directed force is applied to the undersurface of the head with use of the elevator. This maneuver should be done carefully to avoid overreduction or translation of the humeral head. In acute fractures, the head usually reduces very easily and stays in the reduced position after the elevator is removed.

Once the head fragment is reduced, it is fixed in that position with percutaneously placed 2.5-mm terminally threaded pins. Two retrograde anterolateral pins are usually sufficient. The first pin is placed on the skin, its relationship to the humerus is visualized radiographically, and the entry site is located. The pin enters the arm midway between the anterior and lateral surfaces. After the skin incision is made, a hemostat

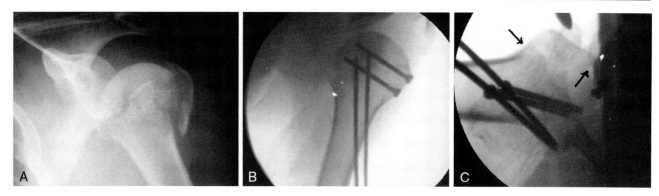

Figure 13 A, AP radiograph of a four-part humeral head fracture. **B,** AP fluoroscopic view of the fracture after reduction and fixation of the head and greater tuberosity fragments. **C,** Axillary fluoroscopic view of the fracture with mild residual displacement of the lesser tuberosity fragment.

is used to spread the soft tissues bluntly until the bone is identified. This lessens the risk of injury to the axillary nerve. The pin is placed on the anterolateral surface of the humerus and advanced to within 1 cm of the subchondral surface of the head under fluoroscopic guidance. Accurate pin placement typically requires angling of the pin 45° medially and 30° posteriorly (Figure 12). A second pin is placed parallel and slightly superior or inferior to the first one. At least 1 cm should separate the pins at their site of entry into the bone. Accurate placement of the pins and the quality of the reduction are evaluated by rotating the humerus in a 90° arc of motion while continuously visualizing the humerus under fluoroscopy.

The greater tuberosity is often found to be anatomically reduced after the head has been reduced. If the tuberosity is anatomically reduced and is stable with motion (as assessed fluoroscopically), it should not need additional fixation. If reduction and fixation of the greater tuberosity is required, a 5-mm incision is made at the midpart of the acromion, approximately 2 to 3 cm distal to the lateral acromial border. A reduction hook or a small elevator is placed through this

incision, through the deltoid, and down to the tuberosity surface. The tuberosity is reduced by pulling it forward and slightly distally. A guidewire from a small cannulated-screw set is then placed percutaneously through the greater tuberosity approximately 1 cm inferior to its most superior edge. The guide-wire is then passed across the humerus and into the subchondral bone of the humeral head at an approximately 90° angle with the shaft. Accurate placement of the guide-wire is verified radiographically in two planes (by rotating the humerus). After measurement of the length of the screw, an appropriately sized cannulated screw is placed. Initial predrilling and tapping of the humerus usually is not necessary. A second, parallel screw is placed in a similar fashion approximately 1.5 cm distal to the first. Accurate screw placement is verified fluoroscopically.

The lesser tuberosity is visualized by rotating the C-arm, without moving the humerus. Residual displacement of the lesser tuberosity is better tolerated than is residual displacement of the greater tuberosity; therefore, it is important to visualize these relationships accurately[1,2] (Figure 13). A nonanatomic relationship between

the lesser tuberosity and the articular surface may be misinterpreted as displacement of the tuberosity rather than residual displacement of the head. If the problem is residual displacement of the head, the relationship between the shaft and the lesser tuberosity will be normal, despite displacement between the head and the lesser tuberosity. Under these circumstances, it is probably better to accept a small (0.5- to 1.0-cm) amount of residual head displacement than to redo the previously placed fixation. If there is residual displacement of the lesser tuberosity, reduction is achieved with a reduction hook placed through the previously made anterolateral incision. Percutaneous screw fixation can be achieved through an anterior incision. Two parallel AP screws are placed with use of the same technique as used for the greater tuberosity.

The pins are cut under the skin, and the wounds are closed in a standard fashion. Pendulum exercises are instituted the next day. Passive flexion and external rotation with the patient supine are begun during the third postoperative week. The pins are removed at 3 to 4 weeks. More aggressive passive stretching and strengthening are instituted at 6 weeks after reduction.

Open Reduction and Internal Fixation Open reduction and internal fixation usually is not required for acute four-part fractures, except when an acceptable reduction could not be attained percutaneously. Under these circumstances, the patient and the C-arm are positioned as described above. The fracture is exposed through a standard deltopectoral incision. The head is then reduced by placing an elevator through the intertubercular fracture line under direct visualization. Percutaneously placed pins are then used as described above to fix the head and shaft fragments. Next, the tuberosities are sutured to themselves with interfragmentary nonabsorbable sutures.

Subacute fractures more than 10 days but less than 4 months old are routinely treated with open reduction and internal fixation. Patient and C-arm positioning is identical to that described above. The fracture is exposed through a standard deltopectoral approach. The intertubercular fracture line is identified and may need to be recreated with an osteotome. The greater and lesser tuberosities are levered open to make them more mobile and to allow access to the undersurface of the valgus impacted head fragment. A small osteotome is used to score the medial junction of the head fragment and the shaft. Care is taken to avoid complete perforation of the medial cortex. The head is then elevated with a small elevator. In the subacute situation, there is a tendency for the head to redisplace into valgus. Therefore, allograft cancellous chips are packed under the elevated head. Fixation of the head can be performed with several devices. A humeral blade-plate is an excellent option in this setting be-

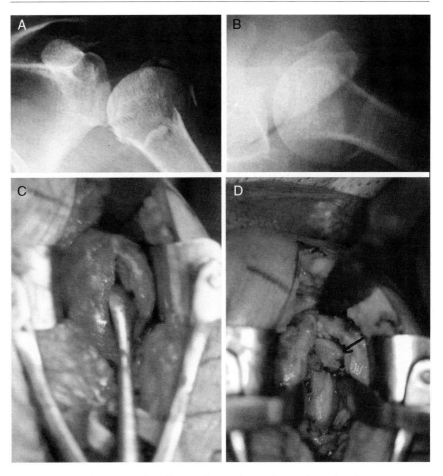

Figure 14 A and **B,** AP and axillary radiographs made 16 days after the patient sustained a subacute valgus impacted fracture. **C,** A Cobb elevator is used to reduce the humeral articular fragment. **D,** A corticocancellous bone graft was placed to maintain the reduction and fill the void. Then, an AO humeral blade-plate was inserted above the graft into the articular fragment, and the side-plate was fixed to the humeral shaft with screws.

cause of its rigidity (Figure 14).

Pendulum exercises are instituted on the first postoperative day. Passive flexion and external rotation exercises with the patient supine are added at 7 to 10 days. More aggressive stretching and strengthening exercises are started at 6 weeks after surgery.

References

1. Neer CS II: Displaced proximal humeral fractures: II. Treatment of three-part and four-part displacement. *J Bone Joint Surg Am* 1970;52:1090-1103.

2. Mouradian WH: Displaced proximal humeral fractures: Seven years' experience with a modified Zickel supracondylar device. *Clin Orthop* 1986;212:209-218.

3. Resch H, Beck E, Bayley I: Reconstruction of the valgus-impacted humeral head fracture. *J Shoulder Elbow Surg* 1995;4:73-80.

4. Resch H, Hubner C, Schwaiger R: Minimally invasive reduction and osteosynthesis of articular fractures of the humeral head. *Injury* 2001;32(suppl 1): SA25-SA32.

5. Resch H, Povacz P, Frohlich R, Wambacher M: Percutaneous fixation of three- and four-part fractures of the proximal humerus. *J Bone Joint Surg Br* 1997;79:295-300.

6. Neer CS II: Displaced proximal humeral fractures: I. Classification and evaluation. *J Bone Joint Surg Am* 1970;52:1077-1089.

7. Flatow EL, Cuomo F, Maday MG, Miller SR, McIlveen SJ, Bigliani LU: Open reduction and internal fixation of two-part displaced fractures of the greater tuberosity of the proximal part of the humerus. *J Bone Joint Surg Am* 1991;73:1213-1218.

8. Beredjiklian PK, Iannotti JP, Norris TR, Williams GR: Operative treatment of malunion of a fracture of the proximal aspect of the humerus. *J Bone Joint Surg Am* 1998;80:1484-1497.

9. Norris TR, Green A, McGuigan FX: Late prosthetic shoulder arthroplasty for displaced proximal humerus fractures. *J Shoulder Elbow Surg* 1995;4:271-280.

10. Siebenrock KA, Gerber C: The reproducibility of classification of fractures of the proximal end of the humerus. *J Bone Joint Surg Am* 1993;75:1751-1755.

11. Sidor ML, Zuckerman JD, Lyon T, Koval K, Cuomo F, Schoenberg N: The Neer classification system for proximal humeral fractures: An assessment of interobserver reliability and intraobserver reproducibility. *J Bone Joint Surg Am* 1993;75:1745-1750.

12. Gerber C, Warner J: Alternatives to hemiarthroplasty for complex proximal-humeral fractures, in Warner JJ, Iannotti JP, Gerber C (eds): *Complex and Revision Problems in Shoulder Surgery*. Philadelphia, PA, Lippincott-Raven, 1997, pp 215-243.

13. Bohler J: Les fractures recentes de l'epaule. *Acta Orthop Belg* 1964;30:235-242.

14. Jaberg H, Warner JJ, Jakob RP: Percutaneous stabilization of unstable fractures of the humerus. *J Bone Joint Surg Am* 1992;74:508-515.

15. Cuomo F, Flatow EL, Maday MG, Miller SR, McIlveen SJ, Bigliani LU: Open reduction and internal fixation of two- and three-part displaced surgical neck fractures of the proximal humerus. *J Shoulder Elbow Surg* 1992;1:287-295.

16. Banco SP, Andrisani D, Ramsey M, Frieman B, Fenlin JM Jr: The parachute technique: Valgus impaction osteotomy for two-part fractures of the surgical neck of the humerus. *J Bone Joint Surg Am* 2001;83(suppl 2):38-42.

17. Hawkins RJ, Bell RH, Gurr K: The three-part fracture of the proximal part of the humerus: Operative treatment. *J Bone Joint Surg Am* 1986;68:1410-1414.

18. Hawkins RJ, Kiefer GN: Internal fixation techniques for proximal humeral fractures. *Clin Orthop* 1987;223:77-85.

19. Esser RD: Open reduction and internal fixation of three- and four-part fractures of the proximal humerus. *Clin Orthop* 1994;299:244-251.

20. Esser RD: Treatment of three- and four-part fractures of the proximal humerus with a modified cloverleaf plate. *J Orthop Trauma* 1994;8:15-22.

21. Cofield RH: Comminuted fractures of the proximal humerus. *Clin Orthop* 1988;230:49-57.

22. Kristiansen B, Christiensen SW: Plate fixation of proximal humeral fractures. *Acta Orthop Scand* 1986;57:320-323.

23. Lee CK, Hansen HR: Post-traumatic avascular necrosis of the humeral head in displaced proximal humeral fractures. *J Trauma* 1981;21:788-791.

24. Paavolainen P, Bjorkenheim JM, Slatis P, Paukku P: Operative treatment of severe proximal humeral fractures. *Acta Orthop Scand* 1983;54:374-379.

25. Svend-Hansen H: Displaced proximal humeral fractures. A review of 49 patients. *Acta Orthop Scand* 1974;45:359-364.

26. Habermeyer P, Schweiberer L: Corrective interventions subsequent to humeral head fractures. *Orthopade* 1992;21:148-157.

27. Jakob RP, Miniaci A, Anson PS, Jaberg H, Osterwalder A, Ganz R: Four-part valgus impacted fractures of the proximal humerus. *J Bone Joint Surg Br* 1991;73:295-298.

Indications for Prosthetic Replacement in Proximal Humeral Fractures

Wesley P. Phipatanakul, MD
Tom R. Norris, MD

Abstract

Prosthetic replacement is a good treatment option in osteoporotic patients with four-part fractures, fracture-dislocations, head-split fractures with more than 40% articular surface involvement, anatomic neck fractures, dislocations present for longer than 6 months, and selected three-part fractures. Early prosthetic replacement of proximal humeral fractures has a better outcome than late reconstructive prosthetic management. Prosthetic design features specific for fracture care have led to a reduction in complications. Techniques will continue to improve as prosthetic design features specific for fractures evolve.

Most fractures of the proximal humerus are relatively nondisplaced and can be treated nonsurgically. Displaced two-part fractures and many three-part fractures generally are not considered for prosthetic replacement because good results are achieved with osteosynthesis. Certain fracture patterns often preclude the ability to use internal fixation techniques to reconstruct the proximal humerus, particularly in elderly patients with osteoporosis. This problem is compounded in patients with comminution and poor bone quality. The literature supports prosthetic replacement as a definitive treatment option in patients with four-part fractures and fracture-dislocations, head-split fractures with greater than 40% articular surface involvement, anatomic neck fractures, dislocations present for 6 months or longer in which the cartilage has softened, and selected three-part fractures in patients with osteopenia that precludes secure internal fixation.[1-3]

The preferred concept is to perform the most reliable procedure in the initial management. The idea of treating all fractures initially with internal fixation with the thought of prosthetic management as the salvage procedure is not a recommended algorithm. Malunions are very difficult to treat. Reconstruction of malunions is one of the most challenging procedures and is associated with a higher rate of complications.[1,4] The literature clearly shows that early prosthetic replacement of proximal humeral fractures has a better outcome than late prosthetic management.[5-11] In addition, late prosthetic surgery for failed early treatment is more technically difficult. Factors to consider in surgical decision making include the risk of nonunion, malunion, or osteonecrosis, bone quality, time from injury, and the need for future surgery and revision.

Anatomic Neck Fracture

Anatomic neck fractures are quite rare. In fact, there are no series in the literature dealing exclusively with this fracture pattern; therefore, much of the management is based intuitively. The fracture location is medial to the rotator cuff insertion and thus the humeral head is devoid of soft-tissue attachment. It is logical to conclude a higher rate of osteonecrosis in this rare fracture pattern. In cadaver studies, it has been shown that displaced anatomic neck fractures completely disrupt the blood flow to the articular portion of the humeral head.[12] Hertel and associates[13] in a recent study identified factors that predict humeral head ischemia following proximal humeral fractures. Their classification scheme divided fractures into 12 types based on five basic fracture planes that can be identified by answering the following questions: Is there a fracture between the greater tuberosity and either the head and/or shaft? Is there a fracture between the lesser tuberosity and the head and/or shaft? Is there a fracture between the lesser and the greater

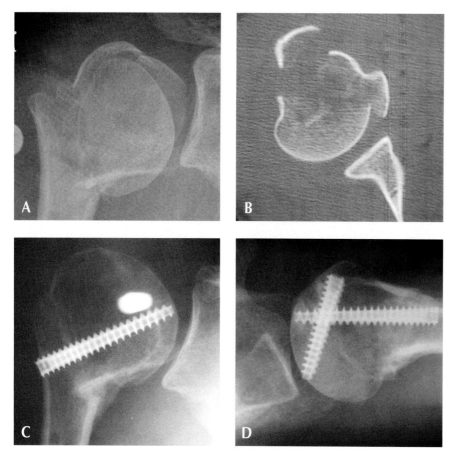

Figure 1 AP radiograph (**A**) and axial CT scan (**B**) demonstrating a four-part proximal humeral fracture with a head-splitting component in a 32-year-old woman. **C** and **D,** Follow-up radiographs demonstrating healed fracture without humeral head collapse. Osteosynthesis should be considered in young patients provided an anatomic reduction can be achieved.

tuberosity? They found that the most relevant predictors of ischemia were the length of the dorsomedial metaphyseal extension with the humeral head; the integrity of the medial hinge; and the basic fracture type determined with the binary description system. In particular, those types with fracture planes between the humeral head and other anatomic structures, that is, variations of the anatomic neck fracture, were at highest risk. By combining the above criteria (anatomic neck, short calcar, disrupted hinge), positive predictive values for ischemia of up to 97% could be obtained. Moderate and poor predictors of ischemia, in descending order, were fractures consisting of four fragments, angular dis-

placement of the head, the amount of dislocation of the tuberosities, glenohumeral dislocation, head-split components, and fractures consisting of three fragments.[13] Acute prosthetic replacement is an appropriate treatment option in this fracture pattern where solid fixation may be difficult to achieve in addition to a high likelihood of head collapse. Attempts at internal fixation should be reserved for the younger population (Figures 1 and 2).

Three-Part Fractures

Good results with internal fixation of three-part fractures have been reported.[14] However, osteosynthesis of three-part fractures in elderly patients has revealed

poorer results. A series of elderly patients were randomized to either conservative treatment or tension band osteosynthesis.[15] No differences in functional outcomes were observed between the two groups. Major complications occurred in the surgically treated group only. Prosthetic management of three-part fractures should be considered in the older patient with osteoporotic bone that prevents stable fixation. A prosthesis may provide immediate stability and decrease the need for secondary procedures because of hardware failure or fracture nonunion/malunion. Head collapse is not the major issue in three-part fractures. In fact, it is unusual to develop osteonecrosis in a three-part fracture because the intact lesser tuberosity preserves the arcuate artery by keeping the intertubercular groove intact. The fracture pattern is usually posterior to the groove and involves the greater tuberosity and the surgical neck. The arcuate artery is a branch off the anterior circumflex artery that supplies the majority of the blood supply to the humeral head and has been shown to have a constant insertion point in the groove.[16]

Four-Part Fractures and Fracture-Dislocation

Treatment of four-part fractures remains controversial. This fracture pattern is much more problematic than the three-part fracture. The articular portion is completely separated from its blood supply.[12] Neer[17,18] found a 75% incidence of osteonecrosis in four-part fractures. Internal fixation of these fracture types in the past has generally been poor.[17,19] Mild osteonecrosis does not necessarily preclude a good outcome. Gerber and associates[20] reviewed 25 patients with post-traumatic osteonecrosis analyzed at 7.5 years follow-up. The patients were divided into two groups: those with anatomic reduction versus those with malunions. Those with anatomic reduction fared significantly better; 62% had good function-

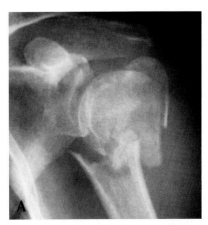 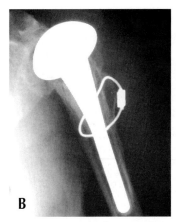 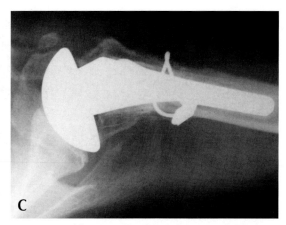

Figure 2 A, Radiograph showing a fracture pattern suggestive of a three-part fracture in a 73-year-old patient. **B** and **C,** Follow-up radiographs with the prosthetic component in place. Intraoperatively, a four-part fracture with head split was discovered. With this same fracture pattern in an older patient with poorer bone quality, a prosthetic replacement is a good treatment option.

al results versus 16% in the other group. When committing to osteosynthesis of a proximal humeral fracture, obtaining an anatomic or near-anatomic reduction, especially in three- and four-part fractures, is paramount. If the fracture pattern doesn't allow for achievement of this goal, then prosthetic replacement should be considered. Recently, one series documented 87% good results using the Constant score with open reduction and internal fixation.[21] However, the patients in that series were younger (average age 48 years), and nearly half of the patients were excluded either because they died or because they required conversion to arthroplasty as a result of failed osteosynthesis. Despite their enthusiasm with osteosynthesis, the authors recommended considering prosthetic replacement for the elderly. Others have found primary prosthetic replacement in four-part fractures to be superior to osteosynthesis.[22]

The results of percutaneous treatment have also been disappointing. One study reported a 75% poor result with this technique secondary to osteonecrosis, and thus concluded that percutaneous pinning is not a good option in four-part fractures.[23] With poor outcomes with surgical fixation of four-part fracture, multiple series documenting improved

results with prosthetic management have emerged. Satisfactory results range mostly in the 60% to 90% range, with good pain relief in about 80% to 85%.[5,6,11,24-28] A joint dislocation further complicates the blood supply. The incidence of osteonecrosis is higher in this situation. A recent report found a 39% incidence of osteonecrosis in three-part fracture-dislocation, and 89% in four-part fracture-dislocation.[21] Another series found that internal fixation in four-part fracture-dislocation resulted in 100% failure and recommended prosthetic management.[29] Patients must be informed that prosthetic treatment is designed to be a pain-relieving operation. Multiple reports document excellent pain relief with functional gains less predictable.[6,25,30,31] Therefore, acute prosthetic management of four-part fractures in the elderly is recommended, particularly because the literature has shown reliable reproducible results in several series using this technique (Figure 3). This indication extends to both the three- and four-part fracture-dislocations in the elderly. Prosthetic replacement in the younger patient causes concern about the longevity of the implant. Recent studies have shown good survivorship of the prosthesis in a fracture situation, over 90% at 10 years.[32]

Osteosynthesis should be reserved for the younger patient. However, when considering osteosynthesis as the initial treatment, it should be remembered that functional outcomes of acute prosthetic replacement are better than those of replacement for either delayed or failed internal fixation.[10] One report found prosthetic replacement within 4 weeks of injury to produce superior results,[5] whereas others have found intervention within 2 weeks to be better.[8,11] Thus, although it is prudent to proceed with treatment sooner rather than later, a 2- to 4-week time period allows enough time for surgical planning and patient optimization.

Impression Fracture and Chronic Dislocation
Impression fractures are often associated with dislocation. More than 40% to 50% involvement of the articular surface can be considered a contraindication to osteosynthesis. In one series it was determined that a head-split fracture with more than 40% articular involvement was an appropriate indication for prosthetic management.[2] Another report recommended arthroplasty if the head involvement was more than 45% or dislocation was present for longer than 6 months.[3]

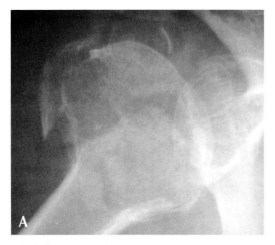

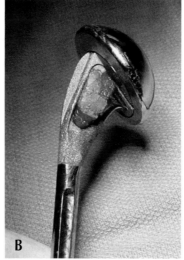

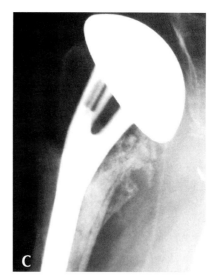

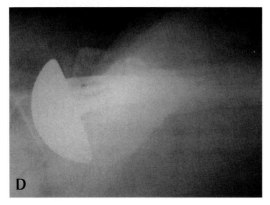

Figure 3 A, An AP radiograph demonstrates a proximal humeral fracture in an elderly patient. **B,** Photograph of a fracture-prosthesis with a bone graft from the patient's removed articular segment in place. **C** and **D,** Follow-up radiographs demonstrate consolidation of the tuberosities with the prosthesis in place.

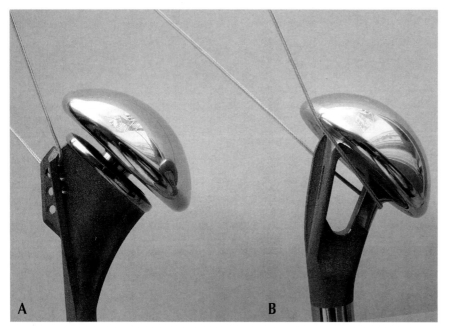

Figure 4 A, This fracture-prosthesis has a smooth medial collar, which facilitates placement of circumferential cerclage sutures without a stress riser. Biomechanical data have found that this configuration is more stable compared with placing sutures through a hole in a prosthetic fin (**B**).

Valgus Impacted Four-Part Fracture

This fracture pattern behaves differently than the true four-part fracture and must be distinguished because this can change the treatment options. The humeral head is impacted without lateral displacement, and thus the periosteum medially leading up to the humeral head is intact and preserves the blood supply for the most part. This is a unique four-part fracture not necessarily requiring prosthetic replacement. Good results are reported with open reduction, bone grafting, and limited internal fixation. However, functional outcome is correlated with obtaining an anatomic reduction.[33]

Summary

Prosthetic replacement of acute proximal humeral fractures is a good treatment option. Osteosynthesis is a poor choice if

the fracture environment precludes stability and an anatomic reduction. It is
important to initially perform the procedure that will provide the most predictable outcome, because secondary
surgery is more technically demanding
with outcomes clearly inferior to primary
treatment. The literature supports that
prosthetic management is a good indication in the older population with complex fracture patterns. When surgical
treatment is indicated, early management
has produced superior results, with pain
relief more predictable than functional
gains. The treatment of the younger population is not as clear. Factors associated
with lower functional scores included
increasing patient age, alcohol and tobacco use, neurologic deficit, and a poorly
positioned prosthesis.[32] Although these
factors do not preclude prosthetic use,
this information can help better inform
patients on outcome expectations.
Changes in the technical aspect of prosthetic surgery will continue to affect the
indications for its use. A recent report
demonstrated that the most significant
factor associated with poor result of
humeral head replacement for acute fracture was tuberosity migration.[34] This has
led to modifications of the prosthetic
design specific for fracture care (Figure
4). These changes include less metal at
the proximal part of the prosthesis and a
smooth medial calcar to allow placement
of a circumferential medial cerclage.
These changes facilitate tuberosity
osteosynthesis. Biomechanical data have
shown that a circumferential medial
cerclage adds significant stability to
the tuberosity construct, while incorporating sutures into a prosthetic fin did
not.[35] These prosthetic design changes
have led to a reduction in tuberosity
migration by a factor of two.[36] Techniques
will continue to improve as prosthetic
design features specific for fractures
evolve and prevention of tuberosity
dehiscence diminishes.

References

1. Antuna SA, Sperling JW, Sanchez-Sotelo J, Cofield RH: Shoulder arthroplasty for proximal humeral malunions: Long-term results. J Shoulder Elbow Surg 2002;11:122-129.

2. Compito CA, Self EB, Bigliani LU: Arthroplasty and acute shoulder trauma: Reasons for success and failure. Clin Orthop 1994;307:27-36.

3. Hawkins RJ, Neer CS II, Pianta RM, Mendoza FX: Locked posterior dislocation of the shoulder. J Bone Joint Surg Am 1987;69:9-18.

4. Beredjiklian PK, Iannotti JP, Norris TR, Williams GR: Operative treatment of malunion of a fracture of the proximal aspect of the humerus. J Bone Joint Surg Am 1998;80:1484-1487.

5. Bosch U, Skutek M, Fremerey RW, Tscherne H: Outcome after primary and secondary hemiarthroplasty in elderly patients with fractures of the proximal humerus. J Shoulder Elbow Surg 1998;7:479-484.

6. Dimakopoulos P, Potamitis N, Lambiris E: Hemiarthroplasty in the treatment of comminuted intraarticular fractures of the proximal humerus. Clin Orthop 1997;341:7-11.

7. Becker R, Pap G, Machner A, Neumann WH: Strength and motion after hemiarthroplasty in displaced four-fragment fracture of the proximal humerus: 27 patients followed for 1-6 years. Acta Orthop Scand 2002;73:44-49.

8. Demirhan M, Kilicoglu O, Altnel L, Eralp L, Akalin Y: Prognostic factors in prosthetic replacement for acute proximal humerus fractures. J Orthop Trauma 2003;17:181-189.

9. Frich LH, Sojbjerg JO, Sneppen O: Shoulder arthroplasty in complex acute and chronic proximal humeral fractures. Orthopedics 1991;14:949-954.

10. Norris TR, Green A, McGuigan FX: Late prosthetic shoulder arthroplasty for displaced proximal humerus fractures. J Shoulder Elbow Surg 1995;4:271-280.

11. Moeckel BH, Dines DM, Warren RF, Altchek DW: Modular hemiarthroplasty for fractures of the proximal part of the humerus. J Bone Joint Surg Am 1992;74:884-889.

12. Brooks CH, Revell WJ, Heatley FW: Vascularity of the humeral head after proximal humeral fractures: An anatomical cadaver study. J Bone Joint Surg Br 1993;75:132-136.

13. Hertel R, Hempfing A, Stiehler M, Leunig M: Predictors of humeral head ischemia after intracapsular fracture of the proximal humerus. J Shoulder Elbow Surg 2004;4:427-433.

14. Hawkins RJ, Bell RH, Gurr K: The three-part fracture of the proximal part of the humerus: Operative treatment. J Bone Joint Surg Am 1986;68:1410-1414.

15. Zyto K, Ahrengart L, Sperber A, Tornkvist H: Treatment of displaced proximal humeral fractures in elderly patients. J Bone Joint Surg Br 1997;79:412-417.

16. Gerber C, Schneeberger AG, Vinh TS: The arterial vascularization of the humeral head: An

17. Neer CS II: Displaced proximal humeral fractures: II. Treatment of three-part and four-part displacement. J Bone Joint Surg Am 1970;52:1090-1103.

18. Neer CS II: Displaced proximal humeral fractures: I. Classification and evaluation. J Bone Joint Surg Am 1970;52:1077-1089.

19. Kristiansen B, Christensen SW: Proximal humeral fractures: Late results in relation to classification and treatment. Acta Orthop Scand 1987;58:124-127.

20. Gerber C, Hersche O, Berberat C: The clinical relevance of posttraumatic avascular necrosis of the humeral head. J Shoulder Elbow Surg 1998;7:586-590.

21. Wijgman AJ, Roolker W, Patt TW, Raaymakers EL, Marti RK: Open reduction and internal fixation of three and four-part fractures of the proximal part of the humerus. J Bone Joint Surg Am 2002;84:1919-1925.

22. Schai P, Imhoff A, Preiss S: Comminuted humeral head fractures: A multicenter analysis. J Shoulder Elbow Surg 1995;4:319-330.

23. Soete PJ, Clayson PE, Costenoble VH: Transitory percutaneous pinning in fractures of the proximal humerus. J Shoulder Elbow Surg 1999;8:569-573.

24. Tanner MW, Cofield RH: Prosthetic arthroplasty for fractures and fracture-dislocations of the proximal humerus. Clin Orthop 1983;179:116-128.

25. Goldman RT, Koval KJ, Cuomo F, Gallagher MA, Zuckerman JD: Functional outcome after humeral head replacement for acute three- and four-part proximal humeral fractures. J Shoulder Elbow Surg 1995;4:81-86.

26. Boileau P, Trojani C, Walch G, Krishnan SG, Romeo A, Sinerton R: Shoulder arthroplasty for the treatment of the sequelae of fractures of the proximal humerus. J Shoulder Elbow Surg 2001;10:299-308.

27. Boss AP, Hintermann B: Primary endoprosthesis in comminuted humeral head fractures in patients over 60 years of age. Int Orthop 1999;23:172-174.

28. Zyto K, Wallace WA, Frostick SP, Preston BJ: Outcome after hemiarthroplasty for three- and four-part fractures of the proximal humerus. J Shoulder Elbow Surg 1998;7:85-89.

29. Darder A, Darder A Jr, Sanchis V, Gastaldi E, Gomar F: Four-part displaced proximal humeral fractures: Operative treatment using Kirschner wires and a tension band. J Orthop Trauma 1993;7:497-505.

30. Kay SP, Amstutz HC: Shoulder hemiarthroplasty at UCLA. Clin Orthop 1988;228:42-48.

31. Wretenberg P, Ekelund A: Acute hemiarthroplasty after proximal humerus fracture in old patients: A retrospective evaluation of 18 patients followed for 2-7 years. Acta Orthop Scand 1997;68:121-123.

32. Robinson CM, Page RS, Hill RM, Sanders DL, Court-Brown CM, Wakefield AE: Primary hemiarthroplasty for treatment of proximal

humeral fractures. *J Bone Joint Surg Am* 2003;85:1215-1223.

33. Resch H, Beck E, Bayley I: Reconstruction of the valgus-impacted humeral head fracture. *J Shoulder Elbow Surg* 1995;4:73-80.

34. Boileau P, Kirshnan SG, Tinsi L, Walch G, Coste JS, Mole D: Tuberosity malposition and migration: Reasons for poor outcomes after hemiarthroplasty for displaced fractures of the proximal humerus. *J Shoulder Elbow Surg* 2002;11:401-412.

35. Frankle MA, Ondrovic LE, Markee BA, Harris ML, Lee WE III: Stability of tuberosity reattachment in proximal humeral hemiarthroplasty. *J Shoulder Elbow Surg* 2002;11:413-420.

36. Boileau P: Prosthetic shoulder replacement for fracture: Results of the multicentre study, in Walch G, Boileau P, Mol D (eds): *2000 Shoulder Prostheses: Two to Ten Year Follow Up.* Paris, France, Sauramps Medical, 2001, pp 561-569.

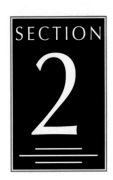

SECTION 2

Lower Extremity Trauma

Lower Extremity Trauma

Lower extremity trauma is common, yet these injuries are often complex alone or in association with other severe conditions. Recent advances in surgical technique and implant design have substantially improved treatment of these injuries. For these reasons, this selection of articles taken from the American Academy of Orthopaedic Surgeons' *Instructional Course Lectures* should be both interesting and of critical importance to all surgeons who care for patients with fractures.

Our aging population has resulted in a steady increase in the number of patients with osteoporotic hip fractures. Three of the articles in this section focus on treatment of this important group of patients. Femoral neck and intertrochanteric fractures are described in separate chapters. The other article is dedicated entirely to prevention of hip fractures, addressing both medical management of osteoporosis and strategies for fall and fracture prevention. Improvements in both automobile safety and critical care medicine have contributed to decreased mortality associated with high-energy mechanisms of injury. Thus, the article that focuses on the care of severe foot and ankle injuries is especially relevant because survival among high-speed motor vehicle crash victims with severe floor board injuries continues to increase. Three articles discuss tibia fractures: open tibial shaft fractures, closed tibial shaft fractures, and distal tibia fractures. The final two articles address two subsets of femur fractures—those that occur in children and those that occur about hip arthroplasty stems.

Andrew Schmidt and associates provide a comprehensive review of nearly all aspects of treatment of femoral neck fractures. Their article begins with a description of appropriate preoperative clinical, radiographic, and laboratory evaluations. Next, perioperative orthopaedic, anesthetic, and medical management strategies, including discussions of thromboprophylaxis and postoperative rehabilitation, are outlined. The principal focus of the article, however, is surgical management. The rationale for each surgical option is discussed in the context of the unique structural and anatomic variances seen in the femoral neck region of elderly patients. Current controversies associated with internal fixation, hemiarthroplasty, and total hip arthroplasty are specifically addressed. The authors provide guidance regarding the technical aspects of internal fixation, specifically the preferred type, number, and geometric location of screws and the role of compression hip screws, with or without a derotation screw. Data justifying the correct choice of unipolar or bipolar hemiarthroplasty or total hip arthroplasty are also analyzed.

In their article on reducing complications associated with surgical treatment of intertrochanteric fractures, David Templeman and associates concisely summarize current treatment options. They correctly point out that stable intertrochanteric, unstable intertrochanteric, reverse obliquity, and subtrochanteric fractures require individualized treatment. Tactics for reducing commonly associated complications such as implant failure, nonunion or malunion, and peri-implant fracture are described, as are reduction techniques for treatment using a fracture table and with the patient in the lateral decubitus position. In this context, the authors review the role of compression hip screw devices, the Medoff sliding plate, adjuvant use of trochanteric stabilization plates, and various intramedullary devices for treating complex fracture patterns. They remind us of the importance of proper surgical technique, especially placement of lag screws into the femoral head in a position to minimize the tip apex distance. Historical data are referenced, but results using modern implants and techniques are the basis for this review.

Julie Lin and Joseph Lane discuss prevention of hip fractures, a topic that may seem outside the scope of orthopaedic practice. However, the topic is critically important given the steadily increasing prevalence of these injuries and the projections that they could reach near-epidemic proportions in the coming decades. The pharmacologic mechanisms of different agents used in the treatment and prevention of osteoporosis are briefly discussed in practical terms. Results and proper use of specific agents such as bisphosphonates, estrogen, selective estrogen receptor modulators, calcitonin, and parathyroid hormone are discussed. The section on prevention of hip fractures is quite comprehensive. Strategies for effective fall prevention are described, beginning with assessment of risk and patient education and continuing with interventions such as physical therapy, withdrawal of psychotropic medications, and home safety modifications, each of which has been shown to reduce the risk of falls. The authors conclude by discussing hip protectors, including explanations of theory, results (up to an eightfold reduction in risk of hip fractures), compliance, and cost-effectiveness. All physicians who care for patients with osteoporotic hip fractures, especially orthopaedic surgeons, will benefit from reading this article. Recent data indicate that patients who sustain a hip fracture are at a particularly high risk for a second fracture. Orthopaedic surgeons are critically important in managing these fractures and ultimately helping to reduce the risk of these potentially devastating injuries.

The initial approach to the treatment of severe foot and ankle injuries sometimes can be overwhelming. Multiple fractures, dislocations, and soft-tissue injuries must be managed simultaneously. Judith Baumhauer and Arthur Manoli provide a rational approach to these difficult injuries. The article begins logically with a discussion of patient evaluation and is followed by a comprehensive strategy to evaluate soft-tissue, vascular, and long bone injuries; assessment of limb viability is also described. The authors emphasize the importance of early realignment and stabilization of associated fractures and dislocations. These goals should not be achieved, however, at the expense of the soft-tissue envelope. External fixation can

be useful to restore and maintain alignment and length. Percutaneous reduction is often used in conjunction with Kirschner wire fixation. Definitive fixation, when required, can follow once the soft-tissue envelope is restored. The authors also provide specific fixation strategies for forefoot, midfoot, hindfoot, and ankle injuries; they also discuss the role of primary arthrodesis.

Little controversy exists regarding intramedullary nailing as the preferred surgical treatment of closed tibial shaft fractures. The utility of Andrew Schmidt and associates' article on closed tibial fractures, however, is the discussion of closed treatment methods and management strategies for proximal and distal tibia fractures. Although the role of casting tibial shaft fractures is indisputable, recent surveys indicate that even nondisplaced tibial shaft fractures are now more commonly treated with intramedullary nailing. The article not only outlines modern indications for nonsurgical treatment but also details the proper techniques for cast treatment. Casting techniques are rapidly becoming a lost art; therefore, this section is invaluable. Proximal tibial shaft fractures are difficult to treat with intramedullary nails. Valgus and apex anterior angulation are seen as common deformities. The authors describe the use of blocking screws as an adjunct to intramedullary nailing to help minimize malalignment of proximal tibia fractures. Although at the time this article was published, the results and relative advantages of locked plating were just beginning to be known, and the authors

correctly included plate fixation as a viable option for both proximal and distal tibia fractures. External fixation is much more commonly used for open than for closed tibia fractures. However, the authors remind us that external fixation is a viable choice in certain patient populations, such as those with extremely small canals, associated end segment tibia fractures, and in children.

Open fractures of the tibial shaft remain one of the most challenging of musculoskeletal injuries. Although intramedullary nailing usually can be used to adequately stabilize the fracture, uncomplicated fracture union and soft-tissue healing can be very difficult to achieve. Steve Olson and Emil Schemitsch present the current evidence on the best way to minimize these common complications. The authors correctly devote equal emphasis to soft-tissue management and fracture stabilization. The role of both systemic and local antibiotics is discussed, including alternative local delivery vehicles such as PMMA, antibiotic powder, and antibiotic-coated nails. The authors also correctly point out that débridement of contaminated tissues is the most important step in the initial management of open tibial fractures. However, the optimal technique for débridement remains controversial. They also present recent data comparing the effectiveness of high- and low-pressure pulsatile irrigation with solutions such as povidone-iodine, bacitracin, saline solution, and soap to remove adherent bacteria while preserving maximum bone structure and function. Although the severity of soft-tissue and bone injuries is the most critical factor impacting the outcome, controversy remains regarding whether the type, method, or timing of skeletal stabilization actually affects outcome. The relative roles of intramedullary nailing and external fixation to minimize infection are explored, as are the biologic and clinical effects of reaming. Finally, the optimal timing for and the type of wound closure are discussed.

Minimally invasive techniques are now well accepted for fracture fixation in many anatomic areas, but nowhere is the impact of these techniques to minimize soft-tissue complications greater than at the distal tibia. In their article, David Helfet and Michael Suk review the history, supply a detailed description of the surgical technique, and present Dr. Helfet's previously unpublished clinical results. Retrospectively, the authors reviewed 17 patients treated with a staged protocol of external fixation and open reduction and internal fixation of the fibula followed by definitive percutaneous plate fixation. All patients achieved union without soft-tissue complications. The use of specifically designed low profile plates in conjunction with such a staged procedure has become the most rational protocol for these demanding injuries.

Pediatric femur fractures have a long history of successful nonsurgical treatment. However, the combination of newer surgical techniques and implants specifically designed for this indication have made surgical treatment of pediatric fractures preferred in certain clinical situations. Paul Sponseller reviews the current indications for surgical treatment, including reduction techniques, pin care strategies, weight-bearing recommendations, the role of implant removal, and the socioeconomic cost of various treatments. The principal focus of the article is the technical descriptions of specific surgical techniques, including external fixation, rigid and flexible intramedullary rods, and plate fixation, along with their respective advantages and disadvantages. Dr. Sponseller points out that in contrast to adult femoral fractures, there are many ways to treat such injuries in children. Surgeons should be familiar with at least one option for each age range.

As the population of patients with total hip arthroplasties continues to grow, the number of periprosthetic fractures continues to grow as well. Sung-Rak Lee and Mathias Bostrom review current strategies for treating these challenging injuries. Their article focuses on treatment modalities and is organized based on the Vancouver classification of fracture type. Type A fractures (ie, those involving the greater trochanter) are associated with little controversy, perhaps due to generally good results and a paucity of published data. The optimal construct for type B1 fractures (defined as those at the tip of a well-fixed prosthesis without bone loss) is more controversial and is discussed in terms of both biomechanics and clinical results. Note, however, that this article was published in 2004, before more recent data were presented supporting treatment of these fractures using modern biologic plating techniques with a single lateral plate without allograft. Type B2 and B3 fractures usually require revision arthroplasty, and the optimal implants for such reconstructions are discussed. Type C fractures (ie, those distal to the tip of the prosthesis) can be treated independently of the arthroplasty. The authors point out the importance of avoiding stress risers between the stem tip and the proximal end of the fracture fixation device. For this reason, strong consideration should be given to extending the length of the plate fixation to overlap the region of the hip prosthesis to minimize the risk of subsequent fracture.

By covering the most common and most demanding lower extremity injuries, the following articles will help any surgeon, whether treating fractures is an interest or an obligation, to achieve the universal goal of optimal patient outcomes.

William M. Ricci, MD
Associate Professor
Department of Orthopaedic Surgery
Washington University School of
    Medicine at Barnes-Jewish Hospital
St. Louis, Missouri

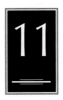

Femoral Neck Fractures

Andrew H. Schmidt, MD
Stanley E. Asnis, MD
George J. Haidukewych, MD
Kenneth J. Koval, MD
Karl-Göran Thorngren, MD, PhD

Abstract

Despite the tremendous advances in the science and practice of orthopaedic surgery, anesthesia, and perioperative care, repair of displaced fractures of the neck of the femur is still associated with complications in up to one third of patients. The risk of nonunion and osteonecrosis in particular is virtually the same today as in the 1930s. Recent data from well-designed outcome studies now indicate that the most predictable, durable, and cost-effective procedure for an active elderly patient with a displaced femoral neck fracture is total joint arthroplasty; however, not all patients are candidates for this procedure, and the potential complications of arthroplasty, including mortality, may be more difficult to manage and more severe than those associated with internal fixation. The laudable goal of obtaining fracture healing and maintenance of a viable femoral head can be successfully achieved in a number of patients.

The femoral neck fracture is an increasingly common and still imperfectly treated injury that is associated with significant morbidity and mortality. The incidence of femoral neck fractures has reached epidemic proportions with profound implications for public health policy. In one recent article, the authors estimated that (assuming the age- and gender-specific incidence of fractures remains constant) the number of fractures in South Australia would increase by approximately 66% by the year 2021 and 190% by 2051.[1] In the United States, the average orthopaedist will treat an estimated 15 to 25 femoral neck fractures each year. It is possible that the health care costs associated with this injury alone will overwhelm the health care system.

In 1935, Speed[2] noted that the fixation of femoral neck fractures was associated with complications in up to 36% of patients. Recently published meta-analyses report that this complication rate is essentially unchanged today.[3] Two comparative studies published in 2002 came to opposite conclusions about the best treatment. In a randomized study of 455 patients, Parker and associates[4] concluded that hemiarthroplasty is preferable to internal fixation. In contrast, Partanen and associates[5] reported a matched-pairs analysis of 714 patients and recommended internal fixation. Thorough economic analyses of the cost of treatment of femoral neck fractures have clearly indicated that the cost of treatment is largely influenced by the cost of treating complications, which are not only expensive to treat but significantly impact patient function.[6] In general, arthroplasty for femoral neck fracture is associated with a dramatically lower complication rate than internal fixation, and the lower risk of revision after arthroplasty more than offsets the higher initial cost of this procedure.[7] Long-term outcome studies demonstrate that arthroplasty, especially total hip replacement, affords the best and most durable function.[7] Increasingly, surgeons are turning toward total hip arthroplasty as the best solution for the fit, active patient with a femoral neck fracture.

When treating a patient with a fracture of the femoral neck, the physician must consider patient age and expectations and choose the procedure that will provide an appropriate degree of function with minimal risk of complications. Most importantly, revisions must be prevented. For each age group, there are many unanswered questions and ongoing controversy about treatment. In the young to middle-aged patient with a femoral neck fracture, immediate anatomic reduction and internal fixation is warranted. Yet even among these healthy patients, approximately one third will experience nonunion or osteonecrosis, and a significant number will eventually require conversion to total joint arthroplasty.[8] The challenge in treating the young patient with a femoral neck fracture is to improve techniques of reduction and fixation to reduce these complication rates.

There is no real consensus regarding the treatment of active, elderly patients. Medicare data suggest that for persons older than 65 years, most patients with femoral neck fractures are treated with some form of prosthetic replacement. No one knows what the ideal proportion of patients receiving arthroplasty should be. Robinson and associates[9] demonstrated that the application of a standard decision-making algorithm based on a scoring system can significantly reduce the rate of complications after internal fixation in patients age 65 to 85 years. In the less active older patient, there is more general agreement that hemiarthroplasty is appropriate, but controversy exists regarding the use of unipolar versus bipolar femoral heads.

To practice true evidence-based medicine, one must turn to the literature for guidance. However, there is a dearth of high-level evidence available regarding femoral neck fractures. Although nearly 300,000 articles can be found in a Medline search for "femoral neck fracture," only a few dozen represent prospective randomized clinical trials. Most of these studies are comparisons of different variations of internal fixation or cover different aspects of the perioperative medical care of these patients; they are of limited value in deciding the best surgical approach for treatment of a fractured hip. Nevertheless, even for aspects of care with high-level evidence, such as the use of prophylactic anticoagulation, prophylactic antibiotics, and regional anesthesia, wide variations in care exist.[10]

Prevention is key in managing the impending epidemic of femoral neck fractures. Fall prevention, improved diag-

nosis of osteoporosis, and possibly the use of trochanteric pads may all contribute to a decrease in the incidence of femoral neck fractures.[11]

In this chapter, the basic evaluation, medical care, and rehabilitation of the patient with a femoral neck fracture, and treatment methods of internal fixation and arthroplasty will be reviewed. A review of the changing treatment of displaced femoral neck fractures in Europe adds a different perspective to the American experience.

Treatment Principles for Femoral Neck Fractures
General Principles
The primary goal of fracture treatment is to return the patient to the preinjury level of function. There is nearly universal agreement that this level of function can best be achieved with surgery.[12] Historically, nonsurgical treatment has resulted in excessive rates of medical morbidity and mortality, as well as malunion and nonunion. Nonsurgical treatment is appropriate only for selected nonambulators who experience minimal discomfort from their injury.[13,14] These patients should be rapidly mobilized to avoid the complications of prolonged recumbency—decubitus ulcers, atelectasis, urinary tract infection, and thrombophlebitis.

Clinical Evaluation
The clinical presentation of patients with a fracture of the femoral neck can vary widely depending on injury type, severity, and/or etiology. Displaced fractures are usually symptomatic; such patients cannot stand or ambulate. Patients who have a nondisplaced or impacted femoral neck fracture may be ambulatory and experience minimal pain.

It is important to determine the mechanism of injury. Most femoral neck fractures in the elderly are the result of a low-energy fall, whereas in young adults they are more often caused by high-ener-

gy trauma, such as from a motor vehicle accident. In high-energy trauma patients, associated head, neck, chest, and abdominal injuries should be assessed. Although patients with a femoral neck stress fracture usually deny specific trauma, they should be questioned about any recent changes in the type, duration, or frequency of physical activity. When trauma can reasonably be ruled out (such as in sedentary individuals with no history of injury), pathologic fracture must be considered.

The timing of the injury must be determined whenever possible. In elderly individuals who live alone, hospital presentation may be delayed hours or even days, by which time these patients are often dehydrated and confused; determining the exact day or time when the fracture occurred may be difficult. In addition, the potential for dehydration mandates evaluation of fluid and electrolyte status in these patients.

A careful, thorough medical history is important because of the impact of preexisting medical comorbidities on both treatment and prognosis. Cardiopulmonary disease (congestive heart failure, intermittent myocardial ischemia, or chronic obstructive pulmonary disease) is a common preexisting medical condition that impacts fracture management in the elderly, affecting the patient's ability to tolerate prolonged recumbency, undergo surgery, and participate in rehabilitation. Cardiopulmonary disease history is also a major determinant of the rating system used by the American Society of Anesthesiologists to assess surgical risk.[15] Injuries resulting from falls by these patients may cause further deterioration of already compromised cardiopulmonary function.

Neurologic conditions such as Parkinson's disease, Alzheimer's disease, and the residual effects of a previous cerebrovascular event must also be considered during treatment. Clinical manifestations in patients with Parkinson's disease range from mild tremors to complete incapacitation with severe contractures; well-controlled disease generally will not impact treatment decisions. Patients who have had a prior stroke are at increased risk for fracture secondary to residual balance and gait problems as well as osteopenia of the paretic limb.[16,17] Treatment of these patients may be complicated by the presence of osteopenia, spasticity, and/or contracture. The degree of involvement, as in Parkinson's disease, ranges from minimal to severe spasticity with contracture. For patients with Alzheimer's disease and severe cognitive dysfunction, a treatment plan requiring a high degree of patient cooperation would be inappropriate.

Radiographic Evaluation

The standard radiographic examination of the hip includes an AP view of the pelvis and an AP and cross-table lateral view of the involved proximal femur. The AP pelvic view allows comparison of the involved side with the contralateral side and can help to identify nondisplaced and impacted fractures. The lateral radiograph can help to assess posterior comminution of the femoral neck and proximal femur; a cross-table lateral view is preferred to a frog-lateral view because the latter requires abduction, flexion, and external rotation of the affected lower extremity and involves a risk of fracture displacement. An internal rotation view of the injured hip may be helpful to identify nondisplaced or impacted fractures. Internally rotating the involved femur 10° to 15° offsets the anteversion of the femoral neck and provides a true AP view of the proximal femur. A second AP view of the contralateral side can be used for preoperative planning. If a pathologic fracture is suspected on the basis of the patient's medical history or the appearance of the fracture, full-length AP and lateral radiographs of the entire femur should be obtained.

When a hip fracture is suspected but not apparent on standard radiographs,

MRI scans should be obtained. MRI has been shown to be at least as accurate as bone scanning in identification of occult fractures of the hip and can be performed within 24 hours of injury.[18,19] MRI within 48 hours of fracture does not, however, appear to be useful for assessing femoral head viability/vascularity or predicting the development of osteonecrosis or healing complications.[20,21]

Laboratory Indices

Selective preoperative laboratory tests should be ordered for patients with confirmed fractures of the proximal hip. In the older patient, a complete blood cell count, electrolyte assessment with blood urea nitrogen and creatinine levels, electrocardiogram, and chest radiograph are probably sufficient. An arterial blood gas (as a baseline) is also probably warranted in older patients as well as in any patient with a history of a pulmonary disorder. Studies have demonstrated that the yield of nonselective laboratory testing to find clinically important abnormalities is low.[22] Additional laboratory studies should be ordered based on the medical history.

Initial Patient Management

All patients with a femoral neck fracture should be admitted to the hospital and maintained on bed rest. In the past, patients were routinely placed in 5 lb of Buck's skin traction to prevent further fracture displacement or additional soft-tissue injury that could compromise the vascular supply to the femoral head. Most authors currently advocate maintenance of the leg in a position of comfort—usually slight hip flexion and external rotation, supported by pillows under the knee. Several studies have shown that the extended position that results from Buck's traction increases intracapsular pressure, thereby diminishing femoral head blood flow.[23,24] Conversely, the position of external rotation and flexion allows for maximum capsular volume.

Surgical Timing

In general, hip fracture surgery should be performed as soon as possible after stabilization of all comorbid medical conditions; particular attention must be given to cardiopulmonary problems and fluid and electrolyte imbalances. In a series of 399 hip fracture patients, Kenzora and associates[25] reported that a surgical delay of less than 1 week to stabilize medical problems was not associated with increased mortality. Interestingly, they found that even healthy patients who underwent surgery within 24 hours of hospital admission had a 34% mortality rate at 1-year follow-up compared with a 5.8% mortality rate for those who underwent surgery between days 2 and 5. Conversely, Sexson and Lehner[26] found that relatively healthy hip fracture patients (with up to two comorbid conditions) who had surgery within 24 hours of admission had a higher survival rate than similar patients who had surgery after 24 hours. However, patients with three or more comorbid conditions had a poorer survival rate when undergoing surgery within 24 hours than those undergoing surgery after 24 hours. In a prospective series of 367 elderly patients with hip fracture, Zuckerman and associates[27] reported that a surgical delay of more than 2 calendar days from hospital admission roughly doubled the risk of the patient dying before the end of the first postoperative year.

Anesthetic Considerations

Although much has been written on the risks and benefits of the different anesthetic techniques, no significant difference in survival rates has been found in elderly patients with hip fracture who undergo surgery under regional versus general anesthesia.[28,29] Many anesthesiologists, internists, and surgeons believe that patients "look better" following regional anesthesia. However, studies have documented no difference in postoperative mental status in patients following regional or general anesthesia.[28,29] Studies have demonstrated the efficacy of regional anesthesia (spinal and epidural) in the prophylaxis of deep venous thrombosis (DVT) and pulmonary embolus.[30] Because pulmonary embolism is a significant cause of morbidity and mortality in this population, regional anesthesia may be preferable, especially if the patient is at increased risk for thromboembolic complications and there are other medical factors that compromise use of thromboprophylaxis.

Thromboprophylaxis

The rates of total and proximal DVT after hip fracture without prophylaxis, derived from prospective studies in which venography was performed, are approximately 50% and 27%, respectively.[31-44] Fatal pulmonary embolism has been reported in the range of 1.4% to 7.5% within the first 3 months after hip fracture.[45-47] In an autopsy study of 581 patients who died after hip fracture in a British hospital from 1953 to 1992, pulmonary embolism was the fourth most common cause of death, accounting for 14% of all deaths.[48] Factors that appear to further increase the risk of thromboembolism after hip fracture include increasing age, surgical delay, and the use of general (versus regional) anesthetic.[46,48-51]

Symptomatic thrombophlebitis and fatal pulmonary embolism can be prevented by use of thromboprophylaxis following hip fracture.[52] Thromboprophylaxis should be provided to all patients who sustain a fracture of the proximal femur. Two approaches might be considered to prevent fatal pulmonary embolism: (1) early detection of subclinical venous thrombosis by screening high-risk patients, and (2) primary prophylaxis using either drugs or physical methods that are effective for preventing DVT and pulmonary embolism. Several prophylactic measures have been recommended, including subcutaneous heparin, low-molecular-weight heparin, intra-venous dextran, warfarin sodium, aspirin, intermittent pneumatic compression of the foot or leg, and various combined modalities.

Oral anticoagulant prophylaxis has been shown to be effective and safe in patients who sustain a fracture of the proximal femur. A randomized trial compared postoperative warfarin with aspirin or no prophylaxis.[41] The DVT rates in these three groups were 20%, 41%, and 46%, respectively ($P = 0.005$), whereas the proximal DVT rates were 9%, 11%, and 30%, respectively ($P = 0.001$). Rates of bleeding were similar across the three groups. Pooled results from three studies of adjusted-dose oral anticoagulant prophylaxis showed a reduction in relative risk of DVT of 61% (66% for proximal DVT) compared with no prophylaxis.[33,36,41] The reported bleeding rates for oral anticoagulant prophylaxis range from 0 to 47%,[33,36,41] with the most recent and largest trial finding no difference in bleeding compared to placebo.[41]

Low-molecular-weight heparin has been shown to lower the risk for DVT and proximal DVT after hip fracture.[32,34,37,39,44] Two studies found no significant difference in bleeding when low-molecular-weight heparin was compared with placebo[37] or with low-dose heparin,[39] although the sample sizes were small.

A recent review of prophylaxis methods after hip fracture included 31 trials and 2,958 patients.[53] Both unfractionated low-dose heparin and low-molecular-weight heparin were shown to protect against DVT (combined risk reduction was 40% compared with no prophylaxis) without increasing the risk for wound hematoma.

The synthetic pentasaccharide fondaparinux, a selective factor Xa inhibitor, has been investigated in patients after hip fracture.[34,54] Eriksson and associates[34] randomized 1,711 hip fracture patients to receive either subcutaneous enoxaparin (40 mg once daily started 12 to 24 hours postoperatively) or subcutaneous fondaparinux (2.5 mg started 4 to 8 hours after surgery). Preoperative initiation of enoxaparin or fondaparinux occurred in 26% and 11% of patients, respectively. The incidence of thromboembolism by postoperative day 11 was 19.1% (119 of 624 patients) in the enoxaparin group and 8.3% (52 of 626 patients) in the fondaparinux group ($P < 0.001$). Proximal DVT rates were also significantly reduced in the fondaparinux group (4.3% vs 0.9%; $P < 0.001$).

A meta-analysis has suggested that antiplatelet agents are effective in preventing postoperative thromboembolism after hip fracture.[55] None of the studies included in this meta-analysis, however, used routine contrast venography as an outcome measure. In the Pulmonary Embolism Prevention Trial, 13,356 hip fracture surgery patients in five countries were randomized to receive either prophylaxis with 160 mg of enteric-coated aspirin or placebo started before surgery (in 82%) and continued for 35 days.[56] Additional thromboembolic prophylaxis was allowed at the discretion of the attending physician and was done with graduated compression stockings, low-molecular-weight heparin, or low-dose heparin in 18%, 26%, and 30% of patients, respectively. Although the study's authors concluded that fatal pulmonary embolism and DVT were both significantly reduced by the addition of aspirin, the confounding and inconsistent use of other means of prophylaxis, as well as possible differences in anesthetic technique, make the conclusions of even this large trial open to criticism.

Elastic stockings are inexpensive, simple to use, and can be used in conjunction with other prophylactic measures. However, there is little evidence that graduated compression stockings provide any thromboprophylaxis when used alone. Intermittent pneumatic compression of the legs is an attractive form of prophylaxis that is effective in patients undergoing general surgery, neurosurgery, and prostatic surgery. Prophylaxis with intermittent pneumatic compression is virtually free of adverse effects and carries no risk of bleeding. External pneumatic compression overcomes venous stasis by intermittently squeezing the leg, and it also enhances fibrinolysis. Thus, intermittent compression has both a physical and a pharmacologic effect. At some institutions, an ultrasound of the venous system of both lower extremities is performed before placement of the external pneumatic compression devices to exclude the presence of preexisting thrombophlebitis. The role of intermittent pneumatic compression in patients undergoing hip surgery remains uncertain because of a lack of data concerning its effectiveness when used alone. One prospective, randomized study of 304 patients with hip and pelvic fractures compared pneumatic sequential compression devices to no specific prophylaxis.[57] As determined by follow-up venous Doppler duplex scans and ventilation perfusion scans, a statistically significant reduction in DVT and/or pulmonary embolism was found overall (11% in control patients and 4% in the experimental group; $P = 0.02$). When the results were stratified by fracture type (hip fracture compared with pelvic fracture), the sequential compression devices remained effective in the patients with hip fractures but were not effective in those with pelvic fractures.[57] Although the total DVT and pulmonary embolism rate may be lowered by mechanical compression devices, this study did not distinguish between proximal and distal DVT. A meta-analysis of total hip arthroplasty patients suggests that sequential compression devices may not be as effective in preventing proximal DVT compared with distal DVT.[58] This is a very real concern because even the combination of graduated compression stockings and subcutaneous low-molecular-weight heparin was found not to be effective in

preventing proximal DVT in 644 patients with hip fractures.[59] The authors of this study recommend screening Doppler ultrasonography in all hip fracture patients to identify DVT.[59] Therefore, although these devices may contribute to a lower overall risk of thromboembolism, especially in patients in whom anticoagulation is contraindicated, the physician must still be vigilant for the development of thromboembolism despite the use of sequential compression devices.

Use of intermittent compression of the plantar venous plexus (foot pumps) for deep vein thromboprophylaxis has garnered recent interest. The pneumatic bladder of this device straps around the patient's foot in the region of the longitudinal arch. Although there are no data describing the efficacy of plantar compression in patients with hip fractures, Westrich and Sculco[60] performed a prospective, randomized study to assess the efficacy of foot pumps for prophylaxis against DVT after total knee arthroplasty. A group of 122 patients (164 knees) were randomized to receive thromboprophylaxis with either aspirin alone or foot pumps in conjunction with aspirin. The prevalence of DVT was significantly less in the foot pump group compared with patients managed with aspirin alone (27% versus 59%, $P < 0.001$). No proximal thrombi were noted in any patient who used the foot pump device, whereas the prevalence of proximal thrombosis in the popliteal or femoral veins was 14% in the group treated with aspirin alone ($P < 0.01$). No adverse effects were noted in any patient who used the foot pump device. The authors concluded that the use of foot pumps in conjunction with aspirin was a safe and effective method of thromboprophylaxis after total knee arthroplasty. However, the applicability of this method for hip fracture patients remains unknown.

Recently, the Seventh American College of Chest Physicians Conference on Antithrombotic and Thrombolytic

Therapy was held.[61] Using evidence-based methodology, this group does not recommend the use of aspirin alone for thromboprophylaxis for any patient group. For patients undergoing surgery for repair of a hip fracture, the group recommends the routine use of either fondaparinux, low-molecular-weight heparin, warfarin (target International Normalized Ratio, 2.5; range 2.0 to 3.0), or low-dose unfractionated heparin.[61]

Rehabilitation

Early mobilization out of bed after hip fracture surgery is important for the general well-being of the patient; it reduces the risk of DVT, pulmonary complications, skin breakdown, and decline in mental status. Mobilization also inspires confidence and encourages the patient to recover. In addition to early mobilization and ambulation training, treatment goals for the physical therapist include patient training in transfers, improving strength, maintaining balance, and maintaining range of joint motion.

Ambulation training should be initiated on the first or second day after surgery. Most patients who have sustained a femoral neck fracture and were treated with either internal fixation or prosthetic replacement should be allowed to bear weight as tolerated. Elderly patients with decreased upper extremity strength and occasionally those with associated upper extremity fractures may find it difficult to comply with a non–weight-bearing or even a partial weight-bearing protocol. Another important consideration is that even partial weight bearing involves the generation of considerable force across the hip by the lower extremity musculature.[62]

Internal Fixation of Femoral Neck Fractures

Femoral neck fractures can be surgically treated by internal fixation or femoral head replacement. Impacted femoral neck fractures are usually treated by

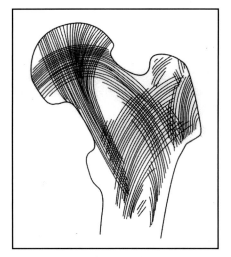

Figure 1 A trabecular network of bone supports the femoral neck and head. The center of the head, where the primary compressive and tension trabeculae coalesce, has the greatest density. The superior dome of the head has the second greatest density. (Reproduced with permission from Asnis SE, Kyle RF: Intracapsular hip fractures, in Asnis SE, Kyle RF (eds): *Cannulated Screw Fixation: Principles and Operative Techniques.* New York, NY, Springer-Verlag, 1996, p 52.)

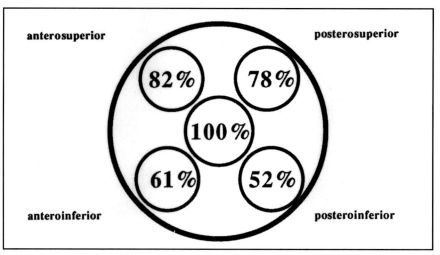

Figure 2 Bone density of cadaveric femoral heads. The middle and superior portions of the femoral head are more dense than the inferior portions.[69] (Reproduced with permission from Asnis SE, Kyle RF: Intracapsular hip fractures, in Asnis SE, Kyle RF (eds): *Cannulated Screw Fixation: Principles and Operative Techniques.* New York, NY, Springer-Verlag, 1996, p 52.)

internal fixation. The goal of this chapter is not to convince the surgeon to favor fixation, but rather when fixation is chosen, to do it properly. The quality of reduction and integrity of the newly constructed "bone-screw complex" can be significant. The quality of the bone, security of the bone-to-bone contact, number of screws, and position of the screws in the femoral neck and head all can be factors in obtaining osteosynthesis of the fracture and minimizing osteonecrosis.

Structural Anatomy and Aging

The male and female adult's neck-shaft angle is approximately $130° \pm 7°$ and the femoral neck anteversion is $10° \pm 7°$.[63,64] The femoral head is slightly oblong[65] with an average size of 40 to 60 mm. The hip capsule is attached anteriorly at the intertrochanteric line, whereas posteriorly the lateral half of the femoral neck is extracapsular.[66] The portion of the neck

that is intracapsular has no periosteum, and fractures must heal by endosteal union. In 1838, Ward[67] described a trabecular network that supported the femoral head and neck. The primary compression trabeculae concentrate at the medial femoral neck and then fan out under the superior dome of the femoral head (Figure 1). The primary tensile trabeculae make an arch from the fovea medially to the lateral femoral cortex just distal to the greater trochanter laterally. Secondary compressive and tensile trabeculae orient themselves according to Wolff's law to increase the structural strength. Singh and associates[68] found that with aging and osteopenia a progressive sequential loss of these trabeculae takes place, thus decreasing structural strength. The trochanteric and secondary compression and tensile trabeculae are lost first. As osteopenia continues, the primary tension trabeculae become interrupted and lost, followed last by the loss of primary compression trabeculae. Because those patients with intracapsular hip fractures usually represent a more osteopenic population, femoral head and neck bone density are most important in

fixation. The trabecular bone within the femoral neck is often of very low density and is unable to support the fixation device alone, necessitating use of the femoral neck cortical bone for support. Bone density studies of cadaveric femoral heads have demonstrated that the bone in the middle and superior femoral head provides better support than the weaker bone of the inferior head[63,69] (Figure 2). These findings are consistent with those in studies assessing trabecular patterns. The densest bone is in the central head, whereas the posterior inferior quadrant is usually the weakest.[69]

The geometry of placement of fixation screws is determined by the anatomy of the femoral head and neck. The bone density within the femoral neck is typically very low, so that screws traversing the center of the femoral neck have very little support (as if they were in a hollow tube). Unlike a dynamic compression hip screw and sideplate, cannulated screw heads buttress against the femoral cortex and the threads lock in the femoral head. If forces are applied to direct the head fragment inferiorly or posteriorly and the screw shafts are apart from the endosteal

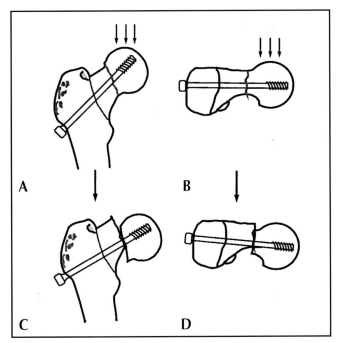

Figure 3 When forces are applied directly to the top of the femoral head in standing (**A**), the head fragment may fall inferiorly until the screw shaft rests on the medial femoral neck endocortex (**B**). Anterior forces on the femoral head, such as those applied when going from a sitting to standing position (**C**), can cause the head fragment to displace posteriorly until the screw shaft rests on the posterior femoral neck endocortex (**D**). (Reproduced with permission from Asnis SE, Kyle RF: Intracapsular hip fractures, in Asnis SE, Kyle RF (eds): *Cannulated Screw Fixation: Principles and Operative Techniques*. New York, NY, Springer-Verlag, 1996, p 53.)

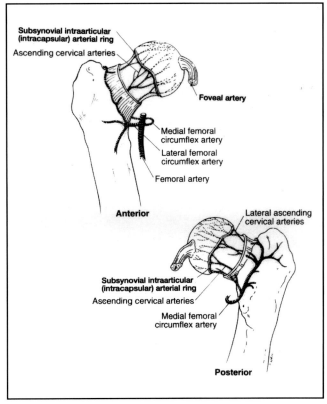

Figure 4 The arterial supply of the femoral head. (Reproduced with permission from Asnis SE, Kyle RF: Intracapsular hip fractures, in Asnis SE, Kyle RF (eds): *Cannulated Screw Fixation: Principles and Operative Techniques*. New York, NY, Springer-Verlag, 1996, p 54.)

cortical femoral neck, the femoral head and screws may drift until a screw's shaft comes to rest against the endosteal cortex[70,71] (Figure 3). Screw thread fixation in the head itself is dependent on the density of the trabecular bone; screw threads placed in the middle and superior head have better holding power than those in an inferior position.

Vascular Anatomy

Three major groups of vessels supply blood to the femoral head: (1) an extracapsular ring located at the base of the femoral neck; (2) ascending cervical branches on the surface of the femoral neck; and (3) arteries of the ligamentum teres, or foveal arteries[72,73] (Figure 4). A large branch of the medial circumflex artery posteriorly and branches of the lateral circumflex artery anteriorly form an extracapsular arterial ring at the base of the femoral neck. From this ring arise the ascending cervical branches that are anatomically described as the anterior, posterior, medial, and lateral groups. The lateral ascending cervical arteries appear to provide most of the blood supply to the superior femoral head and lateral neck. The ascending cervical vessels then go into a less distinct vascular ring at the articular cartilage-neck junction known as the subsynovial intra-articular arterial ring.[74] From this ring, vessels penetrate the femoral head and are then referred to as the epiphyseal arteries. The lateral epiphyseal artery is believed to supply most of the blood to the weight-bearing area of the femoral head. The lateral epiphyseal artery system passes within the posterior retinaculum of Weitbrecht.[73,75-78] More simply—and probably just as clinically relevant and accurate—Swiontkowski describes the lateral epiphyseal artery as the terminal branch of the medial circumflex artery supplying the weight-bearing surface of the femoral head in 90% of adults.[79] The terminal branch of the lateral circumflex artery supplies the inferior portion of the femoral head. The artery of the ligamentum teres is a branch of the obturator or medial circumflex artery. These vessels are believed to supply a substantial portion of the femoral head in only one third of patients.[80] However, these vessels may be important in revascularization of the femoral head after fixation. A very limited amount of blood is supplied through intraosseous vessels that come directly from the marrow below.

In a nondisplaced fracture, the risk of direct damage to epiphyseal arteries is far less. Bleeding into a capsule that has not been disrupted, however, may cause increased pressure and decreased blood supply by tamponade. The benefits of aspiration and capsulotomy during the procedure are still being debated, but may be beneficial in the patient with a nondisplaced fracture.[23,81-84] Significant intracapsular hematomas were not seen in a 1994 study of preoperative MRI of 20 patients with displaced fractures.[20] In the displaced fracture, a tear in the capsule may dissipate the hematoma. Instead, displaced fractures are likely to have direct arterial injury by disruption or kinking. The potential for vascular injury may be greater among Garden IV fractures than in Garden III fractures. The Garden IV fracture is believed to tear the posterior retinaculum of Weitbrecht and thus sustain a greater vascular insult. Early reduction and fixation may play a positive role by unkinking intact vessels, but this is still speculative.

Classification

Although several classification schemes exist for femoral neck fractures, the Garden classification will be discussed in this chapter. Garden's classification,[85-87] based on the degree of displacement of the fracture, is functional and appears to be the classification most widely used today. A Garden I fracture is an incomplete or an impacted fracture. A Garden II fracture is a complete fracture without displacement. A Garden III fracture is a complete fracture with displacement. The retinaculum of Weitbrecht remains intact and maintains continuity between the proximal and distal fragments. By being displaced and yet tethered by the retinaculum, the femoral head becomes tilted in the acetabulum and thus the tra-

becular pattern of the femoral head does not line up with that of the acetabulum. A Garden IV fracture is a completely displaced fracture with all continuity between the proximal and distal fragments disrupted. The femoral head can spin free, and its trabecular pattern usually lines up with that of the acetabulum. Many surgeons find it difficult to differentiate between Garden III and Garden IV fractures. In the Garden IV fracture, the femoral head may be rotated in the acetabulum because of the impingement of the distal fragment on the proximal fragment from the way the subject is positioned during the radiograph. Several surgeons have simply combined Garden I and II fractures into nondisplaced fractures and grouped Garden III and IV as displaced fractures.

The nondisplaced or Garden I and II fractures are fixed in situ. The valgus-impacted fractures are left in place and fixed. A capsulotomy may be considered for tamponade. Full weight bearing is permitted immediately after fixation. The incidence of nonunion is rare and because the vessels are intact, the occurrence of osteonecrosis should be low. The displaced or Garden III and IV fractures are expected to have a higher complication rate. Theoretically, the Garden III fracture has a better prognosis for two reasons. The posterior retinaculum of Weitbrecht is intact and the lateral epiphyseal artery system is more likely to be intact. A good reduction is also more readily obtainable. With the patient in traction and the posterior retinaculum intact, internal rotation reduces the fracture. The posterior retinaculum acts similar to the binding of a book as it is closed. Full weight bearing is generally permitted immediately after surgery if there is a good reduction with bone-to-bone support. Six weeks of partial weight bearing should be considered when the stability of the reduction or fixation is uncertain. Physical therapy is given for ambulation training, but range-of-motion exercises,

particularly rotational exercises, should be avoided.

Treatment Controversy

In the displaced fracture in the elderly patient with osteoporosis, the decision between fixation and arthroplasty becomes an issue. Although prosthetic replacement is a more definitive mode of treatment, some studies have shown a higher morbidity and mortality rate than that for internal fixation.[88-92] In the more active individual, a hemiarthroplasty may require conversion to a total hip replacement.[93,94] Immediate total hip arthroplasty has been shown to have a far higher morbidity and mortality rate when done for an acute fracture than in the patient with chronic arthritis.[95,96] Franzen and associates[96] found the age- and sex-adjusted risk of prosthetic failure in total hip arthroplasties performed for femoral neck fracture complication to be 2.5 times higher than after primary arthroplasty performed for osteoarthritis ($P = 0.012$). Many other researchers have reported that the dislocation rate is significantly higher in fracture patients.[97-101] Nilsson and associates[101] compared one group of patients 4 to 12 years after a primary hemiarthroplasty with another group who had a secondary total hip replacement as a salvage procedure for complications of reduction and fixation of femoral neck fractures. The secondary total hip replacement group used walking aids to a lesser extent and experienced fewer problems in several aspects of life. The authors concluded that secondary total hip replacement in patients with healing complications following primary osteosynthesis provided better long-term functional capacity than that obtained with primary hemiarthroplasty.

Reduction and fixation of the intracapsular hip fracture with multiple pins or screws has been reported as a procedure of much lower morbidity and mortality than prosthetic arthroplasty.[88,91,92,102-104] With improved methods of fixation and a tendency toward earlier weight bearing, internal fixation becomes a more attractive mode of treatment—particularly in younger, more active patients. Those patients who develop the complication of nonunion or osteonecrosis can undergo total hip arthroplasty as a delayed elective procedure, with very low morbidity and mortality.[96,105]

Internal fixation of displaced intracapsular hip fractures is advantageous for many patients. Although statistics vary, it appears that the risk of death or major complication is lower following internal fixation than after immediate prosthetic replacement. For the 70% to 75% of patients whose fractures heal without subsequent development of osteonecrosis, their own femoral heads function as well as, or better than, prostheses. For those who have a problem with union or later develop osteonecrosis, a well-planned elective total hip arthroplasty is usually a safe procedure. The risks of medical complications appear far lower when the procedure is delayed rather than performed immediately after the fracture. The complications of internal fixation, namely osteonecrosis or nonunion, are much easier to deal with than complications of a failed hemiarthroplasty.

In the more active individual, a primary hemiarthroplasty does not perform as well as a total hip replacement. Primary total hip arthroplasty right after fracture has a higher complication rate and may not function as well as a delayed total hip procedure, which is required only in that group of patients who have complications after internal fixation.

Indications for Internal Fixation
The indication for cannulated screw fixation includes all nonpathologic nondisplaced or Garden I and II fractures. Age is not a factor. The displaced or Garden III and IV fractures can be treated by reduction and internal fixation or hemiarthroplasty or total hip arthroplasty. It is the

authors' preference to perform reduction and fixation for all patients other than those in whom a primary prosthetic replacement is required. Prosthetic replacement is indicated for (1) failure to achieve a satisfactory reduction other than in the younger patient; (2) fracture of the femoral head or dislocation of the femoral head with fracture of the femoral neck; (3) fractures more than 5 days old; (4) pathologic fractures; (5) fractures in an abnormal hip, that is, the rheumatoid or osteoarthritic hip; (6) fractures with significant femoral neck comminution with a butterfly fragment of 1 cm or more; and (7) a Garden IV fracture in a patient older than 75 years and a Singh classification of III or less.

In the younger patient (younger than 55 years), all attempts are made to obtain a satisfactory reduction. If this is not possible or there is posterior neck comminution, then open reduction and a bone grafting procedure should be considered.[106]

Potential Complications of Internal Fixation
Problems in Healing Multiple cannulated parallel screws were introduced for the fixation of femoral neck fractures in 1980 in an attempt to increase the accuracy of fixation and decrease complications.[107-109] Although it appears that the rate of successful osteosynthesis has improved significantly with this technique, the incidence of osteonecrosis may be unchanged. In a long-term follow-up study of 141 patients treated with cannulated screws, only 5 had a loss of position or nonunion;[108] this resulted in a 96% chance of successful osteosynthesis. However, internal fixation of the displaced femoral neck fracture is not a simple procedure. A stable reduction is essential and the fixation screws must be placed accurately.

Osteonecrosis Osteonecrosis remains the main complication following internal fixation of femoral neck fractures. A displaced femoral neck fracture has a devas-

tating effect on the blood supply of the femoral head. Following autoradiograms of femoral head specimens of patients given phosphorus 32(P32) before prosthetic arthroplasty for acute femoral neck fractures, Calandruccio and Anderson[110] reported that 22% of the femoral heads were completely vascular, 32% were completely avascular, and 47% were partially avascular. Catto's[111,112] meticulous histologic studies of whole femoral heads obtained at least 16 days after transcervical fracture showed 34% of the femoral heads to be completely vascular, 55% partially avascular, and 11% totally avascular. Sevitt's[113] arteriographic and histologic necropsy of the femoral heads with femoral neck fractures showed total or partial necrosis in 84% of the specimens. Apparently, most patients sustain a significant vascular injury at the time of the fracture, yet only 20% to 30% of patients who undergo internal fixation develop radiographic evidence of osteonecrosis with clinical segmental collapse. Most displaced femoral neck fractures probably undergo significant revascularization following internal fixation. During this period, the fracture heals and most patients function well even though a significant area of the femoral head may still be partially avascular. Many of the original studies on femoral neck fractures gave rates of osteonecrosis based on the false assumption that most segmental collapse would be evident by 2 years. However, it appears that revascularization for the femoral head is a very slow process and in some patients is never complete. In one long-term follow-up study of 141 patients treated with cannulated screws, a 9% rate of osteonecrosis at 2 years was followed by an overall 18% incidence after an average follow-up of 8 years (minimum follow-up 5 years); 3 of the patients first developed clinical symptoms and segmental collapse after 5 years.[104] Although segmental collapse may develop long after the initial fracture, function of the patient is the prima-

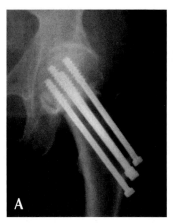
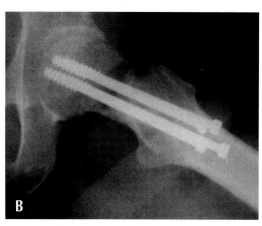

Figure 5 Fixation of a femoral neck fracture with four parallel 6.5-mm screws in a diamond configuration. **A,** The AP radiograph shows the head well supported by the femoral neck. The stable "hat hook" position with the impaction of the superior femoral neck beneath the subchondral bone of the superior femoral head is shown. The most distal screw shaft lies along the medial neck, preventing the femoral head from falling into varus. **B,** The posterior screw shaft lies along the posterior femoral neck, preventing the femoral head from displacing posteriorly.

ry goal of treatment. Many patients have excellent function and no symptoms even though the femoral head is partially avascular. Frequently, symptoms appear only after the ultimate development of segmental collapse. Once symptoms do appear, elective total hip arthroplasty appears safe and extremely effective, with results equivalent to those of total hip replacement in patients with primary osteoarthritis.

Reduction

The most important objective in the treatment of the displaced femoral neck fracture is to obtain stable bony support of the femoral head on the femoral neck. The fixation is used to increase stability by compressing the fracture and then maintaining the reduction by neutralizing forces acting on the hip. Even if a patient is not bearing weight, going from a sitting to a standing position creates three times as much force across the hip as does weight bearing.[114] The factors that decrease stability are comminution of the posterior femoral neck and poor reduction.[115] Major comminution of the femoral neck is a contraindication for

reduction and fixation, and hemiarthroplasty usually becomes the preferred treatment; however, as stated earlier, in the younger patient an open reduction and bone graft should be considered.[106]

The Garden Index is an expression of the angle of the compression trabeculae on the AP radiograph over the angle of the compression trabeculae on the lateral radiograph. A perfect anatomic reduction is therefore expressed as 160/180. Thus, the goal of reduction is a position as close as possible to a Garden Index of 160/180 (AP/lateral).[85-87] On the AP radiograph, the primary compression trabeculae should ideally be at an angle of 160° to the longitudinal axis of the femoral shaft, whereas on the lateral radiograph these compression trabeculae should lie in a straight line or 180° with the femoral shaft axis. In a good reduction, the medial femoral head and neck fragment are well supported by the medial neck of the femur. The position should be either anatomic or with the head and neck fragment in slight lateral translation in relation to the supporting femoral neck. Although slight valgus is acceptable, varus is not. Slight valgus with the supe-

rior femoral neck impacted beneath the subchondral bone of the superior femoral head usually provides a very stable configuration.[64] This acts as a "hat hook" and transforms the downward force of the body weight onto the femoral head into a force that enhances compression of the fracture (Figure 5). On the lateral view, alignment is again important, with the posterior neck of the distal fragment supporting that of the head and neck fragment.[116]

Reduction can be accomplished with traction on a fracture table with the leg in neutral flexion, neutral rotation, and 10° of abduction. The leg is then internally rotated as far as possible, and then backed off into a position of 15° of internal rotation. The medial neck spike of the fragment should be well supported by the femoral neck of the femur. With a cannulated screw system, some overdistraction at the time of the initial reduction is permissible because the fracture can later be guided into a good position and compressed once the parallel guide pins are in place or with the lag of the parallel screws. In most patients without major femoral neck comminution, this maneuver will yield a satisfactory and stable position. In very rare instances, an open reduction may be necessary before fixation.

Fixation Screws

The purposes of the fixation screws are to (1) lock the fracture in a position in which the femoral neck gives bone-against-bone support to the femoral head-neck fragment; (2) prevent posterior and varus migration of the femoral head; and (3) be parallel in order to maintain bone-on-bone support as the fracture settles in the healing period. In a cannulated screw system, the smaller diameter guide pins can be used to accurately determine the screw position as well as the length, and the accuracy of screw placement is improved with jigs for placement of guide pins. With parallel screws, excellent compression can be produced atraumatically by the lag effect of the screws.

Geometry of Screw Position in the Femoral Neck and Head

To prevent femoral head migration, screw positioning is critical. The most distal single screw passes through the femoral cortex, with its shaft resting on the supporting medial neck, and its threads fixing the inferior femoral head (Figure 6). For the femoral head to fall into varus, this screw's threads must first cut through the femoral head. In the lateral plane, a second screw should be placed posteriorly so that it rests on the posterior neck of the distal fragment at the midhead level on the AP plane. For posterior head migration to occur, its threads must cut through the head (Figure 6). The positioning of these two screws is crucial. Martens and associates[70] demonstrated that internal fixation using multiple Knowles pins had a high rate of failure unless the most distal screw rested on the cortical bone of the medial aspect of the femoral neck (Figure 3). Lindequist[71] evaluated 87 patients who had internal fixation of femoral neck fractures with two von Bahr screws. He found that the posterior placement of the proximal screw and the inferior placement of the distal screw improved the rate of fracture union. Studies in Sweden using fixation with only two hooked pins in these key locations gave fair clinical results.[117,118]

Deyerle[119] found that multiple pins placed around the periphery of the femoral neck compressing the fracture provided rotatory stability. Three or four parallel cannulated screws placed peripherally around the femoral neck compressing the fracture are equally atraumatic and also yield excellent rotatory stability.

Following these principles, it is the authors' preference to place two screws—the first along the endocortex of the femoral neck in the distal position and then the second along the endocortex in

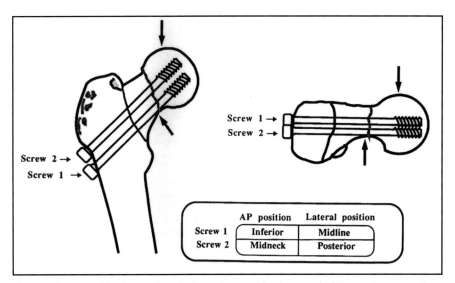

Figure 6 Screw positioning. In the AP plane, the most distal screw shaft (screw 1) rests on the medial femoral neck. A second screw (screw 2) should be at the midhead level on the AP projection and should rest on the posterior femoral neck in the lateral plane. (Reproduced with permission from Asnis SE, Kyle RF: Intracapsular hip fractures, in Asnis SE, Kyle RF (eds): *Cannulated Screw Fixation: Principles and Operative Techniques*. New York, NY, Springer-Verlag, 1996, p 60.)

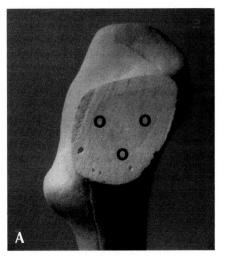 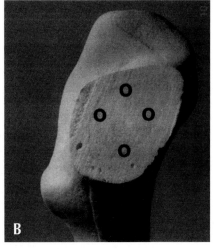

Figure 7 Cross-section showing the position of the screws in the femoral neck. **A,** Three-screw inverted triangle configuration. **B,** Four-screw diamond configuration.

the posterior position. In Garden I and II fractures, a third screw at the midhead level on the AP view and in an anterior position on the lateral view provides additional stability (Figures 7, *A*, and 8). In the Garden III and IV fractures, a fourth screw superiorly on the AP view and midline in the lateral view further supplements fixation (Figures 5 and

7, *B*). Studies by Swiontkowski and associates[120] and Springer and associates[121] have suggested that the fourth screw added little in additional fixation; however, both of these teams used models that represented a Garden II fracture and not the Garden III or IV fracture with some comminution. In a biomechanical study conducted in 1999 by Kauffman and

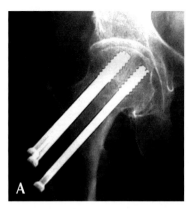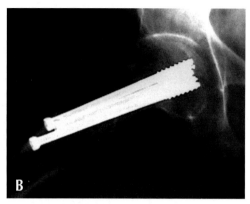

Figure 8 Fixation of an femoral neck fracture with three parallel 6.5-mm screws in an inverted triangle configuration. **A,** The AP radiograph shows the most distal screw shaft resting on the medial neck. The proximal two screws are placed slightly above the midhead level. **B,** The posterior screw shaft lies along the posterior femoral neck.

associates,[122] the fourth screw was shown to add significant fixation.[108,109]

The inverted triangle and diamond patterns of screw placement also fit well into the shape of the femoral neck (Figure 7). Although most mechanical models show the head loaded in the standing position, studies have shown that the hip bears three times the force when going from sitting to standing than when walking.[114] The triangle and diamond patterns adapt well to the different forces applied to the hip in different body positions.

The distal screw should not enter the femoral cortex below the level of the lesser trochanter. No more than one screw hole (either with a screw present or left empty) should ever be made at the level of the lesser trochanter. Because there is no sideplate, weakness at this level can lead to a subtrochanteric fracture.[123] Two distal screws at the level of or distal to the lesser trochanter must be used with caution. Iatrogenic fractures can occur at this level, propagating from a crack between the distal holes. No subtrochanteric fractures occurred in one series of 141 patients.[108]

Femoral Head Bone Density and Fixation Geometry

Fixation of the femoral head is also dependent on the holding power of the screw threads in the trabecular bone of the femoral head. Crowell and associates[69] and Benterud and associates[63] designed screw pull-out models in which they found the previous recommendations of screw placement in the inferior and posteromedial portions of the femoral head for better stability to be incorrect. In each of these studies, screws were placed in different quadrants of femoral heads collected at autopsy and pull-out tests were performed. The inferior portions of the femoral heads were consistently less dense, with significantly lower screw pull-out strength ($P < 0.05$). The increased trabecular density of the central and superior femoral head gave far better fixation (Figure 2). Evidence of better fixation was noted in patient radiographs. The center of the head, where the tension and compression trabeculae both pass, appears most dense, followed by the compression trabeculae in the superior femoral head. In a fracture patient with osteoporosis and/or osteopenia, the inferior head often clearly demonstrates the lack of trabeculae and minimal cancellous bone density. The data strongly favor the inverted triangle and diamond patterns for improved fixation.

Preferred Surgical Technique: Parallel Cannulated Screws

The authors' preference is a system using a 3.2-mm guide pin and a cannulated 6.5-mm self-tapping screw.[107,109] The 3.2-mm guide pin is stiff enough not to bend easily and can reliably be used through guide jigs. The 6.5-mm screw with a 20-mm threaded tip has very good holding power, and the 20-mm thread does not go across the fracture site as can happen with longer thread lengths.

The patient is placed in a supine position on a fracture table. If the fracture is displaced, traction is applied with the leg in neutral flexion, 10° of abduction, and neutral rotation. The leg is then internally rotated as far as possible with moderate force, and then backed off to a position of 15° of internal rotation. The reduction is confirmed by fluoroscopy. If satisfactory alignment but some distraction is present, the internal fixation is performed and the fracture impacted with the parallel guide pins in place or with the lag of the screws.

A 6-cm straight lateral incision is made, starting at the flare of the greater trochanter and extending distally. The fascia lata and fascia of the vastus lateralis are cut in line with the incision and the vastus lateralis is bluntly split. The lateral femoral cortex is visualized. A percutaneous procedure can be used, but in this procedure there is probably as much soft-tissue trauma beneath the skin as that of a small muscle-splitting approach. The open procedure provides the added advantage of direct visualization of the lateral femoral cortex so that the cortical bone entrance holes can be more precise. The cortex can also be visualized as the screws are tightened and the head buttresses against the bone with compression.

The most distal guide pin is placed first. A drill hole is made with a 3.2-mm drill 3 cm to 4 cm distal to the vastus externus tubercle, usually at the level of the lesser trochanter, and midway between the anterior and posterior femoral cortices. This is the only hole that is predrilled for the guide pin because the cortex may be very dense at this location.

The 3.2-mm guide pin is then passed through this hole, along (and almost resting on) the medial femoral neck, across the fracture, and into the femoral head. On the lateral view, this pin should stay in the midline of the femoral neck and head. Pin position is confirmed by fluoroscopy. If a correction is to be made, use of the same cortical hole is attempted. Extra holes at this level of the femoral shaft may weaken the femur at the subtrochanteric level.

A fixed guide with a selection of triangles or diamonds is then selected (Figure 9). The appropriate sized diamond or triangle can be determined with preoperative radiograph stenciling. If there is a question between two sizes, the smaller pattern is used. The use of three screws in an inverted triangle configuration is preferred for Garden I and II fractures, and four screws in a diamond configuration for a Garden III or IV fracture. The fixed jig is placed over the already positioned guide pin, and the remaining two or three guide pins are placed (Figures 10 and 11). These guide pins are driven by power directly through the cortex, up the femoral neck, and into the femoral head. Predrilling is usually not necessary.

The direct reading depth gauge is then used to determine screw length. If the measured length is between sizes, the shorter length is used. If the fracture is to be compressed, a screw 5 mm to 10 mm shorter than measured is chosen. This will leave room for the threads to advance in the femoral head as the screw lags and the fracture compresses.

The self-cutting/tapping cannulated screw of the selected length is then placed over its guide pin and driven through the cortex and across the fracture with the cannulated power screwdriver. When the head is 10 mm from the femoral cortex, the power driver is removed. The screw

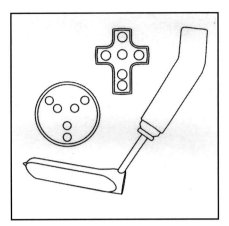

Figure 9 Fixed guides for the triangle or diamond patterns. (Courtesy of Stryker Howmedica Osteonics, Allendale, NJ.)

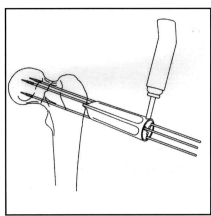

Figure 10 AP projection of the placement of three parallel guide pins. (Courtesy of Stryker Howmedica Osteonics, Allendale, NJ.)

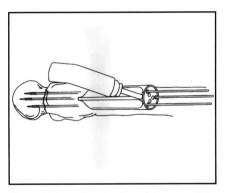

Figure 11 Lateral projection of three parallel guide pins. (Courtesy of Stryker Howmedica Osteonics, Allendale, NJ.)

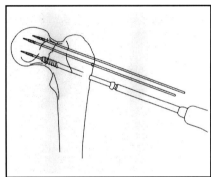

Figure 12 The 6.5-mm cannulated screws of appropriate length are passed over the guide pins. (Courtesy of Stryker Howmedica Osteonics, Allendale, NJ.)

is then driven the remainder of its path with the hand screwdriver (Figure 12). The remaining screws are placed and the guide pins removed. Compression can be obtained by gently tightening the screws (Figure 13). When the screws are tightened, occasionally the inferior screw will spin in the osteoporotic patient because the bone in the inferior head is the weakest. The remaining screws in the middle and upper portions of the head will achieve excellent hold of the femoral head. The lower screw will still deter inferior motion of the head fragment as the screw rests on the endosteum of the femoral neck.

When a screw is removed after frac-

ture healing, the screw thread must recut its way through the healed femoral cortex. Many types of cannulated screws have reverse cutting flutes for this purpose. If the oblique angle (approximately 135°) of the screw to the femoral shaft is not changed, the reverse cutting flutes are not in an optimal position to cut into the cortex. When the thread meets the endocortex, the screw can be pulled into a perpendicular position to the bone with a screwhead retractor, thus permitting the reverse cutting flutes to position themselves properly and facilitate screw removal. A worn or damaged screwdriver should never be used because of the danger of stripping the recess socket.

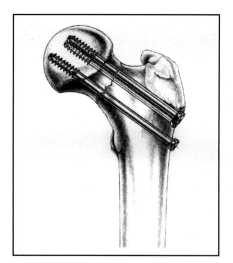

Figure 13 The cannulated screws are placed, the fracture compressed by gently tightening the screws, and the guide pins are removed. (Courtesy of Stryker Howmedica Osteonics, Allendale, NJ.)

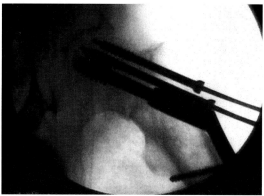

Figure 14 A dynamic hip compression screw and sideplate can be used with one or two derotational screws. The guide pins are placed before inserting the dynamic hip compression screw bolt. After the dynamic hip compression screw and sideplate are applied, cannulated screws are place over their guide pins and the pins removed.

Dynamic Hip Compression and a Parallel Derotational Cannulated Screw

An alternate method of fixation uses a dynamic hip compression screw with a two-hole sideplate. On occasion, when additional fixation may be required (for example, in a patient with Parkinson's disease or certain neurologic disorders), a dynamic hip compression screw and two-hole sideplate is used. The hip is reduced on the fracture table and the dynamic hip compression screw guide pin is placed, followed by one or two guide pins from the 6.5-mm cannulated screw set. The bolt is placed in the center of the femoral head or slightly distal to allow room for the derotational screws. Enough distance is left between the guide pins to allow room for the cannulated screw heads to clear the dynamic hip compression screw plate proximally on the lateral femoral shaft. The derotational guide pins stabilize the head fragment to prevent rotation during the reaming, taping, and placement of the dynamic hip compression screw bolt. After the sideplate of the dynamic hip compression screw is added

and compression applied, the depth gauge is used over the guide pins of the cannulated screw system. The appropriate cannulated screw length is chosen and the screws are placed (Figure 14).

Clinical Results of a Long-Term Follow-up of Parallel Cannulated Screws for Femoral Neck Fractures

In one retrospective study of the results of stabilizing nonpathologic femoral neck fractures with parallel cannulated screws from 1980 through 1985,[108] 50 of the 141 patients (35%) had nondisplaced fractures (Garden I and II), whereas 91 (65%) had displaced fractures (Garden III and IV). The median age was 68 years (range, 24 to 95 years). There were 112 white females (79%) with a median age of 67 years (range, 30 to 90 years) at the time of fracture and 29 white males (21%) with a median age of 69 years (range, 24 to 95 years). The proportion of displaced and nondisplaced fractures was approximately equal by gender and side of fracture. No deaths or wound infections occurred during the fracture hospitalization, and the mean follow-up was 8 years.

Eleven patients, six males and five females (median age, 75 years), died within the first year after surgery. Twenty-nine patients (median age, 75 years) died within 5 years. Fifty percent of the entire group of patients had at least one major concomitant medical disease.

Of the 29 patients who died, only three had no major initial medical disorder. Mortality was related more to the medical condition of the patient than to the fracture episode itself. The mortality rate of this patient group was compared with a control cohort group matched for age, sex, and race. This group was from the population at large and medical illness was not taken into consideration. The survival curve of the cohort group remained within the 95% confidence interval limit of the fracture group for the entire length of the study (Figure 15). Although a trend of increased mortality existed for the first 2 years following fracture, this was not significant. The men and women were separated and compared with each other as well as each with their own control cohort group. The female patients' survival curve followed that of their control cohort group. The survival curve for the males shows a much poorer prognosis than the females ($P < 0.0001$) (Figure 16), and the survival curve for the male patients was significantly poorer than that of their control cohort group.

Five of the 141 patients (4%)—two with Garden III and three with Garden IV fractures—experienced a loss of position or nonunion by 6 months after surgery. All five patients were women. Two of the five patients underwent total hip replacement, and one had a hemiarthroplasty.

Thirteen patients (9%) were found to have histologic or radiographic evidence of osteonecrosis within 2 years of treatment. Ten of these patients had initially displaced fractures. Another 13 cases of osteonecrosis were diagnosed after 2 years; 8 were initially displaced fractures. Twenty-five of the 26 osteonecrosis patients were females. Four of them first developed segmental collapse 5 to 8 years after their fracture. The prevalence of osteonecrosis was therefore 18% with a mean follow-up of 8 years. Osteonecrosis was present in 8 of 39 patients with a Garden II, 6 of 30 patients with a Garden III, and 12 of 40 patients with a Garden IV fracture. Sixteen of the 26 patients with osteonecrosis underwent a total hip replacement at a mean of 2 years following their fracture.

By a minimum 5-year follow-up, 30 patients were lost to follow-up. In 55 patients, fracture healing was free of complications and the patients were found to be functioning well after 5 years (average follow-up 8 years). Using Kaplan-Meier survival rates, this study demonstrated greater than 71% implant survival 7 years following the fracture (Figure 17). Forty-four of these patients had an average Harris Hip Score of 94 (range, 58 to 100) from 5 to 11 years after their procedure.

Multiple cannulated screw fixation represents a procedure with low surgical mortality and morbidity and a very high rate of fracture union (96%). An increased mortality rate was found for the male patients; however, this appeared to be related to the concomitant medical disorders rather than the surgery. The male patient has a poorer survival rate following hip fracture than the female patient. Osteonecrosis remains the major surgical complication following the fixation of the femoral neck fracture and can continue to present itself years after fracture healing. The female patient has a far higher incidence of nonunion or osteonecrosis than the male patient.

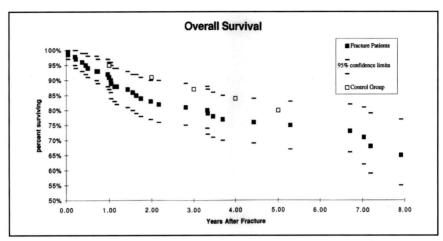

Figure 15 The overall survival curve for the fracture patient group compared with a cohort group matched for age, sex, and race. (Reproduced with permission from Asnis SE, Wanek-Sgaglione L: Intracapsular fractures of femoral neck: Results of cannulated screw fixation. *J Bone Joint Surg Am* 1994;76:1793-1803.)

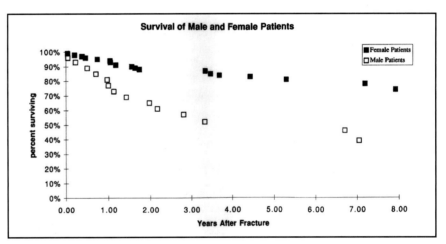

Figure 16 The survival curve following femoral neck fracture shows a much poorer prognosis for the male patients than the female patients. (Reproduced with permission from Asnis SE, Wanek-Sgaglione L: Intracapsular fractures of femoral neck: Results of cannulated screw fixation. *J Bone Joint Surg Am* 1994;76:1793-1803.)

Segmental collapse can be treated with a well-planned elective total hip replacement at a medically safer time. Those patients in whom the fracture heals without osteonecrosis maintain excellent function long after their injury.

Arthroplasty Options for Femoral Neck Fractures

Much controversy surrounds decision making regarding hip arthroplasty for the treatment of acute displaced femoral neck fractures. Controversial topics include the decision as to when prosthetic replacement instead of open reduction and internal fixation is appropriate, which type of prosthesis to choose (monopolar, bipolar, or total hip arthroplasty), and the method of prosthetic fixation (cemented or cementless). This section will review the indications, results, and potential complications of

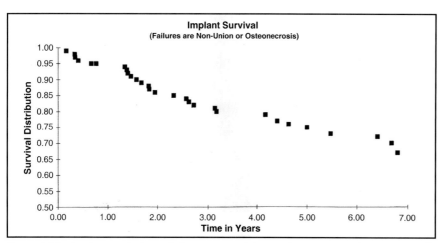

Implant Survival
(Failures are Non-Union or Osteonecrosis)

Figure 17 The implant survival rate defines a successful screw fixation as one functioning well or that functioned well until the death of a patient. A failure is defined as either a failure of fixation, failure to heal satisfactorily, or development of osteonecrosis. This study demonstrated 71% implant survival 7 years following the fracture. (Reproduced with permission from Asnis SE, Wanek-Sgaglione L: Intracapsular fractures of femoral neck: Results of cannulated screw fixation. *J Bone Joint Surg Am* 1994;76:1793-1803.)

prosthetic replacement for the treatment of acute displaced femoral neck fracture.

Justification for Prosthetic Replacement

Many older patients may benefit from an attempt at internal fixation.[124,125] Chronologic age alone should not be the only factor considered when determining the best therapeutic option for the patient with a displaced femoral neck fracture. Robinson and associates[9] recommended a protocol wherein all patients younger than 65 years or those with nondisplaced fractures were treated with internal fixation. Patients older than 85 years were treated with hemiarthroplasty. For those between 65 and 85 years of age, decision making was individualized, taking into account activity, general health, cognitive status, and bone quality compiled into a "physiologic score." Revision was necessary in only 5% of patients. This study underscores the importance of individualizing treatment methods rather than simply using chronologic age. Other authors have identified certain fracture characteristics such as fracture verticality,

perceived difficulty of reduction, or varus reduction as predictive of fixation failure.[126-129] Although many surgeons still favor an attempt at open reduction and internal fixation[108] and reserve arthroplasty for fixation failure, a recent study by McKinley and Robinson[130] documented better outcomes for primary arthroplasty than for arthroplasty performed after fixation failure. Multiple studies have demonstrated hip arthroplasty to be an effective method of salvage of fixation failure.[96,101,131-135]

Many factors contribute to the justification for primary prosthetic replacement over an internal fixation attempt in elderly patients with acute displaced femoral neck fractures. These patients typically have low functional demands, poor medical health, and osteopenia. Many patients can have associated neurologic disease (mild dementia, Parkinson's disease, or sequelae of a previous cerebrovascular accident) and therefore need to be mobilized quickly with a single predictable procedure that carries a low rate of failure and revision. Several challenges face the surgeon attempting successful

internal fixation of a displaced femoral neck fracture in the elderly patient. The main limiting factor to the success of any construct, of course, is the bone quality in the proximal fragment. These fractures can be comminuted and have vertical fracture lines and extremely osteopenic bone; this renders predictable, stable internal fixation of the proximal fragment difficult, if not impossible.

Several retrospective and prospective studies have compared open reduction and internal fixation to primary prosthetic replacement for displaced femoral neck fractures in elderly patients.[125,136,137] Soreide and associates[138] compared open reduction and internal fixation to prosthetic replacement in a prospective, randomized study. Patients treated with prosthetic replacement had fewer complications and better hip scores. Sikorski and Barrington[139] prospectively studied 218 patients older than 70 years treated by three methods: open reduction and internal fixation, cemented hemiarthroplasty through an anterolateral approach, and a cemented hemiarthroplasty through a posterolateral approach. Mortality rates were lower for patients treated through the anterior approach. The technical results were worse with open reduction and internal fixation. Bray and associates[140] compared internal fixation to primary bipolar hemiarthroplasty in a prospective, randomized comparison and found that patients treated with prostheses had less pain, fewer complications, and greater mobility. In a large meta-analysis of displaced femoral neck fractures in elderly patients, Lu-Yao and associates[3] found an overall nonunion rate of 33% with internal fixation in this cohort, and osteonecrosis in 16%. The need for revision was found to be 20% to 36% for those patients treated with internal fixation versus 6% to 18% for those treated with arthroplasty. They demonstrated a 66% decrease in the risk of revision with arthroplasty. In a more recent meta-analysis comparing open reduction and internal fixation with arthroplasty for displaced femoral neck fractures, Bhandari and associates[141] found that arthroplasty reduced the risk of revision by 77%. However, arthroplasty was associated with more blood loss, longer surgical times, more infections, and greater early mortality.[141] Ravikumar and Marsh[7] randomized 290 patients age 65 years and older to receive treatment with internal fixation, hemiarthroplasty, or total hip arthroplasty. Open reduction and internal fixation demonstrated a 33% rate of revision. There was no difference in mortality between those patients treated with arthroplasty and those treated with internal fixation. Johansson and associates[142] randomized 100 patients age 75 years and older with displaced fractures to undergo either open reduction and internal fixation with two screws or total hip arthroplasty. There was no increase in morbidity or mortality in patients treated with arthroplasty. Functional scores were better with total hip arthroplasty. Finally, Rogmark and associates[143] randomized 409 patients older than 70 years to undergo either internal fixation or arthroplasty. After a mean follow-up of 2 years, treatment with internal fixation failed in 43%, whereas arthroplasty treatment failed in only 6%. Of particular importance, there was no difference in mortality between the two groups, and function was generally better with arthroplasty.

For displaced acute femoral neck fractures in elderly patients, arthroplasty offers lower revision rates, generally better function, and no clear increase in morbidity or mortality compared with patients treated with internal fixation. Despite contemporary methods of internal fixation, failure rates of approximately 30% to 40% continue to be consistently reported in the literature. Because internal fixation in this elderly cohort remains unpredictable, primary prosthetic replacement may, in fact, be the treatment of choice for this cohort.

Hemiarthroplasty: General Considerations and Fixation Options

In the United States, hemiarthroplasty has been the traditional treatment of displaced femoral neck fractures in elderly patients because of predictably lower revision rates, a relatively low complication rate, and reasonable function.[89,144-159] Most patients with a displaced femoral neck fracture have normal acetabular cartilage. Additionally, dislocation rates for hemiarthroplasty in general have been approximately 2% or lower, which is much lower than rates reported across several studies for total hip arthroplasty.[160-162] When determining the ideal hemiarthroplasty implant type for each patient, factors such as bone quality, age, and activity level must be individualized, and other potential comorbidities that may make the use of cemented fixation hazardous must be taken into account. First-generation one-piece cementless hemiarthroplasties of the Austin-Moore type should be reserved for the most minimally ambulatory or nonambulatory patients, such as those with severe dementia or prohibitive medical comorbidities. These designs probably function more as spacers, and it is unlikely that they ever achieve enough bony stability to allow prolonged pain-free ambulation. Concerning rates of acetabular erosion and revision have been reported when these designs have been used in active patients.[163-166] Newer designs offer improved metaphyseal geometries allowing fit and fill of the proximal femur and provide modularity to facilitate better restoration of leg length and soft-tissue balancing. Data on the performance of these designs, however, are lacking. Lu-Yao and associates[3] noted that cemented hemiarthroplasty has demonstrated functional results superior to cementless hemiarthroplasty.[167] This is not surprising because cement offers immediate secure fixation in bones that are often capacious and osteopenic.[168] However, the major

concern when performing cemented arthroplasty in this setting is the fact that these patients are frail and may have multiple cardiopulmonary comorbidities and therefore less "reserve." Embolization of the typically fatty marrow contents that are found in large femoral canals can lead to intraoperative hemodynamic instability caused by embolization. Parvizi and associates[169] recently reviewed the intraoperative mortality during hip arthroplasty. Of the 23 patients who died during surgery, 13 were being treated for acute hip fractures, and all died during the cementation process. Bone marrow microemboli were found on autopsy in the pulmonary vasculature. Ereth and associates[170] and Esemenli and associates[171] reported on a "bone-cement implantation syndrome" consisting of hypotension, hypoxemia, arrhythmias, and cardiac arrest at the time of prosthetic insertion. This was observed most frequently in patients undergoing cemented arthroplasty.[172,173] Accordingly, thorough lavage and drying of the canal is recommended with gentle, if any, pressurization during cementation in more frail patients. In general, cement seems to provide better clinical results but should be used with caution.

Bipolar Versus Monopolar Hemiarthroplasty

Once a hemiarthroplasty has been chosen, further controversy surrounds the selection of either a unipolar (fixed head) or a bipolar bearing. The design rationale of the bipolar bearing, developed in 1974,[174] centers on an additional metal and polyethylene bearing surface that theoretically diminishes stress on the articular cartilage of the acetabulum and possibly decreases the rates of acetabular erosion noted in monopolar designs.[175-186] Multiple evaluations of whether any motion occurs at the bipolar bearing over time have been published.[187,188] Although earlier studies with older designs showed unpredictable motion at the inner bearing, a more recent study using contemporary implants demonstrated preservation of motion at the inner bearing in 93% of 177 hips evaluated fluoroscopically at a mean of 47 months postoperatively.[189] Additionally, the motion did not seem to deteriorate with time. Inner bearing motion may be successful in reducing the incidence of acetabular wear, as the developers of the prostheses theorized. However, none of these studies can accurately evaluate motion along the center of rotation of the femoral neck, such as is common with walking or sitting. In theory, even small amounts of motion could unload the acetabular cartilage and perhaps contribute to the longevity of the native acetabular articular surface. Although the controversy regarding preservation of motion will continue, what is most important is to know whether bipolar designs provide long-term pain-free ambulation with a low rate of acetabular protrusio or revision for acetabular wear. Several studies have compared bipolar and monopolar designs, and the literature is somewhat confusing. Beckenbaugh and associates[190] reported 92% survivorship in 51 patients with a cemented unipolar prosthesis, with a minimum age of 70 years and a 3-year follow-up. Cabanela and Van Demark[191] reported on 58 patients with 59 cemented Bateman bipolar prostheses and noted no revisions at a minimum follow-up of 2 years. Yamagata and associates[192] compared 682 fixed-head and 319 bipolar prostheses implanted for various diagnoses, using cemented and cementless techniques. The mean age of the patients was 73 years. They concluded that the revision rates were higher in the patients with fixed-head prostheses (12.5%) than for the patients with bipolar prostheses (7.2%). They also showed a significantly higher survivorship rate for cemented implants, regardless of head type. The Harris Hip Scores were better for the patients with bipolar prostheses. Marcus and associates[193] retrospectively compared 100 cementless Austin Moore–type prostheses to 80 cementless and cemented bipolar prostheses and found no difference in hip scores at 2 years. Lu-Yao and associates[3] examined the rates of revision comparing bipolar and unipolar designs with a minimum 7-year follow-up. The revision rate for the unipolar hemiarthroplasty was 20% and was 10% for the bipolar hemiarthroplasty. This is not surprising because patients who live longer are probably more active and will place more stress on the remaining articular surface.

Much of the literature on cementless unipolar prostheses presents alarming rates of failure. Kofoed and Kofod[164] followed 71 patients treated with a cementless unipolar device with a mean age of 82.5 years for 2 years. Overall, 37% of patients had poor results and required total hip arthroplasty. Of active patients, 55% required total hip arthroplasty. Acetabular degeneration was the most common reason for failure. These authors concluded that active patients, regardless of age, should not be treated with an Austin Moore–type implant. Other investigators also found problems with the Austin Moore–type implant with regard to revision rates and function. The data for cemented unipolar prostheses also have been reported. D'Arcy and Devas[194] studied a series of 354 cemented Thompson (fixed-head) hemiarthroplasties in patients with a mean age of 81 years. Of the 156 survivors available for review at 3 years, the failure rate was 18.9%. The most common reason for failure was acetabular erosion (11%).[194] Maxted and Denham[165] reported on 92 patients treated with cemented Thompson prostheses with a mean follow-up of 4 years. They reported an age-dependent 19% revision rate, with younger patients having more failures.[165]

When reviewing the literature comparing bipolar and unipolar hemiarthroplasties, patient age and the length of follow-up are important considerations because acetabular wear is a time-dependent phenomenon. It is unlikely that any differences will be noted among low-demand patients with short-term follow-up. However, if patients live longer and are more active, the differences will probably become clear. This remains one of the major challenges in prosthesis selection because the surgeon must attempt to estimate the patient's future activity level and life expectancy. Wathne and associates[195] compared 92 patients treated with a cemented bipolar prosthesis and 48 patients treated with a cemented modular unipolar prosthesis and found no difference in function at 1 year. Calder and associates[196] compared cemented unipolar to cemented bipolar prostheses in patients older than 80 years; at 2 years no difference was noted. Kenzora and associates[197] reported on 270 patients older than 65 years, comparing cementless unipolar to cementless bipolar and cemented bipolar prostheses; the best function was noted with a cemented bipolar prosthesis. Ong and associates[198] compared cemented bipolars and cemented unipolars with a mean follow-up of 4 years in 149 patients. There was no difference in functional outcome, mortality, or complications between the two groups. Haidukewych and associates[162] reported on 212 bipolar prostheses in patients with a mean age of 79 years at a mean follow-up of 6 years for the entire group; follow-up was 12 years for surviving patients. Only 10 hips underwent revision (4.7%). The most common reason for revision was femoral loosening, not acetabular wear. Most importantly, only one revision was performed for acetabular erosion. Therefore, the 10-year survivorship rate in this cohort free of revision for acetabular wear was 99.4%, and 96% of patients reported no pain or slight pain at follow-up. The dislocation rate was 1.9%.

In summary, there is justification in the literature for the use of both unipolar and bipolar bearings. In general, cemented fixation appears to provide better results and the choice of unipolar versus bipolar bearings should be based on surgeon preference, estimated patient activity, and life expectancy. It is the authors' preference to use cemented stems with unipolar bearings for minimally ambulatory patients, and patients who are community ambulators are treated with cemented stems that have bipolar bearings. Cementless Austin Moore-type prostheses are reserved for essentially nonambulatory patients who have dementia and prohibitive medical comorbidities.

The Role of Total Hip Arthroplasty

Historically, total hip arthroplasty has been reserved for patients with displaced femoral neck fractures and concomitant symptomatic degenerative changes of the hip. This combination of pathology is extremely rare, probably because patients with degenerative arthritis typically have stiff, thick hip capsules and will tend to fracture in the intertrochanteric region, not in the femoral neck. Recently, the indications for total hip arthroplasty have been broadened to include active elderly patients with acute femoral neck fractures. This has been based largely on the improved functional outcomes documented in multiple studies comparing total hip arthroplasty to hemiarthroplasty.[93,97,199-202] Pain relief is, in all likelihood, more predictable with total hip arthroplasty. However, dislocation is the main concern when performing total hip arthroplasty for acute femoral neck fractures. Dislocation rates have averaged approximately 10% across multiple studies,[93,97,199-202] with approximately 25% of those dislocations becoming recurrent and chronic. A recent meta-analysis documented a 7% dislocation rate for total hip arthroplasty.[141] With the large number of hip fractures treated annually, the potential societal and economic impact of such complications is substantial. Several reasons have been postulated for this increased dislocation rate in this patient

cohort. First, because these patients do not have the stiff hips so common in patients with osteoarthritis, they are likely to regain motion quickly and experience impingement and dislocatation. Additionally, these elderly patients may frequently have adduction and flexion contractures, poor muscle tone, poor balance leading to frequent falls, and difficulty complying with hip precautions. Despite the relatively high dislocation rate, most studies have demonstrated better function and pain relief with a total hip arthroplasty, and importantly, no increase in mortality or morbidity when comparing total hip arthroplasty to hemiarthroplasty or internal fixation. In one study considering the cost of revision and complications over a 2-year period, the most cost-effective method for treating patients with displaced femoral neck fracture was with cemented total hip arthroplasty.[6] Keating and associates[203] recently randomized 301 patients with a mean age of 60 years to undergo either open reduction and internal fixation, cemented bipolar hemiarthroplasty, or total hip arthroplasty. In this multicenter study involving 46 different surgeons, the internal fixation failure rate was 29%. The revision rate for patients treated with bipolar hemiarthroplasty was 5% and for total hip arthroplasty the rate was 8.5%. Three patients treated with total hip arthroplasty experienced dislocation. Total hip arthroplasty demonstrated the best functional outcome. Therefore, it can be concluded from the available literature that function appears to be generally superior with total hip arthroplasty, and there appears to be no increase in morbidity, mortality, or cost in performing a total hip arthroplasty compared with hemiarthroplasty or internal fixation. The main technical hurdle to overcome, therefore, is dislocation. With recent developments in cross-linked polyethylene and the trend to use larger diameter femoral heads in high-risk patients, dislocation rates may be potentially decreased.

Additionally, selection of approaches that historically have demonstrated a lower dislocation rate, such as the anterolateral approach, may be prudent.[204] This may be especially advantageous to patients who have mild adduction and flexion contractures and spend most of their time in a seated position. Additional data are needed to determine whether these strategies will decrease dislocation rates.

In summary, total hip arthroplasty is a reasonable alternative for the treatment of displaced femoral neck fractures in the more active elderly cohort because of generally superior functional outcome. The surgeon and the patient should both be cognizant, however, that dislocation remains problematic and the selective use of larger diameter femoral heads, elevated lipped liners, and approaches that have been associated with a lower dislocation rate may be wise.

Prosthetic replacement remains an effective treatment option for the elderly patient with displaced femoral neck fracture. Revision rates have been shown to be consistently lower than those published for internal fixation, and in general, complication rates are low and functional results are good. The choice of prosthesis and fixation method should be individualized based on surgeon preference and patient characteristics such as bone quality, activity, medical comorbidity, and estimated life expectancy. Age alone should not be used to determine the ideal treatment method for the patient with a displaced femoral neck fracture. Additional research is needed to clearly document which prosthetic choice is superior.

International Comparisons of Hip Fracture Treatment
The Demographic Problem
Scandinavia and North America have already experienced a sizeable increase in the total number and incidence of hip fractures. The World Health Organization has estimated that 1.7 million hip

fractures occurred worldwide in 1990, and the amount has been predicted to grow to over 6 million by year 2050. This increase is primarily the result of an increasing elderly population in Asia, Africa, and the Eastern Mediterranean region. The number of individuals in the world age 65 years or older now living will increase from 323 million to an estimated 1.55 billion by the year 2050.[205] This increase will have a dramatic influence on the number of patients with hip fractures that must be treated each year. Demographic changes alone will cause the annual number of hip fractures in the United States to more than double, from 238,000 in 1986 to 512,000 in the year 2040.

In Sweden, with a population of about 9 million, about 60,000 patients sustain an osteoporotic fracture each year; 18,000 of these fractures are of the hip. It is estimated that at the age of 50 years, every second Swedish woman has the risk of some type of osteoporotic fracture some time during her remaining lifetime. The risk for men is about half that for women. The risk has increased gradually over the decades, especially in individuals older than 80 years. Most of the more extensive fractures occur in the elderly, who often have coexisting diseases but still expect to live an independent, mobile, and pain-free life. A hip fracture can trigger a series of problems and treatments at different levels of care. The lifetime risk of sustaining a hip fracture for a woman in Sweden is estimated at 23% and for a man 11%.[206] This total increase in hip fractures is a potential threat to hospital resources and overall health economy. However, the prognosis for individual patients has improved over the decades because of improved treatment including optimized osteosynthesis and active rehabilitation. Many patients with hip fractures can rapidly return to their own homes, continue the rehabilitation there, and achieve the same level of function as before the fracture.[116,207-211] A few recent studies have reported a trend-break in hip fracture incidence,[212-215] particularly for women, whereas numbers continue to increase for trochanteric fractures in men.[215] However, large age cohorts of those vulnerable to fracture will override the lower incidence trend and will result in an overall increase of the number of hip fractures during the coming decades.

The incidence rates for hip fractures are higher in white populations than other populations and vary by geographic region. Age-adjusted incidence rates of hip fracture by gender are higher in Scandinavia than in North America, and lower in the countries of Southern Europe.[216,217] The absolute number of hip fractures in each region is determined not only by ethnic composition, but also by the size of the population and its age distribution. Consequently, about one third of all hip fractures in 1990 occurred in Asia, despite lower incidence rates among Asians. Almost half of the fractures occurred in Europe, North America, and Oceania, even though the population was smaller, because the population was older than average and composed largely of whites.[218] In Sweden, three of four patients with hip fractures are women.[103] This preponderance is explained because women outnumber men as age increases, and there is an increased incidence of osteoporosis during the postmenopausal period. Hip fractures are rare in patients younger than 50 years and constitute only 2% of the total.[219] The risk of hip fracture increases exponentially in patients age 50 years and older. The mean age of patients with a hip fracture in Sweden is now 81 years. Men have the same exponential increase as women in fracture risk with increasing age, but in men the fractures occur approximately 5 to 10 years later through the age range.

National Registration

In Sweden, a national registration of hip fracture treatment (RIKSHÖFT) was initiated in 1988.[220] This registration has attracted international interest and also resulted in the development of a comparable database within Europe, called Standardised Audit of Hip Fractures in Europe. The philosophy behind national registration is to improve the quality of care in all parts of the country and, through comparisons of everyday practice, to achieve a high treatment standard. In some years, the Swedish National Board of Health and Welfare and the Swedish Association of County Councils have provided financial support to these so-called "National Quality Registers." Through the registration, the orthopaedic departments also participate in a large prospective study; the magnitude of patients has scientific impact and supplements randomized studies with the broad application perspective of new and established methods.

In Sweden, the distribution of fracture types in approximately 80,000 registered patients was nondisplaced cervical fractures (Garden I and II) in 16.2%; displaced cervical fractures (Garden III and IV) in 37.0%; basicervical fractures in 3.5%; trochanteric two-fragment fractures in 22.6%; trochanteric multifragment fractures in 15.2%; and subtrochanteric fractures in 5.5%.

The two main groups are the cervical fractures and the trochanteric fractures. With increasing age, the proportion of trochanteric fractures increases. A geographical difference also exists. In Sweden and Norway, the ratio is close to 1:1, whereas Iceland and Finland have shown a higher proportion of cervical fractures.[221]

The costs of hip fractures are considerable.[218,222] In Sweden, the cost of treatment during the first year following hip fractures has been calculated to be around $420 million annually. Based on RIKSHÖFT data, the total annual cost including nursing care during the first 4 months after the hip fracture amounts to $140 million. In the United States, the

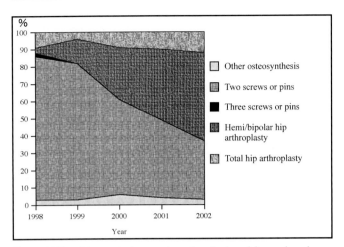

Figure 18 Trend in surgical procedures for displaced femoral neck fractures in Sweden from 1998 to 2002.

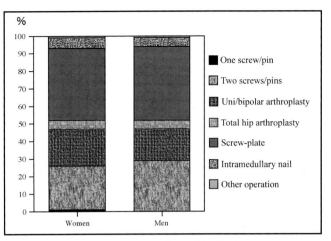

Figure 19 Surgical treatment methods used for hip fractures in women and men during 2002 in Sweden.

annual cost of treating hip fractures has been estimated to be nearly $10 billion. The high number of patients with hip fractures and the increasing costs of treatment make it necessary to optimize treatment. For femoral neck fractures, an optimized selected choice for the primary operation would decrease the need for revisions and diminish the overall treatment costs. This is the goal for future developments.

International Treatment Options
The best method to treat cervical (femoral neck) fractures has been disputed for decades. Different traditions prevail in different parts of the world. In Scandinavia, particularly in Sweden and Norway, virtually all cervical hip fractures have been treated with a primary osteosynthesis, whereas on the European continent, in Great Britain, and in the United States, most patients older than a certain age have been treated with arthroplasty, usually hemiarthroplasty.

In 2002, 27% of the patients in Sweden have been treated with osteosynthesis with two hook pins or two screws. Use of three or more screws or pins is rare (0.4%). Hemiarthroplasty was performed in 19% of the hip fractures, and total hip arthroplasty in 5%. These meth-

ods were mainly used for the femoral neck fractures. Telescoping screw-nail was used in 41%, and an intramedullary nail in 6%; these were primarily trochanteric fractures. Only 0.2% of the hip fracture patients did not have surgery. Since 1998, the trend in Sweden has been increased use of hemiarthroplasties for the displaced femoral neck fractures (Figure 18). For the displaced cervical neck fractures (Garden III and IV), hemiarthroplasties were performed in 3% in 1998 and in 51% of the patients in 2002. If total hip replacements are included, the arthroplasty use was 12% in 1998 and increased to 63% in 2002. This change is the result of several randomized studies. For trochanteric fractures, a screwplate has been the dominating treatment method. In 1998, 91% of the two-part trochanteric fractures were treated with a screwplate; this percentage has remained comparatively unchanged, with 94% performed in 2002. For the multifragment trochanteric fractures, 86% of the fractures were treated with a screwplate procedure in 1998, dropping slightly to 83% in 2002. In 2002, 15% of the multifragment fractures were treated with an intramedullary nail. There is little difference in the surgical treatment choice for women and men (Figure 19). However,

men had somewhat more osteosynthesis with two pins or screws and somewhat fewer arthroplasties; the use of screwplates was the same. There was likewise little difference in the fracture pattern between the sexes (Figure 20).

Based on close to 80,000 hip fractures surgically treated in Sweden from 1988 to 1997 before the trend toward increased use of arthoplasty, 21% of the total were operated with two screws, 24% with hook-pin osteosynthesis, 38% with telescoping screwplate, and fewer than 5% with some type of arthroplasty. The rest were treated with a variety of osteosynthesis methods. The screwplates are used for the trochanteric and sometimes the basicervical fractures as well as some of the subtrochanteric fractures.[223] Two hook-pins or two screws have been used for the cervical hip fractures, together with a minority of arthroplasties (Figure 21).

Improved techniques can now aid the surgeon in more accurate reduction of the fracture and placement of the internal fixation devices, thereby optimizing the stabilization of the fracture. The image intensifier is an indispensable tool. A biplanar apparatus is preferred because of better precision and shorter surgery times (Figure 22). The advantage of a biplanar

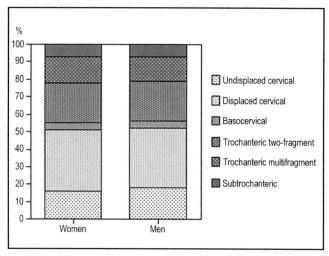

Figure 20 Hip fracture patterns in women and men in Sweden during 2002.

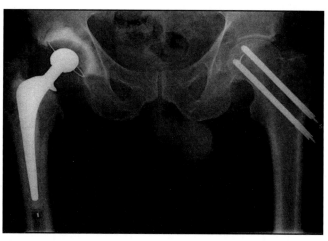

Figure 21 Radiograph of a patient demonstrating a healed femoral neck fracture on the patient's left side after hook-pin osteosynthesis and a cemented total hip arthroplasty without signs of loosening on the patient's right side.

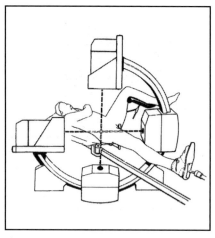

Figure 22 Positioning of the patient on the traction table with biplanar image intensifier. The horizontal x-ray tube (lateral view) is to the left of the surgeon. Images are shifted with a foot pedal.

image intensifier is that after positioning of the equipment, no further movements of the standard tube are necessary, which avoids jeopardizing the draping and thereby the sterility. Shifting between the views on the monitor is accomplished with a foot pedal, which saves considerable surgery time. Furthermore, the easy, rapid shifting between the positions increases the precision in the placement

of the osteosynthesis material. The importance of a minimally invasive surgical technique to the circulation of the femoral head has been proved.[224] The channels should be predrilled, and the hammering in of osteosynthesis material is to be avoided. In addition, impaction of the fracture by hammering decreases the circulation to the femoral head. The best way to achieve compression in the fracture is by the patient's own muscle forces in weight bearing. For cervical fractures, parallel hook-pins or screws are usually used. To prevent these devices from sliding out during healing, they are either reinforced with hooks (hook-pins) or threaded in the end as screws. The most important factors for good healing have proved to be the fracture type, the positioning of the bony parts after reposition, and the positioning of the osteosynthesis material[225] (Figure 23). Criteria for acceptable reduction were no varus, maximum displacement of 2 mm, and valgus alignment of 0° to 15° on the AP view, and on the lateral view, a maximum displacement of 2 mm while allowing 20° of ventral and 10° of dorsal angular displacement. The hook-pin is a cannulated blunt pin (nail) with a diameter of

6.5 mm. It has a thin blade (hook) inside, which is driven out of the tip of the pin during the procedure. Criteria for the acceptable placement of the device were positioning of the distal pin close to the calcar on the AP view and centrally on the lateral view. The proximal pin should be close to the calcar on the lateral view and central on the AP view.

In Sweden, most orthopaedic departments use hook-pins.[117] In a consecutive prospective series of over 600 cervical fractures treated with hook-pin osteosynthesis and followed for 2 years clinically with radiographs, 23% of the original patients showed healing complications.[117] After 2 years, 31% of the patients without hip problems had died from other diseases. Among the surviving patients, the total healing complications amounted to 32%. The need for revision with a secondary total hip arthroplasty for healing disturbance was 13% for the total number of patients and 19% among the survivors. Similar results have been achieved with optimized screw osteosynthesis by dedicated surgeons. A randomized study in Norway between different osteosynthesis methods has demonstrated the importance of repositioning and place-

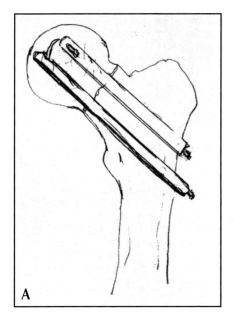
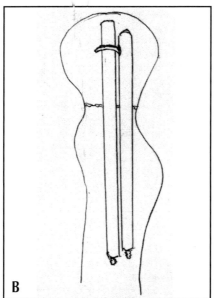
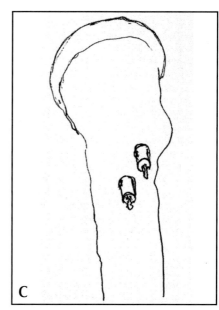

Figure 23 Schematic representation of positioning of hook-pin osteosynthesis. **A,** AP view. **B,** Lateral view of femoral neck. **C,** Lateral view of femoral shaft and pin entrance.

ment of the osteosynthesis material.[225] Osteosynthesis as the sole method for surgical treatment of all cervical hip fractures was successful in 78% of patients. Screws showed higher risk of drill penetration of the femoral head and more femoral head necrosis than the hook-pin method. Thus, osteosynthesis can provide on average 80% of the patients a definitive good treatment of the hip fracture. After 2 years, these patients either have a healed fracture without change of the femoral head (50% of patients) or the patients have died from other diseases in the meantime without healing problems from the hip (30% of patients). If both the reduction of the fracture and the placement of the osteosynthesis material were rated as good according to the criteria given above and no drill penetration had occurred, a successful 2-year outcome was achieved in 86% of the screw group and in 89% of the hook-pin group.

The previous tradition in some areas to treat all cervical fractures regardless of type by a primary arthroplasty has been modified during recent years, and there is now a general agreement that nondis-

placed fractures should be treated with osteosynthesis.[226-228] Many centers now also advocate osteosynthesis for younger patients with displaced fractures, and the age limit for arthroplasty has been shifted more toward the elderly. It is the physiologic age that is important. The recommendation given by Parker and Pryor in Great Britain[226] is an age limit of 70 years. Kyle[227] from the United States advocates a physiologic age of 75 years or older for prosthetic replacement, whereas closed reduction and internal fixation is recommended for younger patients. The recommendations for the type of prosthetic replacement differ. Some advocate the same type for all patients, whereas Kyle[227] recommends an Austin Moore-type prosthesis for minimal ambulators, a bipolar prosthesis for nursing home ambulators or low-level community ambulators, and a total hip replacement for patients with concomitant osteoarthrosis of the fractured hip, rheumatoid arthritis, tumor, or failed pinning.

The rationale for primary arthroplasty is that no healing complication can appear if the fracture has been taken away

and the femoral head is substituted with a metal one. This reasoning, however, overlooks the fact that many of these fractures would have healed if treated with primary osteosynthesis. In this instance, the desire to overcome future healing complications leads to increased time in surgery, greater blood loss, and a greater wound compared with the use of percutaneous pinning. Other potential complications are also introduced, such as displacement of the arthroplasty and, in the long run, loosening. After replacement of only the femoral head with a hemiarthroplasty, the articular cartilage in the acetabulum will wear away over time. Conversely, it has been postulated that elderly patients have less risk of reaching this stage because of other concomitant diseases and expected average mortality. However, with a primary arthroplasty, the trauma from surgery is greater and the mortality reported in the literature is higher.[5,141,219,229-233] There is a great need for randomized studies that compare osteosynthesis and arthroplasty for primary treatment of cervical fractures. Importantly, there is a need for studies comparing treatment methods now used on a large scale in different parts of the world as the primary method. This point was also recently emphasized in a meta-analysis of randomized studies that compared internal fixation and arthroplasty for displaced fractures of the femoral neck.[141]

Since 1998 in Sweden, attempts to find the patients best suited for arthroplasty have intensified. Randomized studies have been initiated, and on the basis of new results, the treatment policy has changed. On average, half of the patients with displaced fractures are treated primarily with an arthroplasty, whereas the other half are still treated with a primary osteosynthesis.[142,156,234,235] For the nondisplaced fractures, it is undisputed internationally that all should be treated with a primary osteosynthesis. The current indication for a primary arthroplasty is a clearly displaced cervical fracture if the patient is walking before the injury and has a biologic age of 70 to 75 years or older, according to the Swedish National Guidelines for the treatment of hip fracture patients.[236] Thus, patients with moderately displaced cervical fractures and biologically younger patients undergo primary osteosynthesis. Also, patients who could not walk before their fracture are determined to not need major arthroplasty, and patients with dementia who have undergone arthroplasty have an increased risk of dislocation. Although the optimum proportions of osteosynthesis and arthroplasty are being sought, the Scandinavian experience clarifies that there is no reason to "behead all because some fail."

Summary

Femoral neck fractures constitute an epidemic, and successful management of these injuries is important to society as well as to the individual patient. All patients with hip fractures should be treated with thromboembolic prophylaxis, prophylactic antibiotics, and nutrition-

al support. The options for management of the displaced femoral neck fracture are well defined; the challenge lies in defining the ideal patient for each intervention. There is a general consensus that repair of the fracture with anatomic reduction and multiple screw fixation, performed as expeditiously as possible, is the treatment of choice in younger, healthy, and active individuals. Internal fixation should be performed with careful attention to detail. Nonanatomic reduction increases the risk of failure; open reduction should be considered for all patients to decompress intracapsular hematoma as well as maximize the opportunity to achieve perfect fracture reduction. Augmentation of bone density with calcium phosphate ceramics or other materials may decrease the risk of fixation failure in the future.

There is a decreasing use of bipolar hemiarthroplasty and increasing use of both unipolar hemiarthroplasty and total joint arthroplasty. Mounting evidence exists that total joint arthroplasty provides the best and most durable function for very active patients; it is also cost-effective when the cost of treating complications after internal fixation is considered. Total joint arthroplasty also is associated with an increased rate of revision surgery. Recent advances in hip arthroplasty, such as the increased use of large-diameter heads and the availability of constrained acetabular liners, may further expand the indications for total joint arthroplasty.

References

1. Chipchase LS, McCaul K, Hearn TC: Hip fracture rates in South Australia: Into the next century. *Aust N Z J Surg* 2000;70:117-119.

2. Speed K: The unsolved fracture. *Surgery Gynecology Obstetrics* 1935;59: 341-352.

3. Lu-Yao GL, Keller RB, Littenberg B, Wennberg JE: Outcomes after displaced fractures of the femoral neck: A meta-analysis of one hundred and six published reports. *J Bone Joint Surg Am* 1994;76:15-25.

4. Parker MJ, Khan RJK, Crawford J, Pryor GA: Hemiarthroplasty *versus* internal fixation for displaced intracapsular hip fractures in the

elderly: A randomized trial of 455 patients. *J Bone Joint Surg Br* 2002;84:1150-1155.

5. Partanen J, Saarenpää I, Heikkinen T, Wingstrand H, Thorngren K-G, Jalovaara P: Functional outcome after displaced femoral neck fractures treated with osteosynthesis of hemiarthroplasty: A matched-pair study of 714 patients. *Acta Orthop Scand* 2002;73:496-501.

6. Iorio R, Healy WL, Lemos DW, Appleby D, Lucchesi CA, Saleh KJ: Displaced femoral neck fractures in the elderly: Outcomes and cost effectiveness. *Clin Orthop* 2001;383:229-242.

7. Ravikumar KJ, Marsh G: Internal fixation versus hemiarthroplasty versus total hip arthroplasty for displaced subcapital fractures of the femur: 13 year results of a prospective randomized study. *Injury* 2000;31:793-797.

8. Kofoed H: Femoral neck fractures in young adults. *Injury* 1982;14:146-150.

9. Robinson CM, Saran D, Annan IH: Intracapsular hip fractures: Results of management adopting a treatment protocol. *Clin Orthop* 1994;302:83-91.

10. March LM, Chamberlain AC, Cameron ID, et al: How best to fix a broken hip: Fractured Neck of Femur Health Outcomes Project Team. *Med J Aust* 1999;170:489-494.

11. Kannus P, Parkkari J, Niemi S, et al: Prevention of hip fracture in elderly people with use of a hip protector. *N Engl J Med* 2000;343:1506-1513.

12. Zuckerman J, Schon L: Hip fractures, in Zuckerman J (ed): *Comprehensive Care of Orthopaedic Injuries in the Elderly*. Baltimore, MD, Urban & Schwarzenberg, 1990, pp 23-111.

13. Koval KJ, Zuckerman JD: Hip fractures: I. Overview and evaluation and treatment of femoral neck fractures. *J Am Acad Orthop Surg* 1994;2:141-149.

14. Winter WG: Nonoperative treatment of proximal femoral fractures in the demented nonambulatory patient. *Clin Orthop* 1987;218:97-103.

15. Owens WD, Felts JA, Spitznagel ELJ: ASA physical status classifications: A study of consistency ratings. *Anesthesiology* 1978;49:239-243.

16. McClure J, Goldsborough S: Fractures neck of femur and contra-lateral intracerebral lesions. *J Clin Pathol* 1986;39:920-922.

17. Soto-Hall R: Treatment of transcervical fractures complicated by certain common neurological conditions, in *Lectures AIC*. St Louis, MO, CV Mosby, 1960, pp 117-120.

18. Guanche CA, Kozin SH, Levy AS, Brody LA: The use of MRI in the diagnosis of occult hip fracture in the elderly: A preliminary report. *Orthopedics* 1994;17:327-330.

19. Rizzo PF, Gould ES, Lyden JP, Asnis SE: Diagnosis of occult fractures about the hip: Magnetic resonance imaging compared with bone scanning. *J Bone Joint Surg Am* 1993;75:395-401.

20. Asnis SE, Gould ES, Bansal M, Rizzo PF, Bullough PG: Magnetic resonance imaging of the hip after displaced femoral neck fractures. *Clin Orthop* 1994;298:191-198.

21. Speer KP, Spritzer CE, Harrelson JM, Nunley JA: Magnetic resonance imaging of the femoral head after acute intracapsular fracture of the femoral neck. *J Bone Joint Surg Am* 1990;72:98-103.

22. Karp A: Preoperative medical evaluation, in Koval K, Zuckerman J (eds): *Fractures in the Elderly.* Philadelphia, PA, Lippincott-Raven, 1998, pp 35-39.

23. Drake JK, Meyers MH: Intracapsular pressure and hemarthrosis following femoral neck fracture. *Clin Orthop* 1984;182:172-176.

24. Melberg PE, Korner L, Lansinger O: Hip joint pressure after femoral neck fracture. *Acta Orthop Scand* 1986;57:501-504.

25. Kenzora JE, McCarthy RE, Lowell JD, Sledge CB: Hip fracture mortality: Relation to age, treatment, preoperative illness, time of surgery, and complications. *Clin Orthop* 1984;186:45-56.

26. Sexson SB, Lehner JT: Factors affecting hip fracture mortality. *J Orthop Trauma* 1988;1:298-305.

27. Zuckerman JD, Skovron ML, Koval KJ, Aharonoff G, Frankel VH: Postoperative complications and mortality associated with operative delay in older patients who have a fracture of the hip. *J Bone Joint Surg Am* 1995;77:1551-1556.

28. Davis FM, Laurenson VG: Spinal anaesthesia or general anaesthesia for emergency hip surgery in elderly patients. *Anaesth Intens Care* 1981;9:352-358.

29. Valentin N, Lomholt B, Jensen JS, Hejgaard N, Kreiner S: Spinal or general anesthesia for surgery of the fractured hip? *Br J Anaesth* 1986;58:284-291.

30. Modig J, Borg T, Karlstrom G, Maripuu E, Sahlstedt B: Thromboembolism after total hip replacement: Role of epidural and general anesthesia. *Anesth Analg* 1983;62:174-180.

31. Agnelli G, Cosmi B, DiFilippo P, et al: A randomised, double-blind, placebo-controlled trial of dermatan sulphate for prevention of deep vein thrombosis in hip fracture. *Thromb Haemost* 1992;67:203-208.

32. Barsotti J, Gruel Y, Rosset P, et al: Comparative double-blind study of two dosage regimens of low-molecular weight heparin in elderly patients with a fracture of the neck of the femur. *J Orthop Trauma* 1990;4:371-375.

33. Borgstrom S, Greitz T, van der Linden W, et al: Anticoagulant prophylaxis of venous thrombosis in patients with fractured neck of the femur: A controlled clinical trial using venous phlebography. *Acta Chir Scand* 1965;129:500-508.

34. Eriksson BI, Bauer KA, Lassen MR, Turpie AG: Fondaparinux compared with enoxaparin for the prevention of venous thromboembolism after hip-fracture surgery. *N Engl J Med* 2001;345:1298-1304.

35. Gent M, Hirsh J, Ginsberg JS, et al: Low-molecular-weight heparinoid Orgaran is more effective than aspirin in the prevention of venous thromboembolism after surgery for hip fracture. *Circulation* 1996;93:80-84.

36. Hamilton HW, Crawford JS, Gardiner JH, Wiley AM: Venous thrombosis in patients with fracture of the upper end of the femur: A phlebographic study of the effect of prophylactic anticoagulation. *J Bone Joint Surg Br* 1970;52:268-289.

37. Jorgensen PS, Strandberg C, Wille-Jorgensen P, et al: Early preoperative thromboprophylaxis with Klexane® in hip fracture surgery: A placebo-controlled study. *Clin Appl Thromb Hemost* 1998;4:140-142.

38. Lowe GDO, Campbell AF, Meek DR, Forbes CD, Prentice CR: Subcutaneous ancrod in prevention of deep-vein thrombosis after operation for fractured neck of femur. *Lancet* 1978:698-700.

39. Monreal M, Lafoz E, Navarro A, et al: A prospective double-blind trial of a low molecular weight heparin once daily compared with conventional low-dose heparin three times daily to prevent pulmonary embolism and venous thrombosis in patients with hip fracture. *J Trauma* 1989;29:873-875.

40. Moskovitz PA, Ellenberg SS, Feffer HL, et al: Low-dose heparin for prevention of VTE in total hip arthroplasty and surgical repair of hip fractures. *J Bone Joint Surg Am* 1978;60:1065-1070.

41. Powers PJ, Gent M, Jay RM, et al: A randomized trial of less intense postoperative warfarin or aspirin therapy in the prevention of venous thromboembolism after surgery for fractured hip. *Arch Intern Med* 1989;149:771-774.

42. Rogers PH, Walsh PN, Marder VJ, et al: Controlled trial of low-dose heparin and sulfinpyrazone to prevent venous thromboembolism after operation on the hip. *J Bone Joint Surg Am* 1978;60:758-762.

43. Snook GA, Chrisman OD, Wilson TC: Thromboembolism after surgical treatment of hip fractures. *Clin Orthop* 1981;155:21-24.

44. TIFDED Study Group: Thromboprophylaxis in hip fracture surgery: A pilot study comparing danaparoid, enoxaparin and dalteparin. *Haemostasis* 1999;29:310-317.

45. Haake DA, Berkman SA: Venous thromboembolic disease after hip surgery: Risk factors, prophylaxis, and diagnosis. *Clin Orthop* 1989;242:212-231.

46. Schroder HM, Andreassen M: Autopsy-verified major pulmonary embolism after hip fracture. *Clin Orthop* 1993;293:196-203.

47. Todd CJ, Freeman CJ, Camilleri-Ferrante C, et al: Differences in mortality after fracture of hip: The East Anglian audit. *BMJ* 1995;310:904-908.

48. Perez JV, Warwick DJ, Case CP, Bannister GC: Death after proximal femoral fracture: An autopsy study. *Injury* 1995;26:237-240.

49. Sorenson RM, Pace NL: Anesthetic techniques during surgical repair of femoral neck fractures: A meta-analysis. *Anesthesiology* 1992;77:1095-1104.

50. Hefley WF, Nelson CL, Puskarich-May CL: Effect of delayed admission to the hospital on the preoperative prevalence of deep-vein thrombosis associated with fractures about the hip. *J Bone Joint Surg Am* 1996;78:581-583.

51. Zahn HR, Skinner JA, Porteous MJ: The preoperative prevalence of deep vein thrombosis in patients with femoral neck fractures and delayed operation. *Injury* 1999;30:605-607.

52. Sevitt S, Gallagher NG: Prevention of venous thrombosis and pulmonary embolism in injured patients: A trial of anticoagulant prophylaxis with phenindione in middle-aged and elderly patients with fractured necks of femur. *Lancet* 1959;ii:981-989.

53. Handoll HH, Farrar MJ, McBirnie J, Tytherleigh-Strong G, Milne AA, Gillespie WJ: Heparin, low molecular weight heparin and physical methods for preventing deep vein thrombosis and pulmonary embolism following surgery for hip fractures. *Cochrane Database Syst Rev* 2002;(4):CD000305.

54. Eriksson BI, Lassen MR, PENTasaccharide in Hip-FRActure Surgery Plus (PENTHIFRA-Plus) Investigators: Duration of prophylaxis against venous thromboembolism with fondaparinux after hip fracture surgery: A multicenter, randomized, placebo-controlled, double-blind study. *Arch Intern Med* 2003;163:1337-1342.

55. Antiplatelet Trialists' Collaboration: Collaborative overview of randomised trials of antiplatelet therapy-III: Reduction in venous thrombosis and pulmonary embolism by antiplatelet prophylaxis among surgical and medical patients. *BMJ* 1994;308:235-246.

56. Pulmonary Embolism Prevention (PEP) Trial Collaborative Group: Prevention of pulmonary embolism and deep vein thrombosis with low dose aspirin: Pulmonary Embolism Prevention (PEP) trial. *Lancet* 2000;355:1295-1302.

57. Fisher CG, Blachut PA, Salvian AJ, Meek RN, O'Brien PJ: Effectiveness of pneumatic leg compression devices for the prevention of thromboembolic disease in orthopaedic trauma patients: A prospective, randomized study of compression alone versus no prophylaxis. *J Orthop Trauma* 1995;9:1-7.

58. Freedman KB, Brookenthal KR, Fitzgerald RH, Williams S, Lonner JH: A meta-analysis of thromboembolic prophylaxis following elective total hip arthroplasty. *J Bone Joint Surg Am* 2000;82:929-938.

59. Lieberman D, Lieberman D: Proximal deep vein thrombosis after hip fracture surgery in elderly patients despite thromboprophylaxis. *Am J Phys Med Rehabil* 2002;81:745-750.

60. Westrich G, Sculco T: Prophylaxis against deep vein thrombosis after total knee replacement. *J Bone Joint Sur Am* 1996;78:826-834.

61. Geerts WH, Pineo GF, Heit JA, et al: Prevention of venous thromboembolism: The Seventh ACCP Conference on Antithrombotic and Thrombolytic Therapy. *Chest* 2004;126:338S-400S.

62. Nordin M, Frankel VH: Biomechanics of the hip, in Nordin M, Frankel VH (eds): *Basic Biomechanics of the Musculoskeletal System.* Malvern, PA, Lea and Febiger, 1989, pp 135-151.

63. Benterud JG, Husby T, Graadahl O, Alho A: Implant holding power of the femoral head. *Acta Orthop Scand* 1992;63:47-49.

64. Brunner CF, Weber BG: *Special Techniques in Internal Fixation.* Berlin, Germany, Springer-Verlag, 1982, p 34.

65. Hoaglund FT, Low WD: Anatomy of the femoral neck and head, with comparative data from Caucasians and Hong Kong Chinese. *Clin Orthop* 1980;152:10-16.

66. Pankovich AM: Primary internal fixation of femoral neck fractures. *Arch Surg* 1975;110:20-26.

67. Ward FO: *Human Anatomy.* London, England, Renshaw, 1838.

68. Singh M, Nagrath AR, Maini PS: Changes in the trabecular pattern of the upper end of the femur as an index of osteoporosis. *J Bone Joint Surg Am* 1970;52:457-467.

69. Crowell RR, Edwards WT, Hayes WC: Pullout strength of fixation devices in trabecular bone of the femoral head. *Trans Orthop Res Soc* 1985;10:189.

70. Martens M, Van Audekercke R, Mulier JC, Stuyck J: Clinical study on internal fixation of femoral neck fractures. *Clin Orthop* 1979;141:199-202.

71. Lindequist S: Cortical screw support in femoral neck fractures: A radiographic analysis of 87 fractures with a new mensuration technique. *Acta Orthop Scand* 1993;64:289-293.

72. Crock HV: A revision of the anatomy of the arteries supplying the upper end of the human femur. *J Anat* 1965;99:77-88.

73. Crock HV: An atlas of the arterial supply of the head and neck of the femur in man. *Clin Orthop* 1980;152:17-27.

74. Chung SMK: The arterial supply of the developing end of the human femur. *J Bone Joint Surg Am* 1976;58:961-970.

75. Claffey TJ: Avascular necrosis of the femoral head: An anatomical study. *J Bone Joint Surg Br* 1960;42:802-809.

76. Harty M: Blood supply of the femoral head. *Br Med J* 1953;2:1236-1237.

77. Sevitt S, Thompson RG: The distribution and anastamoses of arteries supplying the head and neck of the femur. *J Bone Joint Surg Br* 1965;47:560-573.

78. Tucker FR: Arterial supply to the femoral head and its clinical importance. *J Bone Joint Surg Br* 1949;31:82-93.

79. Browner BD, Jupiter JB, Levine AM, Trafton PG (eds): *Skeletal Trauma.* Philadelphia, PA, WB Saunders Company, 1992, vol 2, p 1370.

80. Wertheimer LG, Fernandez Lopes SDL: Arterial supply of the femoral head. *J Bone Joint Surg Am* 1971;53:545-556.

81. Crawfurd EJP, Emery RJH, Hansell DM, Phelan M, Andrews BG: Capsular distention and intracapsular pressure in subcapital fractures of the femur. *J Bone Joint Surg Br* 1988;70:195-198.

82. Holmberg S, Dalen. N: Intracapsular pressure and caput circulation in nondisplaced femoral neck fractures. *Clin Orthop* 1987;219:124-126.

83. Strömqvist B, Nilsson LT, Egund N, Thorngren KG, Wingstrand H: Intracapsular pressures in undisplaced fractures of the femoral neck. *J Bone Joint Surg Br* 1988;70:192-194.

84. Wingstrand H, Strömqvist B, Egund N, Gustafson T, Nilsson LT, Thorngren KG: Hemarthrosis in undisplaced cervical fractures: Tamponade reversible femoral head ischemia. *Acta Orthop Scand* 1986;57:305-308.

85. Garden RS: Low-angle fixation in fractures of the femoral neck. *J Bone Joint Surg Br* 1961;43:647-663.

86. Garden RS: Malreduction and avascular necrosis in subcapital fractures of the femur. *J Bone Joint Surg Br* 1971;53:183-197.

87. Garden RS: Reduction and fixation of subcapital fractures of the femur. *Orthop Clin North Am* 1974;5:683-712.

88. Arnold WD, Lyden JP, Minkoff J: Treatment of intracapsular fracture of the femoral neck. *J Bone Joint Surg Am* 1974;56:254-262.

89. Eiskjaer S, Ostgard SE: Risk factors influencing mortality after bipolar hemiarthroplasty in treating fractures of the femoral neck. *Clin Orthop* 1991;270:295-300.

90. Holmberg S, Conradi P, Kalen R, Thorngren KG: Mortality after cervical hip fracture: 3002 patients followed for 6 years. *Acta Orthop Scand* 1986;57:8-11.

91. Hunter GA: A comparison of the use of internal fixation and prosthetic replacement for fresh fractures of the neck of the femur. *Br J Surg* 1969;56:229-232.

92. Hunter GA: Should we abandon primary prosthetic replacement for fresh displaced fractures of the neck of the femur? *Clin Orthop* 1980;152:158-161

93. Gebhard JS, Amstutz HC, Zinar DM, Dorey FJ: A comparison of total hip arthroplasty and hemiarthroplasty for treatment of acute fracture of the femoral neck. *Clin Orthop* 1992;282:123-131.

94. Salvati EA, Artz T, Aglietti P, Asnis SE: Endoprostheses in the treatment of femoral neck fractures. *Orthop Clin North Am* 1974;5:757-777.

95. Coates RL, Armour P: Treatment of subcapital fractures by primary total hip replacement. *Injury* 1979;11:132-135.

96. Franzen H, Nilsson LT, Strömqvist B, Johnsson R, Herrlin K: Secondary total hip replacement after fractures of the femoral neck. *J Bone Joint Surg Br* 1990;72:784-787.

97. Dorr LD, Glousman R, Sew AL, Vanis R, Chandler R: Treatment of femoral neck fractures with total hip replacement versus cemented and noncemented hemiarthroplasty. *J Arthroplasty* 1986;1:21-28.

98. Gregory RJH, Gibson MJ, Moran CG: Dislocation after primary arthroplasty for subcapital fracture of the hip. *J Bone J Surg Br* 1991;73:11-12.

99. Johnsson R, Bendjelloul H, Ekelund L, Persson BM, Lidgren L: Comparison between hemiarthroplasty and total hip replacement following failure of nailed femoral neck fractures focused on dislocations. *Arch Orthop Trauma Surg* 1984;102:187-190.

100. Sim FH, Stauffer RN: Management of hip fractures by total hip replacements. *Clin Orthop* 1980;152:191-197.

101. Nilsson LT, Pekka J, Franzen H, Niinimaki T, Strömqvist B: Function after primary hemiarthroplasty and secondary total hip arthroplasty in femoral neck fracture. *J Arthroplasty* 1994;9:369-374.

102. Garcia A Jr: Displaced intracapsular fractures of the neck of the femur: Mortality and morbidity. *J Trauma* 1961;1:128-132.

103. Holmberg S, Thorngren KG: Statistical analysis of femoral neck fractures based on 3053 cases. *Clin Orthop* 1987;218:32-41.

104. Holmberg S, Kalen R, Thorngren KG: Treatment and outcome of femoral neck fractures: An analysis of 2418 patients admitted from their own homes. *Clin Orthop* 1987;218:42-52.

105. Nilsson LT, Strömqvist B, Thorngren KG: Nailing of femoral neck fracture: Clinical and sociologic 5-year follow-up of 510 consecutive hips. *Acta Orthop Scand* 1988;59:365-371.

106. Meyers MH, Harvey JP Jr, Moore TM: Treatment of displaced subcapital and transcervical fractures of the femoral neck by muscle-pedicle bone graft and internal fixation. *J Bone Joint Surg Am* 1973;55:256-274.

107. Asnis SE: The guided screw system in intracapsular fractures of the hip. *Contemp Orthop* 1985;10:33-42.

108. Asnis SE, Wanek-Sgaglione L: Intracapsular fractures of femoral neck: Results of cannulated screw fixation. *J Bone Joint Surg Am* 1994;76:1793-1803

109. Asnis SE, Kyle RF: Intracapsular hip fractures, in Asnis SE, Kyle RF (eds): *Cannulated Screw Fixation: Principles and Operative Techniques.* New York, NY, Springer-Verlag, 1996, pp 51-71.

110. Calandruccio RA, Anderson WE: Post-fracture avascular necrosis of the femoral head: Correlation of experimental and clinical studies. *Clin Orthop* 1980;152:49-84.

111. Catto M: The histological appearances of late segmental collapse of the femoral head after transcervical fracture. *J Bone Joint Surg Br* 1965;47:777-791.

112. Catto M: Histological study of avascular necrosis of the femoral head after transcervical fracture. *J Bone Joint Surg Br* 1965;47:749-776.

113. Sevitt S: Avascular necrosis and revascularization of the femoral head after intracapsular fractures: A combined arteriographic and histological necropsy study. *J Bone Joint Surg Br* 1964;46:270-296.

114. Hodge WA, Fijan RS, Carlson KL, Burgess RG, Harris WH, Mann RW: Contact pressures in the human hip joint measured in vivo. *Proc Natl Acad Sci USA* 1986;83:2879-2883.

115. Rubin R, Trent P, Arnold W, Burstein A: Knowles pinning of experimental femoral neck fractures: A biomedical study. *J Trauma* 1981;21:1036-1039.

116. McElvenny R.: The importance of the lateral x-ray film in treating intracapsular fracture of the femur. *Am J Orthop* 1962;212-215.

117. Strömqvist B, Nilsson LT, Thorngren K-G: Femoral neck fracture fixation with hook pins: 2-year results and learning curve in 626 prospective cases. *Acta Orthop Scand* 1992;63:282-287.

118. Strömqvist B, Hansson I, Nilsson LT, Thorngren KG: Hook-pin fixation of femoral fractures: A two year follow-up study of 300 cases. *Clin Orthop* 1987;218:58-62.

119. Deyerle WM: Impacted fixation over resilient multiple pins. *Clin Orthop* 1980;152:102-122.

120. Swiontkowski MF, Harrington RM, Keller TS, VanPatten PK: Torsion and bending analysis of internal fixation techniques for femoral neck fractures: The role of implant design and bone density. *J Orthop Res* 1987;5:433-444.

121. Springer ER, Lachiewicz PF, Gilbert JA: Internal fixation of femoral neck fractures: Comparative biomechanical study of Knowles pins and 6.5-mm screws. *Clin Orthop* 1991;267:85-91.

122. Kauffman JI, Simon JA, Kummer FJ, Pearlman CJ, Zuckerman JD, Koval KJ: Internal fixation of femoral neck fractures with posterior comminution: A biomechanical study. *J Ortho Trauma* 1999;13:155-159.

123. Howard CB, Davies RM: Subtrochanteric fracture after Garden screw fixation of subcapital fractures. *J Bone Joint Surg Br* 1982;64:565-567.

124. Jain R, Koo M, Kreder HJ, Schemitsch EH, Davey JR, Mahomed NN: Comparison of early and delayed fixation of subcapital hip fractures in patients sixty years of age or less. *J Bone Joint Surg Am* 2002;84:1605-1612.

125. Swiontkowski MF: Current concepts review: Intracapsular fractures of the hip. *J Bone Joint Surg Am* 1994;76:129-138.

126. Alho A, Benterud JG, Solovieva S: Internally fixed femoral neck fractures: Early prediction of failure in 203 elderly patients with displaced fractures. *Acta Orthop Scand* 1999;70:141-144.

127. Chua D, Jaglal SB, Schatzker J: Predictors of early failure of fixation in the treatment of displaced subcapital hip fractures. *J Orthop Trauma* 1998;12:230-234.

128. Estrada LS, Volgas DA, Stannard JP, Alonso JE: Fixation failure in femoral neck fractures. *Clin Orthop* 2002;399:110-118.

129. Hudson JI, Kenzora JE, Hebel JR, et al: Eight-year outcome associated with clinical options in the management of femoral neck fractures. *Clin Orthop* 1998;348:59-66.

130. McKinley JC, Robinson CM: Treatment of displaced intracapsular hip fractures with total hip arthroplasty: Comparison of primary arthroplasty with early salvage arthroplasty after failed internal fixation. *J Bone Joint Surg Am* 2002;84:2010-2015.

131. Hagglund G, Nordstrom B, Lidgren L: Total hip replacement after nailing failure in femoral neck fractures. *Arch Orthop Trauma Surg* 1984;103:125-127.

132. Mabry T, Prpa B, Haidukewych GJ, Berry DJ: Long term follow-up of Charnley total hip arthroplasty for femoral neck nonunion. *69th Annual Meeting Proceedings.* Rosemont, IL, American Academy of Orthopaedic Surgeons, 2002.

133. Mehlhoff T, Landon GC, Tullos HS: Total hip arthroplasty following failed internal fixation of hip fractures. *Clin Orthop* 1991;269:32-37.

134. Tabsh I, Waddell JP, Morton J: Total hip arthroplasty for complications of proximal femoral fractures. *J Orthop Trauma* 1997;11:166-169.

135. Turner A, Wroblewski BM: Charnley low-friction arthroplasty for the treatment of hips with late complications of femoral neck fractures. *Clin Orthop* 1984;185:126-130.

136. Hui AC, Anderson GH, Choudhry R, Boyle J, Gregg PJ: Internal fixation or hemiarthroplasty for undisplaced fractures of the femoral neck in octogenarians. *J Bone Joint Surg Br* 1994;76:891-894.

137. van Vugt AB, Oosterwijk WM, Goris RJ: Osteosynthesis versus endoprosthesis in the treatment of unstable intracapsular hip fractures in the elderly: A randomized clinical trial. *Arch Orthop Trauma Surg* 1993;113:39-45.

138. Soreide O, Molster A, Rangstad TS: Internal fixation versus primary prosthetic replacement in acute femoral neck fractures: A prospective, randomized clinical study. *Br J Surg* 1979;66:56-60.

139. Sikorski JM, Barrington R: Internal fixation versus hemiarthroplasty for the displaced subcapital fracture of the femur: A prospective, randomized study. *J Bone Joint Surg Br* 1981;63:357-361.

140. Bray TJ, Smith-Hoefer E, Hooper A, Timmerman L: The displaced femoral neck fracture: Internal fixation versus bipolar endoprosthesis. Results of a prospective, randomized comparison. *Clin Orthop* 1988;230:127-140.

141. Bhandari M, Devereaux PJ, Swiontkowski MF, et al: Internal fixation compared with arthroplasty for displaced fractures of the femoral neck. *J Bone Joint Surg Am* 2003;85:1673-1681.

142. Johansson T, Jacobsson SA, Ivarsson I, Knutsson A, Wahlström O: Internal fixation versus total hip arthroplasty in the treatment of displaced femoral neck fractures: A prospective randomized study of 100 hips. *Acta Orthop Scand* 2000;71:597-602.

143. Rogmark C, Johnell O, Carlsson Å, Sernbo I: Primary arthroplasty versus internal fixation in displaced femoral neck fractures: A randomized study of 450 patients, 5-year results. *70th Annual Meeting Proceedings.* Rosemont, IL, American Academy of Orthopaedic Surgeons, 2003.

144. Bochner RM, Pellicci PM, Lyden JP: Bipolar hemiarthroplasty for fracture of the femoral neck. *J Bone Joint Surg Am* 1988;70:1001-1010.

145. Broos PLO: Prosthetic replacement in the management of unstable femoral neck fractures in the elderly: Analysis of the mechanical complications noted in 778 fractures. *Acta Chir Belg* 1999;99:190-194.

146. Drinker H, Murray WR: The universal proximal femoral endoprosthesis. *J Bone Joint Surg Am* 1979;61:1167-1174.

147. Eiskjaer S, Ostgard SE: Survivorship analysis of hemiarthroplasty. *Clin Orthop* 1993;286:206-211.

148. Emery RJH, Broughton NS, Desai K, Bulstrode CJK, Thomas TL: Bipolar hemiarthroplasty for subcapital fracture of the femoral neck. *J Bone Joint Surg Br* 1991;73:322-324.

149. Gallinaro P, Tabasso G, Negretto R, Brach Del Prever E: Experience with bipolar prosthesis in femoral neck fractures in the elderly and debilitated. *Clin Orthop* 1990;251:26-30.

150. Giliberty RP: Hemiarthroplasty of the hip using a low-friction bipolar endoprosthesis. *Clin Orthop* 1983;175:86-92.

151. Goldhill VB, Lyden JP, Cornell CN, Bochner RM: Bipolar hemiarthroplasty for fracture of the femoral neck. *J Orthop Trauma* 1991;3:318-324.

152. Moshein J, Alter AH, Elconin KB, Adams WW, Isaacson J: Transcervical fractures of the hip treated with the Bateman bipolar prosthesis. *Clin Orthop* 1990;251:48-53.

153. Nather A, Seow CS, Iau P, Chan A: Morbidity and mortality for elderly patients with fractured neck of femur treated by hemiarthroplasty. *Injury* 1995;26:187-190.

154. Rae PJ, Hodgkinson JP, Meadows TH, Davies DRA, Hargadon EJ: Treatment of displaced subcapital fractures with the Charnley-Hastings hemiarthroplasty. *J Bone Joint Surg Br* 1989;71:478-492.

155. Rogalski R, Huebner J, Goulet J, Kaufer H: Two-year follow up of bipolar hemiarthroplasty. *Orthopedics* 1993;16:759-765.

156. Rogmark C, Carlsson Å, Johnell O, Sernbo I: Primary hemiarthroplasty in old patients with displaced femoral neck fracture: A 1-year follow-up of 103 patients aged 80 years or more. *Acta Orthop Scand* 2002;73:605-610.

157. Van Dortmont LM, Wereldsma JC: Complications of hemiarthroplasty. *Int Surg* 1996;81:200-204.

158. Wada M, Imura S, Baba H: Use of Osteonics UHR hemiarthroplasty for fractures of the femoral neck. *Clin Orthop* 1997;338:172-181.

159. Wetherell RG, Hinves BL: The Hastings bipolar hemiarthoplasty for subcapital fractures of the femoral neck. *J Bone Joint Surg Br* 1990;72:788-793.

160. Barnes CL, Berry DJ, Sledge CB: Dislocation after bipolar hemiarthroplasty of the hip. *J Arthroplasty* 1995;5:667-669.

161. Eiskjaer S, Gelineck J, Soballe K: Fractures of the femoral neck treated with cemented bipolar hemiarthroplasty. *Orthopedics* 1989;12:1545-1550.

162. Haidukewych GJ, Israel TA, Berry DJ: Long-term survivorship of cemented bipolar hemiarthroplasty for fracture of the femoral neck. *Clin Orthop* 2002;403:118-126.

163. Gill DRJ, Wilson PDG, Cheung BYK: Southland Hospital's experience with the Austin Moore hemiarthroplasty. *N Z Med J* 1995;108:173-174.

164. Kofoed H, Kofod J: Moore prosthesis in the treatment of fresh femoral neck fractures: A critical review with special attention to secondary acetabular degeneration. *Injury* 1983;14:531-540.

165. Maxted MJ, Denham RA: Failure of hemiarthroplasty for fractures of the neck of the femur. *Injury* 1983;15:224-226.

166. Sharif KM, Parker MJ: Austin Moore hemiarthroplasty: Technical aspects and their effects on outcome, in patients with fractures of the neck of femur. *Injury* 2002;33:419-422.

167. Faraj AA, Branfoot T: Cemented versus uncemented Thompson's prostheses: A functional outcome study. *Injury* 1999;30:671-675.

168. Overgaard S, Toftgaard T, Bonde G, Mossing NB: The uncemented bipolar hemiarthroplasty for displaced femoral neck fractures. *Acta Orthop Scand* 1991;62:115-120.

169. Parvizi J, Holiday AD, Ereth MH, Lewallen DG: Sudden death during primary hip arthroplasty. *Clin Orthop* 1999;369:39-48.

170. Ereth MH, Weber JG, Abel MD, Lemmon RL, Lewallen DG, Ilstrup DM: Cemented versus noncemtned total hip arthroplasty: Embolism, hemodynamics, and intrapulmonary shunting. *Mayo Clin Proc* 1992;67:1066-1074.

171. Esemenli TB, Toker K, Lawrence R: Hypotension associated with methylmethacrylate in partial hip arthroplasties: The role of femoral canal size. *Orthop Rev* 1991;7:619-623.

172. Lennox IAC, McLauchlan J: Comparing the mortality and morbidity of cemented and uncemented hemiarthroplasties. *Injury* 1993;24:185-186.

173. Pitto RP, Blunk J, Kößler M: Transesophageal echocardiography and clinical features of fat embolism during cemented total hip arthroplasty: A randomized study in patients with a femoral neck fracture. *Arch Orthop Trauma Surg* 2000;120:53-58.

174. Bateman JE: Single-assembly total hip prosthesis: Preliminary report. *Clin Orthop* 1990;251:3-6.

175. Dalldorf PG, Banas MP, Hicks DG, Pellegrini VD: Rate of degeneration of human acetabular cartilage after hemiarthroplasty. *J Bone Joint Surg Am* 1995;77:877-882.

176. Devas M, Hinves B: Prevention of acetabular erosion after hemiarthroplasty for fractured neck of femur. *J Bone Joint Surg Br* 1983;65:548-551.

177. James SE, Gallanaugh SC: Bi-articular hemiarthroplasty of the hip: A 7-year follow-up. *Injury* 1991;22:391-393.

178. LaBelle LW, Colwill JC, Swanson AB: Bateman bipolar hip arthroplasty for femoral neck fractures. *Clin Orthop* 1990;251:20-25.

179. Lestrange NR: Bipolar arthroplasty for 496 hip fractures. *Clin Orthop* 1990;251:7-19.

180. Lo WH, Chen WM, Huang CK, Chen TH, Chiu FY, Chen CM: Bateman bipolar hemiarthroplasty for displaced intracapsular femoral neck fractures. *Clin Orthop* 1994;302:75-82.

181. Long JW, Knight W: Bateman UPF prosthesis in fractures of the femoral neck. *Clin Orthop* 1980;152:198-201.

182. Malothra R, Arya R, Bhan S: Bipolar hemiarthroplasty in femoral neck fractures. *Arch Orthop Trauma Surg* 1995;114:79-82.

183. Mannarino F, Maples D, Colwill JC, Swanson AB: Bateman bipolar hip arthroplasty: A review of 44 cases. *Orthopedics* 1986;9:357-360.

184. Meyer S: Prosthetic replacement in hip fractures: A comparison between the Moore and Christiansen endoprosthesis. *Clin Orthop* 1981;160:57-62.

185. Nottage WM, McMaster WC: Comparison of bipolar implants with fixed-neck prostheses in femoral neck fractures. *Clin Orthop* 1990;251:38-43.

186. Phillips TW: Thompson hemiarthroplasty and acetabular erosion. *J Bone Joint Surg Am* 1989;71:913-917.

187. Chen SC, Badrinath K, Pell LH, Mitchell K: The movements of the components of the Hastings bipolar prosthesis: A radiographic study in 65 patients. *J Bone Joint Surg Br* 1989;71:186-188.

188. Mess D, Barmada R: Clinical and motion studies of the Bateman bipolar prosthesis in osteonecrosis of the hip. *Clin Orthop* 1990;251:44-47.

189. Izumi H, Torisu T, Itonaga I, Masumi S: Joint motion of bipolar femoral prostheses. *J Arthroplasty* 1995;10:237-243.

190. Beckenbaugh RD, Tressler HA, Johnson EW: Results after hemiarthroplasty of the hip using cemented femoral prosthesis. *Mayo Clin Proc* 1977;52:349-353.

191. Cabanela ME, Van Demark RE: Bipolar prosthesis, in *The Hip: Proceedings of the Twelfth Open Scientific Meeting of the Hip Society.* St Louis, MO, CV Mosby, 1984, pp 68-82.

192. Yamagata MD, Chao EY, Ilstrup DM, Melton LJ, Coventry MB, Stauffer RN: Fixed-head and bipolar hip endoprostheses: A retrospective clinical and radiographic study. *J Arthroplasty* 1987;2:327-341.

193. Marcus RE, Heintz JJ, Pattee GA: Don't throw away the Austin Moore. *J Arthroplasty* 1992;7:31-36.

194. D'Arcy J, Devas M: Treatment of fractures of the femoral neck by replacement with the Thompson prosthesis. *J Bone Joint Surg Br* 1976;58:279-286.

195. Wathne RA, Koval KJ, Aharonoff GB, Zuckerman JD, Jones DA: Modular unipolar versus bipolar prosthesis: A prospective evaluation of functional outcome after femoral neck fracture. *J Orthop Trauma* 1995;9:298-302.

196. Calder SJ, Anderson GH, Jagger C, Harper WM, Gregg PJ: Unipolar or bipolar prosthesis for displaced intracapsular hip fracture in octo-genarians: A randomized prospective study. *J Bone Joint Surg Br* 1996;78:391-394.

197. Kenzora JE, Magaziner J, Hudson J, et al: Outcome after hemiarthroplasty for femoral neck fractures in the elderly. *Clin Orthop* 1998;348:51-58.

198. Ong BC, Maurer SG, Aharonoff GB, Zuckerman JD, Koval KJ: Unipolar versus bipolar hemiarthroplasty: Functional outcome after femoral neck fracture at a minimum of thirty-six months of follow-up. *J Orthop Trauma* 2002;16:317-322.

199. Delamarter R, Moreland JR: Treatment of acute femoral neck fractures with total hip arthroplasty. *Clin Orthop* 1987;218:68-74.

200. Greenough CG, Jones JR: Primary total hip replacement for displaced subcapital fracture of the femur. *J Bone Joint Surg Br* 1988;70:639-643.

201. Lee BPH, Berry DJ, Harmsen WS, Sim FH: Total hip arthroplasty for the treatment of acute fracture of the femoral neck: Long-term results. *J Bone Joint Surg Am* 1998;80:70-75.

202. Sim GH, Stauffer RN: Management of hip fractures by total hip arthroplasty. *Clin Orthop* 1980;152:191-197.

203. Keating JF, Masson M, Scott N, Forbes J, Grant A: Randomized trial of reduction and fixation versus bipolar hemiarthroplasty versus total hip arthroplasty for displaced subcapital fractures in the fit older patient. *70th Annual Meeting Proceedings.* Rosemont, IL, American Academy of Orthopaedic Surgeons, 2003, pp 582-583.

204. Woo RY, Morrey BF: Dislocations after total hip arthroplasty. *J Bone Joint Surg Am* 1982;64:1295-1306.

205. Assessment of fracture risk and its application to screening for postmenopausal osteoporosis: Report of a WHO Study Group. *World Health Organ Tech Rep Ser* 1994;843:1-129.

206. Odén A, Dawson A, Dere W, Johnell O, Jonsson B, Kanis JA: Lifetime risk of hip fractures is underestimated. *Osteoporos Int* 1998;8:599-603.

207. Ceder L, Thorngren KG: Rehabilitation after hip repair (letter). *Lancet* 1982;2:1097-1098.

208. Jarnlo G-B, Ceder L, Thorngren K-G: Early rehabilitation at home of elderly patients with hip fractures and consumption of resources in primary care. *Scand J Prim Health Care* 1984;2:105-112.

209. Holmberg S, Thorngren K-G: Rehabilitation after femoral neck fracture: 3053 patients followed for 6 years. *Acta Orthop Scand* 1985;56:305-308.

210. Borgqvist L, Nordell E, Lindelöw G, Wingstrand H, Thorngren KG: Outcome after hip fracture in different health care districts: rehabilitation of 837 consecutive patients in primary care 1986-88. *Scand J Prim Health Care* 1991;9:244-251.

211. Thorngren K-G: Fractures in older persons. *Disabil Rehabil* 1994;16:119-126.

212. Melton LJ: Downturn in hip fracture incidence. *Public Health Rep* 1996;111:146-150.

213. Naessén T, Parker R, Persson I, Zack M, Adami HO: Time trends in incidence rates of first hip fracture in the Uppsala health care region, Sweden, 1965-1983. *Am J Epidemiol* 1989;130:289-299.

214. Rogmark C, Sernbo I, Johnell O, Nilsson JA: Incidence of hip fractures in Malmö, Sweden 1992-1995: A trend-break. *Acta Orthop Scand* 1999;70:19-22.

215. Löfman O, Berglund K, Larsson L, Toss G: Changes in hip fracture epidemiology: Redistribution between ages, genders and fracture types. *Osteoporos Int* 2002;13:18-25.

216. Melton LJ III: Differing patterns of osteoporosis across the world, in Chestnut CH III (ed): *New Dimensions in Osteoporosis in the 1990s*. Hong Kong, China, Excerpta Medica Asia, 1991, pp 13-18.

217. Johnell O, Gullberg B, Allander E: Kanis JA, MEDOS Study Group: The apparent incidence of hip fracture in Europe: A study of national register sources. *Osteoporos Int* 1992;2:298-302.

218. Thorngren K-G: Epidemiology of fractures of the proximal fracture, in Kenwright J, Duprac J, Fulford P (eds): *European Instructional Course Lectures*, 1997, Vol 3, pp 144-153.

219. Berglund-Rödén M, Swierstra BA, Wingstrand H, Thorngren K-G: Prospective comparison of hip fracture treatment, 856 cases followed for 4 months in the Netherlands and Sweden. *Acta Orthop Scand* 1994;65:287-294.

220. Thorngren K-G: Experience from Sweden, in *Medical Audit: Rationale and Practicalities*. Oxford, England, Cambridge University Press, 1993, pp 365-375.

221. Thorngren K-G: Optimal treatment of hip fractures. *Acta Orthop Scand* 1991;62:31-34.

222. Borgqvist L, Lindelöw G, Thorngren K-G: Costs of hip fracture: Rehabilitation of 180 patients in primary health care. *Acta Orthop Scand* 1991b;62:39-48.

223. Ahrengart L, Törnkvist H, Fornander P, et al: A randomised study of the compression hip screw and gamma nail in 426 fractures. *Clin Orthop* 2002;401:209-222.

224. Strömqvist B: Femoral head vitality after intracapsular hip fracture: 490 cases studied by intravital tetracycline labeling and Tc-MDP radionuclide imaging. *Acta Orthop Scand Suppl* 1983;200:1-71.

225. Lykke N, Lerud PJ, Stromsoe K, Thorngren K-G: Fixation of fractures of the femoral neck: A prospective randomised trial of three Ullevaal hip screws versus two Hansson hook pins. *J Bone Joint Surg Br* 2003;85:426-430.

226. Parker MJ, Pryor GA: *Hip Fracture Management*. Oxford, England, Blackwell Scientific Publications, 1993.

227. Kyle RF: Fractures of the proximal part of the femur. *J Bone Joint Surg Am* 1994;76:924-950.

228. Parker MJ, Pryor GA, Thorngren K-G: *Handbook of Hip Fracture Surgery*. Oxford, England, Butterworth-Heinemann, 1997.

229. Nilsson LT, Strömqvist B, Thorngren K-G: Secondary arthroplasty for complications of femoral neck fracture. *J Bone Joint Surg Br* 1989;71:777-781.

230. Nilsson LT, Strömqvist B, Thorngren K-G: Function after hook-pin fixation of femoral

neck fractures: prospective 2-year follow-up of 191 cases. *Acta Orthop Scand* 1989;60:573-578.

231. Jalovaara P, Berglund-Rödén M, Wingstrand H, Thorngren K-G: Treatment of hip fracture in Finland and Sweden. Prospective comparison of 788 cases in three hospitals. *Acta Orthop Scand* 1992;63:531-535.

232. Heikkinen T, Wingstrand H, Partanen J, Thorngren K-G, Jalovaara P: Hemiarthroplasty or osteosynthesis in cervical hip fractures: Matched-pair analysis in 892 patients. *Arch Orthop Trauma Surg* 2002;122:143-147.

233. Cserháti P, Fekete K, Berglund-Rödén M, Wingstrand H, Thorngren K-G: Hip fractures in Hungary and Sweden: Differences in treatment and rehabilitation. *Int Orthop* 2002;26:222-228.

234. Neander G, Adolphson P, von Sivers K, Dahlborn M, Dalén N: Bone and muscle mass after femoral neck fracture: A controlled quantitative computed tomography study of osteosynthesis versus primary total hip arthroplasty. *Arch Orthop Trauma Surg* 1997;116:470-474.

235. Tidermark J, Ponzer S, Svensson O, Söderqvist A, Törnkvist H: Internal fixation compared with total hip replacement for dislocated femoral neck fractures in the elderly: A randomised controlled study. *J Bone Joint Surg Br* 2003;85:380-388.

236. Thorngren K-G, Dolk T, Jarnlo G-B, Strömberg L: *Socialstyrelsens riktlinjer för vård och behandling av höftfraktur.* 2003, pp 1-137.

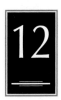

Reducing Complications in the Surgical Treatment of Intertrochanteric Fractures

David Templeman, MD
Michael R. Baumgaertner, MD
Ross K. Leighton, MD
Ronald W. Lindsey, MD
Berton R. Moed, MD

Abstract

The increasing number of hip fractures in the elderly constitutes a health care burden. The subset of unstable intertrochanteric hip fractures is important because the treatment of these fractures continues to be hampered by a moderate complication rate. Osteoporosis, fracture geometry, and the success of surgical treatment are strong predictors of outcome. The surgeon is in control of fracture reduction, implant selection, and implant placement, all of which must be optimized to ensure the success of surgical intervention.

The increasing number of hip fractures resulting from the aging of the North American population is estimated to cost as much as $3 billion per year in the United States and $300 million per year in Canada.[1] Approximately 250,000 hip fractures occur each year, a number that is expected to double by the year 2040.[2] Intertrochanteric hip fractures comprise about half of hip fractures and occur at an annual rate of 63 per 100,000 in elderly women and 34 per 100,000 in elderly men.

Complications after intertrochanteric hip fractures are common and are related to medical comorbidities and factors specific to the fracture. The overall mortality rate is approximately 20% within the first year after the fracture and then returns to standard age- and sex-matched rates.[2-4] Medical comorbidities, dementia, malnutrition, and nursing home residence are correlated with mortality. Because of the increased morbidity and costs caused by complications, it is important to direct efforts toward improving the successful treatment of intertrochanteric fractures.

Internal fixation is the preferred treatment of all but the most seriously ill patients. Most fractures can be successfully treated with various forms of internal fixation, but certain fracture patterns have fixation failure rates as high as 56%.[5] Factors that affect the strength of fixation include the quality of the bone, geometry of the fracture, and surgical technique.[3,6-8]

Although several classification systems are used to describe intertrochanteric fractures, the most important feature of classification is to determine whether fractures have stable or unstable patterns. Stability is determined by the reduction and maintenance of the medial cortex of the proximal femur. Unstable fracture patterns include fractures with a comminuted posterior medial cortex, reverse oblique intertrochanteric fractures, and intertrochanteric fractures with a subtrochanteric extension.[6,9-11]

Unstable fractures are common. In a series of 622 intertrochanteric hip fractures, Kyle and associates[12] documented that 43% were unstable. The fact that unstable fractures have a higher complication rate is well documented and directs attention to avoiding complications caused by unstable fracture patterns. Simple in concept but frequently difficult to achieve, the surgeon-controlled factors include the quality of the reduction and the choice and placement of the implant.[3]

Reduction

The deformity observed after an unstable intertrochanteric fracture includes varus, shortening, flexion, and external rotation. Because anatomic reduction is correlated with improved results, all forms of fixa-

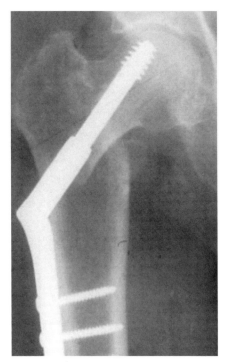

Figure 1 Radiograph showing a varus malreduction, which leads to an increased lever arm and predisposes the patient to cutout of the compression hip screw. Note the high (and incorrect) placement of the compression screw in the femoral head.

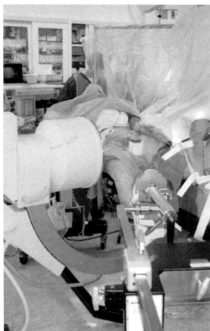

Figure 2 Photograph of a fracture table with the patient in the supine position. The two legs are scissored (the "well" leg is down) to facilitate reduction yet allow for a lateral image of the femoral head and neck.

tion must include a strategy to achieve reduction and maintain stable fixation of the fracture.[3]

A fracture table with the patient in the supine position is widely used for the surgical treatment of intertrochanteric fractures. Less commonly, patients are placed in the lateral decubitus position, which is sometimes used for the surgical treatment of intertrochanteric fractures with subtrochanteric extension. The lateral decubitus position can be used either with or without a fracture table. Whichever position is used, fluoroscopy is required to assess the accuracy of the reduction and guide the positioning of the implant. AP images are usually easier to obtain than lateral images. Careful preoperative positioning and imaging are done to ensure that accurate intraoperative projections can be obtained.

Varus malreductions are a common complication of the treatment of intertrochanteric fractures (Figure 1). A varus malreduction leads to an increased load on the proximal femur by increasing the moment arm on the implant, which in turn increases the probability of a fixation failure. Varus malalignment and shortening may also predispose patients to postoperative abductor weakness by effectively lengthening the abductor mechanism.

Because of the small visible field size provided by intraoperative fluoroscopy, it is frequently difficult for surgeons to determine whether the appropriate valgus alignment between the femoral neck and femoral shaft has been restored. Two guides that assist in assessing the reduction are a radiograph of the opposite hip and the restoration of Shenton's line during the manipulation of the proximal femur. To improve the lateral radiograph-ic image, the two legs can be scissored relative to one another, usually lowering the uninjured leg to improve the lateral radiographic image of the femoral head (Figure 2). This is essential for center-center and deep positioning of the cephalic screw. Apex posterior angulation of the proximal femur (posterior-sag) is associated with supine positioning of the patient. It can be observed with the lateral radiographic image and frequently requires additional manipulation to achieve an accurate reduction.

Implants

The compression hip screw has been the most frequently used implant for the fixation of intertrochanteric hip fractures. Despite its popular use, reported failure rates are as high as 25% for the fixation of unstable fractures.

Sliding hip screws provide controlled collapse and impaction of the intertrochanteric fracture and help achieve a position of stability while maintaining a constant neck-shaft angle (Figures 3 and 4). Most of this collapse is observed in the first 6 weeks after surgery. The usual mechanism of failure occurs when the neck-shaft angle collapses into varus and leads to cutout of the screw from the femoral head. Factors that correlate with varus cutout include the age of the patient, quality of the bone, pattern of the fracture, stability of the reduction, and angle and position of the implant.[13-16]

The Medoff sliding plate was designed to reduce cutout by replacing the side plate of the compression hip screw with a sliding component that allows the fracture to impact parallel to the longitudinal axis of the femur. This creates a controlled biaxial compression by allowing both collapse of the sliding hip screw and longitudinal sliding of the side plate.[17-21]

Watson and associates[21] performed a prospective randomized study of 160 patients that compared the failure rates of compression hip screws with fixed side plates to those of the Medoff sliding plate. Stable fracture patterns united in both groups without complications. However, unstable fractures had an overall failure rate of 9.6% (14% failure rate with the compression hip screw and 3% failure rate with the Medoff sliding plate). The authors concluded that the Medoff sliding plate was associated with a significant decrease in the rate of implant-related failures compared with compression hip screws for the stabilization of unstable intertrochanteric fractures. The disadvantages of using the Medoff sliding plate were a longer surgical time and greater blood loss because of the more extensive surgical dissection required to insert the device. As a result, the authors concluded that the compression hip screw was the preferred implant for stable fracture patterns and the Medoff sliding plate was the preferred implant for unstable fracture patterns.

The trochanteric stabilization plate is another modification of the compression hip screw. The trochanteric stabilization plate is added to the compression hip screw and forms a proximal buttress that prevents lateralization of the greater trochanter and excessive coapts of the compression hip screw. In studies, the use of the trochanteric side plate was associated with lower rates of collapse and medialization (9%) in comparison to the use of a compression hip screw alone (34%). However, the use of the trochanteric side plate requires a more extensive surgical dissection and is associated with greater blood loss and longer surgery times. Additional studies found no differences between the Medoff plate, dynamic hip screw, or use of the trochanteric stabilization plate in regard to walking ability or the rate of fixation failures.

The importance of proper screw positioning in the femoral head is well established. The proper position of the screw depends on two factors: the location of the screw within the femoral head

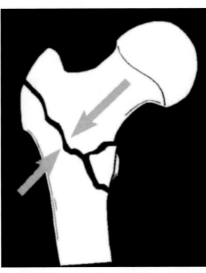

Figure 3 Illustration of a stable fracture pattern. Controlled collapse of the fracture (in the direction of the two arrows) has a high success rate in the treatment of stable fracture patterns. Controlled collapse can be achieved with compression hip screws.

(center-center position) and the depth of screw insertion with respect to the articular surface.[6,2,16]

Baumgaertner and associates[6] describe a simple technique for measuring the placement of the lag screw within the femoral head. The tip-apex distance (TAD) summarizes the position and the depth of the lag screw seen on both AP and lateral radiographs into a single number, in millimeters. In a series of patients treated with lag screw devices, the authors found that none of 120 screws with a TAD of 25 mm or less experienced cutout, but there was a strong statistical relationship between an increasing TAD and the rate of cutout. When the TAD was applied to a prospective series of patients (surgeons were attempting to achieve lag screw placement within 25 mm of the articular surface), the cutout rate was reduced from a historical control rate of 8% (16 of 198 patients) to 0% (0 of 118 patients), which is a statistically significant difference. A secondary finding was that there were fewer poor

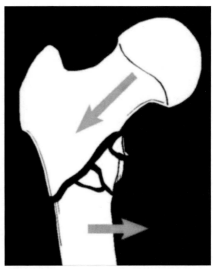

Figure 4 Illustration of a reverse oblique intertrochanteric hip fracture. The fracture plane is inherently unstable when treated using compression hip screws because the fracture plane impacts with the sliding hip screw.

reductions in the study group (Figure 5). Therefore, in the fixation of unstable intertrochanteric hip fractures, only with screw placement along the central axis of the femoral neck can the screw be placed deep enough into subchondral bone to prevent cutout, yet still avoid potential unrecognized joint penetration.

Intramedullary devices were developed for the fixation of intertrochanteric hip fractures because of perceived clinical and mechanical advantages. When intramedullary devices are placed during a percutaneous procedure, the small incisions used for inserting them are associated with less blood loss and reduced muscle stripping. Smaller incisions may also provide for more rapid rehabilitation, earlier weight bearing, and earlier discharge from acute care settings.[13,14,22-29]

The potential mechanical advantages of the intramedullary fixation of intertrochanteric fractures relate to a reduced lever arm on the implant and limiting the amount of collapse of the fracture. The amount that the fracture

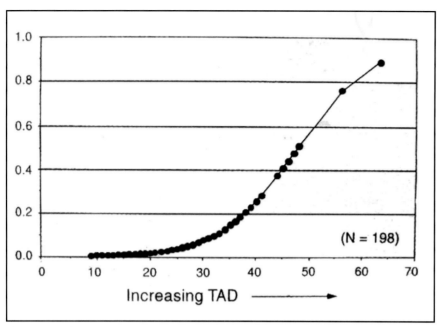

Figure 5 Graph illustrating the probability of the failure of fixation when the TAD exceeds 25 mm.

can impact is related to the proximal portion of the intramedullary nail. Loch and associates[30] describe this as a protruding strut that can act as a buttress to obstruct the sliding of the proximal bone fragment. This feature of intramedullary hip screw design may provide a possible advantage in that it can limit the amount of collapse in patients with unstable fracture patterns. Because the sliding of screws in the barrels of intramedullary devices is determined by the amount of the screw engaged in the barrel and the angle of the barrel, intramedullary devices have two key differences compared with compression hip screws.

First, the angle of the screw through the intramedullary nail is restricted by anatomic factors and the nail itself. Angles of 130° and 135° are common with intramedullary hip screws because these angles allow the screw to pass through the nail and be placed into a center-center position in the femoral head. Higher angle screws will slide easier, but because of the combination of the nail design and anatomy of the proximal femur, higher angled devices are not practical.

The second factor that relates to ease of sliding is the amount of the screw that is engaged in the barrel of the device. For most intramedullary hip screws, the distance over which the screw is engaged in the nail is shorter than the distance engaged within a compression hip screw. In a biomechanical model, Loch and associates[30] found that higher forces were needed to generate sliding in second-generation nails than compression hip screws. When compared with screws, the clinical implication is that second-generation intramedullary devices will require higher loads to initiate sliding and to generate compression of fracture surfaces.

Improvements in surgical techniques for intramedullary fixation of intertrochanteric fractures continue to reduce the complications associated with the use of these devices. Most intramedullary hip screws are placed with patients in the supine position on a fracture table. Fluoroscopy provides unobstructed AP and lateral views to confirm reduction of the fracture and accurate insertion of the intramedullary hip screw.[3,16]

Guide pins are inserted through the tip of the greater trochanter. A common mistake with guide pin insertion is allowing the guide pin and subsequent reaming to drift too far lateral on the slope of the trochanter, which leads to a more eccentric starting portal, varus malalignment, and increased offset. Although reaming assemblies vary, as a general rule it is better to ensure that adequate reaming is done, which allows for a more gentle insertion of the nail. The nails should be inserted gently, without the use of a mallet. Resistance to insertion of the nails should be carefully studied to determine whether the nail passage is being blocked by soft tissues or whether there is a bony block caused by inadequate reaming or malalignment of the nail and fracture site. A common problem is impingement of the nail on the anterior cortex of the femur, in which instance additional reaming should be done or a smaller diameter nail selected. It is important to remember that it is not necessary to fill the canal with an intramedullary hip screw.[16]

When using intramedullary hip screws to treat subtrochanteric fractures and intertrochanteric fractures with subtrochanteric extension, percutaneous and limited open reduction aids are often helpful. These devices allow access to the proper entrance site as well as reduction and stability of the major fracture fragments without devitalizing the fracture zone. (Figure 6). Apex anterior fracture angulation is usually present after an intertrochanteric fracture with subtrochanteric extension. This can be frequently reduced with the use of an intramedullary alignment guide.

As with compression hip screws, it is important to achieve a TAD of less than 25 mm.[6] An AP image is used to help the surgeon center the guidewire in the femoral head and a lateral image is used to evaluate placement. Posterior sag can be corrected at this point by elevating the jig or shaft of the femur and correcting the anteversion of the hip screw by rotating the jig.

Although the role of distal interlocking bolts with intramedullary hip screws is not firmly established, reports of postoperative femoral shaft fractures suggest that stress risers in the proximal femur can be caused by the interlocking bolts. After the nail and compression screw are inserted, it is possible to assess the stability of the fracture to determine whether sufficient fixation has been achieved without the use of distal interlocking bolts. Stability is tested by releasing traction and moving the fracture construct while observing with fluoroscopy. One interlocking bolt is recommended for treating rotational instability, and two interlocking distal bolts are recommended for treating length instability.

Results

In a meta-analysis of randomized trials comparing the gamma nail to the compression hip screw (1,794 patients), it was found that the gamma nail had a 2.4-fold higher rate of postoperative femoral shaft fractures and a 3.4-fold higher rate of postoperative revision surgeries.[31] Analysis of these complications implicated the forceful insertion of implants, the routine use of two interlocking bolts, and nail designs with large diameter nails that were shaped with nonanatomic angles. It is important to note that these results were reported during the initial use of intramedullary hip screws before 1996. From this experience, modifications in nail design and surgical technique have been made to improve the results of using intramedullary fixation to treat intertrochanteric fractures.

Recent studies report improved results and reduced complication rates with the use of intramedullary hip screws. Since 1998, randomized trials (comparing compression hip screws and intramedullary hip screws) and prospective series (comparing long and short

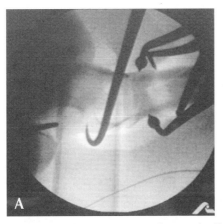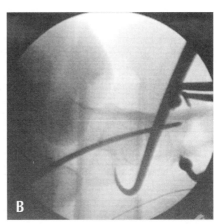

Figure 6 A and **B**, Fluoroscopic photographs illustrating the use of percutaneously placed bone hook and very limited approach (tensor split) to apply pointed bone clamps to improve the reduction and accurate placement of the guide pin.

intramedullary hip screws) document lower complication rates with intramedullary nailing. The most important improvement has been the reduction in the number of postoperative femoral shaft fractures. Several large studies that enrolled between 66 and 981 patients documented a rate of shaft fractures of less than 2%. Additional benefits of the use of intramedullary hip screws are shorter surgical times, less intraoperative blood loss, less collapse of the implant, and a decrease in the degree of limb-length discrepancy.[13,14,16,25,27,29,32]

Reverse Oblique Intertrochanteric Hip Fractures

Several fracture classifications recognize a specific intertrochanteric fracture pattern in which the fracture line extends through the lateral femoral cortex distal to the vastus ridge of the greater trochanter; this pattern is commonly referred to as a reverse oblique intertrochanteric fracture.[5,9,11] Several studies confirm high failure rates when this fracture is stabilized with compression hip screws. Instead of collapse of the hip screw leading to compression of the fracture site, reverse-oblique intertrochanteric fractures exhibit medial displacement of the distal fragment and resultant instability of

the fracture. Haidukewych and associates[5] reviewed the treatment of 1,035 intertrochanteric fractures over a 10-year period and identified 55 (5%) that were reverse oblique intertrochanteric fractures. The overall failure rate for this fracture pattern was 32% (15 of 47 fractures) but the highest failure rate (9 of 16 fractures, 56%) was associated with the use of the compression hip screw. Rosso and associates[33] studied the use of a 95° fixed-angle device used to treat reverse oblique intertrochanteric fractures and documented eight implant failures in a series of 30 patients.

Sadowski and associates[34] performed a prospective study to compare intramedullary fixation and a 95° fixed-angle device for stabilizing reverse oblique intertrochanteric fractures. In the group treated with the fixed-angle device (19 patients), there were six fixation failures and one nonunion. In the group treated with intramedullary fixation (20 patients), there was one nonunion ($P = 0.007$). Other benefits of intramedullary fixation included shorter surgical times, less blood loss, and shorter hospital stays. These results indicate a clear clinical advantage in the use of intramedullary hip screws to treat reverse oblique intertrochanteric fractures[34] (Figure 7).

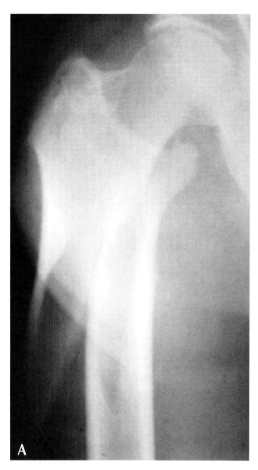
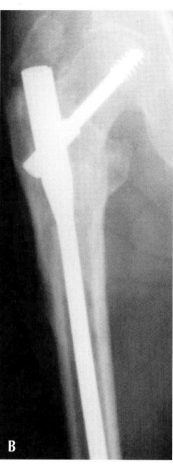

Figure 7 **A**, Preoperative radiograph of a patient with a long reverse oblique intertrochanteric hip fracture with subtrochanteric extension. **B**, Follow-up radiograph. The fracture was stabilized with an intramedullary hip screw and healed uneventfully.

Summary

Several types of implants are available to successfully treat stable intertrochanteric hip fractures. Implants that allow early mobilization and weight bearing should be used. Although studies have not yet documented that the choice of implant for the treatment of stable fractures affects the ultimate clinical outcome, recovery seems to be more dependent on the presence of comorbidities. In treating unstable fractures, the variables of surgical technique and the choice of implant are important to prevent fixation failures. Medoff sliding plates and intramedullary hip screws have reduced fracture-related complications when used in the fixation of unstable fracture patterns. Given the documented very high failure rates associated with a hip screw and side plate, and the statistically significant improved performance over 95° fixed angle devices, there is a clear advantage to the use of intramedullary hip screws in the treatment of reverse oblique intertrochanteric fractures.

References

1. Owen RA, Melton LJ III, Gallagher JC, Riggs BL: The national cost of acute care of hip fractures associated with osteoporosis. *Clin Orthop* 1980;150:172-176.

2. Cummings SR, Rubin SM, Black D: The future of hip fractures in the United States: Numbers, costs, and potential effects of postmenopausal estrogen. *Clin Orthop* 1990;252:163-166.

3. Kyle RF, Cabanela ME, Russell TA, et al: Fractures of the proximal part of the femur. *Instr Course Lect* 1995;44:227-253.

4. Zuckerman JD, Skovron ML, Koval KJ, Aharonoff G, Frankel VH: Postoperative complications and mortality associated with operative delay in older patients who have a fracture of the hip. *J Bone Joint Surg Am* 1995;77:1551-1556.

5. Haidukewych GJ, Israel TA, Berry DJ: Reverse obliquity fractures of the intertrochanteric region of the femur. *J Bone Joint Surg Am* 2001;83:643-650.

6. Baumgaertner MR, Curtin SL, Lindskog DM, Keggi JM: The value of the tip-apex distance in predicting failure of fixation of peritrochanteric fractures of the hip. *J Bone Joint Surg Am* 1995;77:1058-1064.

7. Ellis TJ, Kyle RF: The results of open reduction internal fixation of a highly unstable intertrochanteric hip fracture with a dynamic hip screw, in *67th Annual Meeting Proceedings*. Rosemont, IL, American Academy of Orthopaedic Surgeons, 2000, p 467.

8. Evans EM: The treatment of trochanteric fractures of the femur. *J Bone Joint Surg Br* 1949;31:190-203.

9. Fracture and dislocation compendium: Orthopaedic Trauma Association Committee for Coding and Classification. *J Orthop Trauma* 1996;10(suppl 1):v-ix, 1-154.

10. Jensen JS, Sonne-Holm S, Tondevold E: Unstable trochanteric fractures: A comparative analysis of four methods of internal fixation. *Acta Orthop Scand* 1980;51:949-962.

11. Orthopaedic Trauma Association Committee for Coding and Classification: Fracture and dislocation compendium. *J Orthop Trauma* 1996;10(suppl 1):1-154.

12. Kyle RF, Gustilo RB, Premer RF: Analysis of six hundred and twenty-two intertrochanteric hip fractures. *J Bone Joint Surg Am* 1979;61:216-221.

13. Adams CL, Robinson CM, Court-Brown CM, McQueen MM: Prospective randomized controlled trial of an intramedullary nail versus dynamic screw and plate for intertrochanteric fractures of the femur. *J Orthop Trauma* 2001;15:394-400.

14. Ahrengart L, Tornkvist H, Fornander P, et al: A randomized study of the compression hip screw and Gamma nail in 426 fractures. *Clin Orthop* 2002;401:209-222.

15. Babst R, Renner N, Biedermann M, et al: Clinical results using the trochanter stabilizing plate (TSP): The modular extension of the dynamic hip screw (DHS) for internal fixation of selected unstable intertrochanteric fractures. *J Orthop Trauma* 1998;12:392-399.

16. Baumgaertner MR, Curtin SL, Lindskog DM: Intramedullary versus extramedullary fixation for the treatment of intertrochanteric hip fractures. *Clin Orthop* 1998;348:87-94.

17. Medoff RJ, Maes K: A new device for the fixation of unstable peritrochanteric fractures of the hip. *J Bone Joint Surg Am* 1991;73:1192-1199.

18. Olsson O, Kummer FJ, Ceder L, Koval KJ, Larsson S, Zuckerman JD: The Medoff sliding plate and a standard sliding hip screw for unstable intertrochanteric fractures: A mechanical comparison in cadaver femurs. *Acta Orthop Scand* 1998;69:266-272.

19. Rha JD, Kim YH, Yoon SI, Park TS, Lee MH: Factors affecting sliding of the lag screw in intertrochanteric fractures. *Int Orthop* 1993;17:320-324.

20. Simpson AH, Varty K, Dodd CA: Sliding hip screws: modes of failure. *Injury* 1989;20:227-231.

21. Watson JT, Moed BR, Cramer KE, Kargos DE: Comparison of the compression hip screw with the Medoff sliding plate for intertrochanteric fractures. *Clin Orthop* 1998;348:79-86.

22. Bridle SH, Patel AD, Bircher M, Calvert PT: Fixation of intertrochanteric fractures of the femur: A randomised prospective comparison of the Gamma nail and the dynamic hip screw. *J Bone Joint Surg Br* 1991;73:330-334.

23. Butt MS, Kikler SJ, Nafie S, Ali MS: Comparison of dynamic hip screw and gamma nail: a prospective, randomized, controlled trial. *Injury* 1995;26:615-618.

24. Fornander P, Thorngren K-G, Tornquist H, Ahrengart L, Lindgren U: Swedish experience of the first 209 randomized patients with gamma nails vs. screw-plate. *Acta Orthop Scand* 1992;63(suppl 248):90.

25. Hardy DC, Descamps PY, Krallis P, et al: Use of an intramedullary hip-screw compared with a compression hip-screw with a plate for intertrochanteric femoral fractures: A prospective, randomized study of one hundred patients. *J Bone Joint Surg Am* 1998;80:618-630.

26. Hoffman CW, Lynskey TG: Intertrochanteric fractures of the femur: A randomized prospective comparison of the Gamma nail and the Ambi hip screw. *Aust N Z J Surg* 1996;66:151-155.

27. Lunsjo K, Ceder L, Thorngren KG, et al: Extramedullary fixation of 569 unstable intertrochanteric fractures: A randomized multicenter trial of the Medoff sliding plate versus three other screw-plate systems. *Acta Orthop Scand* 2001;72:133-140.

28. O'Brien PJ, Meek RN, Blachut PA, Broekhuyse HM, Sabharwal S: Fixation of intertrochanteric hip fractures: Gamma nail versus dynamic hip screw. A randomized, prospective study. *Can J Surg* 1995;38:516-520.

29. Radford PJ, Needoff M, Webb JK: A prospective randomized comparison of the dynamic hip screw and the gamma locking nail. *J Bone Joint Surg Br* 1993;75:789-793.

30. Loch DA, Kyle RF, Bechtold JE, Kane M, Anderson K, Sherman RE: Forces required to initiate sliding in second-generation intramedullary nails. *J Bone Joint Surg Am* 1998;80:1626-1631.

31. Parker MJ, Pryor GA: Gamma versus DHS nailing for extracapsular femoral fractures: Meta-analysis of ten randomized trials. *Int Orthop* 1996;20:163-168.

32. Saudan M, Lubbeke A, Sadowski C, Riand N, Stern R, Hoffmeyer P: Peritrochanteric fractures: Is there an advantage to an intramedullary nail? A randomized, prospective study of 206 patients comparing the dynamic hip screw and proximal femoral nail. *J Orthop Trauma* 2002;16:386-393.

33. Rosso R, Babst R, Marx A, Hess P, Heberer M, Regazzoni P: Proximal femoral fractures: Is there an indication for the condylar screw (DCS)? *Helv Chir Acta* 1992;58:679-682.

34. Sadowski C, Lubbeke A, Saudan M, Riand N, Stern R, Hoffmeyer P: Treatment of reverse oblique and transverse intertrochanteric fractures with use of an intramedullary nail of a 95 degree screw-plate: A prospective, randomized study. *J Bone Joint Surg Am* 2002;84:372-381.

Prevention of Hip Fractures: Medical and Nonmedical Management

Julie T. Lin, MD
Joseph M. Lane, MD

Abstract

Hip fractures can have a significant detrimental effect on morbidity and mortality. Medical and nonmedical management approaches both may be used to help decrease the risk of hip fracture. Medical management includes the use of antiresorptive agents such as the bisphosphonates, calcium and vitamin D, selective estrogen receptor modulators, and anabolic agents such as parathyroid hormone, which strengthen bone. Nonmedical management includes fall prevention programs and hip protectors. Physicians caring for patients at risk for hip fracture should be cognizant of these management approaches to most effectively minimize fracture risk.

Of all osteoporotic fractures, hip fractures have the most significant detrimental effect on morbidity and mortality. For example, the cumulative loss of function over time caused by one hip fracture is believed to be equivalent to 4 vertebral fractures or 20 less severe fractures such as distal radius fractures.[1] There are multiple risk factors for hip fracture, including the orientation of the fall, protective responses, bone strength, the fall itself, and local shock absorbers.[2] Both medical and nonmedical management may be used to help decrease fracture risk.

Medical Management

Antiresorptive medications such as the bisphosphonates, calcium and vi-

tamin D, estrogen, selective estrogen receptor modulators such as raloxifene, intranasal calcitonin, and anabolic agents such as parathyroid hormone all have been shown to clearly increase hip bone mineral density. The use of alendronate and risedronate with appropriate amounts of calcium and vitamin D_3, as well as parathyroid hormone can result in significant reductions in hip fracture risk[3] (Table 1).

Studies have shown that calcium and vitamin D can increase bone mineral density and reduce the incidence of hip fractures. Chapuy and associates[4] demonstrated that in 1,634 elderly women, 18 months of vitamin D_3 (cholecalciferol) and calcium supplements resulted in 43%

fewer hip fractures. Proximal femur bone mineral density was increased by 2.7% in a subgroup of patients. Furthermore, serum parathyroid hormone concentration decreased by 44% from baseline, suggesting that the calcium and vitamin D supplements helped to reduce secondary hyperparathyroidism.

The oral bisphosphonates alendronate and risedronate both have been shown to increase hip bone mineral density and decrease the risk of hip fractures. A 10-mg daily dose of alendronate for 3 years increases hip bone mineral density by 5.9% to 7.8%.[5] Hip fracture rates are similarly decreased after 3 years of treatment with alendronate. A 5-mg daily dose of alendronate for 24 months, followed by a 10-mg daily dose for 12 months, results in a relative risk of hip fracture of 0.49.[6] Similarly, after a 2.5-mg or 5.0-mg daily dose of risedronate for 3 years, the incidence of hip fracture is reduced from 3.2% in controls to 1.9% in those receiving risedronate.[7] Increases in hip bone mineral density are seen in those receiving risedronate versus losses seen in controls (1.6% versus 1.2% in the femoral neck and 3.3% versus 0.7%

Table 1

Acceptable Agents Used in the Treatment and Prevention of Osteoporosis

Agent	Class	Dose[†]	Hip Fracture Protection
Calcium and vitamin D	Calcium/vitamin D	1,200 mg elemental calcium and 800 IU of vitamin D daily	Yes
Alendronate	Bisphosphonate (oral)	5 mg daily; 35 mg weekly (prevention) 10 mg daily; 70 mg weekly (treatment)	Yes
Risedronate	Bisphosphonate (oral)	5 mg daily; 35 mg weekly (prevention) 5 mg daily; 35 mg weekly (treatment)	Yes
Pamidronate*	Bisphosphonate (intravenous)	30 mg IV every 3-4 months	?
Zolendronate*	Bisphosphonate (intravenous)	4 mg IV annually	?
Estrogen	Hormone replacement therapy	0.625 mg daily	Yes
Raloxifene	Selective estrogen receptor modulator	60 mg daily	No
Calcitonin (nasal)	Calcitonin analog	200 mg IU alternate nostrils daily	No
Parathyroid hormone	Parathyroid hormone analog (recombinant human parathyroid hormone)	20 µg SQ daily	?

* = Off-label use

† IU = international units; IV = intravenously; SQ = subcutaneous.

in the femoral trochanter, respectively) over 3 years.[8] Hip fracture reduction may be noted as early as within 6 months of treatment with risedronate.[9]

The intravenous bisphosphonates pamidronate and zolendronate have been used off-label in the treatment of osteoporosis in patients unable to tolerate the oral bisphosphonates because of gastrointestinal complications such as esophagitis. Although intravenous bisphosphonates have been shown to increase hip bone mineral density, no hip fracture data have been reported to date. In one study, 30 mg of pamidronate administered every 3 months for a minimum of 18 months resulted in a 4.7% increase in hip bone mineral density.[10] Zolendronate administered in varying doses over 1 year, including a single dose infused annually, resulted in increased bone mineral density in the femoral neck ranging from 3.1% to 3.5%.[11]

Estrogen has been shown to increase bone mineral density as well as decrease hip fracture risk by 35%,[12] with a daily dose of 0.625 mg conjugated estrogen used to prevent bone loss.[13-15] Estrogen appears to be most effective in younger women. A recent meta-analysis of randomized trials demonstrated that the use of hormone replacement therapy results in a relative risk of hip and wrist fractures of 0.60, with a relative risk of 0.45 in women younger than 60 years.[16] Felson and associates[17] demonstrated that estrogen use in women younger than 75 years versus women age 75 years or older resulted in 11.2% versus 3.2% increased bone mineral density compared with controls, respectively. Recently, the Women's Health Writing Group[18] concluded that the overall health risks from estrogen, including coronary heart disease, stroke, pulmonary embolism, and invasive breast cancer, exceeded the positive effects of

its use. Therefore, the use of estrogen as a first-line treatment in the prevention and treatment of hip fractures is currently not recommended.

Selective estrogen receptor modulators, such as raloxifene, have been shown to increase hip bone mineral density. Ettinger and associates[19] demonstrated that raloxifene administered for up to 36 months resulted in increased bone mineral density in the femoral neck ranging from 2.1% in those receiving a 60-mg daily dose to 2.4% in those receiving a 120-mg daily dose. Drawbacks to the use of selective estrogen receptor modulators have included venous thromboembolism and hot flashes[20] and their inability to minimize fracture risk.

Intranasal calcitonin is a calcitonin analog that can increase hip bone mineral density. A meta-analysis including 18 clinical trials demonstrated that calcitonin use resulted in a change in proximal femur bone mineral density of 0.32.[21] Although calcitonin has been shown to reduce the risk of new vertebral fractures by 33%,[22] it has not been shown to similarly reduce the risk of hip fracture.[3]

Recombinant human parathyroid hormone is an anabolic agent recently approved by the Food and Drug Administration for the treatment of osteoporosis. Neer and associates[23] reported that parathyroid hormone administered in a 20-μg subcutaneous daily dose over a median period of 21 months resulted in a 3% increased femoral neck bone mineral density. Although the authors demonstrated that a 40-μg subcutaneous daily dose increased hip bone mineral density 3% more than the 20-μg dose, the 40-μg dose resulted in increased minor adverse effects including headache and nausea. In addition, both doses decrease appendicular and axial fractures. The current recommended daily dose is 20 μg.

Although bisphosphonates and parathyroid hormone can improve bone strength, other factors contributing to fracture risk are generally not addressed. Nonmedical management, such as fall prevention programs and hip protectors, may effectively minimize the fall risk and the risk of hip fracture following the fall, respectively.

Nonmedical Management

Fall Prevention

More than 90% of hip fractures occur as a result of falls.[24,25] It has been estimated that the incidence of falls among nursing home residents is 1.5 falls/person/year, of which there are 0.29 falls/person/year onto the hip. As many as 20% of these falls result in hip fracture.[26] Thirty percent of those older than 65 years fall each year.[27-29] Although falls can directly result in hip fractures and other seri-

ous injuries, they also contribute to less tangible and immediate adverse consequences. One or more falls, with or without serious injury, are associated with declines in basic and instrumental activities of daily living over 3 years in elderly community dwellers.[30] Two or more noninjurious falls are associated with decline in social activities, and at least one injurious fall is associated with a decline in physical activity.[30]

In addition to these adverse effects on quality of life and physical function, falls in general are associated with increased health care costs, which increase with both the frequency and severity of falls.[31] One or more injurious falls have been associated with increased annual hospital costs of over $11,000, nursing home costs of more than $5,000, and total health care costs of more than $19,000.[31]

There are multiple risk factors for falls, which include a patient age of 65 years or older, muscle weakness, gait and balance problems, functional limitations, visual impairment, cognitive impairment, adverse effects of medications, environmental factors, and history of falls.[32] In addition, poor performance on neuromuscular function tests including body sway and gait speed is correlated with falls.[33,34]

Assessment Screening for fall risk in elderly patients may be performed in the office or in any motion analysis center or physical therapy gym if available. A history of falls and the predisposing factors that lead to a fall can provide important information about appropriate interventions. A targeted neurologic examination, such as decreased vibration, may indicate proprioceptive impairment.[35] In addition, simple screening tests may be performed in the office. Assessment of gait, including heel, toe,

and tandem gait, can help to identify specific muscle group deficiencies and unsafe gait patterns. The need for assistive devices such as walkers or canes can be evaluated at this time. The timed single limb stance, performed with the eyes either open or closed, can provide important information about balance because of its good interrater and test-retest reliability.[36,37] In addition, the timed "get up and go" test, in which patients rise from a chair, walk 3 meters, and return to a chair, easily can be performed in the office. In addition to having good interrater and intrarater reliability, this test predicts the patient's ability to go outside alone safely.[38] The functional reach test measures flexibility and balance. Using a fixed base of support, the difference between arm's length and maximal forward reach is documented. This test has been shown to be reliable and precise, a good approximator of stability, and is useful in designing modified environments in elderly persons with balance deficits.[39,40]

Patient Education Educating patients about fall risk and the serious consequences of falls, especially hip fracture, is essential to motivate patients to comply with treatment recommendations. Patients should be informed about the high mortality rate and loss of independence following hip fracture. In addition, specific difficulties with the previously mentioned screening tests can help identify tangible deficiencies in patients who deny they are at increased risk for hip fracture.

Interdisciplinary Approach An interdisciplinary approach in the prevention of falls is necessary to most effectively identify predisposing factors and to reduce risk. The use of strengthening exercises or physical therapy interventions, environmental modifications, assistive devices, balance and gait training, cognitive/behavioral intervention, medication review, and visual assessment all help to minimize risk. Several randomized controlled trials have evaluated interventions such as programs of physical therapy administered by a health professional, tai chi, home hazard assessment and modification, withdrawal of psychotropic medications, and a multidisciplinary, multifactorial, health/environmental risk factor screening and intervention program.[41]

Exercise/Physical Therapy Intervention Specific exercise programs, such as tai chi, as well as physical therapy programs have been documented in several randomized controlled trials to effectively reduce falls. These programs generally improve balance and strengthening, resulting in decreased falls, and are particularly effective in the elderly. Wolf and associates[42] followed 200 elderly community dwellers who received tai chi and computerized balance training. After a 15-week intervention, the authors documented a decreased fear of falling responses. In addition, tai chi was shown to reduce the risk of multiple falls by 47.5%.

Campbell and associates[43] followed 233 elderly community dwellers randomized to an individually tailored physical therapy program in the home compared with the usual care and equal number of social visits. The authors found that after 1 year, the mean rate of falls was lower in the exercise than the control group (0.87 versus 1.34, respectively). In addition, after 6 months, subjects in the exercise group had improved balance.

Robertson and associates[44] assessed the efficacy of a trained nurse individually prescribing a home-based exercise program to reduce

falls in 240 elderly men and women. At 1-year follow-up, falls were reduced by 46%. There were five hospital admissions as a result of injuries caused by falls in the control group, and none in the exercise group. The authors concluded that the program was cost-effective in participants age 80 years and older compared with younger participants.

Home Safety Intervention Cumming and associates[45] followed 530 community dwellers and evaluated whether the occupational therapist home visits targeted at identifying and removing environmental hazards (for example, obstacles in the walker's path, improperly secured throw rugs) and facilitation of necessary home modifications helped to reduce the risk of falls. During a 12-month follow-up period, the authors demonstrated that 36% versus 45% of subjects in the intervention group versus controls, respectively, had at least one fall ($P = 0.05$). The authors concluded that decreased falls in these patients may be a consequence not only of home modifications, but may be secondary to behavioral changes such as increased awareness of surroundings.

Withdrawal of Psychotropic Medications Withdrawal of psychotropic medications has been associated with decreased falls. Campbell and associates[46] performed a randomized controlled trial in 93 elderly patients using psychotropic medications and assessed two interventions: the gradual withdrawal of psychotropic medication versus continuation of psychotropic medication; and a home-based exercise program versus no exercise program. The authors found that after 44 weeks, the relative risk for falls in the medication withdrawal group compared with those taking the original medication was 0.34.

Multifactorial Interventions A multiple risk factor intervention strategy has been shown to result in a significant reduction in fall risk among elderly community dwellers who are not cognitively impaired. One of the best-known fall prevention trials was performed by Tinetti and associates.[47,48] In this study, the authors followed 301 elderly men and women community dwellers possessing risk factors for falling. The subjects were given either a combination of adjustment of their medications, behavioral instructions, and exercise programs aimed at modifying their risk factors; or the usual health care plus social visits. After 1 year, 35% of the intervention group fell, compared with 47% of the control group ($P = 0.04$). Close and associates[49] assessed the benefit of a structured interdisciplinary assessment in elderly community dwellers taken to the emergency department after a fall. Patients in the intervention group received a detailed medical and occupational therapy assessment with referral to relevant services as needed. At 12-month follow-up, there was a reduced risk of falling (odds ratio, 0.39), reduced risk of recurrent falls (odds ratio, 0.33), and the odds of admission to the hospital were lower (odds ratio, 0.61). In addition, there was a greater decline in Barthel score with time in the control group ($P < 0.00001$).

Cognitive status plays an important role in the efficacy of multifactorial interventions, as these interventions have not been shown to be effective in reducing falls in elderly patients with cognitive impairment and dementia. Shaw and associates[50] performed a randomized controlled trial in 274 elderly patients taken to the emergency department after a fall. Intervention consisted of assessment of screening for medical, cardiovascular, gait and balance, and fall hazard risks with corresponding interventions aimed at minimizing these risks. The authors demonstrated no significant differences between intervention and control groups in the proportion of patients who fell after 1-year follow-up; 74% versus 80% of the intervention versus control groups, respectively, sustained falls (relative risk ratio, 0.92).

Hip Protectors

Hip protectors are a simple, efficacious, and cost-effective method to prevent hip fractures if a fall does occur. These orthoses, usually made of polypropylene or polyethylene, are most commonly sewn or placed in undergarments, or may be worn on top of underwear. There are several different types available, with only a handful available for distribution in the United States. Few have been specifically subjected to randomized controlled trials. The most widely used hip protector, the Safehip (Sahvatex-Tytex), is manufactured in Denmark and consists of an outer shield of polypropylene with an inner Plastazote lining. The KPH hip protector, developed in Finland, comprises an undergarment with a pocket in each side into which a removable hip protector is placed. A variant of this hip protector, the KPH2, was used in the largest randomized controlled trial to date, performed by Kannus and associates.[51] The High Impact Protection System (HIPS), made in Denmark, is similar in design to the KPH, consisting of a removable inner and outer shell placed into an undergarment with specially designed pockets. The Hip-Guard is an over-the-clothing hip protector belt made in Canada. Drawbacks to its use include poor cosmesis, as its appearance is bulky

and obvious and cannot be hidden under clothing, unlike the other hip protectors.

Theory of Hip Protectors Most hip fractures are related to direct trauma to the hip and subsequent impact on the greater trochanter. Parkkari and associates[52] demonstrated that in 206 patients with acute hip fractures, 98% of hip fractures resulted from a fall. Fifty-six percent of patients with hip fractures had acute hematomas on their greater trochanter, compared with 6% of control with hematomas. Energy absorption has been suggested to be the main determinant of hip fractures. Therefore, it is hoped that energy-absorbing hip protectors compensate for loss of soft-tissue padding and attenuate forces delivered to the proximal femur.[53] Lauritzen and Askegaard[54] demonstrated that a layer of 29-mm soft tissue could absorb 60% more energy than a 20-mm layer. In a retrospective study evaluating women with and without hip fractures, the authors found that women with hip fractures had an average soft-tissue covering of 22-mm thickness, whereas in those without hip fracture it was an average of 32-mm thickness. Parkkari and associates[55] further demonstrated that hip protectors help maintain forces in the proximal femur below that needed to fracture in the elderly in a series of impact experiments. Using four volunteers with a 40-kg pendulum and 115 joules of energy, the authors demonstrated that none of the volunteers sustained hip fracture or even a hematoma while undergoing the experiments with hip protectors in place.

Randomized Controlled Trials Lauritzen and associates[56] performed a study involving 593 elderly nursing home residents over 11 months. There were 167 women and 80 men

in the hip protector group and 277 women and 141 men in the control group. In addition, a fall register was set up for 45 residents in the treatment group and 76 controls. There were 8 and 31 hip fractures in the intervention and control groups, respectively. None of the eight residents in the intervention group was wearing a hip protector at the time of fracture. Relative risk of hip fracture among women and men in the intervention group was 0.44.

Ekman and associates[57] performed a randomized, controlled trial involving elderly nursing home residents: 302 were offered hip protectors and 442 served as controls. There were 294 and 531 falls in the hip protector and control groups, respectively. There were 4 and 17 hip fractures in the hip protector and control groups, respectively. No hip fractures occurred in patients wearing hip protectors. Relative risk of hip fracture was 0.33, and compliance was 44%.

Villar and associates[58] performed a randomized, controlled trial over a 12-week period in 141 elderly female patients living in nursing homes: 101 were in the treatment group and 40 were in the control group. There were eight falls onto the hip in the treatment group and one in the control group. None of the falls resulted in hip fracture. Compliance was 50% at approximately 1 week, and dropped to 30% at 12 weeks.

The largest randomized, controlled trial involving hip protectors to date was performed by Kannus and associates[51] in 1,801 elderly ambulatory, frail adults. There were 653 falls in the hip protector group and 1,148 in the control group. There were 13 and 67 hip fractures in the hip protector and control groups, respectively. In the hip protector group, 4 hip fractures occurred while the protector was worn (among 1,034 falls) and 9 hip fractures (among 370 falls) without the protector. The compliance rate was 48%. The authors concluded that 41 persons needed to use the hip protector for 1 year or 8 persons for 5 years to prevent one hip fracture.

Chan and associates[59] followed 71 elderly nursing home residents over 9 months. There were 6 fractures and 101 falls in the control group and 3 fractures and 191 falls in the hip protector group. The three fractures in the hip protector group occurred when the pads were not in place. Relative risk of fracture was 0.264. Compliance was 50.3% in the hip protector group.

Cameron and associates[60] performed a randomized controlled trial over 18 months in 174 elderly women living in a residential aged-care facility. They found that there were eight hip fractures in the intervention group and seven in the control group. No hip fractures occurred when hip protectors were being worn as directed. Compliance was 57% over the duration of the study, and 54% at the time of falls in the intervention group.

Harada and associates[61] performed the first hip protector trial in Japan, involving 164 elderly female nursing home residents. There were 131 falls and 1 hip fracture and 90 falls and 8 hip fractures in hip protector wearers and controls, respectively. The authors concluded that the annual hip fracture rate in non-wearers versus wearers was 19.8% versus 2.0%, respectively.

Meyer and associates[62] performed a trial in Germany involving 942 elderly nursing home residents at high risk for falls. Structured education of staff was provided, and residents in the intervention group received three free hip protectors per resident. After a follow-up period of 15 months in the intervention group and 14 months in the control group, there were 21 hip fractures in 21 residents in the intervention group and 42 fractures in 39 residents in the control group (relative risk 0.57).

Hip protectors in association with other interventions have been shown to effectively reduce fall risk. Jensen and associates[63] performed a multifactorial intervention program in 439 elderly residents in residential care facilities to determine whether falls and fall-related injuries would be reduced with an 11-week program. The program involved staff education, environmental modification, exercise programs, reviewing drug regimens, providing hip protectors, guiding staff, supplying and repairing aids, and having post-fall problem-solving conferences. There were 82 falls in the intervention group compared with 109 falls in the control group, with 3 and 12 hip fractures, respectively.

Compliance Although hip protectors are effective in reducing fall risk the compliance rate remains low, typically less than 50%. Some determinants of noncompliance include bulkiness, heat, tightness of waistband, as well as complaints regarding the plastic cover, noises made with movement, and difficulty applying and removing the hip protectors.[64] Other subjects objected to the extra effort needed to wear the orthoses and believed they were not at high risk for falls.[65] Patients also needed additional help with dressing and/or toileting.[66] This was especially true of those with urge incontinence, with additional incontinent episodes noted. Some strategies to improve compliance include patient education, including emphasizing the risks of fall, emphasizing freedom, em-phasizing quality of life, as well as providing constant reinforcement and positive feedback.

Cost-Effectiveness Hip protectors have been demonstrated to be cost effective, especially in elderly patients and those who are institutionalized.[67] Although hip protector use has been shown to result in economic savings, they have also been shown to result in gains in quality-adjusted life years.[68] These gains have been demonstrated in women older than 65 years and in men older than 85 years. On the other hand, biomechanical properties of hip protectors may change with time, rendering them less effective. This is particularly true if the hip protectors are washed in commercial laundries. Furthermore, the costs may be prohibitive for some, as a minimum of three pairs of hip protectors, on average, are recommended per patient per year. Limited distribution of hip protectors may limit procurement. Hip fractures may still occur with the use of hip protectors, and their use cannot prevent all hip fractures.[69]

Quality of Life Quality of life may be compromised secondary to fear of falling and hip fractures in elderly women. Hip protectors can help to improve quality of life related to these fears. Salkeld and associates[70] followed 194 elderly women and rated them on an interval scale between 0 (death) and 1 (full health), a "bad" hip fracture, a good hip fracture, and fear of falling. A "bad" hip fracture was defined as resulting in admission to a nursing home, while a "good" hip fracture was defined as maintaining independent living in the community. The authors found that 80% of women stated they would rather be dead than experience the loss of independence and quality of life associated with a bad hip fracture and admission to a nursing home.

Self-Confidence Several studies have shown that wearing hip protectors can increase self-confidence. Cameron and associates[71] followed 131 elderly women and evaluated the effect of hip protectors on fear of falling and falls self-efficacy, defined as one's belief in his/her ability to avoid falling. At 4-month follow-up, hip protector users had less fear of falling (43% versus 57%, respectively, in hip protector wearers versus controls). In addition, hip protector users had greater improvements in falls self-efficacy. McAughey and McAdoo[72] demonstrated similar findings, and found that hip protector wearers were three times more likely to believe they were offered protection from hip fractures, and that two thirds of patients were more confident about leaving the house.

Summary

Hip fractures are a serious cause of morbidity and mortality worldwide. Both medical and nonmedical interventions can reduce the risk of hip fracture. Medical interventions, including the use of the bisphosphonates alendronate and risedronate as well as the administration of calcium and vitamin D, have been shown to increase hip bone mineral density as well as reduce the risk of hip fracture. Fall prevention and the use of hip protectors can also significantly decrease the incidence of hip fractures. However, compliance is important and remains the main obstacle in the successful use of hip protectors. A multidisciplinary approach to fall prevention can result in significant fall protection as a primary measure. Interventions such as tai chi and exercise training programs, environmental modifications, withdrawal of psychotropic medica-

tions, and a multifactoral intervention program are all effective ways to reduce fall risk. Patient education and close follow-up are necessary to ensure maximal compliance with the medical and nonmedical prevention of hip fractures.

References

1. Kanis JA, Oden A, Johnell O, et al: The burden of osteoporotic fractures: A method for setting intervention thresholds. *Osteoporos Int* 2001;12:417-427.

2. Lauritzen JB, McNair PA, Lund B: Risk factors for hip fractures: A review. *Dan Med Bull* 1993;40:479-485.

3. Hauselmann HJ, Rizzoli R: A comprehensive review of treatments for postmenopausal osteoporosis. *Osteoporos Int* 2003;14:2-12.

4. Chapuy MC, Arlot ME, Duboeuf F, et al: Vitamin D3 and calcium to prevent hip fractures in the elderly women. *N Engl J Med* 1992;327:1637-1642.

5. Liberman UA, Weiss SR, Broll J, et al: Effect of oral alendronate on bone mineral density and the incidence of fractures in postmenopausal osteoporosis. The Alendronate Phase III Osteoporosis Treatment Study Group. *N Engl J Med* 1995;333:1437-1443.

6. Black DM, Cummings SR, Karpf DB, et al: Randomised trial of effect of alendronate on risk of fracture in women with existing vertebral fractures: Fracture Intervention Trial Research Group. *Lancet* 1996;348:1535-1541.

7. McClung MR, Geusens P, Miller PD, et al: Effect of risedronate on the risk of hip fracture in elderly women: Hip Intervention Program Study Group. *N Engl J Med* 2001;344:333-340.

8. Harris ST, Watts NB, Genant HK, et al: Effects of risedronate treatment on vertebral and nonvertebral fractures in women with postmenopausal osteoporosis: a randomized controlled trial: Vertebral Efficacy with Risedronate Therapy (VERT) Study Group. *JAMA* 1999;282(14):1344-1352.

9. Reginster J: Minne HW Sorensen et al: Randomized trial of the effects of risedronate on vertebral fractures in women with established postmenopausal osteoporosis: Vertebral Efficacy with Risedronate Therapy (VERT) Study Group. *Osteoporos Int* 2000;11(1):83-91.

10. Guttmann G, Van Linthoudt D: Efficacy of intravenous pamidronate in osteoporosis, mineralometric evaluation. *Schweiz Rundsch Med Prax* 1999;88(50):2057-2060.

11. Reid IR, Brown JP, Burckhardt P, et al: Intravenous zoledronic acid in postmenopausal women with low bone mineral density. *N Engl J Med* 2002;346:653-661.

12. Kiel DP, Felson DT, Anderson JJ, et al: Hip fracture and the use of estrogens in postmenopausal women: The Framingham Study. *N Engl J Med* 1987;317(19):1169-1174.

13. Genant HK, Cann CE, Ettinger B, et al: Quantitative computed tomography of vertebral spongiosa: A sensitive method for detecting early bone loss after oophorectomy. *Ann Intern Med* 1982;87:699-705.

14. Lindsay R, Hart DM, Clark DM: The minimum effective dose of estrogen for prevention of postmenopausal bone loss. *Obstet Gynecol* 1984;63:759-763.

15. Ettinger B, Genant HK, Cann CE: Postmenopausal bone loss is prevented by treatment with low-dosage estrogen with calcium. *Ann Intern Med* 1987;106:40-45.

16. Torgerson DJ, Bell-Syer SEM: Hormone replacement therapy and prevention of nonvertebral fractures. A meta-analysis of randomized trials. *JAMA* 2001;285(22):2891-2897.

17. Felson DT, Zhang Y, Hannan MT, et al: The effect of postmenopausal estrogen therapy on bone density in elderly women. *N Engl J Med* 1993;329(16):1141-1146.

18. Writing Group for the Women's Health Initiative Investigators: Risks and benefits of estrogen plus progestin in healthy postmenopausal women: Principal results from the Women's Health Initiative randomized controlled trial. *JAMA* 2002;288(3):321-333.

19. Ettinger B, Black DM, Mitlak BH, et al: Reduction of vertebral fracture risk in postmenopausal women with osteoporosis treated with raloxifene: Results from a 3-year randomized clinical trial: Multiple Outcomes of Raloxifene Evaluation (MORE) Investigators. *JAMA* 1999;282(7):637-645.

20. Morello KC, Wurz GT, DeGregorio MW: SERMs: current status and future trends. *Crit Rev Oncol Hematol* 2002;43:63-76.

21. Cardona JM, Pastor E: Calcitonin versus etidronate for the treatment of

postmenopausal osteoporosis: A meta-analysis of published clinical trials. *Osteoporos Int* 1997;7(3):165-174.

22. Chesnut CH, Silverman S, Andriano K, et al: A randomized trial of nasal spray salmon calcitonin in postmenopausal women with established osteoporosis: The prevent recurrence of osteoporotic fractures study. PROOF Study Group. *Am J Med* 2000;109:267-276.

23. Neer RM, Arnaud CD, Zanchetta JR, et al: Effect of parathyroid hormone (1-34) on fractures and bone mineral density in postmenopausal women with osteoporosis. *N Engl J Med* 2001;344(19):1434-1441.

24. Grisso JA, Kelsey JL, Strom BL, et al: Risk factors for falls as a cause of hip fracture in women. *N Engl J Med* 1991;324:1326-1331.

25. Hedlund R, Lindgren U: Trauma type, age and gender as determinants of hip fracture. *J Orthop Res* 1987;5:242-246.

26. Lauritzen JB: Hip fractures: incidence, risk factors, energy absorption, and prevention. *Bone* 1996;18(suppl 1): 65S-75S.

27. Tinetti ME, Speechley M, Ginter SF: Risk factors for falls among elderly persons living in the community. *N Engl J Med* 1988;319:1701-1707.

28. Blake AJ, Morgan K, Bendall MJ, et al: Falls by elderly people at home: Prevalence and associated factors. *Age Ageing* 1988;17:365-372.

29. Campbell AJ, Borrie MJ, Spears GF: Risk factors for falls in a community-based prospective study of people 70 years and older. *J Gerontol* 1989;44:M112-M117.

30. Tinetti ME, Williams CS: The effect of falls and fall injuries on functioning in community-dwelling older persons. *J Gerontol* 1998;53(2):112-119.

31. Rizzo JA, Friedkin R, Williams CS, et al: Health care utilization and costs in a Medicare population by fall status. *Med Care* 1998;36:1174-1178.

32. Rubinstein L: Hip protectors: A breakthrough in fracture prevention. *N Engl J Med* 2000;343(21):1562-1563.

33. Lord SR, et al: Postural stability and associated physiological factors in a population of aged persons. *J Gerontol* 1991;46:69-76.

34. Lord SR, et al: Postural stability, falls, and fractures in the elderly: Results from the Dubbo osteoporosis epidemiology study. *Med J Aust* 1994;160:688-691.

35. Tinetti ME: Clinical practice. Preventing falls in elderly persons. *N Engl J Med* 2003;348(1):42-49.

36. Franchignoni F, Tesio L, Martino MT, et al: Reliability of four simple, quantitative tests of balance and mobility in healthy elderly females. *Aging (Milano)* 1998;10(1):26-31.

37. Birmingham TB: Test-retest reliability of lower extremity functional instability measures. *Clin J Sport Med* 2000;10:264-268.

38. Podsiadlo D, Richardson S: The timed "Up & Go": A test of basic functional mobility for frail elderly persons. *J Am Geriatr Soc* 1991;39(2):142-148.

39. Duncan PW, Weiner DK, Chandler J, et al: Functional reach: A new clinical measure of balance. *J Gerontol* 1990;45(6):M192-M197.

40. Weiner DK, Duncan PW, Chandler J, et al: Functional reach: A marker of physical frailty. *J Am Geriatr Soc* 1992;40(3):203-207.

41. Gillespie LD, Gillespie WJ, Robertson MC, et al: Interventions for preventing falls in elderly people (Cochrane Review), In The Cochrane Library, Issue 4, 2002. Oxford: Update Software.

42. Wolf SL, Barnhart HX, Kutner NG, Mc Neely E, Coogler C, Xu T: Reducing frailty and falls in older persons: An investigation of Tai Chi and computerized balance training. Atlanta FICSIT Group. Frailty and Injuries. Cooperative Studies of Intervention Techniques. *J Am Geriatr Soc* 1996;44(5):489-497.

43. Campbell AJ, Robertson MC, Gardner MM, et al: Randomised controlled trial of a general practice programme of home based exercise to prevent falls in elderly women. *BMJ* 1997;315:1065-1069.

44. Robertson MC, Devlin N, Gardner MM, et al: Effectiveness and economic evaluation of a nurse delivered home exercise programme to prevent falls: 1. Randomised controlled trial. *BMJ* 2001;322:697-701.

45. Cumming RG, Thomas M, Szonyi G, et al: Home visits by an occupational therapist for assessment and modification of environmental hazards: Randomized trial of falls prevention. *J Am Geriatr Soc* 1999;47(12):1397-1402.

46. Campbell AJ, Robertson MC, Gardner MM, et al: Psychotropic medication withdrawal and a home-based exercise program to prevent falls: A randomized, controlled trial. *J Am Geriatr Soc* 1999;47(7):850-853.

47. Cumming RG: Intervention strategies and risk-factor modification for falls prevention: A review of recent intervention studies. *Clin Geriatr Med* 2002;18:175-189.

48. Tinetti ME, Baker DI, McAvay G, et al: A multifactorial intervention to reduce the risk of falling among elderly people living in the community. *N Engl J Med* 1994;331(13):821-827.

49. Close J, Ellis M, Hooper R, et al: Prevention of falls in the elderly trial (PROFET): A randomised controlled trial. *Lancet* 1999;353:93-97.

50. Shaw FE, Bond J, Richardson DA, et al: Multifactorial intervention after a fall in older people with cognitive impairment and dementia presenting to the accident and emergency department: Randomised controlled trial. *BMJ* 2003;326:73-76.

51. Kannus P, Parkkari J, Niemi S, et al: Prevention of hip fracture in elderly people with use of a hip protector. *N Engl J Med* 2000;343(21):1506-1513.

52. Parkkari J, Kannus P, Palvanen M, et al: Majority of hip fractures occur as a result of a fall and impact on the greater trochanter of the femur: A prospective controlled hip fracture study with 206 consecutive patients. *Calcif Tissue Int* 1999;65:183-187.

53. Cummings SR, Nevitt MC: A hypothesis: the causes of hip fractures. *J Gerontol* 1989;44:M107-M111.

54. Lauritzen JB, Askegaard V: Protection against hip fractures by energy absorption. *Dan Med Bull* 1992;39(1):91-93.

55. Parkkari J, Kannus P, Heikkila J, et al: Impact experiments of an external hip protector in young volunteers. *Calcif Tissue Int* 1997;60(4):354-357.

56. Lauritzen JB, Petersen MM, Lund B: Effect of external hip protectors on hip fractures. *Lancet* 1993;341:11-13.

57. Ekman A, Mallmin H, Michaelsson K, et al: External hip protectors to prevent osteoporotic hip fractures. *Lancet* 1997;350:563-564.

58. Villar MTA, Hill P, Inskip H, et al: Will elderly rest home residents wear hip protectors? *Age Ageing* 1998;27:195-198.

59. Chan DK, Hillier G, Coore M, et al: Effectiveness and acceptability of a newly designed hip protector: A pilot study. *Arch Gerontol Ger* 2000;30:25-34.

60. Cameron ID, Venman J, Kurrle SE, et al: Hip protectors in aged-care facilities: A randomized trial fo use by individual

higher-risk residents. *Age Ageing* 2001;30:477-481.

61. Harada A, Mizuno M, Takemura M, et al: Hip fracture prevention trail using hip protectors in Japanese nursing homes. *Osteoporos Int* 2001;12:215-221.

62. Meyer G, Warnke A, Bender R, et al: Effect of hip fractures on increased use of hip protectors in nursing homes: cluster randomised controlled trial. *BMJ* 2002;326:76-80.

63. Jensen J, Lundin-Olsson L, Nyberg L, et al: Fall and injury prevention in older people living in residential care facilities: A cluster randomized trial. *Ann Intern Med* 2002;136:733-741.

64. McAughey JM, McAdoo M: Hip protectors: Acceptability of hip protectors was 35% at six months in the community. *BMJ* 2002;324:1454.

65. Cameron ID, Quine S: Likely noncompliance with external hip protectors: Findings from focus groups. *Arch Gerontol Geriatr* 1994;19:273-281.

66. Becker C, Walter-Jung B, Nikolaus T: The other side of hip protectors. *Age Ageing* 2000;29:183-187.

67. Kumar BA, Parker MJ: Are hip protectors cost effective? *Injury* 2000;31:693-695.

68. Segui-Gomez M, Keuffel E, Frick KD: Cost and effectiveness of hip protectors among the elderly. *In J Tech Assess Health Care* 2002;18:55-66.

69. Cameron ID, Kurrle SE, Cumming RG, et al: Proximal femoral fracture while wearing correctly applied hip protectors. *Age Ageing* 2000;1:57-62.

70. Salkeld G, Cameron ID, Cumming RG, et al: Quality of life related to fear of falling and hip fracture in older women: A time trade off study. *BMJ* 2000;320: 341-346.

71. Cameron ID, Stafford B, Cumming RG, et al: Hip protectors improve falls self-efficacy. *Age Ageing* 2000;29:57-62.

72. McAughey JM, McAdoo M: Acceptability of hip protectors was 35% at six months in the community. *BMJ* 2002;324:1454.

Principles of Management of the Severely Traumatized Foot and Ankle

Judith F. Baumhauer, MD
Arthur Manoli II, MD

Introduction

Traumatic injury of the foot and ankle has several injury mechanisms that produce both bone and soft-tissue disruption requiring a vast array of treatment options. Several treatment principles help guide the surgeon toward the eventual goal of a functional, stable, painless plantigrade foot.

Ten percent to 17% of patients with a severely traumatized limb have associated life-threatening injuries;[1,2] therefore, initial resuscitation efforts with standardized trauma protocols are of primary importance.[3] A patient history that records comorbid conditions affecting life or limb viability is essential. A more specific limb-injury history is investigated. This includes the preinjury status of the limb, such as the patient's occupational demands and recreational and functional activity levels, as well as the time and mechanism of injury, initial care, and any delay of treatment.

Preoperative Evaluation

A thorough evaluation of the traumatized limb is not always possible in the emergency department. The lighting often is poor and the pain control inadequate. In addition, the emotional patient and family interaction are distractions that may disrupt the process of making objective management decisions. The emergency department, therefore, is the staging area to triage and resuscitate patients for a more detailed secondary survey in the operating room.

An emergency department examination of the foot and ankle consists of a bilateral determination of foot sensation, particularly the plantar aspect, as well as palpation of the dorsalis pedis and tibialis posterior pulses, noting their presence or absence and amplitude differences between the limbs. If the pulses are not palpable, then assessment of proximal pulses (femoral/popliteal) and Doppler examination are needed.[4,5] The severity of the soft-tissue injury should be noted, documenting the extent of lacerations and soft-tissue damage on a foot-and-ankle figure in the patient's chart. Probing deep wounds is deferred to the operating room. Exposed or disrupted tendons or joint articulations are noted. The degree of contamination is recorded. Often patients are unable to move the ankle or toes because of the severity of pain; therefore, the absence of motion alone does not indicate motor unit injury and may not be helpful in the initial assessment of a severely traumatized foot and ankle.

After a record is made of all lacerations, a sterile dressing is applied to the wounds. Multiple wound exposures outside the operating room increase the risk of hospital-acquired wound infections.[6-8] In the past, recommendations were made to obtain wound cultures at the time of evaluation in the emergency department.[9,10] Lee,[11] however, found little correlation between the initial wound culture results and subsequent infecting organisms. Emergency department wound cultures are therefore of little value.

A portion of this chapter has been adapted with permission from Baumhauer JF: Mutilating injuries, in Myerson MS (ed): Foot and Ankle Disorders. Philadelphia, PA, WB Saunders, 2000, pp 1245-1264.

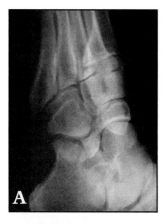
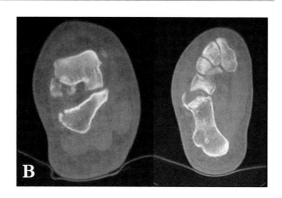
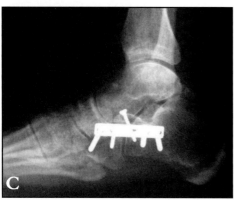
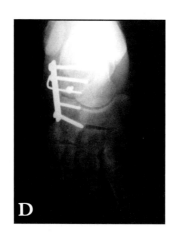

Fig. 1 A, Lateral radiograph of anterior process fracture of calcaneus. **B,** Axial (left) and frontal (right) CT images of the hindfoot demonstrating an impaction of the distal calcaneus and cuboid, with joint incongruity. Postoperative lateral (**C**) and AP (**D**) radiographs of the impaction fracture with an interfragmentary screw and bridge plating across the calcaneocuboid joint. Bone grafting was performed. The bridge plate was removed at 3 months.

Before a plaster splint is placed to immobilize the extremity, radiographic examination of the foot and ankle out of plaster is advisable to evaluate bony injury: 14-cm × 17-cm cassette films of the tibia and fibula in two planes should be obtained to assess the entire tibia and fibula as well as the knee and ankle joints. These views help identify remote fractures caused by rotation, axial load, or a direct blow. In a skeletally immature patient, contralateral foot and ankle radiographs can aid in distinguishing between skeletal injury and physeal injuries. CT is helpful for evaluating the degree of bone injury and displacement in the mid-

foot and hindfoot (Figs. 1 and 2).

The use of antibiotic treatment in open fractures has been clearly demonstrated to decrease infection rates.[6,7,9,10,12-21] In their study of 1,104 open fractures, Patzakis and Wilkins[22] concluded that the rate of infection increased when antibiotics were first administered more than 3 hours after injury. The type of antibiotic chosen should provide broad coverage for gram-positive organisms and gram-negative rods.[1,12,23-25] Typically, a first-generation cephalosporin is used for grade I open fractures, and an aminoglycoside is added for grades II and III.[6,10,13,26] Gross soil contamination necessitates the addition of penicillin

for the coverage of *Clostridium* organisms.[6,9,14,19,27] The recommended duration of antibiotic treatment ranges from 2 to 3 days, with most authors suggesting reinstitution of a 3-day course with each surgical manipulation.[6,7,9,14,15,26,28,29] Routine tetanus prophylaxis also is given.[30]

Limb Salvage Versus Amputation

After the preoperative evaluation, the severity of injury should be discussed with the patient and family. The choice between limb salvage and primary amputation is preferably made at this stage. As multiple authors have commented, protracted limb-salvage attempts may serve only as a demonstration of technical advances in medicine while leaving the patient physically, emotionally, psychologically, and financially in ruin.[2,31-35] Therefore, the surgeon's enthusiasm for limb-salvage procedures must be tempered by the expectations and the functional demands of the injured patient. Amputation should be considered as a positive step toward minimizing overall morbidity in severe injuries and not as a failure of treatment.[35]

Several studies have attempted to identify factors predictive of eventual amputation[2,36-38] (Table 1). A recent study[39] was unable to validate the clinical usefulness of lower extremity injury–severity scoring systems in predicting amputation. Treatment plans based on these grading systems, particularly with respect to amputation, need to be tailored with clinical judgment.

The potential economic impact of limb salvage on the health care system and the patient is significant. Bondurant and associates[31] compared the medical and economic impact of delayed versus primary amputations after severe open fractures of the lower extremity. They reported an

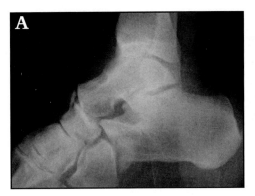

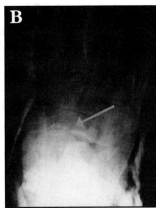

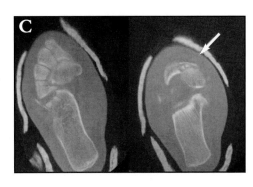

Fig. 2 A, Lateral radiograph demonstrating incongruity of the talonavicular joint and a dorsal bone fragment from the navicular. **B,** AP radiograph depicting a comminuted navicular fracture (arrow) and talonavicular incongruity. **C,** Axial CT images illustrating distal calcaneal impaction fracture at the calcaneocuboid joint (left) and comminuted displaced navicular fracture (right, arrow). AP **(D)** and lateral **(E)** fluoroscopic images of the foot with percutaneous K-wire stabilization of the navicular, bridge plating of the calcaneocuboid joint with bone grafting of the calcaneus and K-wire stabilization, and talonavicular immobilization with K-wire placement to aid in fracture healing. The bridge plate and K-wires were removed at 3 months.

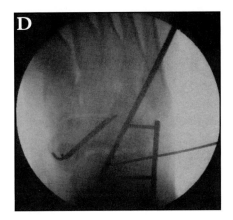

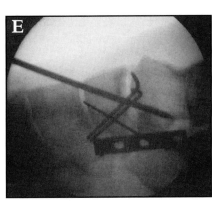

approximately 50% decrease in medical costs with primary amputation compared with delayed amputation. Hansen[33] speculated there may be between 4,000 and 8,000 grade IIIC tibial fractures each year. Extrapolating the $25,000 in hospital costs saved by each primary amputation in this patient population, as much as $100,000,000 to $200,000,000 per year could be saved in hospital costs by performing appropriate primary amputations. Additional factors not considered in this study include the reduction in morbidity and earlier return to gainful employment with primary amputation.

The outcomes of partial foot amputation after trauma have been less commonly studied.[40] Two factors that appear to increase the functional impairment after partial foot amputation are trauma proximal to the ampu-

Table 1
Factors That Influence Outcome and Possible Amputation in Patients With Severe Foot and Ankle Injury
Duration and severity of limb ischemia
Patient age
Presence of shock
Energy of the injury
Degree of contamination (soil)
Nerve disruption
Open or closed injury (Gustilo open-fracture grading system)
Fracture grade, type, level(s)
Delay in fracture fixation
Elevated compartment pressures
Level and type of arterial injury
Delay of revascularization
Injury severity score/associated injuries
Comorbid medical conditions (diabetes mellitus; immunocompromised patients)
Transport time; use of pneumatic antishock garment
Experience of the receiving hospital (trauma center versus community hospital)
Steroid use
Malnutrition
Premature wound closure
Delayed soft-tissue coverage
Operating room time greater than 2 hours
Multiple wound exposures outside the operating room

tation level and a poorly performed amputation with soft-tissue instability, poor durability, and musculotendinous imbalance. Traditional partial foot amputations include digit, ray, transmetatarsal, Lisfranc's (tarsometatarsal), Chopart's (calcaneocuboid-talonavicular), and Syme's (ankle disarticulation) levels. For a successful outcome, extreme attention to detail is needed in performing the amputation, balancing the soft tissues to prevent equinus contractures or equinovarus malalignment, and handling tissue meticulously to avoid delayed wound healing. In traumatic injuries, creative soft-tissue local flap coverage may allow primary closure of wounds while allowing a more distal amputation level. The more distal the amputation level, the less necessary are bracing and shoe modification for ambulation, and the lower the energy needs and oxygen demands.[41]

When primary limb salvage is considered, the goals of surgery need to be carefully identified. The optimal result is a pain-free, functional, plantigrade foot that fits into a conventional shoe or brace. Elements required for the successful outcome of limb salvage include an adequate blood supply to the limb, sufficient bone and joint stability to provide for adequate muscle and tendon function, and a durable soft-tissue envelope to withstand the peak pressures and shear forces of weight bearing.

Initial Trauma Management

All open injuries are treated as surgical emergencies. Surgical intervention should be implemented as soon as possible. A delay in surgical irrigation and débridement of more than 8 hours has been shown to increase the infection rate.[6,7,26,38] Most literature supports the view that the severity of injury parallels the infection rate.[1,6,7,21,22,42-44] This correlation can

be attributed to several factors. The more severe injuries have a greater degree of soft-tissue damage, blood loss, and potential vascular compromise, which increases the amount of necrotic tissue and hypoxic zone of injury. A lower bacterial count is needed to produce an infection in this tissue environment than in a less severe injury.[16,20,22,45]

In a study of more than 1,000 open tibial fractures, Gustilo and Anderson[7] recommended the use of copious amounts of pulsed lavage irrigation, in addition to a thorough débridement of nonviable soft tissue and bone during each surgical event. The wounds should be reevaluated and débrided every 48 to 72 hours until they are devoid of any contaminated or nonviable tissue. The use of antibiotics within the pulsed irrigation has not been proved to be effective in decreasing wound infection rates compared with sterile saline irrigation.[21,46] The use of a tourniquet, electrocautery, and epinephrine are known to increase local soft-tissue ischemia and necrosis; therefore, these are not recommended in open fracture care.[6,10,47]

Fluorescein, a phenolphthalein dye that fluoresces when exposed to ultraviolet light,[48,49] has been used to determine skin viability. The fluorescein is injected systemically and the skin edges are viewed under ultraviolet light. With an intact capillary system, the skin will fluoresce and is considered viable. However, hypersensitivity reactions to the dye have been reported.[48-51] Flourescein use in acute trauma is not recommended.

Stabilization of Fractures and Joints of the Foot and Ankle

After thorough irrigation and débridement, stabilization of the fracture fragments is undertaken. Reduction and stabilization of the fracture fragments

with anatomic restoration of joint surfaces optimize the local conditions for wound healing, leading to decreased infection rates. Realignment and stabilization of the bones and joint surfaces also reduce swelling and eliminate abnormal soft-tissue motion and irritation, thus decreasing trauma to the adjacent neurovascular structures and improving microcirculation within the zone of injury. A less edematous soft-tissue envelope increases the efficacy of cellular and humeral defenses, decreasing infection rates.[44,52] Fracture stabilization allows early patient mobilization, thereby improving pulmonary status and decreasing the incidence of venous congestion and thrombosis while enhancing early rehabilitation.[6,23,26,46,47] Early joint mobility has been shown to improve cartilage nutrition and decrease joint stiffness.[53,54]

With significant soft-tissue trauma, isolated preliminary stabilization through the use of an external fixator to maintain length, stabilize the soft tissues, improve fracture alignment, and maintain joint reduction through ligamentotaxis may be particularly prudent during the acute swelling phase, when additional incisions may compound the zone of injury. The definitive fixation should be done as soon as possible and is dictated by the status of the soft tissues and the need for additional dissection. The principles to follow include careful soft-tissue handling with skin hooks or the retraction of flaps with sutures to avoid additional wound necrosis. The widest possible skin bridges are recommended between incisions, usually 5 cm for the dorsum of the foot and 7 cm at the ankle. Subcutaneous dissection is avoided and full-thickness flaps are raised. Care is taken to avoid denuding the bone fragments of their blood supply by excessive soft-tissue stripping.

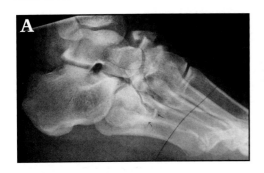

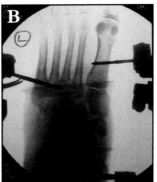

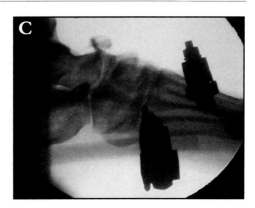

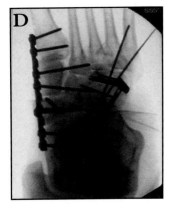

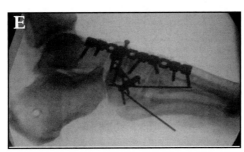

Fig. 3 A, Lateral radiograph of severely comminuted navicular, cuboid, and cuneiform fractures with joint incongruity. AP (**B**) and lateral (**C**) radiographs illustrating the placement of external fixator pins in the first and fifth metatarsals and calcaneus to maintain column length and alignment. AP (**D**) and lateral (**E**) radiographs revealing definitive fixation of complex midfoot fractures, with bridge plating from the first metatarsal to talus to maintain medial column length, and supplemental interfragmentary screw fixation. Miniplate fixation of the cuboid was performed to maintain lateral column length. Bridge plates were removed at 3 months.

The individual hardware recommendations for fracture stabilization depend on the location of the fracture (forefoot, midfoot, or hindfoot), as well as on the degree of comminution. Displaced extra-articular phalangeal fractures, metatarsal fractures, and phalangeal dislocations can be stabilized with Kirschner wires (K-wires) placed either longitudinally or in a crossed configuration.[55,56] Dorsal or plantar displacement of individual metatarsal heads relative to the adjacent metatarsal heads will alter the weight bearing on the plantar foot and create painful callosities.[56,57] These should be reduced. Interarticular phalangeal base fractures or metatarsal head fractures usually are secondary to crush injuries. Provided the toe is well aligned, percutaneous fixation with K-wires or external splint immobilization may be used.[55,56] A crush mechanism creates a severe soft-tissue injury, often leading to significant loss of motion of the small joints in the toes. Additional dissection for anatomic reduction may contribute to more loss of motion as well as the potential for additional wound problems.[58]

If the injury is in the midfoot and hindfoot, the concept of columns of the foot should be considered.[59] The columns of the foot are defined as medial (talonavicular, naviculomedial cuneiform, and first tarsometatarsal joints), middle (second and third tarsometatarsal joints, middle and lateral cuneiform articulations), and lateral (fourth and fifth tarsometatarsal and calcaneocuboid articulations). Maintenance of alignment and length of each of the columns preserves the length:tension ratio for the musculotendinous units and places the appropriate tension on the static soft-tissue structures. In addition, maintaining proper geometric relationships allows the biomechanically complex interrelated articulations of the midfoot, hindfoot, and ankle to function properly.

The fixation of tarsometatarsal fracture-dislocations has been extensively reported.[59-65] For a successful outcome, anatomic restoration of the joint surfaces and articular alignment with screw fixation are recommended. A variety of screw patterns has been suggested. Each emphasizes the need to recognize the fracture pattern, the extent of tarsometatarsal joint injury, and the associated disruption of intercuneiform and cuneiform-navicular relationships. Radiographic guidelines aid in the identification of this injury and are helpful in the intraoperative determination of an adequate reduction.[66-69] In complex injuries to the midfoot, intraoperative clinical assessment of joint stability when the foot is subjected to manual stress may reveal a

Table 2
Compartments of the Foot

Compartment	Muscle/Tendon
Calcaneal compartment	Quadratus plantae
Medial compartment	Abductor hallucis
	Flexor hallucis brevis
Lateral compartment	Abductor digiti minimi pedis
	Flexor digiti minimi brevis pedis
Superficial compartment	Flexor digitorum brevis
	Lumbricales pedis (4)
	Tendons of flexor digitorum longus
Adductor compartment	Adductor hallucis
Interosseous compartment (1)	Interossei
	dorsales pedis
Interosseous compartment (2)	plantares
	dorsales pedis
Interosseous compartment (3)	plantares
	dorsales pedis
Interosseous compartment (4)	plantares
	dorsales pedis
	plantares

more severe injury than is apparent on plain radiographs and also aids in planning screw placement.

The range of motion of the tarsometatarsal joints is small.[70] Hansen[71] suggested that the loss of motion of the flat joints of the midfoot (intertarsal and tarsometatarsal joints) has little effect on overall foot function. Therefore, despite extensive midfoot trauma, even with some bone loss, an external fixator or bridging plates and screws spanning the involved segments that maintain the proper tension and spatial relationship between static and dynamic structures may produce a foot in which late reconstruction can provide a satisfactory long-term outcome.

The hindfoot comprises the talonavicular, calcaneocuboid, and subtalar joints. These articulations join coupled motion segments that play an important role in foot mechanics and determine how the foot meets the floor. When possible, bone and corresponding articulations are anatomically reduced and rigidly fixed. Approaches and fixation for each of these individual hindfoot bones have been described.[55,71] When

extensive comminution precludes anatomic repair, reestablishment of the columns of the foot in both length and hindfoot height is necessary. The use of an external fixator with limited internal fixation, by means of K-wires, screws, or bridging plate fixation, with removal in 3 to 4 months, can aid in achieving these goals (Fig. 3). Circular external fixator frames allow correction of the triplanar alignment of the foot as well as the establishment of height and length. With the exception of displaced fractures that cause excessive pressure and lead to soft-tissue compromise requiring emergency stabilization, delaying the definitive fixation of foot fractures until the acute soft-tissue swelling stage has dissipated has been suggested.

If an external fixator is not used, smooth K-wires can be placed across the affected joints of the hindfoot to maintain joint congruity (Fig. 2). In severe injuries, the soft-tissue structures supporting the joint, including the dorsal and plantar ligaments and capsular structures, are disrupted, leading to joint subluxation or dislocation. The K-wires can

be left outside the skin and pulled in the early postoperative period (4 to 6 weeks).

Primary arthrodesis for severe complex injuries of the foot and ankle is an option when the joint surfaces cannot be reconstructed. Primary arthrodesis of the subtalar joint has been recommended for isolated, severely comminuted calcaneal fractures.[27,72] In severe complex foot and ankle injuries involving not only the hindfoot but also the midfoot, primary arthrodesis is a less attractive option because it will lead to a stiff, nonaccommodative foot at multiple segmental levels. It should be remembered that the goals in treating acute foot trauma are, if possible, to reestablish the intricate articular relationships and the height and length of segments, not to attempt a reconstructive salvage technique in the acute injury setting.

Typical ankle fracture patterns can be stabilized by AO treatment methods,[73,74] that is, by open reduction and internal fixation of the fracture fragments and reestablishment of the ankle mortise. With comminuted distal tibial articular fractures—pilon fractures—the principles of reduction and fixation as reported by Rüedi and Allgöwer[75,76] are appropriate: reestablishment of fibular length and rotation, reduction and fixation of the distal tibial articular surface, bone grafting of metaphyseal defects, and buttress stabilization of the medial aspect of the tibia. Although earlier AO recommendations included anatomic reduction and fixation with plates and screws, currently limited internal fixation of the articular portion of the distal tibia with interfragmentary screws is preferred.[77-80] An external fixator is placed to maintain length, provide ligamentotaxis, and function as the medial buttress to avoid late varus angulation. With a hybrid or ring fixator, the wires can be placed through larger articular fragments for reduction and stabilization, limiting the exposure necessary for interfragmentary lag screws.[81]

Compartment syndrome of the calf is a well-recognized entity, but less attention has been given to the evaluation and treatment of compartment syndrome of the foot. There are nine compartments of the foot[82,83] (Table 2). The current recommendations for evaluation include multistick compartmental pressure measurements. With calcaneal fractures, the calcaneal compartment should be measured.[83] Absolute pressure readings of more than 30 mm Hg are an indication for fascial releases. In a hypotensive patient, 10 to 30 mm Hg less than the diastolic blood pressure may be indicative of a compartment syndrome. Two dorsal incisions and one medial incision will provide exposure of all compartments.[82-84]

After emergent irrigation and débridement, fracture and joint stabilization, and compartment pressure assessment and treatment, the soft-tissue structures of the foot need to be repaired. Failure to repair the long tendons of the foot and ankle may result in biomechanical malalignment and poor foot function because of an unopposed functioning agonist. If possible, primary repair of the tendons crossing the ankle should be done. If tendon substance is lost, then either tenodesis to an adjacent tendon, as is done with the peroneus brevis and longus tendons, or appropriate bracing is done postoperatively. Delayed reconstructive tendon procedures can be done to balance the function of the foot and ankle. Soft-tissue coverage of defects should be done within the first 5 to 10 days after injury.[6,7,9,14,28,48]

Postoperative Care

After significant trauma, the foot and ankle need to be held in the plantigrade position to avoid soft-tissue and joint contractures. This can be accomplished through the use of a plaster cast; however, this makes care of soft-tissue wounds difficult. An external fixator allows the wounds to be examined and the dressings changed as needed. The external fixator can be modified to include pins into the first metatarsal or fifth metatarsal or both to allow the ankle to be brought into dorsiflexion. An alternative option is the use of an outrigger foot plate applied to the external fixator. Care must be taken to examine the plantar skin frequently because these foot plates can apply excessive pressure to the plantar aspect of the foot, causing localized pressure sores and skin necrosis.

References

1. Edwards CC, Simmons SC, Browner BD, Weigel MC: Severe open tibial fractures: Results treating 202 injuries with external fixation. *Clin Orthop* 1988;230:98-115.

2. Lange RH, Bach AW, Hansen ST Jr, Johansen KH: Open tibial fractures with associated vascular injuries: Prognosis for limb salvage. *J Trauma* 1985;25:203-208.

3. Committee on Trauma, American College of Surgeons: *Advanced Trauma Life Support Student Manual*. Chicago, IL, American College of Surgeons, 1989.

4. Keeley SB, Snyder WH III, Weigelt JA: Arterial injuries below the knee: Fifty-one patients with 82 injuries. *J Trauma* 1983; 23:285-292.

5. McCabe CJ, Ferguson CM, Ottinger LW: Improved limb salvage in popliteal artery injuries. *J Trauma* 1983;23:982-985.

6. Gustilo RB, Merkow RL, Templeman D: The management of open fractures. *J Bone Joint Surg Am* 1990;72:299-304.

7. Gustilo RB, Anderson JT: Prevention of infection in the treatment of one thousand and twenty-five open fractures of long bones: Retrospective and prospective analyses. *J Bone Joint Surg Am* 1976;58:453-458.

8. McAndrew MP, Lantz BA: Initial care of massively traumatized lower extremities. *Clin Orthop* 1989;243:20-29.

9. Patzakis MJ: Management of open fracture wounds. *Instr Course Lect* 1987;36:367-369.

10. Patzakis MJ: Management of open fractures. *Instr Course Lect* 1982;31:62-64.

11. Lee J, Goldstein J, Madison M, Chapman MW: The value of pre- and post-debridement cultures in the management of open fractures. *Orthop Trans* 1991;15:776-777.

12. Antrum RM, Solomkin JS: A review of antibiotic prophylaxis for open fractures. *Orthop Rev* 1987;16:246-254.

13. Dellinger EP, Caplan ES, Weaver LD, et al: Duration of preventive antibiotic administration for open extremity fractures. *Arch Surg* 1988;123:333-339.

14. Gustilo RB: Current concepts in the management of open fractures. *Instr Course Lect* 1987;36:359-366.

15. Gustilo RB: Management of infected fractures. *Instr Course Lect* 1982;31:18-29.

16. Merritt K: Factors increasing the risk of infection in patients with open fractures. *J Trauma* 1988;28:823-827.

17. Patzakis MJ, Harvey JP Jr, Ivler D: The role of antibiotics in the management of open fractures. *J Bone Joint Surg Am* 1974;56:532-541.

18. Patzakis MJ: The use of antibiotics in open fractures. *Surg Clin North Am* 1975;55:1439-1444.

19. Tsukayama DT, Gustilo RB: Antibiotic management of open fractures. *Instr Course Lect* 1990;39:487-490.

20. Weigelt JA, Haley RW, Seibert B: Factors which influence the risk of wound infection in trauma patients. *J Trauma* 1987; 27:774-781.

21. Wilkins J, Patzakis M: Choice and duration of antibiotics in open fractures. *Orthop Clin North Am* 1991;22:433-437.

22. Patzakis MJ, Wilkins J: Factors influencing infection rate in open fracture wounds. *Clin Orthop* 1989;243:36-40.

23. Chapman MW: Role of bone stability in open fractures. *Instr Course Lect* 1982; 31:75-87.

24. Dziemian AJ, Herget CM: Physical aspects of primary contamination of bullet wounds. *Mil Surg* 1950;106:294-299.

25. Fischer MD, Gustilo RB, Varecka TF: The timing of flap coverage, bone grafting, and intramedullary nailing in patients who have a fracture of the tibial shaft with extensive soft-tissue injury. *J Bone Joint Surg Am* 1991;73:1316-1322.

26. Gustilo RB: Management of open fractures and complications. *Instr Course Lect* 1982;31:64-75.

27. Sanders R, Fortin P, DiPasquale T, Walling A: Operative treatment in 120 displaced intraarticular calcaneal fractures: Results using a prognostic computed tomography scan classification. *Clin Orthop* 1993;290: 87-95.

28. Gustilo RB, Mendoza RM, Williams DN: Problems in the management of type III (severe) open fractures: A new classification of type III open fractures. *J Trauma* 1984;24:742-746.

29. Sanders R, Swiontkowski M, Nunley J, Spiegel P: The management of fractures with soft-tissue disruptions. *J Bone Joint Surg Am* 1993;75:778-789.

30. Gustilo RB: Management of open fractures, in Gustilo RB, Gruninger RP, Tsukayama DT (eds): *Orthopaedic Infection: Diagnosis and Treatment.* Philadelphia, PA, WB Saunders, 1989, pp 87-117.

31. Bondurant FJ, Cotler HB, Buckle R, Miller-Crotchett P, Browner BD: The medical and economic impact of severely injured lower extremities. *J Trauma* 1988;28:1270-1273.

32. Hansen ST Jr: Overview of the severely traumatized lower limb: Reconstruction versus amputation. *Clin Orthop* 1989; 243:17-19.

33. Hansen ST Jr: Editorial: The type-IIIC tibial fracture: Salvage or amputation. *J Bone Joint Surg Am* 1987;69:799-800.

34. Lange RH: Limb reconstruction versus amputation decision making in massive lower extremity trauma. *Clin Orthop* 1989;243:92-99.

35. Myerson M: Soft-tissue trauma: Acute and chronic management, in Mann RA, Coughlin MJ (eds): *Surgery of the Foot and Ankle,* ed 6. St Louis, MO, Mosby-Year Book, 1993, vol 2, pp 1367-1410.

36. Gregory RT, Gould RJ, Peclet M, et al: The mangled extremity syndrome (M.E.S.): A severity grading system for multisystem injury of the extremity. *J Trauma* 1985;25:1147-1150.

37. Howe HR Jr, Poole GV Jr, Hansen KF, et al: Salvage of lower extremities following combined orthopedic and vascular trauma: A predictive salvage index. *Am Surg* 1987; 53:205-208.

38. Johansen K, Daines M, Howey T, Helfet D, Hansen ST Jr: Objective criteria accurately predicting amputation following lower extremity trauma. *J Trauma* 1990; 30:568-573.

39. Bosse MJ, MacKenzie EJ, Kellam JF, et al: A prospective evaluation of the clinical utility of the lower-extremity injury-severity scores. *J Bone Joint Surg Am* 2001;83: 3-14.

40. Millstein SG, McCowan SA, Hunter GA: Traumatic partial foot amputations in adults: A long-term review. *J Bone Joint Surg Br* 1988;70:251-254.

41. Zachary LS, Heggers JP, Robson MC, Smith DJ Jr, Maniker AA, Sachs RJ: Burns of the feet. *J Burn Care Rehab* 1987;8:192-194.

42. Dellinger EP, Miller SD, Wertz MJ, Grypma M, Droppert B, Anderson PA: Risk of infection after open fracture of the arm or leg. *Arch Surg* 1988;123:1320-1327.

43. Franklin JL, Johnson KD, Hansen ST Jr: Immediate internal fixation of open ankle fractures: Report of thirty-eight cases treated with a standard protocol. *J Bone Joint Surg Am* 1984;66:1349-1356.

44. Rittmann WW, Schibli M, Matter P, Allgower M: Open fractures: Long-term results in 200 consecutive cases. *Clin Orthop* 1979;138:132-140.

45. Swiontkowski MF: Criteria for bone debridement in massive lower limb trauma. *Clin Orthop* 1989;243:41-47.

46. Phillips TF, Contreras DM: Timing of operative treatment of fractures in patients who have multiple injuries. *J Bone Joint Surg Am* 1990;72:784-788.

47. Allgower M, Border JR: Management of open fractures in the multiple trauma patient. *World J Surg* 1983;7:88-95.

48. Papa J, Myerson MS: Soft tissue coverage in the management of foot and ankle trauma: Part 1. *Contemporary Orthopaedics* 1991;22:509-519.

49. Ziv I, Zeligowski A, Mosheiff R, Lowe J, Wexler MR, Segal D: Split-thickness skin excision in severe open fractures. *J Bone Joint Surg Br* 1988;70:23-26.

50. Kalisman M, Wexler MR, Yeschua R, Neuman Z: Treatment of extensive avulsions of skin and subcutaneous tissues. *J Dermatol Surg Oncol* 1978;4:322-327.

51. McCraw JB, Myers B, Shanklin KD: The value of fluorescein in predicting the viability of arterialized flaps. *Plast Reconstr Surg* 1977;60:710-719.

52. Wray JB: Factors in the pathogenesis of non-union. *J Bone Joint Surg Am* 1965; 47:168-173.

53. Mitchell N, Shepard N: Healing of articular cartilage in intra-articular fractures in rabbits. *J Bone Joint Surg Am* 1980;62:628-634.

54. Salter RB, Simmonds DF, Malcolm BW, Rumble EJ, MacMichael D, Clements ND: The biological effect of continuous passive motion on the healing of full-thickness defects in articular cartilage: An experimental investigation in the rabbit. *J Bone Joint Surg Am* 1980;62:1232-1251.

55. DeLee JC: Fractures and dislocations of the foot, in Mann RA, Coughlin MJ (eds): *Surgery of the Foot and Ankle,* ed 6. St Louis MO, Mosby-Year Book, 1993, vol 2, pp 1465-1703.

56. Shields NN, Valdez RR, Brennan MJ, Johnson EE, Gould JS: Metatarsal fractures and dislocations and Lisfranc's fracture-dislocations, in Gould JS (ed): *Operative Foot Surgery.* Philadelphia, PA, WB Saunders, 1994, pp 399-420.

57. Blodgett WH: Injuries of the forefoot and toes, in Jahss MH (ed): *Disorders of the Foot.* Philadelphia, PA, WB Saunders, 1982, vol 2, pp 1449-1462.

58. Johnson VS: Treatment of fractures of the forefoot in industry, in Bateman JE (ed): *Foot Science.* Philadelphia, PA, WB Saunders, 1976, pp 257-265.

59. Myerson MS, Fisher RT, Burgess AR, Kenzora JE: Fracture dislocations of the tarsometatarsal joints: End results correlated with pathology and treatment. *Foot Ankle* 1986;6:225-242.

60. Arntz CT, Veith RG, Hansen ST Jr: Fractures and fracture-dislocations of the tarsometatarsal joint. *J Bone Joint Surg Am* 1988;70:173-181.

61. Goossens M, De Stoop N: Lisfranc's fracture-dislocations: Etiology, radiology, and results of treatment. A review of 20 cases. *Clin Orthop* 1983;176:154-162.

62. Licht NJ, Trevino SG: Lisfranc injuries. *Tech Orthop* 1991;6:77-83.

63. Myerson M: The diagnosis and treatment of injuries to the Lisfranc joint complex. *Orthop Clin North Am* 1989;20:655-664.

64. Resch S, Stenström A: The treatment of tarsometatarsal injuries. *Foot Ankle* 1990;11:117-123.

65. Trevino SG, Baumhauer JF: Lisfranc injuries, in Myerson M (ed): *Current Therapy in Foot and Ankle Surgery.* St Louis, MO, BC Decker, 1993.

66. Foster SC, Foster RR: Lisfranc's tarsometatarsal fracture-dislocation. *Radiology* 1976;120:79-83.

67. Goiney RC, Connell DG, Nichols DM: CT evaluation of tarsometatarsal fracture-dislocation injuries. *AJR Am J Roentgenol* 1985;144:985-990.

68. Norfray JF, Geline RA, Steinberg RI, Galinski AW, Gilula LA: Subtleties of Lisfranc fracture-dislocations. *AJR Am J Roentgenol* 1981;137:1151-1156.

69. Stein RE: Radiological aspects of the tarsometatarsal joints. *Foot Ankle* 1983;3: 286-289.

70. Klaue K, Hansen ST, Masquelet AC: Clinical, quantitative assessment of first tarsometatarsal mobility in the sagittal plane and its relation to hallux valgus deformity. *Foot Ankle Int* 1994;15:9-13.

71. Hansen ST Jr: Foot injuries, in Browner BD, Jupiter JB, Levine AM, Trafton PG (eds): *Skeletal Trauma: Fractures, Dislocations, Ligamentous Injuries.* Philadelphia, PA, WB Saunders, 1992, vol 2, pp 1959-1991.

72. Myerson MS: Primary subtalar arthrodesis for the treatment of comminuted fractures of the calcaneus. *Orthop Clin North Am* 1995;26:215-227.

73. Lauge-Hansen N: Fractures of the ankle: II. Combined experimental-surgical and experimental-roentgenologic investigations. *Arch Surg* 1950;60:957-985.

74. Müller ME, Allgöwer M, Schneider R, Willenegger H (eds): *Manual of Internal Fixation: Techniques Recommended by the AO Group,* ed 2. Berlin, Germany, Springer-Verlag, 1979.

75. Rüedi TP, Allgöwer M: Fractures of the lower end of the tibia into the ankle-joint. *Injury* 1969;1:92-99.

76. Rüedi TP, Allgöwer M: The operative treatment of intra-articular fractures of the lower end of the tibia. *Clin Orthop* 1979;138:105-110.

77. Bonar SK, Marsh JL: Unilateral external fixation for severe pilon fractures. *Foot Ankle* 1993;14:57-64.

78. Bone L, Stegemann P, McNamara K, Seibel R: External fixation of severely comminuted and open tibial pilon fractures. *Clin Orthop* 1993;292:101-107.

79. Saleh M, Shanahan MD, Fern ED: Intra-articular fractures of the distal tibia: Surgical management by limited internal fixation and articulated distraction. *Injury* 1993;24:37-40.

80. Tornetta P III, Weiner L, Bergman M, et al: Pilon fractures: Treatment with combined internal and external fixation. *J Orthop Trauma* 1993;7:489-496.

81. Murphy CP, D'Ambrosia R, Dabezies EJ: The small pin circular fixator for distal tibial pilon fractures with soft tissue compromise. *Orthopedics* 1991;14:283-290.

82. Manoli A II, Weber TG: Fasciotomy of the foot: An anatomical study with special reference to release of the calcaneal compartment. *Foot Ankle* 1990;10:267-275.

83. Myerson M: Diagnosis and treatment of compartment syndrome of the foot. *Orthopedics* 1990;13:711-717.

84. Santi MD, Botte MJ: Volkmann's ischemic contracture of the foot and ankle: Evaluation and treatment of established deformity. *Foot Ankle Int* 1995;16:368-377.

Treatment of Closed Tibial Fractures

Andrew H. Schmidt, MD
Christopher G. Finkemeier, MD, MBA
Paul Tornetta III, MD

Abstract

Closed tibial shaft fractures are common injuries that remain challenging to treat because of the wide spectrum of fracture patterns and soft-tissue injuries. Understanding the indications for surgical and nonsurgical treatment of these fractures is essential for good outcomes. Although cast treatment of stable tibial shaft fractures has traditionally been successful and continues to be widely used, recent clinical studies have shown that intramedullary nails may be more advantageous for fracture healing and function than casting. Surgical treatment (intramedullary nailing, plate fixation, or external fixation) of closed tibial shaft fractures varies depending on multiple factors. Metaphyseal fractures are well suited for plates, although newer intramedullary nail designs provide the option of intramedullary nailing of proximal or distal metaphyseal tibia-fibula fractures. External fixators are well suited for skeletally immature patients with unstable fracture patterns or for patients with unacceptably small intramedullary canals. Interlocking intramedullary nails are the treatment of choice for most unstable tibia-fibula shaft fractures.

Closed tibial shaft fractures are the most common long bone fractures, resulting in approximately 77,000 hospitalizations, 569,000 hospital days (average length of stay, 7.4 days), and 825,000 office visits per year.[1] Closed tibial shaft fractures in young patients are most commonly sport-related injuries, whereas simple falls cause most of the closed tibial shaft fractures in the elderly. The fracture pattern of closed tibial fractures is usually simple, with less severe soft-tissue injury than is seen with open tibial shaft fractures.[2] The more complex fracture configurations are frequently seen in older, less fit patients with osteoporotic bone.[2]

Classification of Tibial Shaft Fractures

There are several ways to classify closed tibial shaft fractures, depending on wheth-er the goal is to communicate the bone injury (fracture pattern) or the soft-tissue injury associated with the fracture. Most surgeons classify tibial shaft fractures with simple descriptive terms such as proximal, middle, or distal in addition to transverse, oblique, spiral, segmental, or comminuted. The benefits of a simple classification such as this are familiarity with the terms and a high degree of understanding of what the terms represent. The disadvantages are ambiguity and subjectivity, which make simple classifications less useful for publication and research purposes.

The two most commonly used classification systems are the AO/OTA classification of bone injury[3] and the Tscherne and Gotzen classification[4] of soft-tissue injury associated with closed tibial shaft fractures. The AO/OTA classification is an alphanumeric system based on the bone involved and the particular region of the bone involved.[3] Generally, the letters A, B, and C are used to designate groups of fractures of increasing severity. These groups are then subdivided, with the numbers 1, 2, and 3 indicating increasing complexity (ie, comminution) within groups.[3] Tscherne and Gotzen described four types of soft-tissue injury (0, 1, 2, and 3) associated with fractures.[4] Type 0 represents minimal soft-tissue damage resulting from an indirect mechanism of injury that has caused a simple bone fracture. A type 1 injury is a superficial abrasion or soft-tissue contusion caused by pressure from the bone injury with a mild to moderately severe fracture pattern. A type 2 injury is typified by a deep contaminated abrasion associated with localized skin and muscle contusion, an impending compartment syndrome, and a high-energy fracture pattern. Finally, a type 3 injury involves extensive skin contusion or crushing, underlying severe muscle damage, a compartment syndrome, and a severe fracture pattern.

Indications for Nonsurgical or Surgical Treatment

To determine the appropriate treatment for these injuries, the surgeon should consider the many factors that lead to disability following a closed tibial shaft fracture, such as delayed union, nonunion, infection, nerve injury, contracture, and angular deformity, and choose the method of treatment that minimizes these problems. Orthopaedic surgeons do not agree on how much deviation from anatomic alignment is acceptable for a good functional outcome.[5] On the basis of a long-term review of the cases of 37 patients with a tibial shaft fracture treated with a cast, Merchant and Dietz[6] concluded that "the clinical and radiographic outcomes were unaffected by the amounts of anterior or posterior and of varus or valgus angulation...." Despite this finding, various standards have been proposed by numerous authors[6-14] as guidelines for "acceptable alignment." Bridgman and Baird[7] found that, depending on the parameters used to define alignment, 4% or 42% of the tibiae in their study would be considered malaligned. Therefore, published alignment parameters are guidelines at best, with no substantiated scientific data to support them. In addition to avoiding factors that lead to disability, surgeons choosing among treatment options must consider other goals, including simple management, early weight bearing, early range of motion of the knee and ankle, early return to work, and cost-effectiveness.

In a survey performed at the OTA meeting in 1997, Khalily and associates[15] asked participants to indicate their preferred method of treatment of a closed, nondisplaced midshaft tibial fracture. Although most respondents favored intramedullary nailing, a large percentage chose cast treatment. Khalily and associates concluded that there was no consensus regarding optimal treatment of closed midshaft tibial fractures, even among trauma experts. Littenberg and associates[16] performed a meta-analysis of the literature on closed tibial shaft fractures in an attempt to determine whether surgical or nonsurgical treatment was more appropriate. Only 19 of 2,372 reports met the authors' strict inclusion criteria, and those studies provided strong comparative data indicating that nonsurgical treatment was more likely to prevent infection and that open reduction and internal fixation was more likely to result in union. There were too few studies available for Littenberg and associates to evaluate intramedullary nailing at the time that they conducted the meta-analysis. Their conclusion was that the data from the published literature were inadequate for decision making with regard to the treatment of closed tibial shaft fractures.

Despite this discouraging lack of guidance from the literature, two classic case series give surgeons some information that can help them to decide between surgical and nonsurgical treatment. In 1995, Sarmiento and associates[12] reported on their extensive experience with functional bracing, which included 1,000 consecutive closed tibial fractures. That experience seemed to indicate that the initial degree of displacement of the fracture is predictive of the degree of final deformity after treatment. On the basis of this premise, patients were selected for functional bracing only if they had a transverse fracture that could be reduced or if they had less than 15 mm of initial shortening. On the average, the duration of treatment with a long leg cast was 3.7 weeks (range, 1.4 to 23 weeks). The fractures healed in a mean of 18.1 weeks (range, 6.7 to 75 weeks). The overall nonunion rate was 1.1%. Although 65% of the tibiae had some shortening, only 10% of them had shortening of more than 1 cm. Nearly half of the tibiae (48%) healed with varus deformity, but only 5% had more than 8° of varus angulation. Nearly one third healed with some degree of either anterior or posterior angulation, but nearly all had less than 10° of sagittal deformity. It was necessary to discontinue brace treatment in 2.4% of the cases because of progressive angulation.

Sarmiento and associates[12] identified several factors that were positively or negatively associated with union. Comminuted and segmental fracture patterns were associated with a longer time to union. Interestingly, the presence of an intact fibula had both positive and nega-tive effects: it was associated with more rapid union, but it was also associated with an increased risk of angulatory deformity. In 1964, Nicoll referred to the concept of the personality of the fracture: "By 'personality' is meant the extent to which each fracture contains in its make up certain factors prejudicial to union— in other words, its inherited criminal tendencies."[17] Four factors that affect the rate of union were identified: (1) displacement: moderate or severe displacement in the absence of other factors increased the rate of delayed union or nonunion from 9% to 27%; (2) comminution: comminution in the absence of other factors increased the rate of delayed union or nonunion from 9% to 15%; (3) associated soft-tissue wounds: in the absence of other factors, associated soft-tissue wounds increased the rate of delayed union and nonunion from 9% to 12%; and (4) infection: this was the most potent, but fortunately the least common, factor; 60% of the infections were associated with delayed union or nonunion.

Nicoll[17] did not find the patient's age or the presence of an intact fibula to be associated with delayed union or nonunion. An interesting finding in his study was the observation that patients with moderate or severe wounds had a prevalence of joint stiffness that was three times higher than that in patients without wounds and that immobilization with a cast for a prolonged period increased joint stiffness only slightly. The worst results occurred when a limb with moderate or severe soft-tissue damage was immobilized for a long period. Taken together, the studies by Nicoll[17] and Sarmiento and associates[12] suggest that fractures, whether open or closed, that are associated with more severe soft-tissue injuries are less likely to do well with cast treatment.

The primary alternative to treatment of closed tibial shaft fractures with a cast or brace is intramedullary nailing. Intramedullary nailing of closed tibial shaft fractures has been reported to be successful in terms of high union and low complication rates.[18] We are aware of two studies comparing the outcome of displaced closed tibial fractures after cast immobilization with that after intramedullary nail fixation. In a 1991 randomized clinical trial, Hooper and associates[19] reported that treatment of displaced tibial fractures with intramedullary nailing resulted in a better outcome, with more rapid union, less malunion, and earlier return to work, than did nonsurgical treatment of such fractures. In a later study, Bone and associates[20] reported the results of a retrospective outcome analysis of 99 patients in whom an isolated displaced fracture of the tibial shaft had been treated with either intramedullary nail fixation or cast immobilization. The two treatment groups were comparable in terms of age, fracture displacement, and tobacco use. The analysis showed that the fractures treated with the intramedullary nailing healed sooner (in 18 weeks compared with 26 weeks) with fewer nonunions (one compared with five) than did the fractures treated with a cast. In a subset of matched pairs of patients who were followed for an average of 4.4 years, those treated with intramedullary nailing were found to have significantly better scores according to the Iowa Knee Score, the Ankle-Evaluation Rating system, and the Short Form-36 ($P < 0.05$). The authors concluded that closed intramedullary nailing might yield better functional results than use of a cast for many patients who have a displaced closed fracture of the tibial shaft. Data on the relative benefits of intramedullary nail fixation and cast immobilization for the treatment of nondisplaced fractures remain controversial, pending the outcome of studies that are currently in progress.

In summary, the advantages of cast immobilization over intramedullary nail fixation include a negligible risk of infection, few problems with knee pain, and no need for hardware removal. However,

the advantages of intramedullary nailing include better control of alignment (including shortening, angulation, and rotation), the ability to institute an early range of motion of the knee and ankle, improved mobility of the patient, the need for less frequent follow-up, and earlier return to work. Currently, the indications for nonsurgical treatment of tibial shaft fractures include low-energy fractures with (1) minimal soft-tissue injury (types 0 and 1 according to the system of Tscherne and Gotzen[4]); (2) a stable fracture pattern, as defined by coronal angulation of less than 5°, sagittal angulation of less than 10°, rotation of less than 5°, and shortening of less than 1 cm; and (3) the ability to bear weight in a cast or functional brace. Conversely, the indications for surgical treatment of tibial shaft fractures include (1) a high-energy fracture; (2) moderate to severe soft-tissue injury; (3) an unstable fracture pattern, as defined by coronal angulation of 5° or more, sagittal angulation of 10° or more, rotation of 5° or more, and shortening of 1 cm or more; (4) an open fracture; (5) compartment syndrome; (6) an ipsilateral femoral fracture; (7) an inability to maintain reduction; and (8) an intact fibula (a relative indication).

Patients must be informed of their choices. The literature suggests that the outcome of intramedullary nailing of displaced tibial fractures may be better than the outcome of nonsurgical treatment of such fractures. If cast treatment is chosen, then the surgeon must be skilled at cast immobilization techniques and the patient must be committed to returning frequently for follow-up and making adjustments during treatment.

Technique of Treatment With a Cast

It has been stated that the technique of applying an immediate weight-bearing cast is as demanding and requires as much motor skill as performing internal fixation.[21] Before choosing closed management, one should be sure that it is indicated for the particular patient and that there is no evidence of a compartment syndrome. If the patient requires manipulative reduction (for example, if he or she has a purely transverse fracture with 100% translation), regional or general anesthesia is helpful to obtain the muscle relaxation necessary for a successful reduction. Intravenous sedation can be used when the fracture does not require manipulative reduction.

The first step in applying a cast for the treatment of a tibial fracture is to wrap a full-contact below-the-knee cast around the leg. A well-padded arm board can be used to dangle the leg over the side of a table (Fig. 1). In this manner, gravity helps to align the fracture and the need

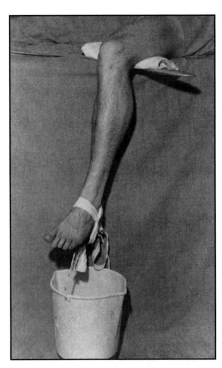

Fig. 1 Position for application of a cast for the treatment of a tibial fracture. An arm-board supports the leg, and traction is obtained by attaching a bucket of water to the ankle with muslin wrapping. (Reproduced with permission from Chapman MW: Fractures of the tibial and fibular shafts, in Evarts CM (ed): *Surgery of the Musculoskeletal System*. New York, NY, Churchill Livingstone, 1983.)

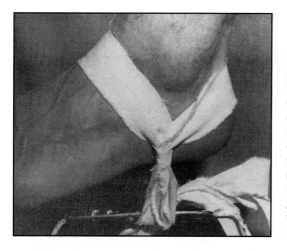

Fig. 2 Example of muslin wrapped around the ankle of a limb with a tibial fracture. A bucket of water can be attached to the muslin around the ankle to provide traction if no assistant is available. (Reproduced with permission from Chapman MW: Fractures of the tibial and fibular shafts, in Evarts CM (ed): *Surgery of the Musculoskeletal System*. New York, NY, Churchill Livingstone, 1983.)

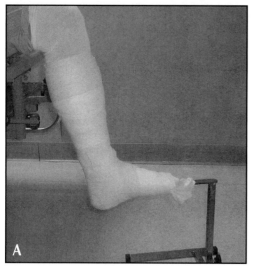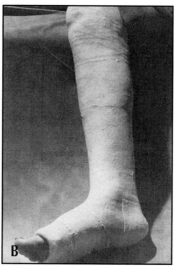

Fig. 3 A, Webril (Kendall Health Care Products, Mansfield, MA) is applied to provide padding with the ankle positioned in neutral. (Reproduced with permission from Chapman MW. Fracture healing and closed treatment, in Chapman MW (ed): *Chapman's Orthopaedic Surgery*, ed 3. Philadelphia, PA, Lippincott-Williams & Wilkins, 2001, p 239.) **B,** Plaster is then wrapped below the knee with the ankle kept in a neutral position. (Reproduced with permission from Chapman MW: Fractures of the tibial and fibular shafts, in Evarts CM (ed): *Surgery of the Musculoskeletal System*. New York, NY, Churchill-Livingstone, 1983.)

for manipulative reduction is minimized. If needed, muslin can be wrapped around the ankle and the ends can be tied to a bucket of water to provide traction and help to hold the leg in the reduced position (Fig. 2). Otherwise an assistant can hold the leg. The cast is applied below the knee, with the ankle positioned in neutral (Fig. 3). When the fracture is stable, the cast is extended to the proximal part of the thigh with the knee slightly flexed so

that weight bearing can be initiated (Fig. 4). Alternatively, when the fracture is less stable, the cast may be applied with the knee flexed 30° to 45° in order to restrict weight bearing. So-called quadrilateral molding must be done in the supracondylar region of the femur to provide a good fit of the cast to the distal part of the thigh (Fig. 4). The cast should then be cut longitudinally in the anterior midline to allow for swelling, and the patient

should be instructed to bear weight as tolerated when the initial pain subsides.

After the initial cast has been applied, radiographs should be made every 1 to 2 weeks for approximately 4 weeks to verify maintenance of the reduction. One should expect (and inform the patient) that any length gained during the reduction will most likely be lost. The fracture will invariably shorten to the position found on the initial radiographs. If coronal or sagittal loss of reduction occurs, a repeat closed reduction with use of cast-wedging techniques will be required.

Once the patient is able to bear weight comfortably and the swelling has decreased, the long leg cast is changed to a patellar tendon-bearing cast or a cast-brace. If the fracture does not meet the criteria for acceptable alignment and more than one or two reductions are required to maintain acceptable alignment, or if the fracture shortens more than a total of 1.5 cm, nonsurgical treatment should be abandoned.

Options for Surgical Treatment of Closed Tibial Shaft Fractures

Many options are available for the surgical management of closed tibial shaft fractures. These include many variations of intramedullary nails, plates, and external fixators, all of which will be discussed in the following sections.

Intramedullary Nails
Indications Many experts consider interlocking intramedullary nails to be the implants of choice for the management of unstable tibial shaft fractures, whether they are open or closed[18,22,23] (Fig. 5). Generally, interlocking nails are preferred because they provide better stability. The issue of reaming has generated much controversy. Although animal models have demonstrated decreased endosteal perfusion after reaming compared with that after no reaming, there is no difference in blood flow within the fracture callus or in the amount of new bone for-

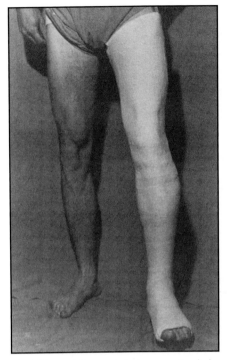

Fig. 4 The padding and plaster are extended above the knee, which is slightly bent (10° to 15°). Careful molding in the supracondylar area of the femur is important to prevent the cast from slipping down. (Reproduced with permission from Chapman MW: Fractures of the tibial and fibular shafts, in Evarts CM (ed): *Surgery of the Musculoskeletal System*. New York, NY, Churchill-Livingstone, 1983.)

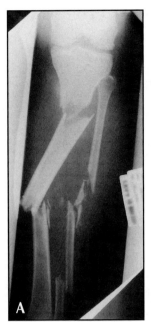
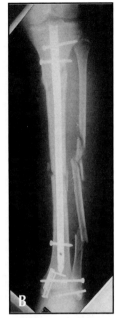

Fig. 5 A, AP radiograph of unstable segmental fractures of the tibial and fibular shafts. A fracture pattern such as this is an excellent indication for interlocking intramedullary nailing. **B,** AP radiograph demonstrating reduction and stabilization of the unstable segmental tibial-fibular fracture with an interlocking intramedullary nail.

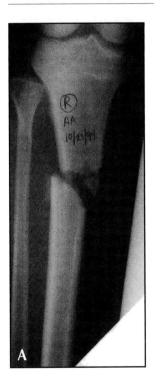
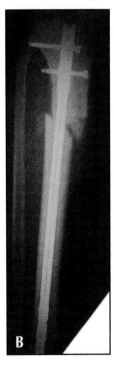

Fig. 6 A, A proximal tibial fracture with valgus angulation. **B,** There was persistent valgus deformity after nailing through a medial approach.

mation.[24,25] Lindström and associates[26] measured leg perfusion before and after nailing in patients randomized to undergo either reamed or unreamed tibial nailing and found no evidence that the type of procedure affected leg perfusion. Clinical studies have confirmed that reamed nailing is safe, even for open tibial fractures, and that it offers the advantage of less hardware breakage and fewer reoperations.[23] When used for the treatment of closed fractures, reamed intramedullary nailing is associated with a lower risk of delayed union and nonunion than is intramedullary nailing without reaming.[23,27] The major problem with small-diameter nails has been the increased prevalence of hardware failure (mostly breakage of interlocking screws).[23,27] This may be less of a problem with newer nail designs; in the personal experience of one of the authors (P.T. III), the rate of failure of these newer nails has been 0.5% over the last 10 years.

Contraindications There are several relative contraindications to reamed intra-medullary nailing. These include the following: (1) An intramedullary canal diameter of less than 6 or 7 mm, which makes excessive reaming necessary. In this situation, plate or external fixation is generally performed. Small tibial medullary canals are not uncommon: up to one third

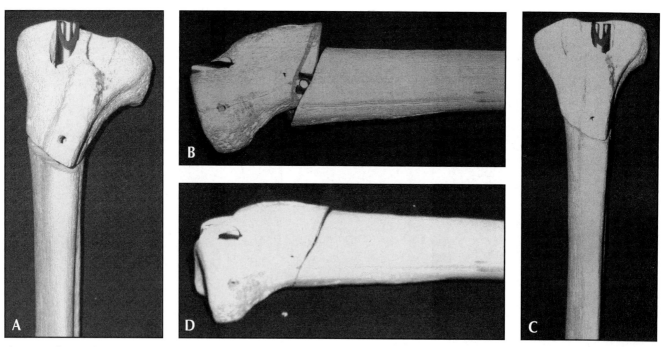

Fig. 7 A and **B,** Sawbones model (Pacific Research Laboratories, Vashon, WA) demonstrating the effect of a medial starting point on the angulation and displacement of a simulated proximal tibial fracture. **C** and **D,** Sawbones model demonstrating that a lateral starting point produces minimal angulation and displacement of a simulated proximal tibial fracture.

of patients have medullary canals of 8 mm or less in diameter.[28] (2) Gross contamination of the canal. (3) Severe soft-tissue injury such that limb salvage is uncertain. (4) Deformity of the canal as a result of a previous injury. (5) Ipsilateral total knee replacement or knee arthrodesis.

Proximal Tibial Fractures The introduction of interlocking tibial nails has extended the indications for nailing to include proximal and distal fractures of the tibia that are well outside the isthmus. However, intramedullary nail fixation of proximal tibial fractures is associated with a much higher rate of complications than intramedullary nail fixation of midshaft fractures.[29] Overall, 12% to 37% of patients have malunion after nailing of a closed tibial fracture,[30,31] and such malunions have been shown to cause substantial disability.[32] Malunion is even more common when the fracture is in the proximal third of the tibia; malunion occurred in 84% of patients who had nailing of such a fracture in the series reported by

Lang and associates.[29] Lang and associates also noted that over one half of the cases had more than 1 cm of displacement at the fracture site and one quarter were complicated by loss of fixation.

Malunion after intramedullary nail fixation of proximal tibial fractures is a consequence of malreduction of these fractures, which results from problems related to the surgical techniques that are commonly used to perform tibial nailing.[29,30] The typical deformities that occur after the nailing of proximal tibial fractures include valgus angulation in the coronal plane, flexion deformity in the sagittal plane, and posterior translation at the fracture site.[29,30,33] The reasons for these deformities are simple to understand and in many cases can be avoided and/or corrected by specific surgical techniques.

Valgus deformity (Fig. 6) results from a mismatch between the axis of the nail insertion in the proximal segment and the anatomic axis of the distal segment that contains the isthmus of the me-

dullary canal.[34] This mismatch is primarily caused by use of a starting point that is located too far medially (Fig. 7, *A* and *B*), but it is also caused to some degree by the shape of the proximal part of the tibia.[34] Typically, when tibial nailing is performed, a medial peripatellar incision is made and the patellar tendon is retracted laterally to expose the entry site. However, when this is done, the entry site remains medial to the axis of the tibial shaft. Furthermore, the anteroposterior width of the tibia is much narrower on the medial side than it is on the lateral side, and the medial cortex of the tibia forces the nail laterally.[35] Finally, the fracture that is most typically seen in the proximal part of the tibia begins in the lateral aspect of the proximal part of the tibia and extends medially and distally. Therefore, often there is no lateral cortex to help guide the nail distally and keep the nail aligned properly. Once the nail engages the distal segment, valgus angulation occurs because of the mismatch

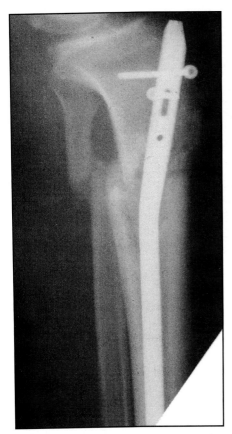

Fig. 8 Flexion of the proximal segment and translation of the fracture.

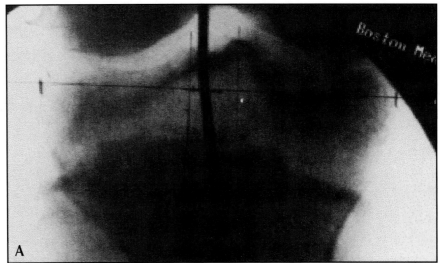

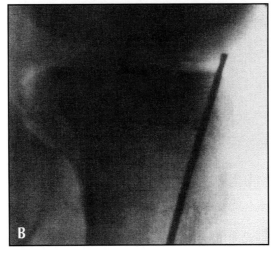

Fig. 9 Assessment of the ideal proximal entry portal on AP (A) and lateral (B) fluoroscopic views. (Reproduced with permission from McConnell T, Tornetta P III, Tilzey J, Casey D: Tibial portal placement: The radiographic correlate of the anatomic safe zone. *J Orthop Trauma* 2001;15:207-209.)

between the so-called nail entrance angle and the tibial canal.[34,36] Additionally, the origin of the musculature of the anterior compartment acts as a tether on the lateral tibial surface proximally, which may contribute to valgus angulation if any gapping of the fracture occurs during the nailing procedure.

Flexion deformity is caused by three factors: the shape of the nail, an eccentric starting point and entrance angle of the nail, and insertion of the nail with the knee flexed. The shape of the nail, specifically the location of the proximal bend, contributes to anterior angulation and posterior translational deformities. When the fracture is proximal to the bend in the nail, it can displace up to 1 cm, with the distal fragment typically translating posteriorly[33] (Fig. 8). In the sagittal plane, the starting point must be placed eccentrically at the edge of the articular surface. This position is anterior to the axis of the medullary canal, so the nail initially must be directed posteriorly to enter the canal. The inability to extend the knee during nail insertion because of the presence of the patella contributes to flexion of the proximal part of the tibia at the fracture site.[37]

There are several potential solutions to the problem of malreduction of proximal tibial fractures during nailing. The most important recommendation is that the entry portal of the nail be made as colinear with the axis of the medullary canal as possible. This is facilitated by use of a lateral portal placed high on the tibia at the edge of the articular surface[35] (Fig. 7, C and D). This places the nail insertion site directly over the medullary canal in the coronal plane and as close as possible to the axis of the canal in the sagittal plane. Furthermore, this entry portal has been shown to reduce the strain within the cortex during nail insertion.[38] The radiographic landmarks that correspond to the ideal insertion point have been recently described[39] (Fig. 9). Several investigators have assessed the relationship of the ideal tibial entry portal to the intra-articular structures of the knee.[40,41] Tornetta and associates[41] reported that the safe zone for nail placement is 9.1 ± 5 mm lateral to the midline of the plateau and 3

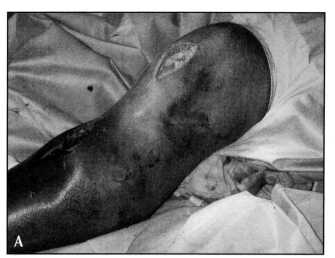 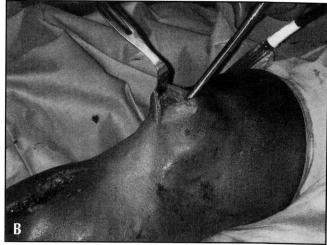

Fig. 10 A and **B,** Clinical photographs showing the semiextended position used for tibial nailing.

mm lateral to the center of the tibial tubercle. The width of the safe zone averaged 22.9 mm and was as narrow as 12.6 mm in their study. In a similar study, Hernigou and Cohen[40] stated that the best position for the insertion of a nail of maximum diameter is 18.7 ± 4.5 mm lateral to the midline or 2.5 ± 1.8 mm lateral to the center of the tibial tubercle. Because of these findings, Hernigou and Cohen advocated a so-called anterior approach to the proximal part of the tibia through the patellar tendon. Tornetta and Collins[37] recommended that a semiextended position with a partial medial knee arthrotomy be used in certain circumstances. This position both neutralizes the deforming force of the quadriceps on the proximal segment and allows the patella to be subluxated laterally, after which the femoral trochlea can be used to guide the nail placement.[37] This approach provides ideal exposure of the ideal entry point without risking knee pain from splitting the patellar tendon (Fig. 10). In order to prevent the proximal tibial fragment from flexing, the nail must be placed as anteriorly in the proximal fragment as possible. The semiextended position allows for easier anterior placement.[36,37]

Another technical contribution to the management of malreduction of tibial fractures is the concept of blocking (Poller) screws as advocated by Krettek and associates[42] and by Cole.[43] This technique, which is simple to perform, involves the placement of bicortical screws into the tibia prior to introduction of the nail. The screws serve to narrow the medullary canal in the tibial metaphysis and have been shown to increase the stability of the bone-nail construct.[44] Because proximal fractures are commonly oriented from distal and anterior to proximal and posterior, nails used in proximal fractures are not forced anteriorly as they are in midshaft fractures. The blocking screw essentially functions as a substitute posterior cortex, keeping the nail close to the anterior cortex as it is maintained in a midshaft fracture. Thus, the blocking screw is placed in the posterior half of the proximal part of the tibia in the sagittal plane, blocking the nail from passing posteriorly and abolishing the flexion and translational forces. Similarly, an anteroposterior screw placed laterally in the metaphyseal region will substitute for the lateral cortex, keep the nail at midline, and prevent valgus deformity. Proximal locking screws from the tibial nail set should be used for the blocking screws, and they may be left in place after the nail is locked. Two proxi-

mal screws that are perpendicular to one another should be used when possible for proximal locking.

Ricci and associates[45] reported the results of the use of blocking screws for 12 consecutive fractures of the proximal third of the tibia. All patients had less than 5° of malalignment, except for one who had a 6° valgus deformity, and a lateral blocking screw had not been used in that patient. Tornetta and associates[46] reported on 73 proximal fractures for which they had used an algorithm to decide if any special techniques were needed to maintain reduction during nailing[46] (Fig. 11). In the operating room, they make a lateral radiograph of the tibia with the knee in flexion. If the fracture goes into anterior angulation, they use a semiextended approach. If posterior translation occurs, a blocking screw is used. If both deformities are present, both techniques are used. Other techniques that have been advocated to prevent malreduction of the proximal part of the tibia include provisional reduction and fixation of the fracture with unicortical plates[47] or a distractor.[35,48,49] The most proximal fractures may need plate fixation.[29] Plate fixation is indicated for the treatment of fractures in the metaphyseal region at or proximal to the tibial tubercle or for fractures with substantial involvement of the articular surface. Intramedullary nailing can be performed when the fracture extends into the diaphysis, but it is difficult and must be accompanied by reduction and separate fixation of the articular fracture (Fig. 12).

Distal Tibial Fractures The management of distal tibial fractures with intramedullary nails has had better clinical success than has nailing of fractures of the proximal fourth of the tibia.[50-54] Mosheiff and associates[52] reported on 52 fractures of the distal tibial metaphysis treated with a small diameter nail without reaming. Twenty of the fractures had intra-articular involvement, 32 had major metaphyseal comminution, and 12 were open. All of the patients underwent nailing with distal interlocking after fixation of the fibula with a plate. Thirteen patients had placement of percutaneous lag screws to repair intra-articular fracture lines before nailing was performed. Fracture union was ultimately achieved in 50 patients (96%) in a mean of 15 weeks, although 22 patients required secondary procedures (dynamization in all 22 and bone grafting in 6). Two nonunions developed in association with a broken nail, and deep infection developed in two patients who had initially had an open fracture. In another series, Dogra and associates[50] reported on 15 fractures (5 of which had intra-articular extension) treated with a larger nail that they shortened by removing the distal centimeter of the nail below the locking screw-holes. These nails were placed after reaming of the tibia and with calcaneal traction. The fibula was not fixed in any of the patients. All of the fractures healed, and all of the patients returned to normal activities.

Malalignment is a concern when distal tibial fractures are treated with intramedullary nailing because of the short distal segment. However, the prevalence of malalignment appears to be low, probably because it is easy to evaluate limb alignment during nail placement. No malu-

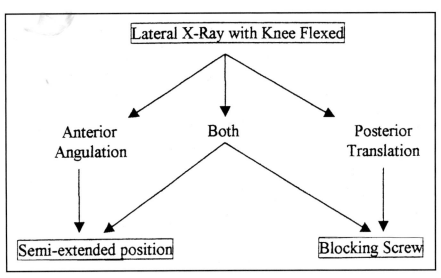

Fig. 11 Algorithm for determining the steps necessary to avoid malalignment during nailing of proximal tibial fractures.[46]

nions were observed in the series reported on by either Mosheiff and associates[52] or Tyllianakis and associates.[54] Interestingly, the surgical protocol used by both of these groups of investigators included routine plate fixation of the fibula. Dogra and associates[50] reported that 3 of the 15 cases in their series had varus or valgus angulation of more than 5°. As noted, those authors did not fix the fibula with a plate. Thus, although fibular fixation seems to have no effect on fracture healing, it may lessen the risk of malunion.

Schmitt and associates[55] described the use of a straight guidewire to help assess the reduction of distal fractures when nailing is performed on a fracture table. If the guidewire is perpendicular to the joint line distally during reaming and nailing, then the fracture will not have a deformity in the coronal plane.[55] Tornetta and associates[46] reported on 81 distal tibial fractures treated with an intramedullary nail. Percutaneous clamps were used in 62 of these cases, and blocking screws were used in 8. A temporary unicortical plate was used for three open fractures. A fracture table was used for the treatment of these fractures. Seven fractures (9%) were nailed with 5° of angu-

lation, and one patient had displacement of an intra-articular fracture. Tornetta and associates[46] warned that, for distal fractures that require secondary procedures, dynamization has a high rate of failure because of shortening, and they recommended exchange interlocking nailing instead.

On the basis of our personal experience and the information available in the literature, we believe that distal tibial fractures with minimal involvement of the ankle can be successfully treated with intramedullary nail fixation. Surgery is performed with the patient supine; a fracture table is not necessary, although the aid of an assistant surgeon or use of a femoral distractor is helpful to maintain reduction during nailing. Fixation of the distal fragment is facilitated by newer nail designs that have three distal interlocking screw-holes and that have holes closer to the end of the nail. It is generally not necessary to shorten the nail, although that remains a simple option if one of the newer nails is not available. Several commercially available nails, with two or three multiplanar holes within 1.5 cm of the end of the nail, are made specifically for distal fractures. **(DVD-52.1)**

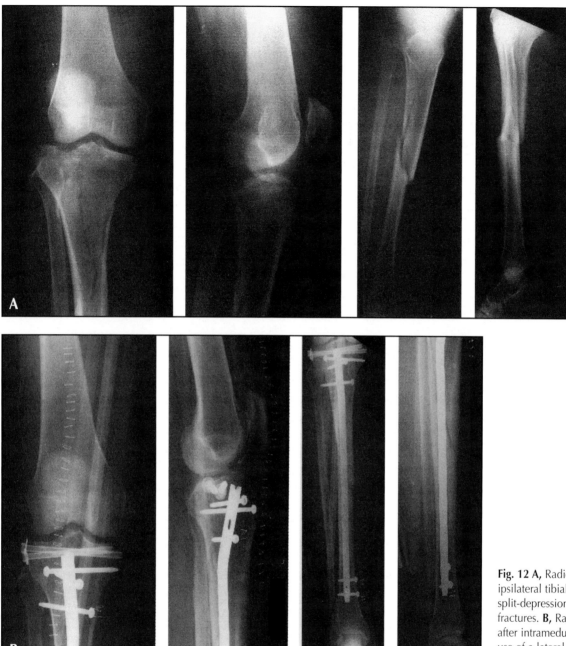

Fig. 12 A, Radiographs showing ipsilateral tibial plateau (lateral split-depression) and tibial shaft fractures. **B,** Radiographs made after intramedullary nailing with use of a lateral arthrotomy and a lateral starting point.

Fibular fixation does not seem to be needed to achieve fracture healing, and fibular fixation may itself contribute to increased morbidity. When the fibular fracture is displaced, fixation of the fibula prior to nailing of the tibia is a useful technique for the restoration of alignment. Fibular fixation is necessary if there is instability of the talus associated with a distal fibular fracture. However, there is not enough information with which to determine the role of fibular fracture fixation.

It is relatively simple to stabilize a fracture that extends to the articular surface. Such fractures are stabilized with percutaneous screws under image intensification. The most important factor in avoiding malreduction of the distal fragment is ensuring that the guidewire is placed in the exact middle of the medullary canal and that it is perpendicular to the ankle plafond. A useful technique for ensuring that the guidewire is properly placed is that described by Schmitt and associates,[55] in which a Kirschner wire is placed into the distal

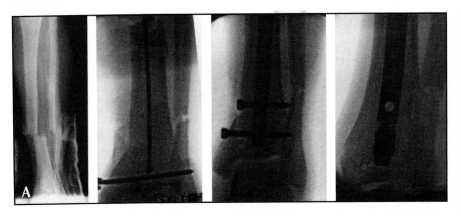

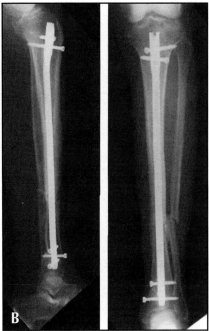

Fig. 13 A, Nailing of a very distal tibial fracture with a Kirschner wire inserted to assist with reduction. **B,** Follow-up radiographs made 3 months postoperatively.

fragment just proximal and parallel to the ankle. With this Kirschner wire as a reference, it is simple to judge the alignment of the guidewire visually as it is advanced to the ankle; the guidewire should appear to meet the Kirschner wire at a right angle. The Kirschner wire can also serve as a tool with which to manipulate the distal fragment (Fig. 13).

Complications There are many potential complications after intramedullary nail fixation; these include anterior knee pain, delayed union or nonunion, malunion, broken hardware (which is related to delayed union), and infection. Complications related to healing are probably the most important problems to consider when comparing different techniques of fracture fixation. Several factors are associated with an increased risk of delayed union or nonunion following intramedullary nail fixation. These factors include placement of a small-diameter nail without reaming, severe soft-tissue injury (either open or closed), bone loss, tobacco use, and infection.

The rationale for the placement of small-diameter nails without reaming

(less vascular insult) may be flawed as it was demonstrated, in a canine model, that tight-fitting nails inserted without reaming cause a loss of endosteal perfusion similar to that seen with reaming.[56] Placement of small diameter nails without reaming has been shown, in several early clinical studies, to be associated with a longer time to weight bearing, return to work, and union.[57,58] This may be due to the fact that small-diameter nails confer less fracture stability than do larger-diameter nails.[59] Furthermore, attempts to insert a nail without reaming may lead to comminution or nail incarceration. More recent clinical studies of unreamed nailing have demonstrated much lower rates of hardware failure and fewer complications related to healing.[60] Recent prospective comparative clinical studies have shown that the results of reamed and unreamed tibial nailing are equivalent.[23]

Several authors have described protocols designed to decrease the prevalence of delayed union after the treatment of a tibial fracture with a small-diameter nail without reaming. Moed and associates[61] used serial ultrasound at 6 and 9 weeks to

determine the presence of callus, and they recommended intervention if evidence of healing was not seen by 9 weeks. Disappearance of the nail signal by 9 weeks after the nailing was predictive of union 97% of the time. Stegemann and associates[62] recommended early bone grafting at 6 weeks, and they reported that this protocol shortened the average time to union from 37 weeks to 24 weeks.[62]

Severe soft-tissue injury and bone loss are factors that the surgeon cannot control, but they have major prognostic importance with regard to fracture healing. These two factors are responsible for the "negative biology" of severe tibial fractures. Successful protocols for the treatment of tibial fractures with soft-tissue injury and/or bone loss all include immediate débridement of soft-tissue and bone and early soft-tissue reconstruction followed by delayed bone grafting.[53] Tobacco use is recognized as another factor that is associated with delayed union of fractures.[63] Patients should be counseled regarding the detrimental effect of tobacco use, and more aggressive

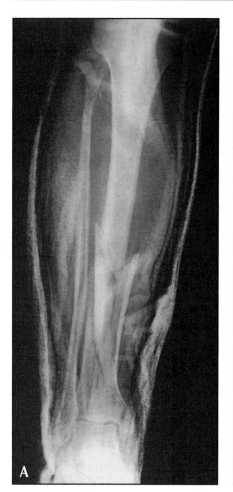
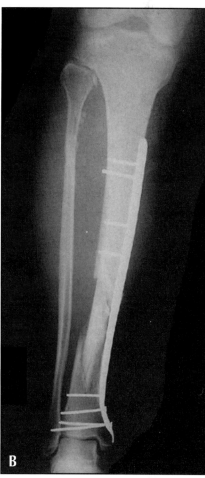

Fig. 14 A, AP radiograph of a comminuted diaphyseal tibial fracture. **B,** Radiograph made after internal fixation with a plate through a percutaneous technique.

Malunion occurs after up to 37% of tibial nailing procedures;[30,31] it can cause substantial disability,[32] and it is particularly common following fractures of the proximal third of the tibia.[29] Angular deformity of midshaft fractures, especially comminuted fractures, can occur if an undersized nail is used. Finally, reduction can be lost following dynamization, especially in fractures of the distal third of the tibia.[66]

Malunion after nailing of tibial shaft fractures can usually be avoided by careful attention to the details of the surgical technique, including careful preoperative planning to determine the correct size (diameter and length) of the nail. One must be aware of magnification errors when using templates.[67] Intraoperative measurements to determine the correct nail length must be made before the nail is implanted. When fractures of the proximal third of the tibia are treated with nailing, more complex techniques such as the use of blocking screws are appropriate.[42]

Anterior knee pain is an often overlooked cause of disability after tibial nailing.[18,68,69] It is thought to be more common when patellar tendon-splitting approaches are used.[69] However, a recent prospective, randomized study demonstrated that knee pain was common regardless of whether a transtendinous or peritendinous procedure had been used.[70] Court-Brown and associates[68] reported knee pain after tibial nailing in 56% of their patients, and Keating and associates[69] noted it in 57% of theirs. Knee pain is more common in younger patients. Although it is typically mild, it can affect function, especially kneeling, squatting, and running, and up to one third of patients may have knee pain at rest.[68] The pain resolves after removal of the nail in one half of patients and decreases in another one fourth.[68] Tibial nailing through a medial peripatellar or a patellar tendon-splitting approach increases patellofemoral contact forces, possibly contributing to chronic patellofemoral

treatment should be considered for patients who smoke.

Infection is also related to problems with healing. Sepsis is usually clinically obvious, but the possibility of a less aggressive infection should always be considered in patients with delayed union or nonunion. C-reactive protein levels and erythrocyte sedimentation rates should be measured, and additional evaluation is warranted if they are elevated. Intraoperative cultures should always be performed when a reoperation is done for the treatment of a healing-related complication. Court-Brown and associates[64] reported that 12 of 13 patients with an infection at the site of a nonunion were treated successfully with reaming of the

tibia and placement of a larger intramedullary nail. The risk of infection associated with titanium nails and solid nails with smooth surfaces may be lower than that associated with hollow nails with rough surfaces or stainless steel nails.

Surgical techniques can reduce the prevalence of healing problems. It is perhaps most important that reamed nailing be used whenever possible because it provides better fracture stability and extraosseous blood flow and it facilitates earlier weight bearing. Reamed nailing may be used safely for both open and closed fractures.[23,65] Patients treated with unreamed nailing should have exchange nailing, bone grafting, or dynamization only if there is evidence of delayed healing.

pain.[71] Tornetta and associates[41] demonstrated the close relationship of the entry portal to the anterior intermeniscal ligament and the menisci. Injury to these structures may contribute to knee pain. As mentioned, Tornetta and associates[41] reported the safe zone for nail placement to be 9.1 ± 5 mm lateral to the midline of the plateau and 3 mm lateral to the center of the tibial tubercle. The width of the safe zone averaged 22.9 mm and was as narrow as 12.6 mm in their study.

Hardware-related problems include breakage of interlocking screws or the nail. Broken hardware, especially screws, is most common when small-diameter nails are used, with a reported prevalence as high as 40%.[72] Small-diameter nails are associated with an increased risk of delayed union and have less mechanical strength, both of which lead to an increased rate of screw failure. To reduce the risk of hardware failure, a large-diameter nail should be used with two distal screws rather than one. Kneifel and associates[73] reported that the rate of screw failure was 59% when a single distal screw had been used compared with 5% when two screws had been used.

Plates

Indications Plates are primarily indicated for metaphyseal injuries. Because of the tenuous soft-tissue coverage of the tibia, plate fixation has typically been associated with an unacceptably high prevalence of wound complications, especially when it has been performed for more severe open fractures.[10,74] Plate fixation of tibial shaft fractures is most successful when the fracture pattern is simple, whereas complications occur in nearly half of patients in whom a comminuted fracture is treated with plate fixation.[10] The recent introduction of percutaneous plate-fixation techniques may lead to a resurgence of plate fixation of long bone fractures. However, the application of plate fixation for the treatment of acute, isolated tibial shaft fractures is limited. Plate fixation is

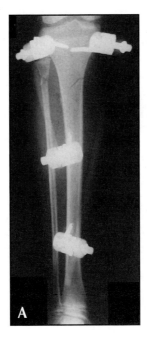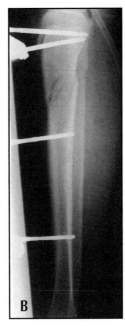

Fig. 15 Anterolateral (**A**) and lateral (**B**) radiographs made after reduction of a proximal metaphyseal fracture in a child with use of an external fixator for immobilization.

a good choice for the management of tibial nonunions.

Contraindications Plate fixation is contraindicated when the soft tissues are compromised, such as in association with an open fracture or a high-energy closed fracture. Extensive comminution of the fracture and a fracture in a patient with osteopenia are relative contraindications to plate fixation.

Technique A plate may be applied to the medial (subcutaneous) or lateral (submuscular) border of the tibia. Lateral application is less likely to result in soft-tissue problems, and it may be better biomechanically because the plate functions as a tension band if the fracture is stable. For percutaneous plate fixation, a prebent plate is applied medially through a small incision. With this technique, a longer plate is used, with screws placed near the fracture and near the ends of the plate (Fig. 14).

Complications Infection and wound-healing complications are the primary problems associated with plate fixation.[58,74] The risk of these adverse events can be lessened when soft-tissue reconstruction is performed at the time of the plate fixation. In general, the risk of

wound problems outweighs the high rate of union and low rate of malunion associated with plate fixation, as other methods (especially reamed nailing) have similarly good results with less risk of wound complications.

External Fixation

Indications External fixation is a versatile technique that can be used for any fracture. Typically, it is chosen for one of two reasons: provisional fixation or definitive fixation. Provisional external fixation is the initial treatment of choice for high-energy closed or open fractures when the viability of the limb is threatened. In these cases, it may be prudent to allow the degree of soft-tissue injury to become apparent before a final decision about limb salvage or fixation is made. Definitive external fixation is usually reserved for patients with unacceptably small medullary canals, children (Fig. 15), or patients with a complex periarticular fracture. In the third case, a ring or hybrid fixator is recommended.

There are no specific contraindications to the use of external fixation for the treatment of closed tibial shaft fractures.

Technique External fixation of tibial shaft fractures is generally accomplished with a unilateral fixator applied to the anteromedial border of the tibia. The pins should be predrilled in order to minimize pin-tract problems. The skin should be released next to each pin to avoid tenting. Four pins are generally sufficient, with two on each side of the fracture. One pin is placed near the fracture (but with avoidance of the fracture hematoma), and the second is placed some distance away. The rigidity of the frame is increased by using two longitudinal bars and placing the bars close to the skin. The system may be progressively dynamized by removing one bar and/or by moving the bars away from the skin. Depending on the configuration of the frame, it may be necessary to reduce the fracture before the fixator is applied.

Complications Pin-loosening and subsequent pin-tract infection are the biggest problems. Pin loosening occurs in nearly every patient. Additionally, if fixation with an intramedullary rod or surface plate is subsequently done, the previous use of an external fixator probably increases the risk of infection. Numerous authors have documented an increased rate of infection when nailing was performed following more than 2 weeks of external fixation.[75] Most authors have recommended that the fixator be removed and all pin sites be allowed to heal before placement of an intramedullary nail.[76] Henry[77] showed that aggressive irrigation and débridement of pin tracks and temporary use of tobramycin-impregnated beads is a successful way to minimize the risk of infection when intramedullary nail fixation is to be done after use of an external fixator.

Summary

Patients with a closed, stable tibial fracture can be treated successfully with a cast. Intramedullary nailing is more convenient, and it may provide superior results, but prospective randomized studies with adequate power need to be done to confirm this. Surgical treatment is recommended for open or closed unstable fractures and for fractures that cannot be held in adequate alignment. Intramedullary nail fixation is the treatment of choice for the majority of tibial fractures that require stabilization.

References

1. Praemer A, Furner S, Rice DP: *Musculoskeletal Conditions in the United States*. Park Ridge, IL, American Academy of Orthopaedic Surgeons, 1992.

2. Court-Brown CM, McBirnie J: The epidemiology of tibial fractures. *J Bone Joint Surg Br* 1995;77:417-421.

3. Fracture and dislocation compendium: Orthopaedic Trauma Association Committee for Coding and Classification. *J Orthop Trauma* 1996;10(suppl 1)1-154.

4. Tscherne H, Gotzen L (eds): *Fractures With Soft Tissue Injuries*. New York, NY, Springer, 1984.

5. Johnson EE: Tibial bracing. *J Orthop Trauma* 2000;14:523-525.

6. Merchant TC, Dietz FR: Long-term follow-up after fractures of the tibial and fibular shafts. *J Bone Joint Surg Am* 1989;71:599-605.

7. Bridgman SA, Baird K: Audit of closed tibial fractures: What is a satisfactory outcome? *Injury* 1993;24:85-89.

8. Haines JF, Williams EA, Hargadon EJ, Davies DR: Is conservative treatment of displaced tibial shaft fractures justified? *J Bone Joint Surg Br* 1984;66:84-88.

9. Harley JM, Campbell MJ, Jackson RK: A comparison of plating and traction in the treatment of tibial shaft fractures. *Injury* 1986;17:91-94.

10. Johner R, Wruhs O: Classification of tibial shaft fractures and correlation with results after rigid internal fixation. *Clin Orthop* 1983;178:7-25.

11. Puno RM, Teynor JT, Nagano J, Gustilo RB: Critical analysis of results of treatment of 201 tibial shaft fractures. *Clin Orthop* 1986;212:113-121.

12. Sarmiento A, Sharpe FE, Ebramzadeh E, Normand P, Shankwiler J: Factors influencing the outcome of closed tibial fractures treated with functional bracing. *Clin Orthop* 1995;315:8-24.

13. Trafton PG: Closed unstable fractures of the tibia. *Clin Orthop* 1988;230:58-67.

14. Weissman SL, Herold HZ, Engelberg M: Fractures of the middle two-thirds of the tibial shaft. *J Bone Joint Surg Am* 1966;48:257-267.

15. Khalily C, Behnke S, Seligson D: Treatment of closed tibia shaft fractures: A survey from the 1997 Orthopaedic Trauma Association and Osteosynthesis International: Gerhard Kuntscher Kreis meeting. *J Orthop Trauma* 2000;14:577-581.

16. Littenberg B, Weinstein LP, McCarren M, et al: Closed fractures of the tibial shaft: A meta-analysis of three methods of treatment. *J Bone Joint Surg Am* 1998;80:174-183.

17. Nicoll EA: Fractures of the tibial shaft: A survey of 705 cases. *J Bone Joint Surg Br* 1964;46:373-387.

18. Court-Brown CM, Christie J, McQueen MM: Closed intramedullary tibial nailing: Its use in closed and type I open fractures. *J Bone Joint Surg Br* 1990;72:605-611.

19. Hooper GJ, Keddell RG, Penny ID: Conservative management or closed nailing for tibial shaft fractures: A randomised prospective trial. *J Bone Joint Surg Br* 1991;73:83-85.

20. Bone LB, Sucato D, Stegemann PM, Rohrbacher BJ: Displaced isolated fractures of the tibial shaft treated with either a cast or intramedullary nailing: An outcome analysis of matched pairs of patients. *J Bone Joint Surg Am* 1997;79:1336-1341.

21. Chapman MW: Fractures of the tibial and fibular shafts, in Chapman MW (ed): *Chapman's Orthopaedic Surgery*, ed 3. Philadelphia, PA, Lippincott-Williams & Wilkins, 2001, pp 755-810.

22. Alho A, Ekeland A, Stromsoe K, Folleras G, Thoresen BO: Locked intramedullary nailing for displaced tibial shaft fractures. *J Bone Joint Surg Br* 1990;72:805-809.

23. Finkemeier CG, Schmidt AH, Kyle RF, Templeman DC, Varecka TF: A prospective, randomized study of intramedullary nails inserted with and without reaming for the treatment of open and closed fractures of the tibial shaft. *J Orthop Trauma* 2000;14:187-193.

24. Schemitsch EH, Kowalski MJ, Swiontkowski MF, Harrington RM: Comparison of the effect of reamed and unreamed locked intramedullary nailing on blood flow in the callus and strength of union following fracture of the sheep tibia. *J Orthop Res* 1995;13:382-389.

25. Schemitsch EH, Turchin DC, Kowalski MJ, Swiontkowski MF: Quantitative assessment of bone injury and repair after reamed and unreamed locked intramedullary nailing. *J Trauma* 1998;45:250-255.

26. Lindström T, Gullichsen E, Lertola K, Niinikoski J: Leg tissue perfusion in simple tibial shaft fractures treated with unreamed and reamed nailing. *J Trauma* 1997;43:636-639.

27. Blachut PA, O'Brien PJ, Meek RN, Broekhuyse HM: Interlocking intramedullary nailing with and without reaming for the treatment of closed fractures of the tibial shaft: A prospective, randomized study. *J Bone Joint Surg Am* 1997;79:640-646.

28. Uhlin B, Hammer R. Attempted unreamed nailing in tibial fractures: A prospective consecutive series of 55 patients. *Acta Orthop Scand* 1998;69:301-305.

29. Lang GJ, Cohen BE, Bosse MJ, Kellam JF: Proximal third tibial shaft fractures: Should they be nailed? *Clin Orthop* 1995;315:64-74.

30. Freedman EL, Johnson EE: Radiographic analysis of tibial fracture malalignment following

intramedullary nailing. *Clin Orthop* 1995;315: 25-33.

31. Williams J, Gibbons M, Trundle H, Murray D, Worlock P: Complications of nailing in closed tibial fractures. *J Orthop Trauma* 1995;9:476-481.

32. Kyro A: Malunion after intramedullary nailing of tibial shaft fractures. *Ann Chir Gynaecol* 1997;86:56-64.

33. Henley MB, Meier M, Tencer AF. Influences of some design parameters on the biomechanics of the unreamed tibial intramedullary nail. *J Orthop Trauma* 1993;7:311-319.

34. Lembcke O, Ruter A, Beck A: The nail-insertion point in unreamed tibial nailing and its influence on the axial malalignment in proximal tibial fractures. *Arch Orthop Trauma Surg* 2001;121:197-200.

35. Buehler KC, Green J, Woll TS, Duwelius PJ: A technique for intramedullary nailing of proximal third tibia fractures. *J Orthop Trauma* 1997;11:218-223.

36. Tornetta P III: Technical considerations in the surgical management of tibial fractures. *Instr Course Lect* 1997;46:271-280.

37. Tornetta P III, Collins E: Semiextended position of intramedullary nailing of the proximal tibia. *Clin Orthop* 1996;328:185-189.

38. Carr JB, Sobba DB, Bear LL: Biomechanics of rigid tibial nail insertion sites. *Am J Orthop* 1996;25:553-556.

39. McConnell T, Tornetta P III, Tilzey J, Casey D: Tibial portal placement: the radiographic correlate of the anatomic safe zone. *J Orthop Trauma* 2001;15:207-209.

40. Hernigou P, Cohen D: Proximal entry for intramedullary nailing of the tibia: The risk of unrecognised articular damage. *J Bone Joint Surg Br* 2000;82:33-41.

41. Tornetta P III, Riina J, Geller J, Purban W: Intraarticular anatomic risks of tibial nailing. *J Orthop Trauma* 1999;13:247-251.

42. Krettek C, Stephan C, Schandelmaier P, Richter M, Pape HC, Miclau T: The use of Poller screws as blocking screws in stabilising tibial fractures treated with small diameter intramedullary nails. *J Bone Joint Surg Br* 1999;81:963-968.

43. Cole JD: Intramedullary nailing of proximal fourth tibia fractures, in the *Final Program of the 1995 Annual Meeting of the Orthopaedic Trauma Association*, 1995, pp 29-30.

44. Krettek C, Miclau T, Schandelmaier P, Stephan C, Mohlmann U, Tscherne H: The mechanical effect of blocking screws ("Poller screws") in stabilizing tibia fractures with short proximal or distal fragments after insertion of smalldiameter intramedullary nails. *J Orthop Trauma* 1999;13:550-553.

45. Ricci WM, O'Boyle M, Borrelli J, Bellabarba C, Sanders R: Fractures of the proximal third of the tibial shaft treated with intramedullary nails and blocking screws. *J Orthop Trauma* 2001;15:264-270.

46. Tornetta P III, Casey D, Creevy WR: Nailing proximal and distal tibia fractures, in the

Orthopaedic Trauma Association 16th Annual Meeting Final Program, 2000, pp 131-132.

47. Matthews DE, McGuire R, Freeland AE: Anterior unicortical buttress plating in conjunction with an unreamed interlocking intramedullary nail for treatment of very proximal tibial diaphyseal fractures. *Orthopedics* 1997;20:647-648.

48. Moed BR, Watson JT: Intramedullary nailing of the tibia without a fracture table: The transfixion pin distractor technique. *J Orthop Trauma* 1994; 8:195-202.

49. Rubinstein RA Jr, Green JM, Duwelius PJ: Intramedullary interlocked tibia nailing: A new technique (preliminary report). *J Orthop Trauma* 1992;6:90-95.

50. Dogra AS, Ruiz AL, Thompson NS, Nolan PC: Dia-metaphyseal distal tibial fractures: Treatment with a shortened intramedullary nail: A review of 15 cases. *Injury* 2000;31:799-804.

51. Konrath G, Moed BR, Watson JT, Kaneshiro S, Karges DE, Cramer KE: Intramedullary nailing of unstable diaphyseal fractures of the tibia with distal intraarticular involvement. *J Orthop Trauma* 1997;11:200-205.

52. Mosheiff R, Safran O, Segal D, Liebergall M: The unreamed tibial nail in the treatment of distal metaphyseal fractures. *Injury* 1999;30:83-90.

53. Robinson CM, McLauchlan GJ, McLean IP, Court-Brown CM: Distal metaphyseal fractures of the tibia with minimal involvement of the ankle: Classification and treatment by locked intramedullary nailing. *J Bone Joint Surg Br* 1995;77:781-787.

54. Tyllianakis M, Megas P, Giannikas D, Lambiris E: Interlocking intramedullary nailing in distal tibial fractures. *Orthopedics* 2000;23:805-808.

55. Schmitt AK, Nork SE, Winquist RA: Intramedullary nailing of distal metaphyseal tibial fractures, in the *Orthopaedic Trauma Association 16th Annual Meeting Final Program*, 2000, pp 133-134.

56. Hupel TM, Aksenov SA, Schemitsch EH: Cortical bone blood flow in loose and tight fitting locked unreamed intramedullary nailing: a canine segmental tibia fracture model. *J Orthop Trauma* 1998;12:127-135.

57. Anglen JO, Blue JM: A comparison of reamed and unreamed nailing of the tibia. *J Trauma* 1995;39:351-355.

58. Coles CP, Gross M: Closed tibial shaft fractures: management and treatment complications: A review of the prospective literature. *Can J Surg* 2000;43:256-262.

59. Fairbank AC, Thomas D, Cunningham B, Curtis M, Jinnah RH: Stability of reamed and unreamed IM tibial nails: a biomechanical study. *Injury* 1995;26:483-485.

60. Lin J, Hou SM: Unreamed locked tight-fitting nailing for acute tibial fractures. *J Orthop Trauma* 2001;15:40-46.

61. Moed BR, Subramanian S, van Holsbeeck M, et al: Ultrasound for the early diagnosis of tibial fracture healing after static interlocked nailing without reaming: Clinical results. *J Orthop Trauma* 1998;12:206-213.

62. Stegemann P, Lorio M, Soriano R, Bone L: Management protocol for unreamed interlocking tibial nails for open tibial fractures. *J Orthop Trauma* 1995;9:117-120.

63. Adams CI, Keating JF, Court-Brown CM: Cigarette smoking and open tibial fractures. *Injury* 2001;32:61-65.

64. Court-Brown CM, Keating JF, McQueen MM: Infection after intramedullary nailing of the tibia: Incidence and protocol for management. *J Bone Joint Surg Br* 1992;74:770-774.

65. Keating JF, O'Brien PI, Blachut PA, Meek RN, Broekhuyse HM: Reamed interlocking intramedullary nailing of open fractures of the tibia. *Clin Orthop* 1997;338:182-191.

66. Templeman D, Larson C, Varecka T, Kyle RF: Decision making errors in the use of interlocking tibial nails. *Clin Orthop* 1997;339:65-70.

67. Krettek C, Blauth M, Miclau T, Rudolf J, Konemann B, Schandelmaier P: Accuracy of intramedullary templates in femoral and tibial radiographs. *J Bone Joint Surg Br* 1996;78: 963-964.

68. Court-Brown CM, Gustilo T, Shaw AD: Knee pain after intramedullary tibial nailing: Its incidence, etiology, and outcome. *J Orthop Trauma* 1997;11:103-105.

69. Keating JF, Orfaly R, O'Brien PJ: Knee pain after tibial nailing. *J Orthop Trauma* 1997;11: 10-13.

70. Toivanen JA, Vaisto O, Kannus P, Latvala K, Honkonen SE, Jarvinen MJ: Anterior knee pain after intramedullary nailing of fractures of the tibial shaft: A prospective, randomized study comparing two different nail-insertion techniques. *J Bone Joint Surg Am* 2002;84:580-585.

71. Devitt AT, Coughlan KA, Ward T, et al: Patellofemoral contact forces and pressures during intramedullary tibial nailing. *Int Orthop* 1998;22:92-96.

72. Cole JD, Latta L: Fatigue failure of interlocking tibial nail implants. *J Orthop Trauma* 1992;6: 507-508.

73. Kneifel T, Buckley RT: A comparison of one versus two distal locking screws in tibial fractures treated with unreamed tibial nails: A prospective randomized clinical trial. *Injury* 1996;27:271-273.

74. Bilat C, Leutenegger A, Ruedi T. Osteosynthesis of 245 tibial shaft fractures: Early and late complications. *Injury* 1994;25:349-358.

75. McGraw JM, Lim EV: Treatment of open tibial-shaft fractures: External fixation and secondary intramedullary nailing. *J Bone Joint Surg Am* 1988;70:900-911.

76. Wheelwright EF, Court-Brown CM: Primary external fixation and secondary intramedullary nailing in the treatment of tibial fractures. *Injury* 1992;70:373-376.

77. Henry SL: Secondary intramedullary nailing of complex open tibia fractures after external fixation: a new protocol. *Am J Orthop* 1999;(suppl): 17-22.

16

Open Fractures of the Tibial Shaft: An Update

Steven A. Olson, MD

Emil H. Schemitsch, MD, FRCSC

Abstract

The treatment of open fractures of the tibial shaft continues to be a challenging problem for the orthopaedic surgeon. The basic principles of treatment for open fractures have changed little over the past decade; urgent wound débridement, early use of antibiotic therapy, skeletal stabilization, and early wound coverage remain the primary goals of treatment. However, the methods used to achieve these goals of treatment have evolved. Recent advances in the treatment of open fractures focus on the treatment of open fractures of the tibial shaft.

The treatment of open fractures present a challenge for the orthopaedic surgeon. Complex injuries, such as open tibial shaft fractures, remain among the most problematic injuries to treat. The medial subcutaneous border, with its minimal soft-tissue coverage, and the frequency of injuries to the tibia caused by motor vehicle crashes make the tibial shaft a common site for high-energy open fractures.[1] The basic tenets of treatment of these open injuries have remained constant and include early and aggressive soft-tissue

One or more of the authors or the departments with which they are affiliated have received something of value from a commercial or other party related directly or indirectly to the subject of this chapter.

débridement, early antibiotic therapy as appropriate, stabilization of the skeletal injury when necessary to facilitate treatment, and timely closure of the soft-tissue envelope.[1,2] However, treatment methods have evolved. Pertinent information and newer emerging techniques for the treatment of these complex injuries will be discussed.

Initial Assessment

The initial treatment of a patient with an open tibial fracture begins with a primary patient survey in the emergency department where an evaluation of airway, breathing, circulation, and the assessment of other potential life-threatening injuries, as outlined by the Advanced Trauma Life Support protocol, are done.[3] Associated musculoskeletal injury also

should be assessed. After the initial assessment and resuscitation of the patient, realignment of the injured limb and the assessment of the adequacy of perfusion and neurologic function in the injured extremity are done.[1,3] Antibiotic therapy should commence at this time.[4-6] The open wound should be inspected and irrigated with a liter of normal saline solution if excessive gross contamination is present or if a delay in surgical débridement of the wound is anticipated. The wound is then covered with a sterile dressing and the extremity is placed in a splint. The dressing should not be removed until the patient is in the operating room for initial débridement. Tscherne[2] reported a substantial increase in infection rate with multiple inspections of the traumatic wound prior to surgical débridement. When many individuals are involved in the treatment of these patients, such as in an academic teaching center, it can be helpful to photograph the traumatic wound for documentation for other team members. Finally, radiographs of the injured extremity should be taken to determine the nature and extent of the skeletal injury prior to surgery.

Wound Contamination

Open fractures expose the deep soft-tissue envelope to contamination, resulting in initial bacterial colonization of the traumatic wound that increases in magnitude with time.[7,8] Traumatic wounds may contain injured or necrotic muscle, a dead space with hematoma, and other poorly vascularized tissue that may predispose the injured area to bacterial growth. Robson and associates[7] showed in an animal model that a traumatic wound would develop a bacterial colony count greater than 10^5 colony-forming units within 5 hours of injury. The implications of these findings are twofold: (1) early wound débridement with removal of necrotic tissue hematoma and dead space management are critical to preventing infection, and (2) the early administration of antibiotic therapy is an important factor in the treatment of open fractures.

Antibiotic Therapy

In 1974, Patzakis and associates[6] reported in a prospective randomized study that the administration of a first-generation cephalosporin antibiotic resulted in lower infection rates (2%) than those found with the use of either the combination of penicillin and streptomycin (10%) or the use of no antibiotics (14%). Braun and associates[4] reported similar results in a prospective randomized study that showed administration of antibiotics to patients with open fractures decreased the infection rate (4.8%) when compared with a placebo (28%). These studies show that early administration of antibiotic therapy is therapeutic even though antibiotic use often is considered prophylactic. As a result of these initial studies, recommendations have been made specifying multidrug therapy as a treatment for patients with severely contaminated wounds. The use of a broad-spectrum cephalosporin such as cefazolin and an aminoglycoside such as gentamicin to provide adequate coverage for a type III open fracture is usually recommended.[1] The addition of anaerobic antibiotic coverage such as penicillin or metronidazole is indicated for wounds with soil contamination to prevent clostridial infections.[8] Patzakis and associates[9] have shown double drug therapy with cefamandole and gentamicin to be superior to single drug therapy with ciprofloxacin in decreasing infection rates in type III open fractures. Studies suggest that a single daily dose of gentamicin (6 mg/kg daily) is equally effective as divided doses of gentamicin without an increase in side effects.[10]

Topical antibiotics recently have been reintroduced for the care of orthopaedic wounds. These antibiotics usually are used after débridement in conjunction with systemic antibiotic therapy. Early studies suggest that adding a powdered form of the antibiotic to powdered polymethylmethacrylate (PMMA) prior to mixing results in elution of antibiotics into the local serum.[11] This cement is usually formed into beads that are either handmade or molded along a suture or wire. The antibiotic bead pouch is discussed in greater detail in chapter 65. Because PMMA beads elute the antibiotic based on the surface area exposed, the smaller and more uniform that the beads are, the more desirable they are for use.[11] Antibiotics used in this process need to be heat stable to avoid desaturation during the curing stage of the PMMA. Tobramycin is often used as an antibiotic with PMMA with a typical dosage of 1.2 g (one vial of tobramycin) per batch of cement.

Antibiotic beads are usually placed in the wound bed after débridement and the wound is then sealed with a transparent film dressing that allows local serum to accumulate in the wound, where elution of the antibiotic from the beads will occur. Eckman and associates[11] reported that this technique resulted in tobramycin levels of up to 80 μg/mL in wound serum, with negligible serum levels. Significant decreases in infection rates in open fractures have been reported with the use of this technique.[12,13] More recently, Miclau and associates[14] evaluated the effect of high levels of aminoglycoside antibiotic on cell function of osteoblasts in tissue culture. Results showed that serum levels of tobramycin of less than 200 micrograms/mL had little or no effect on osteoblast replication, whereas concentrations of 400 micrograms/mL or more caused significant abnormalities in cell replication. Recently, materials other than PMMA have been introduced as carriers for topical antibiotics. Materials such as calcium sulfate and polylactic acid have been used as bioabsorbable carrier vehicles; both have excellent clinical potential although little clinical data are currently available on their use. These bioabsorbable materials allow the incorporation of other antibiotics for local use.[15] Other studies suggest that local levels of vancomycin, up to 1000 μg/mL, and levels of cefazolin, up to 100 μg/mL, have little effect on osteoblast replication.[16]

The addition of antibiotic powder to autogenous bone graft has been shown to be an effective method of delivering antibiotic without compromising the efficacy of the bone graft in animal models.[17] Intramedullary nails coated with an antiseptic combination of chlorhexidine and chloroxylenol recently have been shown to decrease infection rates in animal models.[18]

The duration of antibiotic therapy in the typical open fracture remains controversial. Both Robinson and associates[8] and Patzakis and associates[9] have reported the results of studies that show initial wound cultures, taken in the emergency department or at the time of initial débridement, were not predictive of late infections.[8,19] Therefore, the choice of antibiotic therapy or its duration cannot be based on findings from these initial cultures. Dellinger and associates[5] reported on a prospective study in which a single day (24 hours) of antibiotic therapy produced results equivalent to 5 days of antibiotic therapy. However, most authors continue to recommend a minimum of 3 days of therapy for type I and II fracture wounds with the possibility of up to 5 days of therapy for more highly contaminated type III fracture wounds.[1,20]

Surgical Treatment: The Use of Débridement and Irrigation

The open fracture traumatic wound should be explored in the operating room using débridement and irrigation.[1,21] Meticulous débridement of contaminated soft tissues must be regarded as the most important initial step in the treatment of open tibial fractures. Exploration should be done in a thorough but judicious manner to evaluate the condition of the underlying soft tissues. The wound should be extended so that the full extent of the soft-tissue damage or zone of injury is seen. A limited fasciotomy in the muscular compartment(s) involved in the traumatic injury is often required to view the muscle tissue and fully assess the damage.[1] Retained necrotic muscle is known to have potentially serious systemic side effects, including myoglobinuria and renal failure in addition to increasing the risk for infection.[1]

Débridement should be done in a systematic manner that usually involves inspection of the periphery of the wound and the skin edges around the wound, followed by a similar inspection of the subcutaneous and fatty layers, an additional inspection of the underlying muscular tissue, and finally, an inspection and débridement of the underlying bony tissue. In less severe open injuries, with small wounds, this systematic approach to débridement may seem overly cautious. However, in more complex wounds with extensive lacerations and soft-tissue damage, a systematic method to evaluate the wound is critical in order to assess soft-tissue damage and to ensure that no area remains uninspected during débridement. Tourniquets should be used infrequently.

It is occasionally questioned whether the open fracture with a "pinhole" open wound always requires surgical débridement. It is important to remember that débridement is done to assess the underlying soft-tissue injury. In some cases, it may be possible to adequately anesthetize and surgically prepare the patient's wound outside of the operating room, but it is our opinion that the patient will benefit from a formal débridement in the operating room.

At the time of débridement, the surgeon can be conservative with excision of skin, as potentially viable skin flaps will not compromise the patient's outcome.[1] The surgeon should be more liberal with the débridement of underlying subcutaneous fat and fascia. The classic four Cs of color, consistency, contractility, and capillary bleeding should all be checked and noted for assessment of muscle injury.[1] Although it is clear that débridement of necrotic muscle tissue is beneficial, it is equally clear that it is also beneficial to preserve the integrity of the musculotendinous units so that long-term function for the patient is maintained. Paradoxically, the more extensive the soft-tissue injury, the more conservative the surgeon will want to be in the débridement of the muscular injury. In low-grade open fractures, a relatively radical débridement of a muscle tissue is easily done without significant damage to musculotendinous units. In high-grade open tibial fractures, a radical approach to débridement of injured muscle could result in the eradication of many, if not all, of the musculotendinous units in a given anatomic compartment.[1]

Débridement of bone is equally important. Edwards and associates[22] found that retention of large segments of necrotic cortical bone resulted in a 50% increase in the infection rate in a study of high-grade open tibial fractures treated with external fixation. Segments of cortical bone have no soft-tissue attachment and should be débrided at the time of the initial débridement. Exceptions may be made for segments of the articular surface or important periarticular fracture segments that are important in the salvage of the associated joint injury.[1]

Mechanical débridement of contaminated soft tissues can be done using irrigation in the treatment of open tibial fractures.[1,23-26] The efficacy of high-pressure irrigation in decreasing the bacterial load in soft tissues has been well established in the literature.[27-33] The advent of pulsatile irrigation has further improved bacterial removal from soft tissues.[29,30,33] High-pressure pulsatile irrigation provides a pulse compression phase and an interpulse decompression phase during which soft-tissue recoil occurs, dislodging particulate matter and bacteria. The popularity and effectiveness of high-pressure pulsatile lavage in soft-tissue débridement has been extrapolated to a perceived efficacy in the débridement of bone.

High-pressure pulsatile irrigation for fracture débridement has potential complications.[28,34-37] Dirschl and associates[28] found that high-pressure pulsatile lavage resulted in visible damage at the fracture site and delayed healing in an in vivo study.[28] Bhandari and associates[34] examined the effects of high-pressure pulsatile irrigation on contaminated human tibiae in an in vitro model. They reported that high-pressure irrigation of tibiae resulted in significant macroscopic bony damage and carried surface bacteria into the intramedullary canal. West and associates[36] supported these findings with electron microscopy and showed that high-pressure lavage left vacant interstices of bone devoid of cells.

The optimal technique for bone débridement should achieve maximal effectiveness in the removal of adherent bacteria while preserving bone structure and function. Low-pressure pulsatile irrigation has obvious potential advantages in decreasing the degree of bone damage but its ability to remove adherent bacteria may

Table 1
Classification of Open Fractures

Type	Characteristics
I	Minimal soft-tissue wound (< 1 cm) No comminution Minimal contusion
II	1- to 10-cm wound Minimal comminution Moderate muscle contusion
IIIA	Includes severe open tibial fractures that do not require flap coverage over bone Skin graft is occasionally required
IIIB	Require either local or distant free tissue transfer to cover exposed bone Usually associated with extensive bone devitalization
IIIC	Associated with a vascular injury that requires vascular repair for limb survival Presentation varies from open amputation to tibial fracture and knee dislocation to popliteal artery disruption

be less than optimal. Bhandari and associates[35] have shown that low-pressure irrigation results in significantly less macroscopic and microscopic bone damage and is as effective as high-pressure lavage in removing bacteria within 3 hours of contamination. However, after a 3-hour delay in irrigation, low-pressure lavage is less effective in removing bacteria.

The ability of various solutions to remove adherent bacteria from hard surfaces has been reported in the literature.[38-42] Kaysinger and associates,[43] in a study of the effect of betadine and bacitracin solutions on cultured chick osteoblasts, found that a 2-min exposure to 5% betadine solution resulted in a 30% inhibition of lactate production (a marker of glycolytic energy metabolism) and a 90% inhibition of DNA synthesis (a marker of cell number).

Anglen and associates[39] studied the effect of soap, antibiotic (bacitracin), and normal saline solutions in removing *Staphylococcus aureus* from cortical bone fragments using pressure irrigation. They found that soap solutions, delivered under pressure irrigation, were the most effective method of reducing residual colony counts of bacteria. In a comparison of the effects of various irrigating solutions on osteoblast and osteoclast number and function, and an examina-

tion of their additional efficacy in the removal of adherent bacteria from contaminated bone, Bhandari and associates[44] found that soap solution was the most effective irrigating solution for the preservation of osteoblast number and activity. The addition of soap irrigation with low-pressure lavage resulted in the most efficacious removal of bacteria adherent to bone. Despite these experimental findings, it remains unproven whether the substantially improved efficacy of bacterial removal with soap solution under low-pressure lavage can be extrapolated to the treatment of grossly contaminated open fractures of the tibial shaft.

Classification of Open Fractures

The classification of open fractures is best done at the time of surgical débridement. This provides the best opportunity to understand the actual extent of the bony and soft-tissue injury. The Gustilo classification system, as originally described in 1976 and subsequently modified in 1984, is the most widely used open fracture classification system in North America.[21,45] In the original classification system, the length of the integument wound was associated with the ultimate classification of the fracture. Since that time, the energy dissipated in the mechanism of injury

also has been recognized as an important classification factor. Clearly, a tibial fracture with a small pinhole opening and an underlying severely comminuted fracture is more severe than a typical type I fracture, which is a low-energy injury with a small (< 1 cm) defect in the integument. There is typically no comminution of fracture site and minimal, if any, muscle contusion in a type I injury. A type II fracture is an intermediate injury with a skin laceration of less than 10 cm and moderate comminution and moderate soft-tissue injury.[21] Type III injuries, which are more severe than type I or II, are caused by a variety of injury mechanisms[45] and are characterized by extensive soft-tissue laceration (> 10 cm), severe contamination (such as with soil or water from a public waterway), severe comminution of the fracture or associated compartment syndrome, and all associated conditions that predispose the injury to delayed union and increased risk of soft-tissue infection.[1,21,45] In 1984, Gustilo subdivided the type III injuries into three subtypes[45] (Table 1).

Brumback and Jones[46] reported on the intraobserver reliability of the Gustilo open fracture classification system. More than 200 orthopaedic surgeons were surveyed using a videotaped presentation of open fractures. The average agreement among observers was 60%. The overall agreement on fracture type ranged from 42% to 94%, emphasizing the subjective nature of open fracture classification.

Skeletal Stabilization

The importance of skeletal stabilization in the treatment of open fractures has been widely recognized in recent years.[1] In general, it has been found that the more open the wound and the more unstable the fracture pattern, the greater is the need for skeletal stabilization. The benefits of bony stabilization are the restoration of length and rotation, which decreases dead space by restoring the proper length to the soft-tissue envelope;

improved access to the soft-tissue envelope for wound care; a decrease in the amount of ongoing tissue damage from displaced bony fragments; and the facilitation of early return to function for many patients.[1,24] External fixation was the earliest form of skeletal stabilization to be routinely used in open tibial fractures in North America.[21,24] There is an increasing trend toward the use of intramedullary fixation for skeletal stabilization. In a recent survey of North American orthopaedic surgeons, Bhandari and associates[47] reported that a predominant number of surgeons use intramedullary fixation for type I, II, and IIIA open tibial fractures. There is a nearly equal use of intramedullary fixation and external fixation for type IIIB tibial fractures (Table 2). The efficacy of such treatment is supported by literature suggesting that the use of intramedullary nail fixation provides similar benefits to external fixation regarding the incidence of deep wound infection and timely union, but without the added morbidity of pin tract infections.[1,48-51]

Two prospective randomized studies of open tibial fractures compared the incidence of wound infection using standard half-pin external fixation compared with intramedullary nail fixation.[50,51] Both studies found that the incidence of deep traumatic wound infection and timely union is similar with either method of fixation; the overall incidence of complications was higher in the external fixation group primarily because of associated pin tract morbidity.

Reamed or unreamed intramedullary fixation can be performed. At present, the optimal treatment for tibial shaft fractures with significant associated soft-tissue injury is controversial. Many studies have shown that intramedullary nail insertion interferes with circulation in the diaphyseal cortex.[52-64] This fact is significant because satisfactory tissue response for fracture healing is dependent on an adequate vascular supply. Any

Table 2
Preferences for Fixation of Tibial Shaft Fractures Among North American Surgeons*

Fixation Type	Reamed or Unreamed Intramedullary Fixation	External Fixation
Closed, low energy	96.3	0.5
Closed, high energy	96.0	1.8
Open, type I	94.5	3.4
Open, type II	88.1	11.1
Open, type IIIA	68.4	30.6
Open, type IIIB	48.4	50.5

*Numbers in table denote percentage of responding surgeons (Adapted with permission from Bhandari M, Guyott OH, Swiontkowski MF, et al: Surgeons' preferences for the operative treatment of fractures of the tibial shaft: An international survey. *J Bone Joint Surg Am* 2001;88:1746-1752.)

violation of the intramedullary canal can affect cortical vascularity or viability.[65] Current debate concerns the use of reamed and unreamed intramedullary nailing because both techniques, to varying degrees, negatively affect the circulation of cortical bone;[52-54,59,65-69] controversy exists regarding whether an unreamed nail and a reamed nail are equally responsible for this effect.

Reaming of the bone in patients with an open fracture has significant implications. After reaming, the intramedullary blood supply is destroyed, leading to necrosis of diaphyseal bone. Reaming and insertion of a tight-fitting nail will injure up to 70% of the cortical bone. The vascular system will reconstitute itself in 2 to 3 weeks, during which time the presence of dead bone and an open fracture wound may increase the risk for infection.

The biology of reamed and unreamed nail insertion has been extensively investigated and a number of conclusions can be made that impact the treatment of open tibial shaft fractures. Schemitsch and associates[69] found that the soft-tissue envelope significantly contributes to perfusion following intramedullary nail insertion. Hupel and associates[70] found, in the presence of an intact soft-tissue envelope, intramedullary reaming of the canine tibia has a major effect on increas-

ing circulation to the surrounding muscles. The degree of canal fit of the intramedullary nail and the extent of reaming before nail insertion does not further influence soft-tissue circulation. Schemitsch and associates[61] found that unreamed nail insertion with a loose-fitting nail is superior to reamed nail insertion in preventing devascularization of tibial cortex and encouraging an increase in revascularization. In another study, Schemitsch and associates[60] found that perfusion of callus and early strength of union are similar following intramedullary nailing with or without reaming. In yet another study, Schemitsch and associates[62] found that a more severe injury or overall cortical porosity is associated with reamed nail insertion and that there is no difference between the amount of new bone formation following reamed and unreamed nail insertion. Hupel and associates[56] found that a loose-fitting nail spares cortical perfusion at the time of nail insertion more than a canal-filling nail and allows more complete cortical reperfusion at 11 weeks postnailing. Hupel and associates[57] found that limited reaming spares cortical perfusion when compared with standard reaming at the time of nail insertion, but has no long-term advantage. In another study, Hupel and associates[58] found that limited reaming prior to insertion of a locked intramedullary nail resulted in less cortical bone injury than did passage through the bone of the same nail without prior reaming and with standard reaming prior to nail insertion.

Experimental findings suggest that the ideal implant for use in an open tibial shaft fracture is a loose-fitting, small diameter nail inserted with limited reaming because it provides better cortical vascularity, improved cortical porosity, the same strength of union, and the best stimulation of the extra osseous circulation. These findings agree with those of Keating and associates,[71] who found no difference in infection or nonunion rates in a prospective study using reamed and unreamed nail fixation in open tibial fractures. In our institution, open fractures are reamed minimally. This implies that the fracture is reamed no more than 1 mm past obtaining chatter. In no instance is a nail inserted that is longer than 10 mm.

Although there is a trend toward intramedullary fixation, there is also a role for alternative forms of skeletal stabilization. External fixation can be applied relatively quickly when the time for the initial stabilization is limited.[1,24] External fixation also offers the option of taking the initial fixation apart, allowing for redébridement of the intramedullary canal or access to deeper parts of the wound that could not be reached easily without redisplacement of the fracture.[1,24]

There is an abundance of literature on the secondary conversion of external fixation to intramedullary nail fixation. The initial use of this technique resulted in a relatively high incidence of deep sepsis after intramedullary fixation.[72] However, more recent studies suggest that if the conversion to intramedullary fixation is performed early in the course of the treatment, before pin tract infection can occur, the risk of sepsis with intramedullary fixation is similar to that found with primary intramedullary nailing.[72-74]

The Ilizarov fixation is an alternative form of external fixation. The use of small tension-wire fixation is popular for very proximal or very distal periarticular fracture extension.[75-77] This type of fixation can use small wires entirely, or can be combined with half pins in the diaphysis. In North America, the use of this technique is typically restricted to those fractures with periarticular fracture extension where intramedullary fixation is not easily used.[48] However, authors from other countries have reported the use of Ilizarov fixation in open tibial fractures.[75-77] The benefit of segmental transport with the use of small wire fixators to replace large segments of bone loss is clearly advantageous in some complex open tibial injuries.[76,78] There is little data on the conversion of small-wire fixation to intramedullary fixation. It appears that those physicians who use small-wire fixation as their initial treatment for skeletal stabilization prefer to maintain this type of fixation throughout the course of treatment.

Plate fixation usually is reserved for specific indications in periarticular extension of fractures in the tibial shaft. Treatment using plate fixation for open tibial shaft fractures with the middiaphyseal injury is seldom used in North America.[79]

Soft-Tissue Coverage

The timing of soft-tissue coverage is a subject of controversy. Standard teaching recommends that open fractures remain open until the patient is returned to the operating room for a "second look" débridement to ensure that adequate débridement of necrotic tissue from the wound has been done prior to wound closure.[1,48,80] Delayed primary closure has been recommended at 48 to 72 hours after the traumatic injury, assuming that the wound bed was viable at the time of return to the operating room.[81-83] This recommendation recently has been challenged, with authors advocating primary closure of open wounds in some cases.

Delong and associates[84] reported on the "aggressive treatment" study of open fractures with immediate primary closure of the open fracture wound after a thorough débridement. The authors emphasized the need for an experienced surgeon to participate in the surgical débridement to ensure the adequate removal of necrotic tissue. These authors reported a 7% deep infection rate in 119 open fractures ranging from type I to type IIIB injuries.[84] These results are similar to those of conventional open fracture treatment.

Where either primary or delayed primary wound closure is not possible, the use of flap coverage has gained wide acceptance. In 1982, May and associates[85] introduced the use of the free vascularized flap for the coverage of traumatic tibial defects. Since that time, this technique has been widely accepted. The timing of coverage for these complex injuries, like lesser grade open tibial fractures, continues to be a source of controversy. Most authors currently recommend closure prior to 7 days after the initial treatment.[80,81,83] However, some authors have advocated a more aggressive approach of a "fix and flap," requiring an early wide débridement or necrectomy with removal of all necrotic tissue.[86-89] Primary skeletal stabilization is followed by either immediate free vascularized tissue coverage or wound coverage within 72 hours after injury. Using this approach, Godina[87] reported on the results of the treatment of 532 patients with complex open tibial fractures. He found that in patients who underwent free flap transfer within 72 hours of injury, there was a less than 1% incidence of flap failure and a deep infection rate of 1.5% when compared with a rate of flap failure of 12% with delayed flap coverage and a deep infection rate of 17.5%. Gopal and associates[86] reported on a study of 80 patients with 84 type IIIB open tibial fractures. The authors found a deep infection rate of 6% for patients treated with soft-tissue coverage 72 hours or less after injury compared with a 30% deep infection rate with wound coverage occurring more than 72 hours after injury.[86] Sinclair and associates[89] reported results from a study of 17 consecutive patients with type IIIB open tibial fractures treated with primary stabilization and soft-tissue flap coverage within 72 hours of injury that resulted in a 0% infection rate. Hertel and associates[88] reported on a comparative study of 29 open tibial fractures of which 24 were type IIIB and 5 were type IIIC fractures. Fifteen fractures were treated with fixation followed by delayed soft-tissue coverage, and 14 fractures were treated with primary débridement, bony stabilization, and soft-tissue coverage with an immediate free vascularized tissue transfer. These authors reported a deep infection rate of 27% after delayed soft-tissue coverage compared with no deep infections in the group with primary soft-tissue coverage. The argument for early soft-tissue coverage is supported by findings of Breidenbach and associates[90] who reported that free tissue transfer covering a wound with a bacterial colony count greater than or equal to 10^4 has a significantly higher rate of deep wound sepsis when compared with wounds with lower bacterial colony counts.[90] Earlier (done within 72 hours after initial débridement) soft-tissue coverage may allow coverage of a wound with a relatively decreased bacterial colony count, although this hypothesis remains unproven.

The primary alternative method of tissue coverage other than free tissue transfer is local rotational flap coverage.[1,91] For a tibial shaft fracture, either a gastrocnemius transfer or soleus transfer are the two predominant forms of local flap coverage. Fasciocutaneous flaps have also been advocated in some cases.[92] The use of local rotational flaps for wound coverage in the open tibial fracture presents a risk for damage to the muscle in the zone of injury.[1,91] This concept implies that the muscle to be transferred is itself damaged and may not be as viable

as otherwise healthy muscle in a transposed position. Recently, the Lower Extremity Assessment Project study group reported on 190 patients with 195 injured limbs that required flap coverage, with 6-month follow-up.[93] In this study, the authors reported the successful use of both local rotational flap coverage and free tissue transfers. However, they noted that when the bony injury was an Association for the Study of Internal Fixation/Orthopaedic Trauma Association this classification describes the bony injury only) type C injury, treatment with a local rotational flap was 4.3 times more likely to have a wound complication requiring surgical intervention in those patients treated with a free tissue flap. No difference was found with respect to flap type for limbs that had a lower grade osseous injury.

Recent advances in wound treatment include the antibiotic bead pouch, as discussed earlier in this chapter, and vacuum-assisted closure.[12,94] Vacuum-assisted closure, commonly known as wound vac, is a wound treatment system that uses subatmospheric pressure to help expedite wound healing and granulation tissue formation. Some preliminary findings suggest that this system is excellent in promoting granulation tissue formation and in facilitating the closure of some complex wounds where dead space management may be an issue.[94]

The use of Ilizarov techniques with bone transfer has been widely advocated to help facilitate treatment of open tibial fractures with bone loss. Several reports have advocated the concomitant use of free tissue transfer along with segmental transport.[76,77] Several authors have reported good success with this technique. Isik and associates[95] reported on the delayed use of segmental transport after early free tissue flap coverage of an open wound. These authors found that, in the period of time between initial flap coverage and the undertaking of distraction osteogenesis, the flap significantly

contracts, resulting in the skin curtain dipping into the open wound. In two of seven patients, this resulted in a slough of the muscle flap and required a repeat free tissue transfer.

Summary

Although open fractures of the tibial shaft are difficult to treat, several new advances in antibiotic therapy and skeletal stabilization appear to be influencing the way in which these injuries are treated. In addition, fracture fixation and soft-tissue management techniques continue to evolve. Aggressive and early treatment of open fractures of the tibial shaft will eventually result in an improved outcome.

References

1. Olson SA, Finkemeier CF, Moehring HD: Open fractures, in Bucholz, Heckman (eds): *Fractures in Adults*, ed 5. Philadelphia, PA, Lippincott-Williams & Williams, 2001.

2. Tscherne H: The management of open fractures, in *Fractures With Soft Tissue Injuries*. New York, NY, Springer-Verlag, 1984.

3. Advanced Trauma Life Support (ATLS) American College of Surgeons: Committee on Trauma, Chicago, IL, 2000.

4. Braun R, Enzler MA, Rittmann WW: A double-blind clinical trial of prophylactic cloxacillin in open fractures. *J Orthop Trauma* 1987;1:12-17.

5. Dellinger EP, Caplan ES, Weaver LD, et al: Duration of preventive antibiotic administration for open extremity fractures. *Arch Surg* 1988;123:333-339.

6. Patzakis MJ, Harvey JP Jr, Ivler D: The role of antibiotics in the management of open fractures. *J Bone Joint Surg Am* 1974;56:532-541.

7. Robson MC, Duke WF, Krizek TJ: Rapid bacterial screening in the treatment of civilian wounds. *J Surg Res* 1973;14:426-430.

8. Robinson D, On E, Hadas N, Halperin N, Hofman S, Boldur I: Microbiologic flora contaminating open fractures: Its significance in the choice of primary antibiotic agents and the likelihood of deep wound infection. *J Orthop Trauma* 1989;3:283-286.

9. Patzakis MJ, Bains RS, Lee J, et al: Prospective, randomized, double-blind study comparing single-agent antibiotic therapy, ciprofloxacin, to combination antibiotic therapy in open fracture wounds. *J Orthop Trauma* 2000;14:529-533.

10. Sorger JI, Kirk PG, Ruhnke CJ, et al: Once daily, high dose versus divided, low dose gentamicin for open fractures. *Clin Orthop* 1999;366:197-204.

11. Eckman JB Jr, Henry SL, Mangino PD, Seligson D: Wound and serum levels of tobramycin with the prophylactic use of tobramycin-impregnated

polymethylmethacrylate beads in compound fractures. *Clin Orthop* 1988;237:213-215.

12. Ostermann PA, Seligson D, Henry SL: Local antibiotic therapy for severe open fractures: A review of 1085 consecutive cases. *J Bone Joint Surg Br* 1995;77:93-97.

13. Keating JF, Blachut PA, O'Brien PJ, Meek RN, Broekhuyse H: Reamed nailing of open tibial fractures: Does the antibiotic bead pouch reduce the deep infection rate? *J Orthop Trauma* 1996;10:298-303.

14. Miclau T, Edin ML, Lester GE, Lindsey RW, Dahners LE: Bone toxicity of locally applied aminoglycosides. *J Orthop Trauma* 1995;9:401-406.

15. Burd TA, Anglen JO, Lowry KJ, Hendricks KJ, Day D: In vitro elution of tobramycin from bioabsorbable polycaprolactone beads. *J Orthop Trauma* 2001;15:424-428.

16. Edin ML, Miclau T, Lester GE, Lindsey RW, Dahners LE: Effect of cefazolin and vancomycin on osteoblasts in vitro. *Clin Orthop* 1996;333:245-251.

17. Lindsey RW, Probe R, Miclau T, Alexander JW, Perren SM: The effects of antibiotic-impregnated autogeneic cancellous bone graft on bone healing. *Clin Orthop* 1993;291:303-312.

18. Darouiche RO, Farmer J, Chaput C, Mansouri M, Saleh G, Landon GC: Anti-infective efficacy of antiseptic-coated intramedullary nails. *J Bone Joint Surg Am* 1998;80:1336-1340.

19. Lee J: Efficacy of cultures in the management of open fractures. *Clin Orthop* 1997;339:71-75.

20. Wilkins J, Patzakis M: Choice and duration of antibiotics in open fractures. *Orthop Clin North Am* 1991;22:433-437.

21. Gustilo RB, Anderson JT: Prevention of infection in the treatment of one thousand and twenty-five open fractures of long bones: Retrospective and prospective analyses. *J Bone Joint Surg Am* 1976;58:453-458.

22. Edwards CC, Simmons SC, Browner BD, Weigel MC: Severe open tibial fractures: Results treating 202 injuries with external fixation. *Clin Orthop* 1988;230:98-115.

23. Esterhai JL Jr, Queenan J: Management of soft tissue wounds associated with type III open fractures. *Orthop Clin North Am* 1991;22:427-432.

24. Gustilo RB, Merkow RL, Templeman D: The management of open fractures. *J Bone Joint Surg Am* 1990;72:299-304.

25. Patzakis MJ: Management of open fracture wounds. *Instr Course Lect* 1987;36:367-369.

26. Bhhaskar SN, Cutright D, Runsuck EE, Gross A: Pulsating water jet devices in debridement of combat wounds. *Mil Med* 1971;136:264-266.

27. Brown LL, Shelton HT, Bornside GH, Cohn I Jr: Evaluation of wound irrigation by pulsatile jet and conventional methods. *Ann Surg* 1978;187:170-173.

28. Dirschl DR, Duff GP, Dahners LE, Edin M, Rahn BA, Miclau T: High pressure pulsatile lavage irrigation of intraarticular fractures: Effects on fracture healing. *J Orthop Trauma* 1998;12:460-463.

29. Gross A, Bhaskar SN, Cutright DE, Beasley JD III, Perez B: The effect of pulsating water jet lavage on experimental contaminated wounds. *J Oral Surg* 1971;29:187-190.

30. Gross A, Cutright DE, Bhaskar SN: Effectiveness of pulsating water jet lavage in the treatment of contaminated crushed wounds. *Am J Surg* 1972;124:373-377.

31. Hamer ML, Robson MC, Krizek TJ, Southwick WO: Quantitative bacterial analysis of comparative wound irrigations. *Ann Surg* 1975;181:819-822.

32. Rhodeheaver GT, Pettry D, Thacker JG, Edgerton MT, Edlich RF: Wound cleansing by high pressure irrigation. *Surg Gynecol Obstet* 1975;141:357-362.

33. Sobel JW, Goldberg VM: Pulsatile irrigation in orthopedics. *Orthopedics* 1985;8:1019-1022.

34. Bhandari M, Adili A, Lachowski RJ: High pressure pulsatile lavage of contaminated human tibiae: An in vitro study. *J Orthop Trauma* 1998;12:479-484.

35. Bhandari M, Schemitsch EH, Adili A, Lachowski R, Shaughnessy SG: High and low pressure pulsatile lavage of contaminated tibial fractures: An in vitro study of bacterial adherence and bone damage. *J Orthop Trauma* 1999;13:526-533.

36. West BR, Nichter LS, Halpern DE, Nimni ME, Cheung DT, Zhou ZY: Ultrasound debridement of trabeculated bone: Effective and atraumatic. *Plast Reconstr Surg* 1994;93:561-566.

37. Wheeler CB, Rhodeheaver GT, Thacker JG, Edgerton MT, Edlich RF: Side-effects of high pressure irrigation. *Surg Gynecol Obstet* 1976;143:775-778.

38. Anglen JO, Apostoles S, Christensen G, Gainor B: The efficacy of various irrigation solutions in removing slime-producing Staphylococcus. *J Orthop Trauma* 1994;8:390-396.

39. Anglen J, Apostoles S, Christensen G, Gainor B, Lane J: Removal of surface bacteria by irrigation. *J Orthop Res* 1996;14:251-254.

40. Dirschl DR, Wilson FC: Topical antibiotic irrigation in the prophylaxis of operative wound infections in orthopedic surgery. *Orthop Clin North Am* 1991;22:419-426.

41. Gainor BJ, Hockman DE, Anglen JO, Christensen G, Simpson WA: Benzalkonium chloride: A potential disinfecting irrigation solution. *J Orthop Trauma* 1997;11:121-125.

42. Moussa FW, Gainor BJ, Anglen JO, Christensen G, Simpson WA: Disinfecting agents for removing adherent bacteria from orthopaedic hardware. *Clin Orthop* 1996;329:255-262.

43. Kaysinger KK, Nicholson NC, Ramp WK, Kellam JF: Toxic effects of wound irrigation solutions on cultured tibiae and osteoblasts. *J Orthop Trauma* 1995;9:303-311.

44. Bhandari M, Adili A, Schemitsch EH: The efficacy of low-pressure lavage with different irrigating solutions to remove adherent bacteria from bone. *J Bone Joint Surg Am* 2001;83:412-419.

45. Gustilo RB, Mendoza RM, Williams DN: Problems in the management of type III (severe) open fractures: A new classification of type III open fractures. *J Trauma* 1984;24:742-746.

46. Brumback RJ, Jones AL: Interobserver agreement in the classification of open fractures of the tibia. *J Bone Joint Surg Am* 1994;76:1162-1166.

47. Bhandari M, Guyatt GH, Swiontkowski MF, et al: Surgeons' preferences for the operative treatment of fractures of the tibial shaft: An international survey. *J Bone Joint Surg Am* 2001;83:1746-1752.

48. McGraw JM, Lim EV: Treatment of open tibial-shaft fractures: External fixation and secondary intramedullary nailing. *J Bone Joint Surg Am* 1988;70:900-911.

49. Schandelmaier P, Krettek C, Rudolf J, Kohl A, Katz BE, Tscheme H: Superior results of tibial rodding versus external fixation in grade 3B fractures. *Clin Orthop* 1997;342:164-172.

50. Tornetta P III, Bergman M, Watnik N, Berkowitz G, Steuer J: Treatment of grade-IIIb open tibial fractures. *J Bone Joint Surg Br* 1994;76:13-19.

51. Henley MB, Chapman JR, Agel J, Harvey EJ, Whorton AM, Swiontkowski MF: Treatment of type II, IIIA, and IIIB open fractures of the tibial shaft: A prospective comparison of unreamed interlocking intramedullary nails and half-pin external fixators. *J Orthop Trauma* 1998;12:1-7.

52. Danckwardt-Lillestrom G: Reaming of the medullary cavity and its effect on diaphyseal bone: A fluorochromic microangiographic and histologic study on the rabbit tibia and dog femur. *Acta Orthop Scand* 1969;128:1-153.

53. Danckwardt-Lillestrom G, Lorenzi GL, Olerud S: Intramedullary nailing after reaming: An investigation on the healing process in osteotomized rabbit tibias. *Acta Orthop Scand* 1970;(suppl 134):1-78.

54. Danckwardt-Lillestrom G, Lorenzi L, Olerud S: Intracortical circulation after intramedullary reaming with reduction of pressure in the medullary cavity. *J Bone Joint Surg Am* 1970;52:1390-1394.

55. Grundnes O, Utvag SE, Reikeras O: Restoration of bone flow following fracture and reaming in rat femora. *Acta Orthop Scand* 1994;65:185-190.

56. Hupel TM, Aksenov SA, Schemitsch EH: Cortical bone blood flow in loose and tight fitting locked intramedullary nailing: A canine segmental tibia fracture model. *J Orthop Trauma* 1998;2:127-135.

57. Hupel TM, Aksenov SA, Schemitsch EH: Effect of limited and standard reaming on cortical bone blood flow and early strength of union following segmental fracture. *J Orthop Trauma* 1998;12:400-406.

58. Hupel TM, Weinberg JA, Aksenov SA, Schemitsch EH: Effect of unreamed, limited reamed and standard reamed intramedullary nailing on cortical bone porosity and new bone formation. *J Orthop Trauma* 2001;15:18-27.

59. Rhinelander FW, Baragry RA: Micro-angiography in bone healing: Undisplaced closed fractures. *J Bone Joint Surg Am* 1962;44:1273-1298.

60. Schemitsch EH, Kowalski MJ, Swiontkowski MF, Harrington RM: Comparison of the effect of reamed and unreamed locked intramedullary nailing on blood flow in the callus and strength of union following fracture of the sheep tibia. *J Orthop Res* 1995;13:382-389.

61. Schemitsch EH, Kowalski MJ, Swiontkowski MF, Senft D: Cortical bone blood flow in reamed and unreamed locked intramedullary nailing: A fractured tibia model in sheep. *J Orthop Trauma* 1994;8:373-382.

62. Schemitsch EH, Turchin DC, Kowalski MJ, Swiontkowski MF: Quantitative assessment of bone injury and repair after reamed and unreamed locked intramedullary nailing. *J Trauma* 1998;45:250-255.

63. Utvag SE, Grundnes O, Reikeras O: Effects of degrees of reaming on healing segmental fractures in rats. *J Orthop Trauma* 1998;12:192-199.

64. Kessler SB, Hallfeldt KK, Perren SM, Schweiberer L: The effects of reaming and intramedullary nailing on fracture healing. *Clin Orthop* 1986;212:18-25.

65. Indrekvam K, Lekven J, Engesaeter LB, Langeland N: Effects of intramedullary reaming and nailing on blood flow in rat femora. *Acta Orthop Scand* 1992;63:61-65.

66. Rhinelander FW: Effects of medullary nailing on the normal blood supply of diaphyseal cortex. *Clin Orthop* 1998;350:5-17.

67. Rhinelander FW: The normal microcirculation of diaphyseal cortical and its response to fracture. *J Bone Joint Surg Am* 1968;50:784-800.

68. Rhinelander FW: Tibial blood supply in relation to fracture healing. *Clin Orthop* 1974;105:34-81.

69. Schemitsch EH, Kowalski MJ, Swiontkowski MF: Soft tissue blood flow following reamed versus unreamed locked intramedullary nailing: A fractured sheep tibia model. *Ann Plast Surg* 1996;3:70-75.

70. Hupel TM, Aksenov SA, Schemitsch EH: Muscle perfusion after intramedullary nailing of the canine tibia. *J Trauma* 1998;45:256-262.

71. Keating JF, O'Brien PJ, Blachut PA, Meek RN, Broekhuyse HM: Locking intramedullary nailing with and without reaming for open fractures

of the tibial shaft: A prospective, randomized study. *J Bone Joint Surg Am* 1997;79:334-341.

72. Blachut PA, Meek RN, O'Brien PJ: External fixation and delayed intramedullary nailing of open fractures of the tibial shaft: A sequential protocol. *J Bone Joint Surg Am* 1990;72:729-735.

73. Antich-Adrover P, Marti-Garin D, Murias-Alvarez M, Puente-Alonso C: External fixation and secondary itramedullary nailing of open tibial fractures. *J Bone Joint Surg Br* 1997;79:433-437.

74. Siebenrock KA, Gerich T, Jakob RP: Sequential intramedullary nailing of open tibial shaft fractures after external fixation. *Arch Orthop Trauma Surg* 1997;116:32-36.

75. Agarwal S, Agarwal R, Jain UK, Chandra R: Management of soft-tissue problems in leg trauma in conjunction with application of the Ilizarov fixator assembly. *Plast Reconstr Surg* 2001;107:1732-1738.

76. Schwartsman V, Martin SN, Ronquist RA, Schwartsman R: Tibial fractures: The Ilizarov alternative. *Clin Orthop* 1992;278:207-216.

77. Tukiainen E, Asko-Seljavaar S: Use of the Ilizarov technique after a free microvascular muscle flap transplantation in massive trauma of the lower leg. *Clin Orthop* 1993;297:129-134.

78. Shtarker H, David R, Stolero J, Grimberg B, Soudry M: Treatment of open tibial fractures with primary suture and Ilizarov fixation. *Clin Orthop* 1997;335:268-274.

79. Bach AW, Hansen ST Jr: Plates versus external fixation in severe open tibial shaft fractures: A randomized trial. *Clin Orthop* 1989;241:89-94.

80. Cierny G III, Byrd HS, Jones RE: Primary versus delayed soft tissue coverage for severe open tibial fractures. *Clin Orthop* 1983;178:54-63.

81. Byrd HS, Cierny G III, Tebbetts JB: The management of open tibial fractures with associated soft-tissue loss: External pin fixation with early flap coverage. *Plast Reconstr Surg* 1981;68:73-79.

82. Russell GG, Henderson R, Arnett G: Primary or delayed closure for open tibial fractures. *J Bone Joint Surg Br* 1990;72:125-128.

83. Ostermann PA, Henry SL, Seligson D: Timing of wound closure in severe compound fractures. *Orthopedics* 1994;17:397-399.

84. DeLong WG Jf, Born CT, Wei SY, Petrik ME, Ponzio R, Schwab CW: Aggressive treatment of

119 open fracture wounds. *J Trauma* 1999;46:1049-1054.

85. May JW Jr, Gallico GG III, Lukash FN: Microvascular transfer of free tissue for closure of bone wounds of the distal lower extremity. *New Engl J Med* 1982;306:253-257.

86. Gopal S, Majumder S, Batchelor AG, Knight SL, De Boer P, Smith RM: Fix and flap: The radical orthopaedic and plastic treatment of severe open fractures of the tibia. *J Bone Joint Surg Br* 2000;82:959-966.

87. Godina M: Early microsurgical reconstruction of complex trauma of the extremities. *Plast Reconstr Surg* 1986;78:285-292.

88. Hertel R, Lambert SM, Muller S, Ballmer FT, Ganz R: On the timing of soft-tissue reconstruction for open fractures of the lower leg. *Arch Orthop Trauma Surg* 1999;119:7-12.

89. Sinclair JS, McNally MA, Small JO, Yeates HA: Primary free-flap cover of open tibial fractures. *Injury* 1997;28:581-587.

90. Breidenbach WC, Trager S: Quantitative culture technique and infection in complex wounds of the extremities closed with free flaps. *Plast Reconstr Sur* 1995;95:860-865.

91. Levin SL: Soft tissue principles for orthopaedic surgeons. *Tech Orthop* 1995;10:1-10.

92. Louton RB, Harley RA, Hagerty RC: A fasciocutaneous transposition flap for coverage of defects of the lower extremity. *J Bone Joint Surg Am* 1989;71:988-994.

93. Pollak AN, McCarthy M, Burgess AR: Short-term wound complications after application of flaps for coverage of traumatic soft-tissue defects about the tibia: The Lower Extremity Assessment Project (LEAP) Study Group. *J Bone Joint Surg Am* 2000;82:1681-1691.

94. Morykwas MJ, Argenta LC, Shelton-Brown EI, McGuirt W: Vacuum-assisted closure: A new method for wound control and treatment: Animal studies and basic foundation. *Ann Plast Surg* 1997;38:553-562.

95. Isik S, Guler MM, Selmanpakoglu N: Unexpected, late complication of combined free flap coverage and Ilizarov technique applied to legs. *Ann Plast Surg* 1997;39:437-438.

Minimally Invasive Percutaneous Plate Osteosynthesis of Fractures of the Distal Tibia

David L. Helfet, MD
Michael Suk, MD, JD, MPH

Abstract

Fractures of the distal tibia are notoriously difficult to treat, and traditional methods of fixation are often fraught with soft-tissue complications. With recent emphasis on meticulous handling and preservation of the soft-tissue envelope, minimally invasive percutaneous plate osteosynthesis has become a safe and reliable method of treating these fractures. This technique involves conventional open reduction and internal fixation of the fibula and spanning external fixation of the tibia until the soft-tissue swelling subsides. Subsequently, limited open reduction and internal fixation of displaced articular fragments is performed through small incisions based on CT evaluation. This is followed by minimally invasive percutaneous plate osteosynthesis of the tibia, in which the plafond is attached to the tibial shaft using a variety of commercially available plates.

Fractures of the distal tibia involving the weight-bearing articular surface and metaphysis are notoriously difficult to treat.[1-14] In 1905, Lambotte called such fractures "fractures de l'epiphyse"[3,15] and was perhaps the first to perform an open reduction and internal fixation to treat this type of fracture. In 1911, Destot introduced the term pilon ("hammer").[1,16] In 1950, Bonin used the term plafond ("ceiling")[17] to describe the region of metaphyseal impaction caused by the talus as it is driven up into the tibial articular surface. And most recently, in 1971, Ruoff and Snider[18] coined the term "explosion fracture" to describe the potential complexity of fractures of the distal

tibia. Disturbingly, 10% to 30% of these are open fractures, and most are associated with other injuries.[2,15,19,20] Additionally, the degloving and crushing of the skin that can accompany such injuries frequently leads to necrosis and further complicates treatment.[4,5,16,19,21,22]

Historical Treatment

In 1963, the AO group introduced four principles of open reduction and internal fixation to treat intra-articular fractures of the distal tibia: (1) reestablishment of fibular length and stabilization of the lateral column, (2) reconstruction of the articular surface of the tibia, (3) placement of metaphyseal bone graft, and (4) stab-

ilization of the medial tibia using a plate. Although good to excellent results are frequently reported for closed, low-energy fractures, high-energy and open fractures are accompanied by complications. Poor results, skin slough, wound dehiscence, and infection often are associated with increased fracture severity.[5,7,8,18,19,23-28]

To improve on the poor results traditionally associated with open reduction and plate and screw fixation, minimally invasive techniques were developed to include limited internal and hybrid external fixation.[29] Other investigators have also endorsed the concept of limited surgery to treat severe pilon injuries.[15,25,29-31] From a desire to produce minimal additional insult at surgery, modern biologic principles have evolved that emphasize meticulous soft-tissue dissection, limited stripping of fracture fragments, indirect reduction techniques, and adequate fixation.[9,20,21,32]

Minimally Invasive Percutaneous Plate Osteosynthesis

Minimally invasive percutaneous plate osteosynthesis was developed in response to disappointing results following traditional methods of sur-

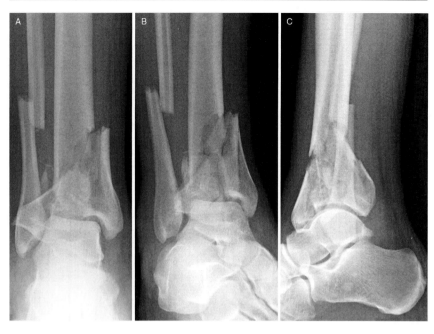

Figure 1 AP (**A**), lateral (**B**), and mortise (**C**) views of a high-energy, right-sided closed pilon fracture sustained by a 39-year-old man who fell 14 feet from a ladder.

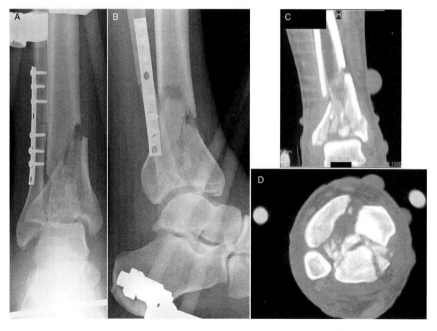

Figure 2 AP (**A**) and lateral (**B**) views after open reduction and internal fixation of the fibula fracture and application of the spanning external fixator of the patient as described in Figure 1. Coronal (**C**) and transverse (**D**) CT scans are shown.

gical stabilization of fractures of the distal tibia and the complications also introduced by the newer methods of limited internal and external fixation.[27] The percutaneous plating technique is advantageous because it minimizes soft-tissue compromise and devascularization of the fracture fragments. Indications for using minimally invasive percutaneous plate osteosynthesis to treat distal tibia fractures include open fractures, displaced intra-articular tibial pilon fractures with sufficient medial soft-tissue coverage to allow percutaneous plating and articular reconstruction, low-energy ankle fractures associated with significant soft-tissue compromise, and unstable metaphyseal/diaphyseal fractures that are located too distally for stabilization with an intramedullary nail.

Surgical Technique

Management of patients with distal tibia fractures includes rapid skeletal stabilization on the day of admission to the hospital with the placement of a triangular ("delta") external fixator from the tibia to the calcaneus. Early placement of an external frame enhances recovery of the soft-tissue envelope and assists in the restoration of length. Two 4.5-mm or 5.0-mm Schanz screws are placed in the anterior aspect of the tibia proximal to the fracture, and a centrally threaded transfixion pin is placed through the tuberosity of the calcaneus in a medial to lateral direction. Two carbon fiber rods are used to connect the Schanz screws, thus completing the triangle. Manual traction is applied to achieve a closed reduction of alignment, length, and rotation through ligamentotaxis before the pin to bar clamps are tightened. For additional stability in the plane of the calcaneal pin, an additional 4.5-mm Schanz pin can be applied to the midfoot across the medial and middle cuneiforms.

If a fibular fracture is present, concurrent open reduction and internal fixation is performed with either a one third tubular plate or a 3.5-mm conventional or locked combination plate (LCDCP or LCP, Synthes, Paoli, PA). Early reduction of the fibular fracture provides lateral stability

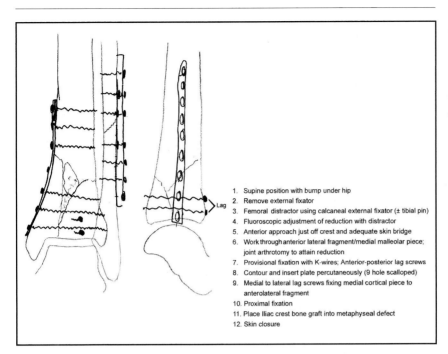

1. Supine position with bump under hip
2. Remove external fixator
3. Femoral distractor using calcaneal external fixator (± tibial pin)
4. Fluoroscopic adjustment of reduction with distractor
5. Anterior approach just off crest and adequate skin bridge
6. Work through anterior lateral fragment/medial malleolar piece; joint arthrotomy to attain reduction
7. Provisional fixation with K-wires; Anterior-posterior lag screws
8. Contour and insert plate percutaneously (9 hole scalloped)
9. Medial to lateral lag screws fixing medial cortical piece to anterolateral fragment
10. Proximal fixation
11. Place Iliac crest bone graft into metaphyseal defect
12. Skin closure

Figure 3 Same patient as described in Figure 1. Preoperative plan for definitive open reduction and internal fixation of the pilon fracture including delta frame removal, fluoroscopic-aided reduction using a femoral distractor, and placement of a bone graft and scallop plate.

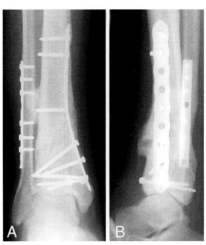

Figure 4 AP (**A**), and lateral (**B**) views of the patient as described in Figure 1, 1 year after percutaneous fixation with a scallop plate.

to the construct and serves as a guide to proper restoration of length of the plafond. Anatomic landmarks are assessed intraoperatively with the use of fluoroscopy to prevent overdistraction through the external frame.

The affected limb is then maintained in a well-padded posterior splint and elevated on a Bohler-Braun frame until such time as the soft-tissue swelling allows further surgery. Definitive surgery is delayed until resolution of the acute phase of soft-tissue edema, typically 7 to 14 days after injury and evidenced by wrinkling of the skin over the medial and anterior aspects of the ankle. Open wounds are treated with serial irrigations and débridement and delayed soft-tissue closure or coverage is obtained within 5 to 7 days of the injury.

For minimally invasive plate osteosynthesis of a distal tibial fracture,

the patient is placed supine on a radiolucent table, a roll is placed beneath the ipsilateral buttock, and a pneumatic tourniquet is applied to the proximal thigh. The ipsilateral iliac crest and entire lower extremity are made ready for surgery in the usual sterile fashion. After exsanguination of the extremity, the tourniquet is inflated to 300 mm Hg.

Initial attention is paid to the fracture lines, which extend into the tibial plafond and are identified by careful evaluation of the CT scan (Figures 1 through 3). Articular fragments are anatomically reduced percutaneously, using fluoroscopy and pointed reduction forceps, or via direct open reduction using small incisions and arthrotomies. Once articular reduction is obtained, the articular fragments are stabilized with either 2.7-mm or 3.5-mm lag screws. An additional T plate, one

third or even smaller plates (Synthes) may be applied through limited approaches to buttress a large metaphyseal defect or act as washer in the face of significant comminution.

Once the articular fragments are stabilized, the metaphyseal fracture is addressed. The appropriate length of the semitubular plate, scallop plate (Synthes), or precontoured periarticular medial distal tibia plate (Synthes; Zimmer, Warsaw, IN) is determined by placing a plate along the anterior aspect of the leg and adjusting it so that under fluoroscopy the distal end of the plate is at the level of the tibial plafond and the proximal end extends at least three screw holes proximal to the proximal extent of the fracture. A 3-cm incision is made along the anteromedial aspect of the tibia and proximal to the fracture. A subcutaneous tunnel is created along the medial aspect of the tibia by blunt dissection using a large Kelly clamp. The plate can then be advanced directly beneath the soft tissues often with a suture to pull the leading edge through the tunnel. The position of the plate is adjusted

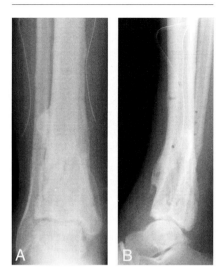

Figure 5 Same patient as described in Figure 1. AP (**A**) and lateral (**B**) views 2 years after hardware removal.

under fluoroscopy in both the coronal and sagittal planes to assure correct length and that it lies along the medial aspect of the tibia.

Cortical screws (3.5 or 4.0 mm) are placed through the plate via small percutaneous stab incisions to achieve an indirect reduction from distal to proximal or proximal to distal, depending on the fracture pattern. The distal metaphyseal articular fragment is indirectly reduced to the proximal fragment in this fashion. Percutaneous lag screws are placed across the fracture planes as needed to maintain the reduction, provide interfragmentary compression, and increase the stability of the construct (Figures 4 and 5). Radiographs are taken in the operating room to assess the overall alignment of the limb and ensure proper placement of the implants. The surgical incisions are irrigated and closed, sterile dressings are applied, and the limb is immobilized in a well-padded posterior and U splint, with the ankle maintained in neutral position.

Clinical Results

The senior author recently reviewed retrospectively 17 patients treated between 1999 and 2001 for tibial plafond fractures, using a newly designed and minimally invasive ultra-slim scallop plate (Synthes). As per protocol, staged surgical treatment with open reduction and fixation of the fibular fracture and application of an external fixator was initially performed in 12 patients. As soon as the soft tissues and swelling allowed, (ie, skin wrinkling occurred), the articular surface was reconstructed and anatomically reduced through a small incision, and the articular block was fixed to the diaphysis using a medially placed, percutaneously introduced flat scallop plate (DL Helfet, MD, unpublished data, 2003).

Hemovac drains were removed when the drainage was less than 20 mL per 8 hours and generally within the first 24 to 48 hours. All patients received 48 hours of perioperative prophylactic antibiotic therapy. Postoperatively, the limb was elevated while the patient was in bed, and ambulation training was begun on postoperative day one with toe-touch weight bearing of 20 lb with crutches. On postoperative day two, gentle range-of-motion exercises of the ankle were begun, the patients were instructed on the use of a theraband, and a fracture boot was applied.

The patients were discharged when able to perform toe-touch weight bearing of 20 lb in their fracture boots. Sutures were removed at 10 to 14 days after surgery. Radiographs including an AP, lateral, and mortise views of the distal tibia and fibula were taken at 2 weeks, 6 weeks, and 3 months postoperatively to assess healing and alignment. Patients were progressed to partial weight bearing and then full weight bearing depending on the results of

clinical and radiographic evaluation.

All patients achieved bony union at an average of 14.1 weeks. Eleven fractures (65%) were high-energy injuries. Two fractures were open. There were no plate failures or loss of fixation or reduction. Two superficial wound-healing problems resolved with local wound care. At an average follow-up of 17 months (range, 6 to 29 months), eight patients (47%) had excellent results, seven (41%) had fair results, and two (12%) had poor results. The average American Orthopaedic Foot and Ankle Society Ankle-Hindfoot Score was 86.1 (range, 61 to 100). Four patients subsequently required hardware removal, and one of these patients required ankle arthrodesis. Most importantly, there were no chronic or deep infections and no soft-tissue sloughs, flaps, etc. Based on initial results, a minimally invasive surgical technique using a new low-profile plate can decrease soft-tissue problems while leading to fracture healing and obtaining results that are comparable to those reported in other more recent series. The new scallop plate is appropriate for the treatment of pilon fractures and should be used in conjunction with a staged procedure in the acute trauma setting.

Summary

Open reduction and internal fixation of fractures of the distal tibia with articular involvement (ie, pilon fractures) has been plagued by complications. In keeping with modern trends for less invasive surgery, the protocol of (1) initial fibula fixation and spanning external fixation to manage the soft-tissue injury; (2) limited open arthrotomies and fixation of the displaced distal tibial articular segment; and (3) percutaneous plate osteosynthesis of the articular segment to the tibial diaphysis has proved efficacious with an acceptably low rate of complications, especially to the soft-tissue envelope.

References

1. Destot EAJ (ed): *Traumatismes du pied et rayons x: Malleoles, Astragale, Calcaneum, Avant-pied*. Paris, France, Masson, 1911.

2. Helfet DL, Koval K, Pappas J, Sanders RW, DiPasquale T: Intra-articular "pilon" fracture of the tibia. *Clin Orthop* 1994;298:221-228.

3. Lambotte A: *Chirurgie operatoire des fractures*. Paris, France, Masson, 1913.

4. Muhr G, Breitfuss H: Complications after pilon fractures, in Tscherne H, Schatzker J (eds): *Major Fractures of the Pilon, the Talus, and the Calcaneus: Current Concepts of Treatment*. Berlin, Germany, Springer-Verlag, 1993, pp 65-67.

5. Ovadia DN, Beals RK: Fractures of the tibial plafond. *J Bone Joint Surg Am* 1986;68:543-551.

6. Ruedi TP, Allgower M: The operative treatment of intra-articular fractures of the lower end of the tibia. *Clin Orthop* 1979;138:105-110.

7. Sanders R, Pappas J, Mast J, Helfet D: The salvage of open grade IIIB ankle and talus fractures. *J Orthop Trauma* 1992;6:201-208.

8. Ruedi T, Allgower M: Fractures of the lower end of the tibia into the ankle-joint. *Injury* 1969;1:92-99.

9. Mast JW, Spiegel PG, Pappas JN: Fractures of the tibial pilon. *Clin Orthop* 1988;230:68-82.

10. Blauth M, Bastian L: Krettek C, Knop C, Evans S: Surgical options for the treatment of severe tibial pilon fractures: A study of three techniques. *J Orthop Trauma* 2001;15:153-160.

11. Borelli J Jr, Ellis E: Pilon fractures: Assessment and treatment. *Orthop Clin North Am* 2002;33:231-245.

12. Moller BN, Krebs B: Intra-articular fractures of the distal tibia. *Acta Orthop Scand* 1982;53:991-996.

13. Ruedi TP: Fractures of the lower end of the tibia into the ankle joint: Results 9 years after open reduction and internal fixation. *Injury* 1973;5:130-134.

14. Sirkin M, Sanders R: The treatment of pilon fractures. *Orthop Clin North Am* 2001;32:91-102.

15. Kellam JF, Waddell JP: Fractures of the distal tibial metaphysis with intra-articular extension: The distal tibial explosion fracture. *J Trauma* 1979;19:593-601.

16. Bone L, Stegemann P, McNamara K, Seibel R: External fixation of severely comminuted and open tibial pilon fractures. *Clin Orthop* 1993;292:101-107.

17. Bonnin JG (ed): *Injuries to the Ankle*, ed 1. London, England, Heinemann, 1950, pp 248-260.

18. Ruoff AC III, Snider RK: Explosion fractures of the distal tibia with major articular involvement. *J Trauma* 1971;11:866-873.

19. Heim U (ed): *The Pilon Tibial Fracture: Classification, Surgical Techniques, Results*. Philadelphia, PA, WB Saunders, 1995.

20. Helfet DL, Shonnard PY, Levine D, Borrelli J Jr: Minimally invasive plate osteosynthesis of distal fractures of the tibia. *Injury* 1997;28(suppl 1):A42-A48.

21. Beck E: Results of operative treatment of pilon fractures, in Tscherne H, Schatzker J (eds): *Major Fractures of the Pilon, the Talus, and the Calcaneus: Current Concepts of Treatment*. Berlin, Germany, Springer-Verlag, 1993, pp 49-51.

22. McFerran MA, Smith SW, Boulas HJ, Schwartz HS: Complications encountered in the treatment of pilon fractures. *J Orthop Trauma* 1992;6:195-200.

23. Bourne RB: Pylon fractures of the distal tibia. *Clin Orthop* 1989;240:42-46.

24. Maale G, Seligson D: Fractures through the distal weight-bearing surface of the tibia. *Orthopedics* 1980;3:517-521.

25. Fitzpatrick DC, Marsh JL, Brown TD: Articulated external fixation of pilon fractures: The effects on ankle joint kinematics. *J Orthop Trauma* 1995;9:76-82.

26. Pierce RO Jr, Heinrich JH: Comminuted intra-articular fractures of the distal tibia. *J Trauma* 1979;19:828-832.

27. Teeny SM, Wiss DA: Open reduction and internal fixation of tibial plafond fractures: Variables contributing to poor results and complications. *Clin Orthop* 1993;292:108-117.

28. Wyrsch B, McFerran MA, McAndrew M, et al: Operative treatment of fractures of the tibial plafond: A randomized prospective study. *J Bone Joint Surg Am* 1996;78:1646-1657.

29. Tornetta P III, Weiner L, Bergman M, et al: Pilon fractures: Treatment with combined internal and external fixation. *J Orthop Trauma* 1993;7:489-496.

30. Allgower M, Muller ME, Willenegger H: *Technik der operativen Frakturbehandlung*. New York, NY, Springer-Verlag, 1963.

31. Marsh JL, Bonar S, Nepola JV, Decoster TA, Hurwitz SR: Use of an articulated external fixator for fractures of the tibial plafond. *J Bone Joint Surg Am* 1995;77:1498-1509.

32. Manca M, Marchetti S, Restuccia G, Faldini A, Giannini S: Combined percutaneous internal and external fixation of type-C tibial plafond fractures: A review of twenty-two cases. *J Bone Joint Surg Am* 2002;84(suppl 2):109-115.

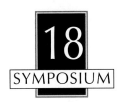

18

SYMPOSIUM

Surgical Management of Pediatric Femoral Fractures

Paul D. Sponseller, MD

Introduction

Pediatric femoral fractures are common injuries that have been treated successfully in a nonsurgical manner since the beginning of medicine. This chapter will review situations in which surgical treatment seems to be advantageous and to describe how to perform these operations safely and successfully.

Indications for Surgical Treatment

The decision to operate is based on the age and size of the patient, the presence of associated injuries, and the surgeon's experience with some of the surgical techniques. Specific associated injuries that may influence the decision include a tibial fracture creating a "floating knee", soft-tissue damage creating an open fracture, a head injury, or polytrauma.[1]

Surgical treatment of a floating knee generally provides a higher percentage of good results in terms of length and angulation than does nonsurgical treatment.[1] Open fractures tend to be better managed surgically because the management of the soft-tissue injury is made easier by access to the skin and ease of movement of the patient. In addition, open injuries take longer to heal, and the greater the soft-tissue injury, the longer the time to healing.[2] In some patients, therefore, surgical management may provide a useful benefit in preventing a long rehabilitation time.

Patients with closed head injuries often have a difficult neurologic recovery, sometimes associated with spasticity. The recovery period can be very difficult if the patient is in a cast or in traction. The angulation and length also are sometimes difficult to control in patients with a head injury. Fractures in the presence of head injuries may heal faster. Nevertheless, immediate surgery is not always safe if the intracranial pressure is unstable.

The polytrauma patient poses multiple and sometimes unpredictable challenges for the entire medical team. Fracture fixation in children has not been shown to decrease morbidity. However, surgical treatment that can control the fracture yet otherwise allow mobilization for the patient may make management and recovery easier.

For each range of patient ages, a specific set of techniques is particularly appropriate. Early spica casting works best in patients age 5 years or younger because these children are light and easy to mobilize, heal quickly, and do not need to be taken out of school.[3] Traction for 10 to 20 days followed by a spica cast is another option. Surgical methods have fewer advantages in this age group than in older children.

For children 6 to 10 years of age a stronger argument can be made for surgical fixation because of patient size, the need to be in school, and the demands of patient adjustment.[3] Flexible intramedullary nails probably provide the best quality of life during recovery.

External fixation also allows mobilization, but with some greater difficulty and discomfort.

For children 11 to 14 years of age, flexible nails may not stabilize the fractures as well as in younger patients, and the use of rigid intramedullary fixation becomes feasible. However, the risk of osteonecrosis has become recognized in the past few years with intramedullary fixation in patients younger than age 14 years (RA Mileski, MD, WW Huurman, MD, unpublished data, 1996). The risk of osteonecrosis can be lessened by making the entry portal through the greater trochanter. The size of these patients allows the use of a rigid nail that can be interlocked and maintains alignment well. An external fixator also is an option, although with external fixation, time to healing increases.

Specific Surgical Techniques
External Fixation

External fixation works much better in children than in adults because of the greater intrinsic healing potential in younger patients. Usually a monolateral fixator with four pins is satisfactory.[4-6] Two pins above and two pins below the fracture are used, except in unusually large patients; three pins above and below may be used for larger patients. The pins should be placed in the midlateral (coronal) plane so that they do not interfere with quadriceps motion any more than is necessary. They should be in the center of the bone so that they do not produce a

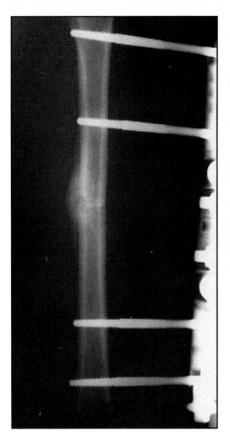

Fig. 1 Radiographic appearance of a femur fixed externally.

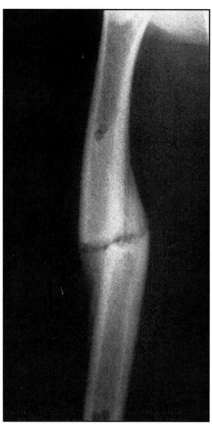

Fig. 2 The callus formed with external fixation is more modest than that with a spica.

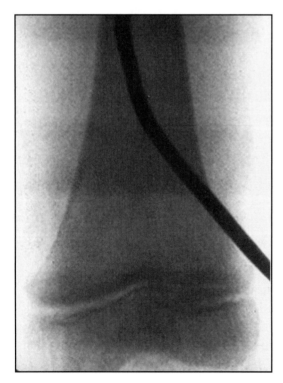

Fig. 3 The flexible nail is making the initial acute bend during retrograde insertion.

stress riser, thus causing refracture. In the operating room, the surgeon should strive for reduction of the fracture with no angulation and less than 1 cm of shortening because there may be some slight loss of position postoperatively (Fig. 1). Whether to attempt an anatomic "end-on" reduction or a bayonet apposition with some intentional shortening is up to the surgeon's discretion.[7] The overgrowth phenomenon does not seem to be exaggerated with the use of external fixation, so an anatomic reduction will produce at most a clinically insignificant 1 to 1.5 cm overgrowth.

After surgery, patients are allowed to bear weight as tolerated.[5] Return to school is possible, but is discouraged by many schools. In most patients, knee range of motion is somewhat limited while the fixator is in place. I do not try to push the range of motion beyond about 10° to 80° of flexion because it often is uncomfortable, and motion will return with removal of the fixator. The only exception to this is in a patient with extensive muscle damage around the knee, in whom the early fibrosis may be hard to reverse. It is helpful to give the family a prescription for oral antibiotics, to be taken in 5-day courses if the pin tracts become red. The occurrence of severe infections requiring intravenous antibiotics is rare, on the order of 1% to 2%.[5]

The fixator usually delays healing beyond that seen with a spica cast. In one large series of patients across the age spectrum, the mean time to healing was 11 weeks.[5] This is 2 to 3 weeks longer than would be expected for children treated in a spica cast. Loading and weight bearing may help this process. Refracture is a problem with external fixation; one study[8] reported a rate of 12%. Refracture rates seem to be highest with transverse or short oblique fractures, which have a lower fracture surface area. The fracture may occur through the original fracture or through a pin site.

The fixator should be removed only when satisfactory callus is definitely present on at least three of the four cortices on AP and lateral films[8] (Fig. 2). If there is any question about the quality of the healing, a simple protective cast consisting of a pelvic band and a thigh cuff, with the hip flexed 45°, may be used for 1 month. The fixator usually is removed with the patient under anesthetic sedation according to the preference of the family, although it can certainly be done in the clinic if the patient prefers.

Flexible Intramedullary Rods

Although they have fallen out of favor for use in femoral shaft fractures in adults, flexible intramedullary rods work well in children. The ideal age group is approximately 6 to 11 or 12 years of age, although flexible nails may be used outside this age group. The reasons for the success of flexible rods in patients in this age range seem to be the smaller canal diameter, lower mechanical stresses, and faster healing time of children. Patient comfort is probably greater with this method than with external fixation.

Flexible nails usually are inserted from distal to proximal.[9] Either a fracture table or a fluoroscopic table may be used. The entry points are approximately 1.5 cm above the distal femoral physis medially and laterally. A drill is used to make an entry hole, then is angled proximally as acutely as possible (Fig. 3). The nail chosen should be about 40% of the diameter of the isthmus of the femur. Options for implants include Rush rods, Ender nails, and elastic titanium implants. Each rod should be contoured in a C shape so that it provides three-point fixation in the femur.[10] Both rods are advanced to the fracture site, which is then reduced using an F-shaped leverage tool (Fig. 4). Rotation should also be reduced. After reduction, the rods are advanced proximally to the level of the calcar of the femur (Fig. 5). They are left about 1.5 cm

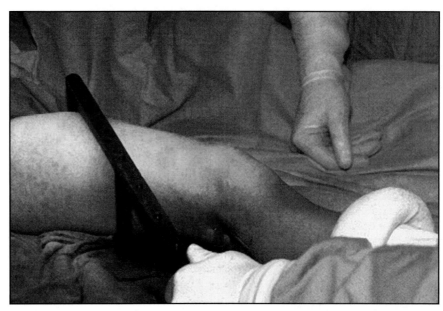

Fig. 4 The "F tool" is used for reduction during flexible nail insertion.

outside the femur distally to facilitate removal.

The most stable fractures to treat with flexible nails are those with a transverse or short oblique pattern. When the fracture is a long spiral or is comminuted, segmental, or very proximal, stability seems to be lessened. If the fracture does not appear to be intrinsically stable, then a protective spica cast can be used for 1 month or longer.

Patients treated with these nails should not bear weight until the fractures have healed. Rod removal is recommended and can be done as soon as the fracture is well healed, usually in 4 to 6 months. If the rods seem to be hard to remove, the process may be eased by waiting until additional growth has occurred and the wider metaphyseal part of the femur has migrated away from the rods. When removing elastic titanium nails, it is essential to have vise-grip pliers with narrow gripping ends.

Problems noted after the use of flexible nails have included angulation, malrotation, shortening, pin tract irritation, and refracture. This list should serve to remind the surgeon that the alignment is

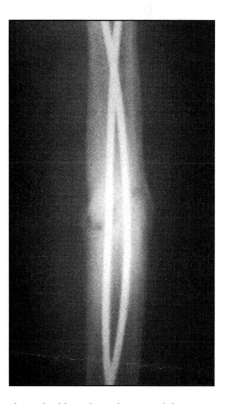

Fig. 5 Flexible nails in place to stabilize a femur fracture in an 8-year-old child.

not as automatic as with rigid rods in adults; therefore, attention to indications and technique is important.

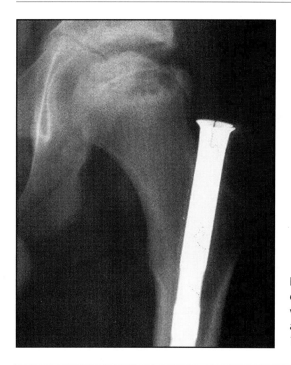

Fig. 6 Osteonecrosis is a potential complication after rigid nailing when the piriformis fossa is used as the entry site, as seen in this 12-year-old child.

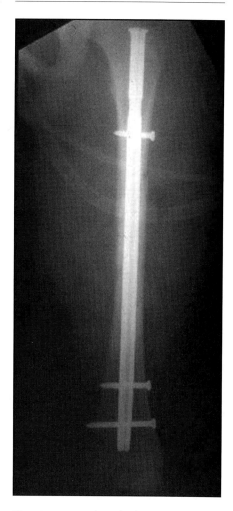

Fig. 7 To prevent the risk of osteonecrosis, the entry site for antegrade nailing may be made through the greater trochanter.

Rigid Intramedullary Nailing

Rigid intramedullary nailing of femoral shaft fractures is attractive because it produces automatic alignment, ease of recovery for patients, and a high union rate. A survey of the Pediatric Orthopaedic Society of North America showed that rigid intramedullary nails inserted through the piriformis fossa in skeletally immature patients carried an approximately 1% risk of osteonecrosis (RA Mileski, MD, WW Huurman, MD, unpublished data, 1996) (Fig. 6). It is hypothesized that this risk results from damage to the lateral ascending cervical arteries that supply the femoral epiphysis.[11] No reports have involved patients older than age 15 years or nails inserted through the greater trochanter.

In an attempt to combine safety with patient comfort, many orthopaedic surgeons use rigid nails inserted through the greater trochanter in patients between approximately 11 or 12 and 15 years of age (Fig. 7). The trochanteric entry technique does not produce any growth disturbance in this age group and requires only a small incision. Because of the non-linear trajectory necessitated by this entry site, some minor modifications are necessary,[12] including using a straight nail and accepting slight varus alignment or using a nail with a slight bend proximally. Implant options include a tibial nail rotated 90° (off-label usage not cleared by the Food and Drug Administration)[13] or one of the pediatric rigid nails now available. In small children, the surgeon should verify that the isthmus can be reamed to accommodate the rod and that the proper length is available in advance. With appropriate interlocking, early weight bearing is possible. Rod removal generally is recommended after healing because of the growth remaining.

Plate Fixation

The use of a plate occasionally is appropriate in children. Examples include polytrauma patients who need rapid stabilization in the absence of fluoroscopy and patients with fractures exposed for vascular repair. Disadvantages of plate fixation include the long incision required and relatively greater blood loss. The largest plate possible should be used, with at least four screws on either side of the fracture. Published studies of patients treated with plates[14,15] all report refracture with plate fatigue. The reported cases involved patients older than age 10 years, and refracture occurred several months after surgery, presumably when the patients began full weight bearing but when fracture healing was insufficient. If a plate is used, the patient should be limited to partial weight bearing until definite healing is seen on radiographs.

Costs of Treatment

With the advent of managed care, containing costs, even with trauma patients, is a concern. The common understanding was that traction for 2 to 3 weeks followed by a spica cast incurred a much higher cost than did surgical methods. However, a recent study[16] showed that, for surgical methods, the day in the operating room was so expensive that it equaled the costs of a long hospitalization, to say nothing of the costs of removing any implants. The only method clearly shown to be less expensive was early application of a spica cast. Costs, therefore, really should not be a major factor in making treatment decisions for pediatric femoral fractures.

Summary

In contrast to adult femoral fractures, there are many ways to treat a child's femoral fracture. The differences mainly involve ease of postoperative care and small rates of various complications. The surgeon should be familiar with at least one of the options for each age range and be adept at performing them to provide the best care for children of all ages.

References

1. Tolo VT: Orthopaedic treatment of fractures of the long bones and pelvis in children who have multiple injuries. *J Bone Joint Surg Am* 2000; 82:272-280.

2. Hutchins CM, Sponseller PD, Sturm P, Mosquero R: Open femur fractures in children: Treatment, complications, and results. *J Pediatr Orthop* 2000;20:183-188.

3. Hughes BF, Sponseller PD, Thompson JD: Pediatric femur fractures: Effects of spica cast treatment on family and community. *J Pediatr Orthop* 1995;15:457-460.

4. Aronson J, Tursky EA: External fixation of femur fractures in children. *J Pediatr Orthop* 1992;12:157-163.

5. Blasier RD, Aronson J, Tursky EA: External fixation of pediatric femur fractures. *J Pediatr Orthop* 1997;17:342-346.

6. Mendelow MJ, Kannellopoulos AD, Mencio GA, Green NE: External fixation of pediatric femur fractures. *Orthop Trans* 1998;21:185-186.

7. Miner T, Carroll KL: Outcomes of external fixation of pediatric femoral shaft fractures. *J Pediatr Orthop* 2000;20:405-410.

8. Skaggs DL, Leet AI, Money MD, Shaw BA, Hale JM, Tolo VT: Secondary fractures associated with external fixation in pediatric femur fractures. *J Pediatr Orthop* 1999;19:582-586.

9. Flynn JM, Hresko T, Reynolds RA, Blasier RD, Davidson R, Kasser J: Titanium elastic nails for pediatric femur fractures: A multicenter study of early results with analysis of complications. *J Pediatr Orthop* 2001;21:4-8.

10. Vrsansky P, Bourdelat D, Al Faour A: Flexible stable intramedullary pinning technique in the treatment of pediatric fractures. *J Pediatr Orthop* 2000;20:23-27.

11. Mileski RA, Garvin KL, Huurman WW: Avascular necrosis of the femoral head after closed intramedullary shortening in an adolescent. *J Pediatr Orthop* 1995;15:24-26.

12. Momberger N, Stevens P, Smith J, Santora S, Scott S, Anderson J: Intramedullary nailing of femoral fractures in adolescents. *J Pediatr Orthop* 2000;20:482-484.

13. Tortolani PJ, Ain MC, Miller NH, Brumback RJ, Sponseller PD: Tibial nails for femoral shaft fractures in adolescents: "Off-label" usage. *Orthopedics* 2001;24:553-557.

14. Fyodorov I, Sturm PF, Robertson WW Jr: Compression-plate fixation of femoral shaft fractures in children aged 8 to 12 years. *J Pediatr Orthop* 1999;19:578-581.

15. Ward WT, Levy J, Kaye A: Compression plating for child and adolescent femur fractures. *J Pediatr Orthop* 1992;12:626-632.

16. Stans AA, Morrissy RT, Renwick SE: Femoral shaft fracture treatment in patients 6 to 16 years. *J Pediatr Orthop* 1999;19:222-228.

Periprosthetic Fractures of the Femur After Total Hip Arthroplasty

Sung-Rak Lee, MD
Mathias P.G. Bostrom, MD

Abstract

The incidence of periprosthetic femur fracture has increased recently, and these fractures have become of a great concern to the reconstructive orthopaedic surgeon. Intraoperative fractures are usually stable. To prevent intraoperative fracture, careful preoperative planning and gentle surgical techniques are essential. In managing unstable intraoperative and late postoperative periprosthetic fractures, the surgeon should know the exact pattern of fracture, prosthesis stability, and bone quality. Loose prostheses should be revised and displaced fractures should be reduced and adequately fixed.

The incidence of complications related to total hip arthroplasty (THA) and revision THA is increasing as the population of patients with hip arthroplasties increases.[1-3] Although Scott and associates[4] reported that periprosthetic fractures occurred too rarely to draw any definite conclusions about the management of these fractures, as their incidence has increased, these fractures have become of great concern to the reconstructive orthopaedic surgeon, especially because of complexity of treatment and poor outcomes.[1-3,5-8]

Periprosthetic fractures of the femur can be divided into intraoperative and postoperative fractures. Intraoperative and early postoperative fractures are mainly related to intraoperative technical errors, whereas late postoperative fractures frequently are associated with loosening or osteolysis.[1,3,5,6,9,10] This chapter will focus on late postoperative periprosthetic fractures of the femur, and treatment approaches used at the Hospital for Special Surgery.

Intraoperative Periprosthetic Femoral Fractures

The incidence of intraoperative periprosthetic fractures is more common in cementless THAs because of the need for a tight press fit.[1,3,5] The incidence varies from 3% to 20% after cementless hip replacement and is much higher at revision surgery.[1,11]

Intraoperative periprosthetic fractures usually occur around the trochanteric area.[1,3] Prevention of these fractures is dependent on careful preoperative planning.[1,3] During THA these fractures can occur during reaming, broaching, or final seating of the implant.[1,9] If the surgeon believes there is a risk of fracture, prophylactic cerclage wires or cables should be used.[1,3] Because fracture can occur during every step of surgery,[6] careful handling of weakened bone is mandatory.

The treatment of recognized intraoperative fractures depends on their location, pattern, and the stability of the implant.[1,3] Fractures at the trochanteric area can be treated with cerclage wiring or cables, and fractures around the stem tip should be treated with a long-stem prosthesis that bypasses the fracture and fixation secured with bone graft.[1,3,5,9] Nondisplaced fractures not recognized during surgery are usually stable and can be treated with limited weight bearing;[1,3,9] however, displaced fractures may require reoperation.

Incidence of Postoperative Periprosthetic Femoral Fractures

Because periprosthetic fractures usually occur late and the follow-up periods differ between centers, the ex-

Table 1

Risk Factors Associated With Periprosthetic Femoral Fracture

General Factors	Local Factors
Osteoporosis	Loose prosthesis
Primary	Localized osteolysis
Secondary	Stress riser within the cortex
Female sex	Cementless prosthesis
Osteopenia	
Rheumatoid arthritis	
Osteomalacia	
Paget's disease	
Osteopetrosis	
Osteogenesis imperfecta	
Thalassemia	
Neuromuscular disorder	
Parkinsonism	
Neuropathic arthropathy	
Poliomyelitis	
Cerebral palsy	
Myasthenia gravis	
Seizures	
Ataxia	

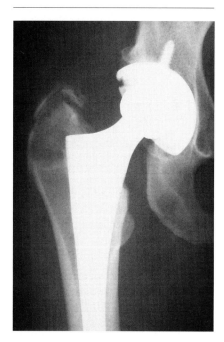

Figure 1 A type A$_G$ fracture.

act incidence of postoperative periprosthetic femur fracture is difficult to determine.[5]

Kavanagh[11] reported that the incidence of periprosthetic femur fracture was less than 1% after primary THA, and 4.2% after revision THA. Lewallen and Berry[2] reported the incidence of periprosthetic femur fracture was 0.6% after 17,597 primary cemented THAs, 2.8% after 3,265 cemented revision THAs, and 1.5% after 1,132 cementless revision THAs during 31 years. Berry[8] reported a 0.1% to 2.1% incidence of periprosthetic femur fracture. Based on these figures, the risk of postoperative periprosthetic femoral fracture can be estimated at between 1% to 4%.[3]

Etiology of Postoperative Periprosthetic Femoral Fractures

Periprosthetic femoral fractures are in actuality pathologic fractures, because there is usually an underlying bone lesion prone to fracture. Thus these fractures occur spontaneously or often in conjunction with minor trauma such as a fall.[5,8,12,13]

There are general and local risk factors related to periprosthetic femoral fracture (Table 1). General risk factors are any conditions causing increased bone fragility. Local risk factors are confined bony deficiencies, which are more important in the development of late periprosthetic femoral fractures.[1,3,5,6] Bethea and associates[14] reported 75% of patients with periprosthetic femoral fracture had underlying stem loosening and emphasized that loosening is a major risk factor of periprosthetic femoral fracture.[6] Therefore, early identification of these risk factors with serial radiographs is paramount.[3]

Classification of Postoperative Periprosthetic Femoral Fractures

In general, any classification system has to have the potential to guide treatment and enable comparison of results in different centers.[15] There are many classification systems of periprosthetic femoral fractures, but they all include the parameters of fracture location, pattern, and timing.[14,16,17] Historically, the Johansson classification has been used most commonly.[3] Type I fractures occur proximal to the stem tip. Type II fractures extend from proximal femoral shaft to beyond the stem. Type III fractures are situated entirely distal to the stem tip.[3]

Because periprosthetic femoral fractures occur around the femoral stem, the status of the stem stability and the bone stock around the stem are important.[3,15] The Vancouver classification is based on the location of fracture, stem stability, and status of the bone stock around the stem. It is the only classification system that has reported reliability and validity.[3,5,15,18] Type A fractures involve the trochan-

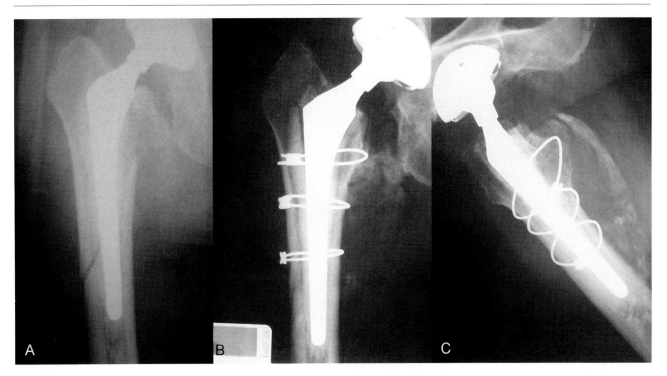

Figure 2 A, A type B1 fracture. **B** and **C,** The fracture was fixed with three cables and revealed fracture union and a stable prosthesis.

teric region and are subclassified as Type A_G fractures, which involve the greater trochanter (Figure 1), and type A_L fractures, which involve the lesser trochanter. Type B fractures occur around the stem of the femoral prosthesis, or extend slightly distal to it and are subclassified based on the stability of the implant and the quality of bone stock. In type B1 fractures (Figure 2), the implant is stable; in type B2 fractures (Figure 3), the implant is unstable or loose. In type B3 fractures, the stem is loose or unstable and the bone stock around the femoral component is inadequate (Figure 4). Bone stock may be inadequate because of severe osteopenia, osteolysis, or fracture comminution.[3,15] Type C fractures are so distal to the stem that the presence of the femoral component may be ignored (Figure 5). Duncan and Masri[3] reported that there were 4% type A, 18.5% type B1, 44.6% type B2, 36.9% type B3, and 9.3% type C

in a review of 75 periprosthetic femoral fractures that occurred between February 1985 and February 1994.

Treatment of Postoperative Periprosthetic Femoral Fractures

Periprosthetic femoral fractures can be difficult to manage and there is a high complication rate. Prosthesis stability and fracture union are issues that affect treatment. Beals and Tower,[19] in an analysis of 93 periprosthetic femoral fractures, reported 41% had complications relating to the fractures and 33% had complications relating to the arthroplasty.

Historically, these fractures were treated nonsurgically. Studies on the results of nonsurgical treatment reveal a high incidence of complications (malunion, delayed or nonunion, early prosthetic loosening, problems of recumbency).[20] Surgery has its own set of complications including the risk

of dislocation and infection;[21] however, in recent studies, surgical treatment is preferred except for nondisplaced fractures.[19,22-24]

The choice of treatment depends on fracture location, prosthesis stability, available bone stock, and age and medical status of the patient.[1] Prosthesis stability and the condition of the periprosthetic bone stock are of the most importance.[3,5,25] In principle, a loose prosthesis should be revised and a displaced fracture should be treated with reduction and secure fixation, which may not be easy to achieve.[3,5,15,22] Treatment must often be individualized with a combination of open reduction and internal fixation (ORIF) techniques (with plate, cable and/or strut allograft), with or without revision surgery.[1,2,5,9,12]

Type A Fracture

Most type A fractures are stable and minimally displaced and can be

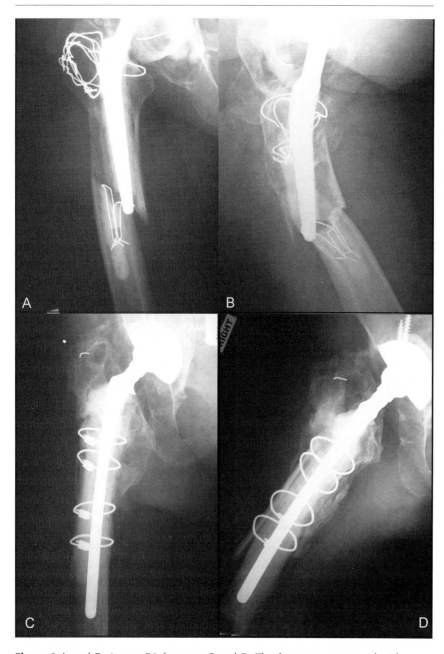

Figure 3 A and **B,** A type B2 fracture. **C** and **D,** The fracture was treated with a cemented long-stem prosthesis and four cables with two strut cortical allografts. The AP and lateral radiographs demonstrate good healing with graft incorporation.

treated nonsurgically.[1,2] When the displacement is widespread, ORIF with trochanteric wiring/cables with or without a trochanteric claw is preferred to maintain abductor function.[3,26] If a greater trochanter fracture is associated with osteolysis and severe polyethylene wear, then an acetabular revision, fixation of the displaced fragment, and bone graft should be considered.[2,3] Recently Claus and associates[27] reported nine cases of wear-related greater trochanteric fractures in 208 THA patients with mean 12.2-year follow-up, and found no correlation be-tween the size of osteolytic lesion and the risk of fracture. They emphasized that cortical erosion is a risk factor for fracture and recommended conservative treatment in case of minimal displacement and mild to moderate osteolysis.

Type B1 Fracture

There has been a high rate of malunion, nonunion, and implant loosening reported with nonsurgical treatment of type B1 fractures.[3,4,14,17,19,21] Therefore, most type B1 fractures should be treated with accurate reduction and secure internal fixation.[1]

Options for fixation are wires or cables, plate and screws and/or cables, cortical onlay allograft, and combined methods.[1-5,9,14,17,19,21] Cerclage wires or cables can be used to treat oblique or spiral fractures as well as for the fixation of plate or cortical strut grafts[1,5,9] (Figure 2). Use of demineralized bone matrix should be considered. If nonunion is present, use of bone morphogenetic protein may be indicated and is now available for this indication. Plates and screws are commonly used. In the proximal segment of the fracture, screw fixation may be difficult, so unicortical screws and/or cables can be used. In a biomechanical study, Dennis and associates[28] compared five options for plate fixation about the femoral stem: plate and cables, plate with proximal cables and distal bicortical screws, plate with proximal unicortical screws and distal bicortical screws, plate with proximal cables plus unicortical screws and distal bicortical screws, and two allograft struts fixed with cables. The plate constructs with proximal unicortical screws and distal bicortical screws or proximal unicortical screws, proximal cables, and distal bicortical screws were significantly more stable

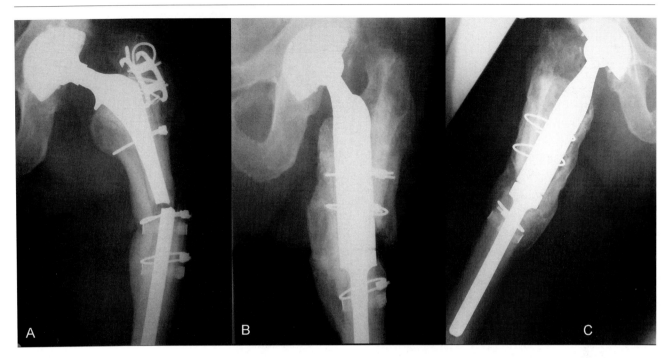

Figure 4 A, The AP radiograph of type B3 fracture reveals a deficient proximal lateral cortex and accompanying prosthesis fracture. **B** and **C,** The AP and lateral radiographs after replacement of the proximal femur. The proximal bone stock was repaired with cables.

in axial compression, lateral bending, and torsional loading than the other constructs.

The most important factors that determined the long-term results of the plate fixation are implant alignment, specifically cases of varus stem alignment with plate fixation result in high rates of late plate failure or implant loosening;[21,29] preservation of periosteal blood supply; and adequacy of stress riser augmentation. ORIF interferes with the extraosseous blood supply. Because of this decreased blood supply, Duncan and Masri[3] recommended routine bone grafting of all periprosthetic femoral fractures treated with ORIF. The reported union rates for plate and screws fixation and fixation with modified plates and cerclage wires range from 90% to 100%.[16,17]

Use of a cortical onlay strut allograft as a biologic plate can restore periprosthetic bone stock and has no

stress shielding effect; however, the time for graft incorporation can be prolonged. There is a possibility of stress fracture and these allografts are a potential source of infection.[5,30] Combination with a metal plate is preferable because of the weak mechanical strength of cortical allograft alone.[31]

Haddad and associates[30] reported the results of 2-year follow-up of cortical onlay allograft with or without plate in 40 patients with periprosthetic femoral fractures. There were no implant loosenings, and union was achieved in 98% (39 patients). Therefore, cortical onlay strut allograft proves to be a useful adjunct to ORIF but in B1 fractures should never be used alone.

Type B2 Fracture

In type B2 fractures, loose stems should be revised with a long-stem prosthesis, and fractures must be

fixed adequately.[1-3,5,9,22,24,26]

The most distal aspect of the fracture should be bypassed by at least two bone diameters with a long-stem prosthesis and fixed with a plate with or without cortical onlay strut allograft. The choice of implant is decided by the surgeon. The cementless prosthesis has the potential for biologic fixation[32] and the difficulty of cement use is avoided, which can prevent fracture union. The disadvantages of cementless femoral revision is that initial stability may be less than could be obtained with a well-fixed cemented prosthesis.[13,33]

In older individuals with limited lifespan and when early ambulation with weight bearing is critical, a cemented implant can be used (Figure 3). However, in young patients, a cementless prosthesis is preferred as long as fixation can be achieved in the isthmus of the femur or more proximally.

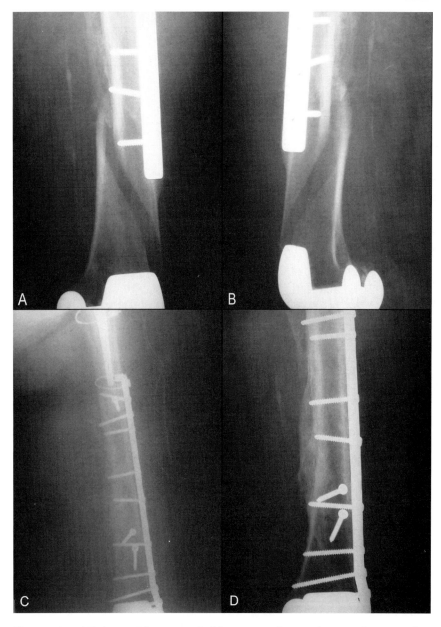

Figure 5 A and **B,** A type C fracture, spiral fracture can be seen between knee prosthesis and plate, which was used for treatment of a B1 periprosthetic fracture previously. **C** and **D,** The fracture was treated with DCS™ Plate (Synthes, Paoli, PA) and bone graft. Immediate postoperative and recent follow-up AP radiographs demonstrate good reduction and healing.

cementless long-stem revision combined with cerclage wiring and/or strut allograft.[10,13,25,33]

When infection is associated with periprosthetic femoral fractures, removal of the loose prosthesis and débridement of all necrotic or infected tissue is critical, followed by fracture stabilization.[9] Hartford and Goodman[37] reported the use of femoral intramedullary nailing as a salvage technique during complicated infected periprosthetic fractures. After removal of the loose infected stem, interim intramedullary nailing provides axial and rotational stability of the femur while maintaining femoral alignment.

Type B3 Fracture

For complex B3 fractures, surgical options include proximal femoral reconstruction or replacement. For proximal femoral reconstruction, impaction bone grafting with cortical onlay strut allograft or structural allografting of the proximal femur can be used.[3]

The choice of proximal femoral reconstruction or replacement is based on patient age, severity of bone defect, and the functional class of patient. In patients who have massive bone loss and a fracture, are older than 70 years of age, and place low demands on the hip, a modular proximal femoral replacement may be used[2] (Figure 4). If a fracture of the proximal femur is associated with circumferential uncontained loss of bone stock, a structural allograft may be indicated.[2,5,37,38]

Type C Fracture

This type of fracture can be treated independently of the arthroplasty according to the fracture treatment principles when there is loosening.[1-3] A frequently used method of fixation is a plate and

In the case of proximal femoral fracture, implant stability using a proximally porous coated stem may be more difficult to obtain[10,25] and proximal porous coated implants are associated with the poorest results and should be avoided.[2,34,35] Extensively coated long-stem curved prostheses that control torsion distally can be used. Fluted long stems can also be used because they have the capability of controlling torsion of the distal fragment.[2,10,12,13,26,36] Recent reports revealed good results with screws and/or cables with or without strut allograft (Figure 5). Retrograde intramedullary nailing is also possible. Because it is important to avoid the creation of any stress risers, the proximal end of the plate should overlap the femoral stem so as not to leave any region of the femur unprotected.[5]

Summary

Late postoperative periprosthetic fractures are challenging to treat. The patients are usually elderly and have multiple medical problems. The most important aspect of treatment is prevention. The creation of stress risers at the primary or revision surgery should be avoided, and pre-existing stress risers should be augmented.

The surgeon should know the exact pattern of fracture, prosthesis stability, and bone quality. According to the Vancouver classification, both aspects of periprosthetic fracture, the arthroplasty and the fracture, must be treated. Loose prostheses should be revised and displaced fractures should be reduced and adequately fixed.

References

1. Garbuz DS, Marsi BA, Duncan CP: Periprosthetic fractures of the femur: Principles of prevention and management. *Instr Course Lect* 1998;47:237-242.

2. Lewallen DG, Berry DJ: Periprosthetic fracture of the femur after total hip arthroplasty: Treatment and results to date. *Instr Course Lect* 1998;47:243-249.

3. Duncan CP, Masri BA: Fractures of the femur after hip replacement. *Instr Course Lect* 1995;44:293-304.

4. Scott RD, Turner RH, Leitzes SM, Aufranc OE: Femoral fractures in conjunction with total hip replacement. *J Bone Joint Surg Am* 1975;57:494-501.

5. Schmidt AH, Kyle RF: Periprosthetic fractures of the femur. *Orthop Clin North Am* 2002;33:143-152.

6. Haddad FS, Masri BA, Garbuz DS, Duncan CP: The prevention of periprosthetic fractures in total hip and knee arthroplasty. *Orthop Clin North Am* 1999;30:191-207.

7. Younger AS, Dunwoody I, Duncan CP: Periprosthetic hip and knee fractures: The scope of the problem. *Instr Course Lect* 1998;47:251-256.

8. Berry DJ: Epidemiology: Hip and knee. *Orthop Clin North Am* 1999;30:183-190.

9. Kelley SS: Periprosthetic femoral fractures. *J Am Acad Orthop Surg* 1994;2:164-172.

10. Moran MC: Treatment of periprosthetic fractures around total hip arthroplasty with an extensively coated femoral component. *J Arthroplasty* 1996;11:981-988.

11. Kavanagh BF: Femoral fractures associated with total hip arthroplasty. *Orthop Clin North Am* 1992;23:249-257.

12. Tower SS, Beals RK: Fractures of the femur after hip replacement: The Oregon experience. *Orthop Clin North Am* 1999;30:235-247.

13. Incavo SJ, Beard DM, Pupparo F, Ries M, Wiedel J: One-stage revision of periprosthetic fractures around loose cemented total hip arthroplasty. *Am J Orthop* 1998;27:35-41.

14. Bethea JS III, DeAndrade JR, Fleming LL, Lindenbaum SD, Welch RB: Proximal femoral fractures following total hip arthroplasty. *Clin Orthop* 1982;170:95-106.

15. Brady OH, Garbuz DS, Marsi BA, Duncan CP: Classification of the hip. *Orthop Clin North Am* 1999;30:215-220.

16. Serocki JH, Chandler RW, Dorr LD: Treatment of fractures about hip prostheses with compression plating. *J Arthroplasty* 1992;7:129-135.

17. Cooke PH, Newman JH: Fractures of the femur in relation to cemented hip prostheses. *J Bone Joint Surg Br* 1988;70:386-389.

18. Brady OH, Garbuz DS, Marsi BA, Duncan CP: The reliability and validity of the Vancouver classification of femoral fractures after hip replacement. *J Arthroplasty* 2000;15:59-62.

19. Beals RK, Tower SS: Periprosthetic fractures of the femur: An analysis of 93 fractures. *Clin Orthop* 1996;327:238-246.

20. Somers JF, Suy R, Stuyck J, Mulier M, Fabry G: Conservative treatment of femoral shaft fractures in patients with total hip arthroplasty. *J Arthroplasty* 1998;13:162-171.

21. Campbell P, McWilliams TG: Periprosthetic femoral fractures. *Curr Orthop* 2002;16:126-132.

22. McLauchlan GJ, Robinson CM, Singer BR, Christie J: Results of an operative policy in the treatment of periprosthetic femoral fracture. *J Orthop Trauma* 1997;11:170-179.

23. Mont MA, Maar DC: Fractures of the ipsilateral femur after hip arthroplasty: A statistical analysis of outcome based on 487 patients. *J Arthroplasty* 1994;9:511-519.

24. Crockarell JR Jr, Berry DJ, Lewallen DG: Nonunion after periprosthetic femoral fracture associated with total hip arthroplasty. *J Bone Joint Surg Am* 1999;81:1073-1079.

25. Macdonald SJ, Paprosky WG, Jablonsky WS, Magnus RG: Periprosthetic femoral fractures treated with a long-stem cementless component. *J Arthroplasty* 2001;16:379-383.

26. Wilson D, Marsi BA, Duncan CP: Periprosthetic fractures: An operative algorithm. *Orthopedics* 2001;24:869-870.

27. Claus AM, Hopper RH Jr, Engh CA: Fractures of the greater trochanter induced by osteolysis with the anatomic medullary locking prosthesis. *J Arthroplasty* 2002;17:706-712.

28. Dennis MG, Simon JA, Kummer FJ, Koval KJ, DiCesare PE: Fixation of periprosthetic femoral shaft fractures occurring at the tip of the stem: A biomechanical study of 5 techniques. *J Arthroplasty* 2000;15:523-528.

29. Tadross TS, Nanu AM, Buchanan MJ, Checketts RG: Dall-Miles plating for periprosthetic B1 fractures of the femur. *J Arthroplasty* 2000;15:47-51.

30. Haddad FS, Duncan CP, Berry DJ, Lewallen DG, Gross AE, Chandler HP: Periprosthetic femoral fractures around well-fixed implants: Use of cortical onlay allografts with or without a plate. *J Bone Joint Surg Am* 2002;84:945-950.

31. Chandler HP, Tigges RG: The role of allografts in the treatment of periprosthetic femoral fractures. *J Bone Joint Surg Am* 1997;79:1422-1432.

32. Jensen JS, Barford G, Hansen D, et al: Femoral shaft fracture after hip arthroplasty. *Acta Orthop Scand* 1988;59:9-13.

33. Kolstad K: Revision THR after periprosthetic femoral fractures: An

analysis of 23 cases. *Acta Orthop Scand* 1994;65:505-508.

34. Berry DJ, Harmsen WS, Ilstrup D, Lewallen DG, Cabanela ME: Survivorship of uncemented proximally porous-coated femoral components. *Clin Orthop* 1995;319:168-177.

35. Malkani AL, Lewallen DG, Cabanela ME, Wallrichs SL: Femoral component revision using an uncemented, proximally coated, long-stem prosthesis. *J Arthroplasty* 1996;11:411-418.

36. Ries MD: Periprosthetic fractures: Early and late. *Orthopedics* 1997;20:798-800.

37. Hartford JM, Goodman SB: The use of femoral intramedullary nailing as an interim or salvage technique during complicated total hip replacement. *J Arthroplasty* 1998;13:467-472.

38. Wong P, Gross AE: The use of structural allografts for treating periprosthetic fractures about the hip and knee. *Orthop Clin North Am* 1999;30:259-264.

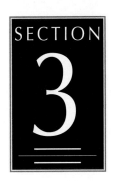

SECTION 3

Pelvic and Acetabular Trauma

Pelvic and Acetabular Trauma

Pelvic fractures are commonly caused by falls and motor vehicle accidents, and although these injuries often can be managed nonsurgically, the natural history of displaced pelvic injuries is associated with a high incidence of back pain, gait abnormalities, and sitting imbalance as a result of pelvic obliquity.

Intense interest in the diagnosis and treatment of pelvic fractures has produced more than 200 publications in the last 10 years. This research has led to the development of reproducible surgical techniques that reliably improve outcomes. This section of *Instructional Course Lectures Trauma* attempts to summarize the current knowledge about and approaches to patients with pelvic fractures. As a way of introduction, the following paragraphs attempt to illuminate both established areas and areas in which further research is needed to resolve ongoing questions regarding the best treatment for pelvic ring injuries.

Despite improvements in surgical techniques, orthopaedic traumatologists clearly do not have uniform indications for surgical stabilization. Professor Emil Letournel described the presence of instability or deformity of the pelvic ring as indications for open reduction and internal fixation. However, the adjectives deformity and instability are problematic when assigned to patients.

The article by Steven Olson and Andrew Burgess defines a stable pelvic ring injury as one that will "withstand the physiological forces incurred with protected weight bearing (and/or bed-to-chair mobilization) without abnormal deformation of the pelvis until bony union or soft-tissue healing can occur." Perhaps most importantly, they note that displacement of the innominate bones and the sacrum typically indicates instability. A detailed explanation of classification systems follows and assists in distinguishing between stable and unstable injuries.

For the small percentage of patients with high-energy injuries, the importance of obtaining skeletal stability as part of the resuscitation effort is not controversial. The correlation of systemic injuries with the pattern of pelvic injury is useful in estimating transfusion requirements and thus identifying patients who are at risk for exsanguination. Several protocols for the management of patients with pelvic ring injuries and hemodynamic instability have been published, and the authors review the advantages and disadvantages of each approach. These authors are especially adept at analyzing different protocols in the context of available resources; this analysis is particularly useful when determining whether a specific approach is either more or less suitable for a specific hospital.

Surgical management of pelvic injuries is potentially complicated and technically demanding. In an article I wrote with Tamara Simpson and Joel Matta, the options for surgical treatment of these injuries are reviewed. Unstable pelvic ring injuries with significant deformity are best treated by open reduction and internal fixation. Obtaining a reduction is paramount because anatomic alignment restores sitting balance and avoids limb-length discrepancy. Established indications for surgical treatment appear to be displacement of the posterior ring of at least 1 cm and sacroiliac fracture-dislocations. Although the indications for the treatment of sacral fractures are not as well defined, those caused by lateral compression injuries and characterized by less than 1 cm of displacement have been reported to be inherently stable. Treatment of these injuries with early protected weight bearing is not associated with further fracture displacement.

The debate surrounding whether open or closed reduction is the best approach to achieve an accurate reduction continues. There are strong advocates for both sides, but no prospective studies comparing the two. The primary problem remains reduction of the deformity, and this should be foremost in the mind of the surgeon. Historically, open reduction has been associated with a high rate of wound complications; however, a recent multicenter study documented a low incidence of wound problems (3.9%).

What are the results of treatment, and what are the expected outcomes for patients with pelvic injuries? Because these injuries frequently are a result of high-energy trauma and often affect multiple systems, these are complex questions. Factors that require consideration include whether the pelvic injury is bony or ligamentous, whether the patient has associated neurologic and urologic injuries, and whether the fracture is displaced.

The anatomic location of the fracture and the quality of the reduction also affect patient outcomes. The quality of reduction has been correlated with outcome; patients with displaced injuries have poorer results at final follow-up. Given the number of variables, however, the study of outcomes can be difficult and, in some reports, even confusing. Scoring systems that attempt to evaluate quality of life are difficult to use in patients with pelvic injuries because many of these patients also have lower extremity injuries, sometimes severe, that may be the key factor affecting quality of life. Examples of these populations include patients with pilon fractures or severe open tibia fractures.

Paul Tornetta and I wrote both a historical and thorough review of expected outcomes after pelvic ring injuries. Associated injuries to the urologic system occur in about 15% of patients with pelvic injuries, and sequelae such as urethral strictures, impotence, and sexual dysfunction occur despite excellent skeletal reduction and fixation. The degree of neurologic injury also has been correlated with ultimate functional outcome. Neurologic injuries are specific both to the pattern of injury and the extent of fracture displacement. Anatomic reduction does not appear to significantly affect recovery because the severity of the injury is believed to occur at the time of the initial insult.

The final two articles in this section focus on treatment of acetabular fractures. The first, by Dana Mears and John Velyvis, reviews primary total hip arthroplasty (THA) after acetabular fracture. David Helfet and Arif Ali address periprosthetic fractures of the acetabulum after THA. Patients with acetabular fractures are at risk for posttraumatic osteoarthritis; therefore, the role of THA and its associated complications is important to understand for long-term care and follow-up of these patients. Mears and Velyvis outline the classification of the numerous problems associated with failed acetabular fracture surgery and present details on the surgical techniques. The article reviews literature that documents the extensive problems with performing THA after acetabular fracture surgery. They also note that there is a group of patients who may benefit from primary THA after acetabular fracture— a point that remains quite controversial because they note it is "only appropriate for a highly selected group of patients."

The aging of the US population and the widespread acceptance of THA will undoubtedly lead to an increased number of periprosthetic fractures of the acetabulum. Helfet and Ali describe both intraoperative and postoperative occurrences of these fractures. One of the critical problems associated with this complication is whether the anterior or posterior column was involved and, more importantly, whether there was fracture union at the time of the planned revision. An algorithm based on the time of the fracture and the stability of the innominate bone should be of great help in the management of this complex problem.

David C. Templeman, MD
Associate Professor
Department of Orthopaedic Surgery
University of Minnesota
Hennepin County Medical Center
Minneapolis, Minnesota

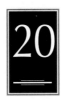

Classification and Initial Management of Patients With Unstable Pelvic Ring Injuries

Steven A. Olson, MD, FACS
Andrew Burgess, MD

Abstract

Unstable pelvic ring injuries in hemodynamically unstable patients are life-threatening emergencies that many orthopaedic surgeons encounter in practice. Therefore, it is important to be up to date regarding current methods of evaluating, assessing, and treating patients with these complex and severe injuries. Surgeons should first determine whether patients have hemodynamic instability and identify the source of the hemorrhage. Patients should then be assessed for stabilization of unstable pelvic ring injuries.

Most pelvic fractures treated by orthopaedic surgeons are stable injuries that occur as the result of either a low-energy mechanism, such as a fall, or a high-energy mechanism, during which little energy is actually transmitted to the pelvis. The management of low-energy pelvic ring injuries is generally nonsurgical, with progressive weight bearing permitted as tolerated. Although true high-energy pelvic ring injuries make up a relatively small percentage of all pelvic ring injuries, they give rise to greater concern among orthopaedic surgeons.

Anatomy

The pelvis is composed of a bony ring made up by the sacrum and the two innominate bones. The two innominate bones meet anteriorly at the pubic symphysis, where they are united by a fibrocartilaginous interpubic disk, which is reinforced from above by the superior pubic ligament and from below by the arcuate pubic ligament.[1] Additional anterior support is provided by the anterior abdominal wall and inguinal ligaments. In the posterior pelvic ring, the innominate bones articulate with the sacrum. The sacrum is roughly triangular when viewed in the frontal plane and trapezoidal when viewed in an axial projection.[1] The configuration of the sacrum reflects its mechanical role in transmitting load from the axial skeleton to the lower extremities. Tile[2] compared the sacrum to the keystone of an arch in that an axially applied load increases the stability of the articulation of the hemipelves, sacrum, and lumbar spine.

The sacroiliac joint is the major articulation between the sacrum and innominate bones. This joint has a relatively small synovial cavity between two large articular surfaces.[1] Schunke[3] described the sacral cartilage as being hyaline in nature but found the iliac articular surface to be nearly always fibrocartilaginous in adults. The articular surface of the sacroiliac joint is irregular in contour, which contributes to its intrinsic stability. The strong posterior ligamentous complex provides most of the mechanical stability to the pelvis.[1,2,4,5] The interosseous ligaments, which originate from the internal surface of the iliac wing posterior to the sacroiliac articulation and run to the dorsal surface of the sacrum, are thought to be the primary stabilizing ligaments of the sacroiliac joint. The long posterior sacroiliac ligaments are oriented longitudinally and blend with the fibers of the sacrotuberous ligament.[1,4] More ventrally, the anterior sacroiliac ligaments represent the anterior part of the fibrous capsule of the sacroiliac joint. This fibrous membrane is thin and relatively weak.[2]

The pelvic floor is supported by the sacrotuberous and sacrospinous ligaments that contribute to the posterior, superior, and rotational stability of the pelvic ring.[1,2,4] The sacrotuberous ligament originates in three locations: from the dorsal surface of the lower three sacral vertebrae, from a posterior portion of the iliac crest in the region between the posterior-superior and posterior-inferior iliac spines, and from the long posterior sacroiliac ligaments.[1] From these origins, the fibers run laterally and inferiorly to form a strong ligamentous attachment at the medial border of the ischial tuberosity. The medial portion of this attachment of the tuberosity blends with the obturator internus membrane as the falciform process. The sacrospinous ligament is thinner and narrower than the sacrotuberous ligament. It is triangular, originates on the lateral border of the sacrum and coccyx, and inserts on the ischial spine. The sacrospinous ligament divides the posterior pelvis into the greater sciatic foramen and lesser sciatic foramen. The pudendal nerve courses posteriorly over the sacrospinous ligament after exiting the greater sciatic notch to enter the lesser sciatic notch, where it courses along the inferior pubic ramus before exiting into the perineum. The anterior surface of the sacrospinous ligament blends with the coccygeus muscle, which is thought to represent a degenerated posterior part of the muscle belly itself.[1]

Superiorly, the iliolumbar ligament arises from the transverse process of the fifth lumbar vertebrae and extends to insert on the inner surface of the ilium just anterior to the sacroiliac joint, blending with the anterior sacroiliac ligaments.[1] With superior or lateral displacement of the hemipelvis, strain on this ligament often results in avulsion fractures of the fifth lumbar transverse processes. These fractures serve as radiographic markers for the severity of the injury.

Pathoanatomy

Pelvic ring injuries have classically been categorized as stable or unstable.[5-7] A stable pelvic ring injury can be defined as one that will withstand the physiologic forces incurred with protected weight bearing (and/or bed-to-chair mobilization without abnormal deformation of the pelvis) until bony union or soft-tissue healing can occur. However, in clinical practice it is displacement of the innomi-

nate bones and sacrum that typically indicates instability.

Tile[2] sequentially sectioned ligaments of anatomic specimen pelves to investigate the ligamentous contributions to pelvic stability. When the pubic symphysis is sectioned without injury to other ligamentous structures, loading of the pelvis results in pubic symphysis diastasis of as much as 2.5 cm. Further opening is inhibited by the sacrospinous and anterior sacroiliac ligaments. If the pubic symphysis and sacrospinous ligaments (pelvic floor) are both sectioned, more than 2.5 cm of pubic symphysis diastasis (external rotation of the hemipelvis) can occur. Recently, however, Vrahas and associates[5] have reported mechanical testing of ligamentous injuries and have shown very minimal contributions of the sacrospinous and sacrotuberous ligaments to overall pelvic stability. Impingement of the posterior iliac spines against the sacrum eventually limits the total amount of hemipelvis external rotation possible. The effect of the abdominal wall on rotational stability of the pelvis has recently been emphasized. Ghanayem and associates[8] reported a substantial increase in injured pelvic volume after laparotomy in a cadaver with an experimentally induced rotationally and vertically unstable pelvic injury. As long as the posterior interosseous and sacroiliac ligaments remain intact, posterior, superior, or inferior migration of the hemipelvis does not occur. In this instance, the pelvis is said to be rotationally unstable.[2,9] The rotationally unstable pelvic injury can be restored to its anatomic integrity by using the intact posterior ligamentous complex as a hinge or tension band.

Tile[2] also found that sectioning of the pubic symphysis, sacrospinous ligament, sacrotuberous ligament, and the posterior sacroiliac ligamentous complex (including interosseous ligaments) created a markedly unstable posterior hemipelvis that allowed posterior and superior translation of the innominate bone relative to

the sacrum in addition to rotational displacement. This posterior-superior complex of instabilities is often referred to as vertical instability of the pelvis.[2,4] With complete disruption of the posterior ligamentous complex in the pelvic ring, the potential displacements of the innominate bone relative to the sacrum are posterior migration, superior migration, internal or external rotation of the innominate bone (rotation in the horizontal plane), and flexion of the innominate bone (rotation in the sagittal plane).

Radiographic Assessment

Radiographic assessment of the pelvis is an essential part of the evaluation of pelvic ring injuries. An AP radiograph of the pelvis is obtained in the resuscitation room for all trauma patients[10] (Figure 1, A). This is a very useful view for identifying pelvic ring injuries that may be potential causes of hemodynamic instability.[2,4,11] Initial assessment for integrity of the pubic rami, pubic symphysis, and posterior structures such as the sacroiliac joints and iliac wings is possible with the AP view. Sacral fractures are often visible on the AP view, although occasionally they are quite difficult to visualize. The additional plain film radiographs used in evaluation of pelvic ring injuries include the inlet (or caudad) projection, the outlet (or cephalad) projection of the pelvic ring, and the lateral view of the sacrum. The inlet view is taken with the patient supine and the tube directed in a caudad direction approximately 40° from vertical[2,4,12] (Figure 1, B). This view is extremely useful for evaluating continuity of the pelvic ring. Displacement of the pelvic ring at the sacroiliac joint can be clearly visualized. This view is also very useful for evaluating rotational deformities of the hemipelvis and for identifying fracture lines that cross the sacral ala or body. The outlet view is taken with the patient supine and the tube directed in a cephalad direction approximately 40° from ver-

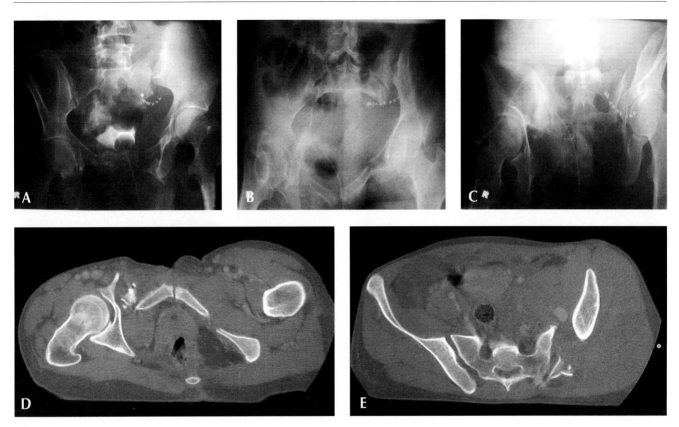

Figure 1 Bucholz type III instability pattern. **A,** AP view of the hemipelvis (slightly rotated) demonstrating obvious disruption of the posterior pelvic ring with superior translation of the iliac segment relative to the sacrum. This is a fracture-dislocation. Note the residual segment of iliac wing with the sacrum. The superior gluteal artery has been embolized in this case. **B,** Inlet view of the hemipelvis demonstrating significant posterior translation of the posterior pelvic ring. Note again the intact segment of iliac wing with the sacrum, indicating that this is a fracture-dislocation. Note also the significant translation of the contralateral anterior pubic ramus segment. **C,** Outlet view demonstrating significant superior translation of the left hemipelvis. Note the difference in the height of the ischial tuberosities relative to the sacrum. **D,** CT scan of an anterior pelvic ring injury. Note the significant amount of soft-tissue disruption and translation of the right-sided anterior pubic ramus segment. **E,** CT scan of a posterior pelvic ring injury. Note the obvious left-sided sacroiliac joint disruption. The innominate bone on the left is at a level just above the acetabulum, whereas the right innominate bone is at the level of the iliac wing. This indicates a significant amount of superior translation on the injured left hemipelvis.

tical[2,4,12] (Figure 1, *C*). This radiographic view is useful for determining superior or inferior displacement and flexion or sagittal plane rotation of the hemipelvis. The sacral foramina are seen best on this view, and this view often offers the best visualization of fractures through the sacrum. The lateral view of the sacrum is useful in identifying transverse sacral fractures and fractures of the coccyx.[13] Transverse sacral fractures at the level of S3 or below do not result in pelvic ring instability, but they can be extremely painful and often are unrecognized without careful inspection of a lateral view.

Bony injuries reflecting associated soft-tissue trauma are frequently visible on the three views (AP, caudad, and cephalad) of the pelvis.[2,4,11,14,15] These include avulsions of the transverse process of the fifth lumbar vertebra (which are associated with disruption of the iliolumbar ligament) and avulsions of the ischial spine or the inferior portion of the sacral cortex (which are associated with disruption of the sacrospinous and sacrotuberous ligaments). The work of Tile[2,9] and others has demonstrated that 1 cm of posterior or superior migration of the hemipelvis on either the AP, cau-

dad, or cephalad view suggests complete posterior and interosseous ligament disruption in the hemipelvis.[2,4,15] Limb-length discrepancies can also be noted by assessing the level of the hip joints on the AP view.[4]

CT continues to play a major role in the evaluation of the posterior pelvic ring. CT is often the best method for determining the exact nature of a posterior pelvic ring injury because it can discriminate between the type and location of injury, whether in the sacrum, sacroiliac joint, or iliac wing; it is also useful as an adjunct in defining associated acetabu-

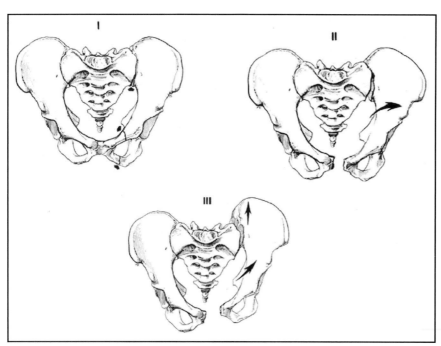

Figure 2 Illustration of the Bucholz fracture classification system. Type I fractures are stable pelvic ring injuries. Type II fractures have partial or rotational instability and are typically open-book type injuries. Type III fractures have complete instability with disruption at both anterior and posterior pelvic ring. (Adapted with permission from Bucholz RW: The pathological anatomy of Malgaigne fracture-dislocations of the pelvis. *J Bone Joint Surg Am* 1981;63:400-404.)

lar injuries[14] (Figures 1, *D* and *E*). CT can also aid in the evaluation of sacroiliac joint instability. Uniform separation of the sacroiliac joint surfaces from anterior to posterior is an indication of disruption of the strong interosseous posterior ligaments, which is typically an indication of a globally unstable injury posteriorly, whereas anterior separation of the sacroiliac joint with posterior apposition of the sacroiliac joint is typically an indication of a more rotationally unstable injury without vertical instability.[4,14]

Most pelvic ring injuries can be characterized via physical and radiographic examination. Those rare injuries for which questions remain regarding the presence of instability can be further assessed by direct examination of the hemipelvis under anesthesia or with the use of push-pull films.[9] Push-pull films are obtained with the patient under gen-

eral anesthesia with traction applied to the leg, ipsilateral to the hemipelvis being assessed. Although any motion in the pelvic ring is abnormal, displacement of 10 mm or greater is generally considered grossly unstable. These studies are contraindicated in the presence of zone 2 or 3 sacral fractures (as categorized by Denis and associates[16]) and in patients who are hemodynamically unstable because this maneuver may exacerbate soft-tissue injury. Instances of late displacement of the hemipelvis despite initial normal push-pull films have been noted (J Kellam, MD, personal communication, 1995). Push-pull films are occasionally used to assess the possibility of obtaining a closed reduction.

Classification

Bucholz[6] reported the findings at autopsy of patients with pelvic ring injuries who

died as a result of associated trauma. His findings provide a clinical correlation to the bench top tests performed by Vrahas and associates[5] and Tile.[2,9] Bucholz[6] devised a classification system describing three basic categories of pelvic ring injuries (Figure 2). Type I injuries have a stable pelvic ring with isolated pubic symphysis disruption or pubic rami fractures without other ligamentous or displaced bony injuries. Bucholz noted that isolated pubic rami fractures are frequently accompanied by an impacted or nondisplaced sacral fracture. Type II injuries are rotationally unstable pelvic ring injuries with either internal or external rotation deformities of the hemipelvis relative to the sacrum. Type III injuries are rotationally and vertically unstable injuries. Vertical instability refers to disruption of the anterior and posterior pelvic ring allowing potential displacement posteriorly, superiorly, and in sagittal plane rotation (flexion) in addition to rotation in the horizontal plane (internal or external rotation).

The Tile classification system categorizes pelvic ring injuries according to severity as type A, B, or C (type A is least severe and type C is most severe). This system, detailed in Table 1, combines both mechanism of injury and potential instability in classifying pelvic ring injuries. Type B injuries are subdivided as B1 injuries (open-book or anterior-posterior compression injuries without posterior ring instability) or B2 injuries (lateral compression injuries). These are both considered rotational instabilities in this classification system. However, B2 injuries can often be treated nonsurgically because they are clinically stable. Thus, the type B category includes injuries with mixed instabilities. The Orthopaedic Trauma Association has adopted an official fracture classification system.[17] For pelvic ring injuries, this is identical to the Tile classification system with the addition of a numeric modifier (61A, 61B, or 61C).

Young and Burgess[11] have developed a modification of the Tile classification system based primarily on mechanism of injury (Figure 3). This classification divides injuries into lateral compression, anterior-posterior compression, vertical shear, and combined mechanical injury categories. Lateral compression and anterior-posterior compression injuries each have three gradations of severity. Anterior-posterior compression type I injuries are essentially stable pelvic ring injuries with isolated pubic symphysis or pubic ramus disruption. Anterior-posterior compression type II injuries are rotationally unstable and are associated with disruption of the pubic symphysis or, less commonly, fracture of the pubic rami and disruption of the sacrotuberous, sacrospinous, and anterior sacroiliac ligaments. Anterior-posterior compression type III injuries are associated with disruption of the posterior sacroiliac ligaments and are rotationally and vertically unstable.[11]

Lateral compression type I injuries produce horizontal fractures of the ischial and pubic rami in the anterior ring and impaction fractures in the sacrum. All major ligamentous structures remain intact, and the pelvis remains grossly stable. A lateral compression type II injury is associated with either a ligamentous disruption of a sacroiliac joint posteriorly or an equivalent bony disruption of the posterior ilium. Because posterior pelvic ring injuries are not stable impactions, rotational instability results. Ligaments of the pelvic floor remain intact, resulting in relative vertical stability. A lateral compression type III injury creates the so-called windswept pelvis. This injury typically results from a rollover mechanism. The site of initial impact usually sustains a lateral compression type II injury with internal rotational displacement, and, as the tire or offending structure crosses the pelvis, the contralateral hemipelvis sustains an external rotational (or anterior-posterior compression) injury. Vertical

Table 1
Tile Classification System for Pelvic Ring Injuries

Type A: Stable pelvic ring injuries	
A1	Fractures not involving the pelvic ring; avulsion injuries
A1.1	Anterior-superior spine
A1.2	Anterior-inferior spine
A1.3	Ischial tuberosity
A2	Stable, minimal displacement
A2.1	Iliac wing fractures
A2.2	Isolated anterior pelvic ring injuries
A2.3	Stable, nondisplaced or minimally displaced fractures of the pelvic ring
A3	Transverse fractures of the sacrum or coccyx
A3.1	Nondisplaced transverse sacral fractures
A3.2	Displaced transverse sacral fractures
A3.3	Coccygeal fractures
Type B: Rotationally unstable, vertically stable pelvic ring injuries	
B1	External rotational instability, open-book injuries
B1.1	Unilateral injury
B1.2	< 2.5 cm displacement
B1.3	> 2.5 cm displacement
B2	Internal rotational instability, lateral compression injuries
B2.1	Ipsilateral anterior and posterior injuries
B2.2	Contralateral anterior and posterior injuries, bucket-handle fracture
B3	Bilateral posterior rotational instability injuries
Type C: Rotationally and vertically unstable pelvic ring injuries	
C1	Unilateral injuries
C1.1	Fractures through ilium
C1.2	Sacroiliac dislocations and/or fracture-dislocations
C1.3	Sacral fractures
C2	Bilateral injury, one-sided rotational instability, one-sided rotational and vertical instability
C3	Bilateral injury, both sides with rotational and vertical instability

(Adapted with permission from Kellam J, Browner B: Fractures of the pelvic ring, in Browner B, Jupiter J, Levine A, Trafton P (eds): *Skeletal Trauma: Fractures, Dislocations, and Ligamentous Injuries.* Philadelphia, PA, WB Saunders, 1992.)

shear injuries are of only one type and are associated with disruption of all major ligamentous constraints, with resultant rotational and vertical instability. Other pelvic ring injuries typically fall into the combined mechanical injury category.[11]

Letournel suggested a classification of pelvic ring injuries based on the anatomic site of injury by dividing sites of injury into anterior and posterior pelvic ring locations[3] (Figure 4). In this classification system, anterior ring injuries include pure symphysis pubis diastasis, vertical fracture lines dividing the obturator ring or adjacent body of the pubis, and acetabular fractures. Posterior pelvic ring injuries include transiliac fractures not involving the sacroiliac joint, fracture-dislocations of the sacroiliac joint with the bony injury extending either through

the sacrum or through the iliac wing (the so-called crescent fracture), pure sacroiliac joint disruption, and transsacral fractures. Denis and associates[16] further characterized sacral fractures based on the anatomic region within the sacrum. In this classification system, zone 1 injuries include fractures to the sacral ala lateral to the sacral foramina that do not cross the sacral foramina or sacral body; zone 2 injuries include fractures extending into the sacral foramina that may begin in the sacral ala and extend to the foramina; and zone 3 injuries include fractures that extend into the central body of the sacrum and can be vertical, oblique, or transverse and cross the sacrum in any number of patterns, all of which involve the sacral body and canal. The classification system of Denis and associates has

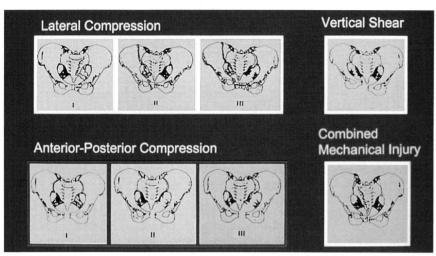

Figure 3 Illustration of the Young-Burgess fracture classification system. This system categorizes pelvic ring injuries based on injury mechanism. (Adapted with permission from Burgess AR: Fractures of the pelvis: Part I. The pelvic ring, in Rockwood CA Jr, Green DP, Bucholz RW (eds): *Rockwood and Green's Fractures in Adults*, ed 4. Philadelphia, PA, Lippincott Williams & Wilkins, 2001, pp 1469-1512.)

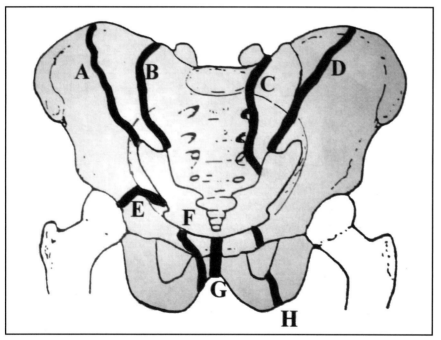

Figure 4 Illustration of the Letournel classification system of pelvic ring injuries. The Letournel classification system is anatomically descriptive and identifies eight types of posterior and anterior pelvic ring injuries. Posterior pelvic ring injuries include iliac wing fractures (A), pure sacroiliac joint dislocations (B), transsacral fractures (C), and iliac fracture-dislocations (D). Anterior pelvic ring injuries include acetabular fractures (E), pubic body fractures (F), pubic symphysis diastasis (G), and pubic rami fractures (H). (Adapted with permission from Kellam J, Browner B: Fractures of the pelvic ring, in Browner B, Jupiter J, Levine A, Trafton P (eds): *Skeletal Trauma: Fractures, Dislocations, Ligamentous Injuries, Volume 1*. Philadelphia, PA, WB Saunders Co, 1992, pp 1117-1179).

proved very useful in predicting the presence of associated neurologic injuries with sacral fractures. It has been noted that the combination of a Denis zone 3 sacral fracture with a Tile type C pelvic ring injury has the highest incidence of neurologic deficit (T Pohlemann, MD, personal correspondence, 1992).

The value of a classification system lies in its ability to assist the surgeon in determining treatment and prognosis of the injury. The combination of the Bucholz classification system, which reflects the general assessment of pelvic stability, and the Letournel classification system, which specifies the anatomic site of injury, is valuable in determining the requirements for surgical stabilization for pelvic ring injuries in hemodynamically stable patients.[2,4] The Young and Burgess[11] classification system has been correlated with fluid resuscitation requirements, associated skeletal and solid organ injury, energy transmission to the victim, the need for acute stabilization of pelvic ring injuries in hemodynamically unstable patients, and patient survival.[18] Anterior-posterior compression type III, lateral compression type III, and vertical shear injuries are all associated with high-energy mechanisms of injury. Anterior-posterior compression type III injuries and vertical shear injuries are associated with the highest transfusion requirements. Each of these classification systems offers useful information to the surgeon treating pelvic ring fractures, and orthopaedic surgeons treating such injuries should be familiar with each of them. Table 2 illustrates how these various classification systems compare.

Initial Orthopaedic Management
Unstable Pelvic Ring Injuries
The focus of management of patients with pelvic ring injuries depends on the time between treatment and injury as well as the physiologic status of the patient on presentation. In the younger patient, hemodynamic stability will typi-

cally be maintained in the presence of ongoing hemorrhage, especially in the first minutes to hours after an injury has occurred. In general, a combination of vital signs, pelvic stability assessment, and knowledge of injury characteristics is key to effective treatment.

The clinician should determine if the physiologic status of the patient is being impacted by an unstable pelvic ring injury. An unstable pelvic fracture and compromised physiologic status are frequently directly related in the multiple-trauma patient, usually as a sequela of hemorrhage. Dalal and associates[18] were able to relate the pelvic fracture type to fluid resuscitation requirements, blood loss, and associated injury patterns in a way that made it possible to develop a risk profile that guides emergency treatment both at the scene and on arrival to the emergency department. In general, treating a grossly disrupted pelvic ring injury by initial stabilization or other interventions is part of the initial resuscitation of the physiologically compromised patient.[19]

To experienced field medical providers, emergency department staff, trauma surgeons, and orthopaedic traumatologists, the mechanism and history of the injury are important.[20] Elements of importance are characteristics of the injury, vehicle occupant restraint history, motorcycle use,[21] and determining whether the patient was a pedestrian or motor vehicle occupant at the time of injury,[22] whether the injury resulted from a fall from a height,[23] or whether the patient has a crush injury. Additional elements of importance include evidence of the energy of injury (velocity of impact or the mass involved in a crush injury). Direction of impact is also useful information.[24] The direction in which the patient was struck, either from the side or head-on is also important because motor vehicle occupants in frontal crashes often incur acetabular fractures associated with posterior fracture-dislocation, whereas lateral impacts tend to cause lateral com-

Table 2
Relationship of Classification Systems for Pelvic Ring Injuries

	Bucholz	Tile	OTA/AO	Young-Burgess	Letournel	Denis
Stable pelvic ring	I	A1, B2	61A, 61B2	Anterior-posterior compression I	*	*
				Lateral compression I		
				Combined mechanical injury*		
Partial instability	II	B1	61B2	Anterior-posterior compression II	*	*
				Lateral compression II		
				Combined mechanical injury*		
				Lateral compression III		
Complete instability	III	C	61C	Anterior-posterior compression III	*	*
				Lateral compression III		
				Vertical shear		
				Combined mechanical injury*		

*Can be associated with all types of instability
OTA = Orthopaedic Trauma Association

pression pelvic ring injuries or displaced acetabular fractures with medial or anterior displacement. Motorcycle collisions with frontal impact at high velocities often cause life-threatening pelvic injuries with open-book or abduction mechanisms, such as anterior-posterior compression type II and III injuries. These injuries often are complicated by open perineal wounds as well. Upon arrival at the hospital, the ABCs (airway, breathing, circulation) of advanced trauma life support are instituted, and the hemodynamic status and pelvic stability of the patient is assessed.

Physical Examination The physical examination of patients with pelvic ring injuries is extremely important. Whether performed in the emergency department or operating room, the basic evaluation is the same. Signs of hemorrhage such as flank or buttock contusions with swelling or discoloration are indicative of clinically significant injuries and underlying bleeding. Scrotal hematomas are often associated with substantial anterior pelvic ring injuries. Palpation of the soft tissues about the pelvis may reveal large hematomas or palpable bony disruptions in areas of fractures or dislocations. Degloving injuries about the pelvis (Morel-Lavallee lesions) are often not

apparent initially, but they typically become evident over time. A high suspicion for injury to the urethra should be maintained with displaced anterior pelvic ring injuries. Inspection for evidence of blood at the urethral meatus as well as evaluation of the prostate to ensure it is in the appropriate position and not high-riding are mandatory before insertion of a Foley catheter. A retrograde urethrogram is recommended before insertion of the Foley catheter when there is high suspicion of urethral injury.[4,10]

Initial evaluation of patients with potential pelvic ring injuries should be directed to identify potential instability and deformity. The bony stability of the pelvis can be evaluated by simultaneously applying pressure through both iliac crests on either side of the pelvis and applying an internal and external rotation stress, anterior-posterior stress, and superior-inferior stress. Any gross motion of the pelvic ring should be considered abnormal. Examination is frequently difficult in the awake patient because of marked discomfort in the pelvic region. This examination is best performed with patients anesthetized or sedated.

Once evidence of gross instability of the pelvis is identified on physical examination, repeat examination is contraindicated. This is especially critical in hemodynamically unstable patients in whom excessive motion of the unstable hemipelvis may exacerbate bleeding. Stabilization of grossly unstable hemipelves in hemodynamically unstable patients is a surgical emergency and should be undertaken as soon as possible. Palpation over the pubic symphysis and sacroiliac joints posteriorly in awake patients can identify areas of tenderness representing occult injury to the pelvic ring. Deformities including limb-length discrepancy and asymmetry in hip rotation from side to side should also be documented.

Careful examination of the soft tissues about the pelvis is required to ensure that an open pelvic fracture is not overlooked. The examining surgeon should carefully inspect the perineum, perirectal areas, and posterior pelvis for soft-tissue defects. Anoscopy is recommended to evaluate the rectum in patients with unstable pelvic ring injuries. In women, a speculum examination of the vaginal vault is mandatory to detect occult open injuries with displaced anterior pelvic ring injuries. A diverting colostomy with mucus fistula should be performed for lacerations that involve the anal sphincter and for significant perineal lacerations that are adjacent to the rectal sphincter.[25] Open fractures of the pelvis are associated with a high incidence of morbidity and mortality. Early aggressive treatment with appropriate resuscitation, immediate débridement of open wounds, stabilization of the bony pelvis, and early colostomy are the fundamental principles of treatment.[25]

Options for Resuscitation An AP radiograph soon after admission can yield valuable information and often is a good guide to resuscitative intervention both for the orthopaedist and general surgeon. Further manipulation is contraindicated once patients have been diagnosed with unstable pelvic ring injuries. Although more detailed studies such as CT inlet and outlet views may define the fine points of injury pathology, the three data points of physiologic status, history (mechanism), and instability and injury pattern will provide the basis for decision making in orthopaedic resuscitative measures. Which resuscitative measures should be applied for unstable patients with unstable pelves and for which indications have been topics of great debate in the literature and have often been determined according to the personal preferences of treating physicians. Additionally, institutional capabilities often seem to play a significant role in determining which interventions are most appropriate and the order in which they will occur.

In a typical scenario, a patient with a high-energy injury arrives in the emergency department. Vital signs and physiologic parameters indicate hemodynamic instability. Because one of the patient's injuries is determined by physical examination to be a high-risk pelvic ring injury (gross instability by examination and/or evidence of a high-risk pattern on radiograph), the decision to begin orthopaedic musculoskeletal intervention should be made at this time. When the patient presents with hemodynamic instability and a grossly unstable pelvis either at the scene of the injury or in the emergency department, what are the risks of inappropriately applying pelvic stabilization? Stabilizing the pelvis in the field or emergency department with a binder or sheet before a radiographic confirmation of fracture type contributes minimal risk. The pelvic fracture may be medially displaced and may maintain that position until radiographs are completed. Patients with lateral compression injuries may also be physiologically unstable from local hemorrhage or associated solid organ or thoracic injury. The pelvis may present as clinically unstable on first assessment.

Possible musculoskeletal interventions for an unstable pelvic ring include immediate stabilization of the pelvic ring, which is often preceded by a reduction maneuver if external rotation and lateral displacement of a hemipelvis is recognized, and surgical intervention to directly control hemorrhage, which has been described previously as exploration and ligation and had been suggested in the past as a management protocol.[26,27] Unfortunately, this intervention was often unsuccessful and frequently disastrous. Review of the earlier experiences suggested this protocol had value primarily when the pelvic injury was caused by penetrating trauma, such as a gunshot, shrapnel, or a stabbing injury.[28] However, in patients who experience blunt high-energy trauma, associated hemorrhage is often caused by disruption of multiple venous and/or small arterial sites as well as bleeding from the bony fracture site itself. In such instances, surgical exploration is usually contraindicated because of the concern that decompression of the retroperitoneum severely compromises any potential for anatomic tamponade of hemorrhage. Interventional angiography has been suggested, both to localize the source of hemorrhage and to treat it. Early success with interventional angiography was reported from academic centers with active and available interventional services that were able to provide such treatment in a timely fashion when emergently necessary.[29] As this modality became more commonly used, it proved most successful when provided in a timely fashion and rapidly available for the trauma patient.[30]

One potential concern is that routinely treating every pelvic fracture with angiographic intervention without clear and appropriate indications regardless of the patient's physiologic status or type of pelvic fracture would result in unnecessarily performed procedures and, therefore, a perceived high success rate in patient survival. Thus, a unique combination of methods has been suggested by trauma surgeons in Europe that includes surgical intervention plus stabilization.[31] The German and Swiss trauma surgeons who developed this method treat selected multiply injured patients with pelvic fractures with pelvic ring fixation and packing of the true pelvic retroperitoneal space. Packs are exchanged at a scheduled revision, which is a damage control procedure similar to that performed for abdominal hemorrhage by general surgeons in North America. This method has demonstrated encouraging results in European centers.[31] Table 3 outlines the methods of interventions available for controlling the unstable hemipelvis in hemodynamically unstable patients.

Emergent pelvic stabilization should be a part of any protocol to treat the unstable pelvis in unstable patients, but exact implementation may vary. Reduction of a laterally displaced hemipelvis reduces the diameter of the true pelvis, thereby decreasing the potential retroperitoneal space and contributing to stability of tamponade. In addition, external stabilization and reduction of pelvic ring fractures stabilizes the local environment and may reduce the fracture fragments, thereby minimizing bleeding from the bony fragments as well as preventing the disruption of clots that have formed. In recent years, immediate stabilization has become synonymous with formal external fixation. However, stabilization may be provided emergently with soft goods, such as with sheets drawn tightly around the pelvis, inflation of military antishock trousers,[32] or use of pelvic binders,[33] which apply a circumferential force about the pelvis. More secure fixation may be achieved with traditional formal external fixation, but surgical experience and considerable institutional commitment are required to make this readily available and efficiently used in the emergency setting.[34] A soft stabilization device may be applied emergently and removed or exchanged for a more definitive external fixation device or definitive fixation as patient stabilize.[35]

Two of these methods are often used in sequence, with external stabilization

Table 3
Advantages and Disadvantages of Interventions for Controlling the Unstable Hemipelvis in Hemodynamically Unstable Patients

Method	Advantage(s)	Disadvantage(s)
Exploration/ligation	Penetrating pelvic trauma	Decompresses retroperitoneal space, increasing hemorrhage in blunt trauma
Interventional angiography	Relatively atraumatic, precise control of arterial bleeding	Requires skilled, timely intervention
Military antishock trousers	Quickly applied, may reduce and stabilize	Skin pressure, limits vascular access at femoral triangle
Exploration, packing pelvic fixation (damage control)	Packing directed at traumatic area, pelvis stabilized	Requires experienced European-type trauma surgeon skilled in both general and orthopaedic surgery
Sheets and pelvic binders	Inexpensive and quickly applied	Skin pressure and limited access to femoral triangle
External fixation	Adequate stabilization with access to perineum, femoral triangle, and abdomen	Difficult to apply quickly by inexperienced surgeon, pin sites may contaminate surgery sites
Pelvic clamps	Packages as a set, appear easy to apply, rotate out of laparotomy field	Posterior use puts skin and sciatic notch contents at risk
Percutaneous fixation	Relatively rigid fixation, minimal blood loss	Requires experienced team for rapid treatment

typically being applied first via a soft-grip binder, which provides mechanical stability of the pelvis when transporting the patient for interventional radiography. There are several advantages to this approach. If the patient is both physiologically and anatomically unstable, a pelvic binder or sheet can be applied early or in the midstages of resuscitation, and the remainder of the resuscitation workup can continue until the patient is stable enough to be transported to the angiography suite. After emergent stabilization, completion of resuscitative efforts (which often includes angiography),[36] and the patient is determined to be stabilized, more definitive pelvic reconstruction can be completed. Pelvic stabilization in the early phases of management in combination with adequate fluid resuscitation and blood transfusion as needed frequently stabilizes hemodynamics.

Another protocol describes the use of two therapeutic methods in the acute phase of management. Acute stabilization is first achieved using soft-good external

binders applied rapidly shortly after admission; within the first 6 to 24 hours, percutaneous fixation is then performed.[37] Efficiently performed percutaneous fixation results in essentially no more blood loss than external fixation, yet it still achieves definitive stability in most patients. Minor malreductions are occasionally acceptable if the overall gross reduction of the pelvic volume is accomplished rapidly. Experienced traumatologists are required to use this technique as an emergent therapy. As experience with elective percutaneous fixation increases and imaging technology improves, this method will likely be used more frequently.

Open Pelvic Fractures
Once open pelvic fractures are diagnosed, two primary clinical issues must be addressed to determine treatment. First, what are the life-threatening characteristics of the injury, especially those regarding hemorrhage? Second, does the injury involve the rectum and is there risk of

external or fecal contamination?[25,38] The risk of significant blood loss is worsened by an open wound that communicates with the pelvic floor. In a small series from a level 1 trauma center, one third of the patients with pelvic fractures and severe perineal lacerations died within a few hours of injury as a result of hemorrhage.[39] Any advantage gained by reduction and stabilization and the resulting tamponade effect is compromised by the venting effect of the open perineal wound. Treatments aimed at reducing hemorrhage should be more aggressive in this patient population, with stabilization applied earlier, aggressive use of interventional angiography, and possibly application of pelvic packing to the open wound.

Packing of an open perineal wound has a limited effect in the absence of stabilization because the packing is forced into an expansile space in an unstable pelvic ring injury. Likewise, stabilization without wound packing is compromised secondary to the venting effect. To maximize the effectiveness of each clinical intervention, emergent stabilization and packing should be applied concurrently.[40]

Shortly after attaining and assuring hemodynamic stability, wound management is undertaken in a second phase to minimize risk of local infection and eventual sepsis. This phase begins with wound exploration, thorough débridement,[41] and diversion of the fecal stream if required.[42] Redébridement will frequently be necessary for these injuries. The adequacy of the débridement is enhanced and the risk of additional hemorrhage is minimized when the pelvis is stabilized temporarily before débridement. This permits patients to be positioned for surgical wound exploration and débridement without risk of additional hemorrhage. The placement of the lower extremities in abduction (lithotomy position) for rectal or perineal débridement in the operating room is facilitated by stabilizing the pelvic ring. Scheduled formal redébridement, even if

it is essentially a thorough dressing change done with the patient under anesthesia, should be part of the management protocol for pelvic ring injuries.[39] Wound care is also facilitated when the pelvis is stabilized.

Summary

Most pelvic ring injuries that are encountered by the orthopaedic surgeon are not associated with hemorrhage. Those less common injuries with severe pelvic instability can have significant risk for life-threatening hemorrhage associated with the injury. The orthopaedic surgeon should provide early care for these patients including advice to the surgical and emergency care physicians regarding the types of pelvic ring injuries that are at risk for hemorrhage, providing early assessment of injury pattern and early bony stabilization with a sheet or binder when appropriate, and providing surgical care when needed to facilitate the patient's early transfer to a tertiary care facility.

References

1. Hollinshead WH: *Anatomy for Surgeons: The Back and Limbs*, ed 3. Philadelphia, PA, Harper and Row Publishers, 1982.

2. Tile M: *Fracture of the Pelvis and Acetabulum*. Baltimore, MD, Williams & Wilkins, 1984.

3. Schunke GB: The anatomy and development of the sacro-iliac joint in man. *Ana Rec* 1938;72:313.

4. Kellam JF, Browner BD: Fractures of the pelvic ring, in Browner B, Jupiter J, Levine A, Trafton P (eds): *Skeletal Trauma*. Philadelphia, PA, WB Saunders, 1992, pp 849-897.

5. Vrahas M, Hern TC, Diangelo D, Kellam J, Tile M: Ligamentous contributions to pelvic stability. *J Orthop* 1995;18:271-274.

6. Bucholz RW: The pathological anatomy of the Malgaigne fracture dislocation of the pelvis. *J Bone Joint Surg Am* 1981;63:400-404.

7. Holdsworth FW: Dislocation and fractures dislocation of the pelvis. *J Bone Joint Surg Br* 1948;30:461-466.

8. Ghanayem AJ, Wilbur JH, Leiberman JM, Mogta AO: The effect of laparotomy and external fixator stabilization on pelvic volume in an unstable pelvic injury. *J Trauma* 1995;38:396-401.

9. Tile M: Pelvic ring fractures: Should they be fixed? *J Bone Joint Surg Br* 1988;70:1-12.

10. Committee on Trauma: American College of Surgeons: *Advanced Trauma Life Support: Instructor Manual*. Chicago, IL, American College of Surgeons, 1993.

11. Young JWR, Burgess AR: *Radiological Management of Pelvic Ring Fractures*. Baltimore, MD, Urban and Schwarzenberg, 1987.

12. Matta JM, Saucedo T: Internal fixation of pelvic ring fractures. *Clin Orthop* 1989;242: 83-97.

13. Doty JR, Rengachary SS: *Surgical Disorders of the Sacrum*. New York, NY, Thieme Medical Publishers, 1994.

14. Mears DC: Fracture dislocation of the pelvic ring, in Chapman MW (ed): *Operative Orthopaedics*. Philadelphia, PA, JB Lippincott Company, 1993, pp 505-538.

15. Pohlemann T, Bosch U, Gansslen A, Tscherne H: The Hannover experience in management of pelvic fractures. *Clin Orthop* 1994;305:69-80.

16. Denis F, Davis S, Comfort T: Sacral fractures: An important problem. *Clin Orthop* 1988;227:67-81.

17. Orthopaedic Trauma Association Committee for Coding and Classification: Fracture and dislocation compendium. *J Orthop Trauma* 1996;10(suppl 1):1-154.

18. Dalal S, Burgess A, Siegel J, et al: Pelvic fracture in multiple trauma: Classification by mechanism is key to pattern of organ injury, resuscitative requirements, and outcome. *J Trauma* 1989;29:981-1002.

19. Burgess AR, Eastridge BJ, Young JW, et al: Pelvic ring disruptions: Effective classification system and treatment protocols. *J Trauma* 1990;30:848-856.

20. Whitbeck MG, Zwally HJ II, Burgess AR: Innominosacral dissociation: Mechanism of injury as a predictor of resuscitation requirements, morbidity, and mortality *J Orthop Trauma* 1997;11:82-88.

21. Ankarath S, Giannoudis PV, Barlow I, Bellamy MC, Matthews SJ, Smit RM: Injury patterns associated with mortality following motorcycle crashes. *Injury* 2002;33:473-477.

22. Eastridge BJ, Burgess AR: Pedestrian pelvic fractures: 5-year experience of a major urban trauma center. *J Trauma* 1997;42:695-700.

23. Richter D, Hahn MP, Ostermann PA, Ekkernkamp A, Muhr G: Vertical deceleration injuries: A comparative study of the injury patterns of 101 patients after accidental and intentional high falls. *Injury* 1996;27:655-659.

24. Gokcen EC, Burgess AR, Siegel JH, Mason-Gonzalez S, Dischinger PC, Ho SM: Pelvic fracture mechanism of injury in vehicular trauma patients. *J Trauma* 1994;36:789-795.

25. Hanson PB, Milne JC, Chapman MW: Open fractures of the pelvis: Review of 43 cases. *J Bone Joint Surg Br* 1991;73:325-329.

26. Goldstein A, Phillips T, Sclafani SJ, et al: Early open reduction and internal fixation of the disrupted pelvic ring. *J Trauma* 1986;26:325-333.

27. Pohlemann T, Paul C, Gansslen A, Regel G, Tscherne H: Traumatic hemipelvectomy:

Experience with 11 cases. *Unfallchirurg* 1996;99:304-312.

28. Ryan W, Snyder W III, Bell T, Hunt J: Penetrating injuries of the iliac vessels: Early recognition and management. *Am J Surg* 1982;144:642-645.

29. Mucha P Jr, Welch TJ: Hemorrhage in major pelvic fractures. *Surg Clin North Am* 1988;68:757-773.

30. Biffl WL, Smith WR, Moore EE, et al: Evolution of a multdisciplinary clinical pathway for the management of unstable patients with pelvic fractures. *Ann Surg* 2001;233:843-850.

31. Ertel W, Keel M, Eid K, Platz A, Trentz O: Control of severe hemorrhage using C-clamp and plevic packing in multiply injured patients with pelvic ring disruption. *J Orthop Trauma* 2001;15:468-474.

32. Frank LR: Is MAST in the past? The pros and cons of MAST usage in the field. *JEMS* 2000;25:38-45.

33. Vermeulen B, Peter R, Hoffmeyer P, Unger PF: Prehospital stabilization of pelvic dislocations: A new strap belt to provide temporary hemodynamic stabilization. *Swiss Surg* 1999;5:43-46.

34. Tucker MC, Nork SE, Simonian PT, Routt ML Jr: Simple anterior external fixation. *J Trauma* 2000;49:989-994.

35. Starr AJ, Walter JC, Harris RW, Reinert CM, Jones AL: Percutaneous fixation of fractures of the iliac wing and fracture dislocations of the sacro-iliac joint (OTA Types 61-B2.2 and 61-B2.3, or Young-Burgess "lateral compression type II" pelvic fractures). *J Orthop Trauma* 2002;16:116-123.

36. Miller PR, Moore PS, Mansell E, Meredith JW, Chang MC: External fixation or arteriogram in bleeding pelvic fracture: Initial therapy guided by markers of arterial hemorrhage. *J Trauma* 2003;54:437-443.

37. Routt ML Jr, Simonian PT, Ballmer F: A rational approach to pelvic trauma: Resuscitation and early definitive stabilization. *Clin Orthop* 1995;318:61-74.

38. Kottmeier SA, Wilson SC, Born CT, Hanks GA, Iannacone WM, Delon WG: Surgical management of soft tissue injuries associated with pelvic ring injury. *Clin Orthop* 1996;329:46-53.

39. Kudsk KA, McQueen MA, Voeller GR, Fox MA, Mangiante EC Jr, Fabian TC: Management of complex perineal soft-tissue injuries. *J Trauma* 1990;30:1155-1159.

40. Beard JD, Davidson CM, Scott DJ, Turner AG: Pelvic injuries associated with traumatic abduction of the leg. *Injury* 1988;19:353-356.

41. Birolini D, Steinman E, Utiyama E, Arroyo A: Open pelviperineal trauma. *J Trauma* 1990;30:492-495.

42. Faringer PD, Mullins RJ, Feliciano PD, Duwelius PJ, Trunkey DD: Selective fecal diversion in complex open pelvic fractures from blunt trauma. *Arch Surg* 1994;129:958-963.

21

Surgical Management of Pelvic Ring Injuries

David C. Templeman, MD
Tamara Simpson, MD
Joel M. Matta, MD

Abstract

Posterior pelvic ring injuries disrupt the weight-bearing function of the pelvis and cause deformity that results in pain and loss of function. The indications for reduction and fixation are the presence of instability and/or deformity. Surgical fixation of the pelvic ring is divided into anterior and posterior ring injuries. In many instances, reduction and fixation of the anterior pelvic ring is not needed after reduction and fixation of the posterior pelvic ring. Although techniques exist for both open and closed reductions, the main difficulty remains achieving anatomic restoration of the pelvis. Whether posterior pelvic ring injuries are best treated using closed reduction and fixation or open reduction and fixation remains a controversial topic.

The indications for reduction and fixation of pelvic ring injuries are the presence of instability and/or deformity of the pelvic ring.[1-8] These factors are determined from the radiographic evaluation of pelvic ring injuries and the use of classification systems that predict the stability of pelvic ring injuries.[1,2,9]

The approach to the surgical treatment of the pelvic ring is divided into anterior and posterior ring injuries. Anterior pelvic ring injuries are usually pubic ramus fractures or disruptions of the pubic symphysis. Most pubic ramus fractures are best managed using nonsurgical treatment because nonunion and symptomatic deformities of the pubic rami are rare. Letournel's "Golden Rule" for the reduction of pelvic ring injuries emphasizes that the initial reduction and fixation of posterior pelvic ring injuries usually results in an acceptable position of the pubic rami fractures.[3,9] In most instances, reduction and fixation of anterior pelvic ring fractures is not needed after reduction and fixation of the posterior pelvic ring.[3,9,10]

Treatment Considerations

Diastasis of the pubic symphysis frequently requires reduction and fixation to restore rotational stability to the pelvic ring. With disruption of the pubic symphysis and external rotation of the innominate bone, one of the sacroiliac joints typically sustains an injury to the anterior capsule and ligaments; with continued displacement, disruption of the sacroiliac ligamentous complex completes the spectrum of possible injury.[1] Diastasis of the pubic symphysis of greater than 2.5 cm indicates both disruption of the sacrospinous ligaments and the presence of rotational instability of

the pelvic ring. An initial symphysis pubis diastasis of greater than or equal to 2.5 cm is an indication for open reduction and internal fixation of the symphysis pubis.[3,6,7,10]

Segmental fractures of the superior pubic ramus are commonly referred to as tilt fractures. These uncommon injuries are treated with reduction and fixation to avoid impingement on the vaginal vault, bladder, and birth canal.[6] Parasymphyseal fractures and other pubic rami fractures that lead to vaginal impingement are also relative indications for fixation of anterior pelvic ring fractures.[6,10]

The appropriate treatment of pelvic ring injuries is determined by radiographic assessment to diagnose pelvic ring deformity and the use of classification systems that predict instability of injuries (see chapter 39 for a detailed description of the various classification systems).[1,2,6] Most evidence supports the reduction and fixation of displaced posterior ring injuries to improve long-term functional outcome.[6,8,11]

Posterior displacement of greater than or equal to 1 cm is a common indication for reduction and fixation. The caudal/inlet radiograph is usually the most sensitive indicator of this displacement. Although lateral compression type II injuries that cause a displaced sacroiliac fracture-dislocation may not exhibit this degree of posterior translation, these injuries are rotationally unstable and require reduction and fixation.[2,12]

Posterior pelvic ring injuries that disrupt the weight-bearing function of the pelvic ring or cause deformity result in considerable pain and loss of function. Letournel identified the following four common posterior pelvic ring injury patterns: transsacral fractures, iliac wing fractures, iliac wing fracture-dislocations, and pure sacroiliac joint dislocations. Of these patterns, sacroiliac dislocations represent the only pattern with a pure ligamentous injury. Because of the absence of bony healing, they typically have the poorest prognosis for functional recovery.[3,9,11]

It is important to differentiate among the four different injuries of the posterior pelvic ring to choose the appropriate fixation construct. Iliac wing fracture-dislocations are in general best treated by open reduction and internal fixation with plate and screw constructs; the use of iliosacral screws alone is associated with the risk of the screws cutting into the fracture plane.[12] The other three injuries are usually stabilized using iliosacral screws.[3,4,13-16]

Many sacral fractures can be treated nonsurgically. Reilly and associates (unpublished data, presented at the Orthopaedic Trauma Association National Meeting, 2000) documented that sacral fractures with less than 1 cm of displacement that are caused by lateral compression injuries are inherently stable. In a group of patients with lateral compression type I sacral fractures that were treated with early protected weight bearing, there were no instances of displacement. Nonsurgical treatment of sacral fractures is indicated when the three pelvic radiographs do not indicate deformity and the CT scan demonstrates impaction of the sacral fracture. Many of these injuries will have a degree of internal rotation of one innominate bone from the lateral compression mechanism of injury.[17]

In contrast, sacral fractures with 1 cm or more of displacement and CT evidence of a diastasis of the fracture plane are considered to be displaced and unstable. This pattern of sacral fractures may be secondary to anterior-posterior compression, vertical shear, or combined mechanism of injury force vectors.[4,8,14,16-19]

Denis and associates[17] have classified sacral fractures into the following three anatomic zones: zone 1 fractures involve the sacral ala, zone 2 fractures involve the foramina, and zone 3 fractures involve the sacral canal. The location of the sacral fracture has a high correlation with the incidence of neurologic injury.

Displaced and unstable sacral fractures are usually stabilized with iliosacral screws. The indications for open reduction versus closed reduction and percutaneous fixation are controversial. Proponents of closed reduction contend that this avoids surgical incisions and possible wound healing complications. Proponents of open reduction cite that this more reliably provides an accurate reduction and more stable internal fixation.[4,8,14,16-19]

Reilly and associates[20] have shown (with cadaver studies) that malalignment of sacral fractures causes a reduction of the area of the fracture plane. This reduces the available area for the insertion of iliosacral screws. The stability of the fracture construct is also reduced with a malreduction because the reduction in the area of the fracture plane reduces the amount of bony interdigitation at the fracture surface and ultimately the stability of the fixation.

The closed reduction and percutaneous fixation of zone 2 sacral fractures is most controversial. The risk of malreduction of the sacral foramina creates the potential for compression of sacral nerve roots if compression is applied across the fracture site.[4,16,18,19,21-25] One series has identified that vertical sacral fractures were prone to postoperative displacement after closed reduction and percutaneous fixation.[14] In contrast, proponents

of open reduction contend that more accurate reductions are achieved, which allows for stronger interfragmentary compression to be applied across the sacral fractures and ultimately improves the stability of the fracture construct.[4,16]

Closed Reduction and Percutaneous Fixation or Open Reduction and Internal Fixation of the Posterior Pelvic Ring

The accuracy of the reduction of the pelvic ring rather than the technique of fixation should be foremost in the mind of the surgeon. Whether posterior pelvic ring injuries are best treated using closed reduction and fixation or open reduction and fixation is controversial. Both methods have strong advocates, and no randomized prospective studies comparing these methods have yet been conducted. The primary problem remains reduction of the deformity rather than the technique of fracture fixation.[3,4,9,10,13,18,22-26]

For most sacroiliac fracture-dislocations, open reduction and internal fixation is needed both to achieve an accurate reduction and appropriate fixation because plate and screw fixation is required to treat this injury pattern. Sacral fractures and sacroiliac dislocations can be stabilized by the percutaneous insertion of iliosacral screws when an accurate reduction is achieved. The success of closed reduction seems to depend on early surgical management and accurate intraoperative imaging.[13,14,21-25,27,28]

Proponents of closed reduction and percutaneous fixation contend that avoiding open surgical approaches avoids the high incidence of soft-tissue complications.[22-25] A multicenter study conducted by Stover and associates (unpublished data presented at the National Meeting of the Orthopaedic Trauma Association, 1998) documented a low incidence of wound problems (3.9%) and no instances of chronic osteomyelitis. All of these surgeries were performed using anatomic dissection of the gluteus maximus as described by Letournel.[3,9] These data indicate that open reduction, when appropriately performed, is not compromised by soft-tissue complications.

The major determinant of performing a successful closed reduction is the ability of the surgeon to achieve an accurate closed reduction. Failure to achieve acceptable reduction compromises both the safe area available for the placement of iliosacral screws and the stability of the fixation construct. In a cadaver model, 1 cm of cranial displacement of sacral fractures resulted in a 50% reduction of the surface area at the fracture site.[20] To achieve successful closed reduction, surgeons must have the ability to accurately assess the intraoperative fluoroscopic images of the pelvis as the closed reduction is performed.[22,24] All series describing this technique also document that varying percentages of fractures required an open reduction because an accurate closed reduction could not always be obtained.

Currently, few data exist regarding the outcomes of patients treated with closed versus open reduction of posterior pelvic ring injuries. The planning for open reduction and internal fixation of posterior ring injuries is complex because many variables must be considered. The timing of the surgery is dependent on the presence of other injuries and the resuscitation of the patient.[29]

Urologic, neurologic, and soft-tissue injuries have a profound effect on the planning of the surgery. Lower urinary tract injuries must be appropriately diagnosed, and adequate diversion of the urinary stream is necessary if any fixation of the anterior pelvic ring is required. Repair of intraperitoneal and extraperitoneal bladder ruptures before fixation of the anterior pelvic ring is preferred to reduce the risk of urosepsis, which can lead to infection of fixation of anterior pelvic ring injuries.

Soft-tissue degloving injuries (Morel-Lavallee lesions) must be diagnosed and taken into account when planning a pos-

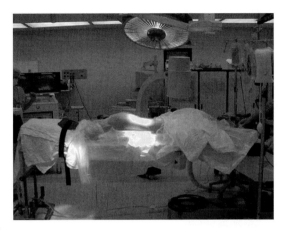

Figure 1 Photograph showing how the prone position of the patient on a radiolucent table provides for excursion of the fluoroscope to obtain both caudal and cephalad views of the pelvic ring.

terior surgical approach. These injuries have a high risk for colonization and infection when not treated. Hak and associates[30] found that culture results for these degloving injuries were positive in 40% of patients. The need for débridement and subsequent wound care must be assessed as part of the surgical strategy. A recent study by Tornetta and Normand (unpublished data presented at the National Meeting of the Orthopaedic Trauma Association, 2002) documented that early percutaneous irrigation and débridement of degloving injuries were successful. Open débridement and later wound closure is another strategy for the treatment of degloving injuries.

Open Reduction and Internal Fixation

Open reduction and internal fixation of posterior ring injuries is done with the patient in the prone position, which requires that associated injuries are considered. Although most patients with multiple injuries can be safely placed in the prone position, the presence of cervical spine injuries, facial fractures, ocular trauma, and closed head injuries occasionally constitute relative contraindications for such placement. As a result of reported instances of blindness after patients were placed in the prone position, it is important to make sure that patients are adequately resuscitated and

that anemia is corrected by transfusions before surgery. This point is emphasized when the use of hypotensive anesthesia is planned.

A careful neurologic examination that includes motor grading and a detailed sensory examination needs to be conducted and the results documented before performing open reduction and internal fixation. Outcome studies indicate that neurologic injuries causing motor deficits are strongly correlated with the level of functional recovery.[16] Patients in whom there is gross disruption of the anterior pelvic ring (particularly males with diastasis of the symphysis pubis) need to be counseled about the possibility of impotence that is associated with the traumatic injury before proceeding with surgery.

Surgical Approach/Patient Positioning

The patient is placed prone on a radiolucent table (Figure 1). Obtaining clear radiographic views is required for the insertion of iliosacral screws.[4,23,24,28] The first step in the procedure after positioning the patient is to check fluoroscopic images. The cephalad/outlet and caudal/inlet views as described are the most important for inserting iliosacral screws with an open technique. An additional lateral image of the sacrum can be obtained, but this is more commonly done for percutaneous

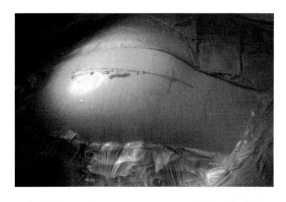

Figure 2 Photograph showing the posterior pelvic incision placed lateral to the posterior-superior iliac spine and extending distally. The patient's head is located to the left of the photograph.

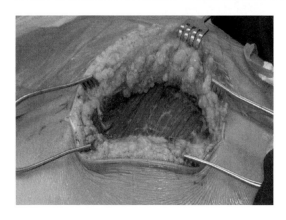

Figure 3 Photograph showing the anatomic dissection of the gluteus maximus muscle.

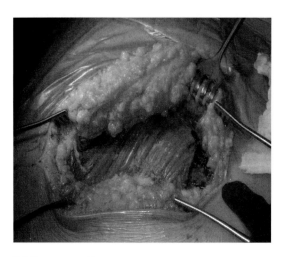

Figure 4 Photograph showing the incision extending far enough distally to expose the inferior aspect of the sacroiliac joint.

section of the gluteus maximus muscle, which is first released from its origin on the iliac crest and then from its aponeurosis over the erector spinae muscle (Figure 3). The gluteus maximus is progressively reflected with a subperiosteal elevation from the external surface of the innominate bone as this dissection progresses from proximal to distal. The dissection exposes the greater sciatic notch just inferior to the posterior-inferior iliac spine. This allows inspection of the inferior aspect of the articular surfaces of the sacroiliac joint and the piriformis muscle, which inserts on the anterior aspect of the sacrum (Figure 4). The piriformis muscle is elevated from the anterior aspect of the sacrum to allow palpation of the anterior aspect of the sacral ala and the sacroiliac joint. Palpation of the anterior aspect of the sacroiliac joint is critical to assessing the reduction of the sacroiliac dislocation. This palpation of the sacroiliac joint assists in correcting both anterior-posterior translation and the rotational component of the reduction.

Reduction

The deformity of the pelvic ring injury determines which vectors need to be applied to achieve reduction. A variety of clamps of different sizes and shapes must be available. Simple widening of the sacroiliac joint, with no translation or cephalad migration of the innominate bone is the easiest deformity to reduce. In this instance, a simple Weber forceps can be placed across the sacroiliac joint with one tine placed on the anterior aspect of the sacrum and the other tine on the outer surface of the innominate bone.[4,31] The reduction is subsequently judged by finger palpation along the anterior aspect of the joint and by radiographic images. When there is cephalad displacement of the innominate bone, one tine can be placed on the iliac crest and one tine on the sacral lamina to reduce the cephalad translation. Once this is done, a second clamp is sometimes needed to improve

iliosacral screw fixation. If there is any doubt about visualization of the posterior sacroiliac complex, the surgery should be postponed. A table that allows wide excursions of the C-arm is required to obtain the cephalad/outlet and caudad/inlet views. Patients are given preoperative antibiotics and a Foley catheter is inserted.

The surgical incision extends approximately 1 to 2 cm lateral to the prominence of the posterior-superior iliac spine and extends from the level of the iliac crest proximally to the greater sciatic notch distally[4,10] (Figure 2). The key to the surgical approach is an anatomic dis-the reduction between the innominate bone and the sacrum. The clamps are placed in varying positions until the appropriate vectors to reduce the injury are obtained. This technique will achieve an accurate reduction for nearly all posterior pelvic ring injuries.[4,31]

Additional reduction tools include Schanz screws inserted into the iliac crest for use as joysticks, or bone screws inserted into the ilium and the lateral iliac crest for the application of either a Farabeuf or pelvic manipulation clamp. Some have recommended the use of an antishock pelvic clamp or external fixator to help reduce the posterior pelvic ring. In general, these additional techniques for reduction are necessary in the correction of chronic deformities.

After the reduction is verified with AP and inlet/outlet radiographs, the iliosacral screws are inserted. The optimal position for insertion of the screws is determined by projecting a line parallel to the crista glutea, which runs from the iliac crest to the greater sciatic notch. The distance between this line and the crista glutea is approximately 15 mm.[4] Screws are inserted on either side of the midpoint of this line. Fluoroscopic guidance is required even when placing the screws via open technique. It is easiest to start with visualizing the outlet projection. The drill bit is placed at or slightly above the level of the S1 foramina and angles slightly upward into the body of S1. For sacroiliac joint screw fixation on the inlet view, the drill bit is angled from slightly posterior to anterior. A drill bit is used in contrast to the use of cannulated guidewires that have terminal threads. When using a drill bit, the surgeon receives direct tactile sense of the drill bit being contained within the bone. Cannulated screws with threaded tips do not provide a reliable sensation when the guidewire has penetrated the bone. Once the drill bit is started in the sacral ala, attention is directed to the inlet view to ensure that the drill bit is appropriately

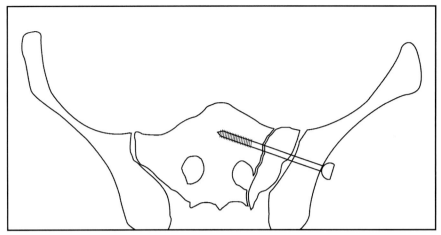

Figure 5 Schematic illustration of the dimensions of the iliosacral corridor for the insertion of iliosacral screws. The average distance from the S1 foramina to the sacral ala is 24 mm.

targeted toward S1. It is not unusual for the surgeon to have to reorient a drill bit before arriving at the appropriate insertion site and angle.[16,32]

Given the small distance between the anterior cortex of the sacral ala and the S1 foramina, trigonometric analysis indicates that the target corridor is plus or minus 4° when an ideal starting point is achieved[13,32] (Figure 5). This analysis indicates that insertion of iliosacral screws is technically demanding. Once the drill bit is placed into the body of S1, it can easily be replaced with a guidewire for a cannulated screw system. In general, 6.5- or 7-mm cannulated screws are inserted with the use of a washer and tightened to achieve excellent compression of the sacroiliac joint. A washer is necessary because without it the screw heads can penetrate between the two tables of the iliac wing. The position of the implants is confirmed with AP and inlet/outlet fluoroscopic projections.

Once reduction and fixation are completed, the wound is irrigated and the gluteus maximus tendon is repaired to its aponeurosis over the erector spinae distally and to the iliac crest proximally. Hemovac drains are inserted, and the subcutaneous and skin layers are then closed.

Closed Reduction and Percutaneous Fixation

Both supine and prone positioning of patients are used for closed reduction and percutaneous fixation of pelvic ring injuries.[15,22] Fluoroscopic imaging is used to assess both the reduction and the placement of iliosacral screws. Various forms of longitudinal traction are used to obtain reduction of the pelvic ring, and the ability to achieve closed reduction is greatly facilitated by early reduction and fixation after the injury. Although not well documented in the literature, centers that predominately use closed reduction techniques are in general able to treat patients earlier compared with centers using open techniques where delayed referrals and treatment seem to be more common. The major challenge of closed reduction is applying external traction and manipulation in the correct vectors to achieve an accurate reduction of the posterior ring injury.

With patients positioned either supine or prone on a radiolucent table, fluoroscopic images of the posterior pelvic ring are obtained. In addition to the cephalad and caudal views described by Matta and Saucedo[4] and Matta and Tornetta,[18] Routt and associates[24] have popularized the use of a lateral sacral view. These authors have documented that the addition of the lateral sacral view avoided misplaced iliosacral screws that were initially encountered when not using lateral sacral imaging. The lateral sacral view helps to avoid exiting the anterior and cephalad surface of the sacrum by displaying the upper sacral slope.

Not all patients can be successfully treated by closed reduction and percutaneous fixation. In an initial series of 177 patients, 38 patients (21.5%) required open reductions.[23] Excluded from this group of patients were patients with certain patterns of sacral fractures and sacroiliac fracture-dislocations that were treated in the prone position with open reductions.

Postoperative Plans

High quality AP and inlet/outlet radiographs are obtained postoperatively. Patients should not bear weight for a minimum of 3 months after open reduction and internal fixation of the sacroiliac joint. This prolonged period is necessary and in contrast to the recovery period of bony injuries that heal more rapidly than the ligamentous injuries of sacroiliac dislocations.

Summary

Unstable pelvic ring injuries are associated with significant deformity and are best treated by reduction and fixation. The treatment of pelvic ring injuries is complicated and technically demanding. Foremost in the treatment of these injuries is obtaining an appropriate reduction. There is continued controversy regarding whether or not open reduction or closed reduction best achieves this objective. Given the spectrum of injuries it is likely that one technique will not be suitable for the treatment of the variety of pelvic ring injuries that are encountered by the orthopaedic surgeon.

References

1. Bucholz RW: The pathological anatomy of Malgaigne fracture-dislocations of the pelvis. *J Bone Joint Surg Am* 1981;63:400-404.

2. Burgess AR, Eastridge BJ, Young JW, et al: Pelvic ring disruptions: Effective classification system and treatment protocols. *J Trauma* 1990;30:848-856.

3. Letournel E: Surgical fixation of displaced pelvic fractures and dislocations of the symphysis pubis (excluding acetabular fractures) [author's transl]. *Rev Chir Orthop Reparatrice Appar Mot* 1981;67:771-782.

4. Matta JM, Saucedo T: Internal fixation of pelvic ring fractures. *Clin Orthop* 1989;242:83-97.

5. Semba RT, Yasukawa K, Gustilo RB: Critical analysis of results of 53 Malgaigne fractures of the pelvis. *J Trauma* 1983;23:535-537.

6. Tile M: *Fractures of the Pelvis and Acetabulum.* Baltimore, Williams and Wilkins, 1984, pp 1-9.

7. Tornetta P III, Dickson K, Matta JM: Outcome of rotationally unstable pelvic ring injuries treated operatively. *Clin Orthop* 1996;329:147-151.

8. Tornetta P III, Matta JM: Outcome of operatively treated unstable posterior pelvic ring disruptions. *Clin Orthop* 1996;329:186-193.

9. Letournel E: Pelvic fractures. *Injury* 1978;10:145-148.

10. Matta JM: Indications for anterior fixation of pelvic fractures. *Clin Orthop* 1996;329:88-96.

11. Holdsworth FW: Dislocation and fracture dislocation of the pelvis. *J Bone Joint Surg Br* 1948;30:461-466.

12. Borrelli J Jr, Koval KJ, Helfet DL: The crescent fracture: A posterior fracture dislocation of the sacroiliac joint. *J Orthop Trauma* 1996;10:165-170.

13. Carlson DA, Scheid DK, Maar DC, et al: Safe placement of S1 and S2 iliosacral screws: The "vestibule" concept. *J Orthop Trauma* 2000;14:264-269.

14. Griffin DR, Starr AJ, Reinert CM, Jones AL, Whitlock S: Vertically unstable pelvic fractures fixed with percutaneous iliosacral screws: Does posterior injury pattern predict fixation failure? *J Orthop Trauma* 2003;17:399-405.

15. Keating JF, Werier J, Blachut P, Broekhuyse H, Meek RN, O'Brien PJ: Early fixation of the vertically unstable pelvis: The role of iliosacral screw fixation of the posterior lesion. *J Orthop Trauma* 1999;13:107-113.

16. Templeman D, Goulet J, Duwelius PJ, Olson S, Davidson M: Internal fixation of displaced fractures of the sacrum. *Clin Orthop* 1996;329:180-185.

17. Denis F, Davis S, Comfort T: Sacral fractures: An important problem: Retrospective analysis of 236 cases. *Clin Orthop* 1988;227:67-81.

18. Matta JM, Tornetta P III: Internal fixation of unstable pelvic ring injuries. *Clin Orthop* 1996;329:129-140.

19. Simonian PT, Routt C Jr, Harrington RM, Tencer AF: Internal fixation for the transforaminal sacral fracture. *Clin Orthop* 1996;323:202-209.

20. Reilly MC, Bono CM, Litkouhi B, Sirkin M, Behrens FF: The effect of sacral fracture malreduction on the safe placement of iliosacral screw. *J Orthop Trauma* 2003;17:88-94.

21. Ricci WM, Padberg AM, Borrelli J: The significance of anode location for stimulus-evoked electromyography during iliosacral screw placement. *J Orthop Trauma* 2003;17:95-99.

22. Routt ML, Kregor PJ, Simonian PT, Mayo KA: Early results of percutaneous iliosacral screws placed with the patient in the supine position. *J Orthop Trauma* 1995;9:207-214.

23. Routt ML Jr, Nork SE, Mills WJ: Percutaneous fixation of pelvic ring disruptions. *Clin Orthop* 2000;375:15-29.

24. Routt ML Jr, Simonian PT, Agnew SG, Mann FA: Radiographic recognition of the sacral alar slope for optimal placement of iliosacral screws: A cadaveric and clinical study. *J Orthop Trauma* 1996;10(3):171-177.

25. Routt ML Jr, Simonian PT, Mills WJ: Iliosacral screw fixation: early complications of the percutaneous technique. *J Orthop Trauma* 1997;11:584-589.

26. Nork SE, Jones CB, Harding SP, Mirza SK, Routt ML Jr: Percutaneous stabilization of U-shaped sacral fractures using iliosacral screws: technique and early results. *J Orthop Trauma* 2001;15(4):238-246.

27. Gautier E, Bachler R, Heini PF, Nolte LP: Accuracy of computer-guided screw fixation of the sacroiliac joint. *Clin Orthop* 2001;393:310-317.

28. Moed BR, Ahmad BK, Craig JG, Jacobson GP, Anders MJ: Intraoperative monitoring with stimulus-evoked electromyography during placement of iliosacral screws: An initial clinical study. *J Bone Joint Surg Am* 1998;80:537-546.

29. Connor GS, McGwin G Jr, MacLennan PA, Alonso JE, Rue LW III: Early versus delayed fixation of pelvic ring fractures. *Am Surg* 2003;69:1019-1023.

30. Hak DJ, Olson SA, Matta JM: Diagnosis and management of closed internal degloving injuries associated with pelvic and acetabular fractures: The Morel-Lavallee lesion. *J Trauma* 1997;42:1046-1051.

31. Moed BR, Karges DE: Techniques for reduction and fixation of pelvic ring disruptions through the posterior approach. *Clin Orthop* 1996;329:102-114.

32. Templeman D, Schmidt A, Freese J, Weisman I: Proximity of iliosacral screws to neurovascular structures after internal fixation. *Clin Orthop* 1996;329:194-198.

Expected Outcomes After Pelvic Ring Injury

Paul Tornetta III, MD

David C. Templeman, MD

Abstract

Pelvic ring injuries are a result of high-energy trauma and are often associated with nonskeletal injuries. Although malunions and nonunions are rare with the use of current techniques of reduction and fixation, outcome studies show that these injuries have long-lasting effects. Associated urologic and neurologic injuries are commonly the determinants of outcome.

Historically, pelvic ring injuries have resulted in high rates of back pain, impaired gait, pelvic obliquity, sitting problems, and neurologic sequelae.[1-5] Poor results have been correlated with initial displacement, displacement at union, anatomic location of the injury, and residual neurologic dysfunction. Interpretation of reported results from older studies is difficult because they categorized what are now considered type II and type III posterior ring injuries together. For example, a mild to moderate symphyseal separation with anterior sacroiliac joint opening (anterior-posterior compression type II fractures) was considered a sacroiliac dislocation.[5] Thus, many early reports underestimate the sequelae of a type III injury by reporting type II and type III injuries together.

This problem is illustrated by the classic and often quoted report of Slatis and Huittinen.[5] Sixty-five patients (163 double vertical fractures) were observed long term with a reported 17% incidence of low back pain, 32% incidence of impaired gait, and 48% incidence of neurologic sequelae. However, only 18% of these patients had hemipelvic displacement. Most injuries were vertically stable, which by today's standards would be considered lateral compression type I or type II injuries.

Similarly, Semba and associates[6] reported on 30 Malgaigne fractures that were observed for 2 to 12 years. Fewer than 50% of fractures had even 5 mm of vertical translation, and all but two were treated nonsurgically. Despite this, only 36% of patients were asymptomatic, with 31% reporting impaired gait and 26% reporting severe low back pain. The authors concluded that greater than 10 mm of combined anterior and posterior displacement of the pelvic ring correlated with pain. In 1948, Holdsworth[1] reviewed 50 patients who were treated with a pelvic sling with or without traction. Again, this group of patients included those with type II and type III pelvic ring injuries. It was reported that sacroiliac dislocations had worse outcomes than

sacral fractures or fractures affecting the iliac wing, and this was one of the first reports to make the differentiation between bony and ligamentous injuries.

In 1966, Raf[4] reported on 101 double vertical fractures of the pelvis (61 patients). Similar to the results of the study by Semba and associates,[6] anterior pelvic displacement was greater than 5 mm in only 66% of patients, and 42% had no craniocaudad displacement. Thus, a maximum of 38% of the fractures were type III injuries. Of the 66 patients observed clinically, 29% reported disabling pain. According to Raf's study, more severe pain occurred in patients with sacral fractures than those with other injuries.

In the context of these earlier studies, it becomes apparent that the factors that require evaluation include whether the injury is bony or ligamentous, the neurologic status of the patient, and the displacement of the fracture. Urologic status and other skeletal injuries are now known to also play an important role.

Surgical Treatment

The indications for open reduction and internal fixation of pelvic ring injuries are discussed in another chapter, and the techniques to gain reduction and stable fixation are also discussed elsewhere. From an outcomes perspective, it is important to understand that the single goal of surgery for pelvic ring injuries is anatomic restoration of the bony alignment and stability to allow for union in this position. Anatomic alignment will restore sitting balance, avoid limb-length discrepancy, and allow for the best possible outcome given the nature of the pelvic injury and any associated injuries.[7,8]

Surgical outcomes must be judged not only by the reduction and stability gained but by the pain patients experience in follow-up, their ability to work, their return to activities of daily living, and their participation in recreational activities as well as by general health outcome measures. Some of these factors require specific evaluation and others can be judged based on scoring systems.

To properly evaluate surgical outcomes many factors must be evaluated. Some of these factors deal with the patient and initial injury and others with the surgery and position of the pelvis at union. The initial injury is quite important because stable injuries are expected to have a better outcome than those that are unstable. Thus, stability needs to be assessed. Fractures can be stable (such as a lateral compression type I injury that is stable in both rotation and vertical translation); rotationally unstable (such as a lateral compression type II injury or an anterior-posterior compression type II injury that is vertically stable); or completely unstable (such as a lateral compression or anterior-posterior compression type III injury which is unstable in rotation and vertical displacement).[9] The anatomic location of the injuries to the ring also have an impact on outcomes. This is true both in the anterior and posterior portion of the pelvic ring. Bony injuries such as fractures of the rami, iliac wing, or sacrum tend to heal quite well, even if only generally apposed. By contrast, ligamentous injuries such as sacroiliac dislocations and symphyseal separations do not heal well unless they are well

aligned. This was demonstrated by Fell and associates[10] who reported on the 7-year follow-up of nonsurgically treated patients with type A, B, and C pelvic injuries. The authors found that there was moderate pain or functional deficit in the type A, B, and C fractures of 40%, 55% and 90% of patients, respectively. Most significantly, the authors found that sacroiliac dislocations that were not well reduced had the worst outcomes.

Pain has also been correlated with displacement at the time of union. Recent studies that include only well-aligned and stably fixed injuries have not demonstrated this difference.[8,11-16] However, in a multicenter study conducted by Kellam,[3] it was reported that for patients treated only with external fixation for completely unstable type III injuries, 50% of those with final displacement of less than 10 mm and 77% of those with union and greater than 10 mm of displacement had significant pain. Overall, 31% of patients were reported to have normal function.

Associated Injuries
Urologic Injuries
Urologic injuries occur in approximately 15% of patients with pelvic fractures, and higher rates of urologic injuries occur in patients with more complex pelvic fractures.[17] Most of these injuries involve either the urethra or bladder. The successful treatment of associated pelvic fractures and urologic injuries requires a team approach to minimize complications and improve functional outcomes.

Because of the relative lengths of the urethra, associated urethral injuries are more common in men than women. Complications include strictures, incontinence, and impotence. After complete urethral disruption, the incidence of stricture is as high as 44% and that of erectile dysfunction as high as 72%. Early repair and primary realignment of complete urethral tears has lowered the incidence of late strictures (18.5%).[17]

A high rate of late genitourinary and reproductive problems has been documented in women with pelvic fractures despite the apparent absence of initial injuries. Copeland and associates[18] documented that 21% of women experience urinary tract problems after pelvic fractures. These problems included stress incontinence, an increased rate of cesarean section, and dyspareunia. It was postulated that subclinical soft-tissue injury to the pelvic floor, including the possibility of both muscular and neurologic injuries, might cause these problems.

An increased incidence of cesarean section in women is observed after pelvic fractures. The indications for cesarean section in this setting are poorly described but seem to depend on fetal factors, obstetrician factors, anatomic changes leading to fetal pelvic disproportion, or physiologic factors. In the absence of clear guidelines, it is prudent for orthopaedic surgeons to give factual information to the patient and her obstetrician regarding the nature of the injury and any residual pelvic ring displacement.

Urinary tract injuries associated with pelvic fracture result in an increased risk of infection. The presence of suprapubic catheters and indwelling Foley catheters within the surgical field increases the risk of associated infection at the fracture site. The risk of infection is increased because of inadequate urinary diversion associated with both extraperitoneal bladder ruptures and urethral disruptions. Routt and associates[17] documented a late infection rate of 4.3% after the early combined treatment of bladder and urethral tears and open reduction and internal fixation of the anterior pelvic ring during the same procedure. The role of long-term antibiotic therapy after internal fixation in the setting of long-term Foley catheter placement after urologic repair has not been documented.

Although blood at the penile meatus or the vaginal introitus are signs of urethral trauma, in many instances these

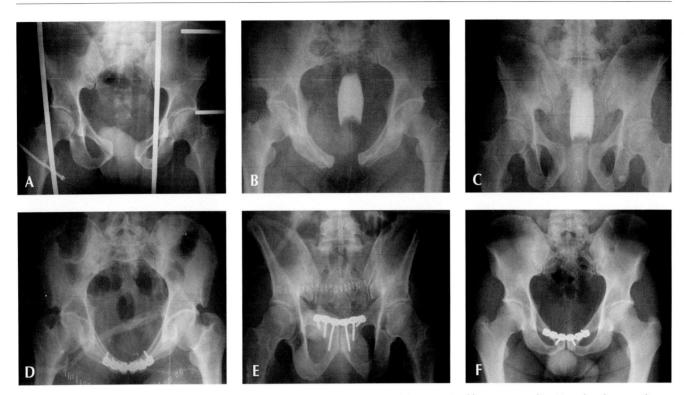

Figure 1 A, Presentation AP radiograph of an anterior-posterior compression type II injury sustained by a motorcyclist. Note that the sacroiliac joints are not vertically displaced, they only open anteriorly. **B,** Inlet view showing sacroiliac joint opening. **C,** Outlet view showing minimal flexor extension deformity. Initial inlet (**D**) and outlet (**E**) views after standard anterior fixation. At 1-year follow-up the patient had returned to work and normal activities with only minimal pain with extremely stressful activity (**F**).

signs are not present. Retrograde urethrograms are recommended before inserting a Foley catheter in male patients; in hemodynamically unstable patients, it is appropriate to attempt to gently pass a catheter. Cystograms should be performed in the presence of hematuria. Because impotence, incontinence, and stricture can significantly impact quality of life, patients should be informed before treatment and appropriate referrals should be made for late problems.

Neurologic Injuries

Neurologic injuries associated with pelvic fractures depend on the severity of the injury and anatomic location. The frequency of injury increases with increasing instability of the pelvic fracture. These facts mandate a careful peripheral neurologic examination and documentation of motor grading in patients with pelvic fractures.

Sacral fractures have the highest rate of neurologic injury, and the rate of injury is correlated with the site of the fracture. The Denis classification of sacral fractures correlates directly with the incidence of nerve injury; for zone 1 alar fractures, the rate of injury is 24%; for zone 2 fractures through the neural foramina, it is 29%; for zone 3 fractures of the central canal, it is 60% to 75%.[19] Zone 1 and zone 2 fractures are usually unilateral, whereas zone 3 fractures are frequently bilateral and may lead to bladder dysfunction.

The role of foraminotomy for decompression of sacral nerve injuries is controversial, and no studies have presented convincing evidence that this procedure improves functional recovery/outcome. However, the presence of bony debris within the sacral foramina is considered by some to be an indication for foraminotomy at the time of open reduction and internal fixation.[11] It is thought that the prognosis of the nerve injury depends on the trauma to the nerve that occurs at the time of the injury; anatomic reduction after these injuries does not appear to have an effect upon the ultimate prognosis of the neural injury.[11] For unstable pelvic ring injuries, as many as 40% of patients present with both sensory and motor deficits. The degree of deficits has been correlated with the ultimate functional outcome of these patients. However, clinical nerve injury does not appear to correlate with posterior pelvic pain.

Skeletal Outcomes

Outcomes with pelvic injuries correlate

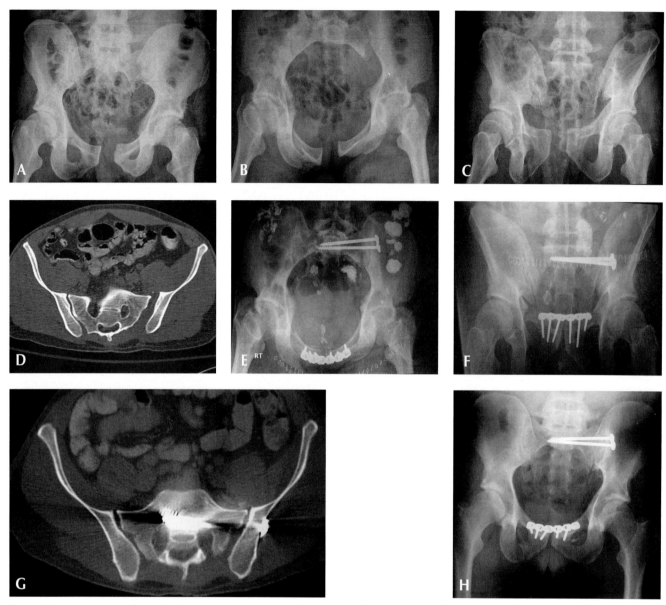

Figure 2 A, Presentation radiograph of a patient with a rotationally and vertically unstable sacroiliac joint. Note the vertical displacement of the left hemipelvis with respect to the right hemipelvis. **B,** The inlet shows significant posterior displacement in the plane of the sacrum of the entire hemipelvis. **C,** The outlet view also shows significant displacement. **D,** The CT scan shows that the sacroiliac joint is open both anteriorly and posteriorly with complete displacement. The initial inlet **(E)** and outlet **(F)** views after open reduction of the symphysis and percutaneous screw fixation of the sacroiliac joint. **G,** The postoperative CT scan shows reduction of the sacroiliac joint. **H,** At 6 months postoperatively, the patient is doing well with minimal pelvic pain. However, the patient had an L5 palsy at the time of injury that did not resolve and requires the use of a brace and restriction on work activities.

with initial displacement, particularly initial instability. Type B injuries, including anterior-posterior compression type II fractures with a symphyseal displacement and anterior sacroiliac joint opening with the posterior tether intact, as well as some lateral compression type II injuries, such as fracture-dislocations, tend to have much better outcomes than type C injuries, which are completely unstable. Pohlemann and associates[12] reported 80% good or excellent results in patients with type B injuries compared with only 27% in those with type C injuries. In a series of 29 patients with anterior-posterior compression type II injuries that were treated with open reduction and internal fixation (anterior pelvic fixation and a near anatomic reduction), it was reported that 96% of patients had good or excellent results, with 83% returning to work in less than 1 year[13] (Figure 1). These results compare favorably with outcomes in patients with type C or completely unstable injuries.[20,21] A multicenter study using various treatments for pelvic injuries demonstrated a 36% incidence of pain overall but a 60% incidence for type III injuries.[22] In a series of 15 patients treated with initial external fixation and delayed open reduction and internal fixation of the posterior pelvic ring, Browner and associates[23] reported that 50% of patients with type III injuries were not working at 1- to 4-year follow-up. The reason for patients not returning to work was evenly divided between pelvic pain and associated skeletal injuries. In this series, 33% had significant posterior pain. Draijer and associates[24] reported similar findings, with 50% of patients with type C injuries requiring a job change. These authors also concluded that functional outcome correlated with the severity of injury and type of instability.

Tornetta and Matta[14] reviewed a series of 69 patients with 76 type III injuries (Figure 2). Forty-six patients with 48 injuries were available for follow-up at an average of 44 months, 13 (30%) of whom had associated acetabular fractures and 17 (38%) had associated neurologic injuries. Patients were evaluated using a questionnaire that assessed return to work, ambulation, and pain. For the overall group, 67% of patients were back to work in an unrestricted capacity, whereas 43% had to change jobs. Of those who changed jobs, less than half had to do so because of pelvic pain, 8% because of neurologic injuries, 8% because of associated injuries, and 2% because of other problems. The largest percentage of patients who changed jobs had pure sacroiliac dislocations. Thirty-five percent of the patients in this series had neurologic injuries, which were most common for patients with sacroiliac joint

dislocations and sacral fractures rather than fracture-dislocations. Overall, 13% of patients had sexual difficulties, including diminished erection, 13% had causalgic type pain, and 27% had weakness of which half required an ankle-foot orthosis for walking. Pain was absent during regular activities in 63% of the patients, 50% had no pain at all, and 13% had pain only with strenuous activity. Thirty-five percent, however, had pain during activities of daily living, approximately half of which were patients with posterior pelvic ring injuries, some of whom required a change in their activities to accommodate the pain. Only 2% of patients had severe and constant pain. No patients in the entire study had anterior pain, possibly because all patients had an adequate reduction. Sixty-three percent of patients ambulated without restriction or the use of a cane. Twelve percent had a limp or required a cane because of posterior pelvic pain, and an additional 25% had diminished ambulation because of associated injuries or neurologic deficit rather than problems specifically related to the pelvis. No patient in this series had any complaints related to pelvic obliquity, malunion, or nonunion. Neither initial displacement nor postoperative reduction was found to correlate with pain. This conclusion, however, is slightly biased because all of the reductions were considered to be good or excellent; therefore, the amount of displacement postoperatively was small in all of the patients. Additionally, all patients had completely unstable injuries.

Several recent studies have looked specifically at posterior pelvic ring injuries. Templeman and associates[11] reported on 30 patients with sacral fractures, all of whom had initial displacement of greater than 1 cm. Forty percent of the patients had neurologic injuries. Patients treated with both open reduction and internal fixation and percutaneous reduction and fixation techniques had a 100% union rate, regardless of the treat-

ment method. The authors found that functional score correlated most closely with neurologic outcomes for patients with displaced sacral injuries. Leighton and Waddell[25] examined 54 patients with pure sacroiliac dislocations that were treated with an anterior approach and plating of the sacroiliac joint. This group of patients clearly demonstrated the importance of achieving an anatomic reduction of an unstable ligamentous posterior pelvic ring injury. Eighty percent of the patients had an anatomic reduction. Twenty-five percent of those patients reported pain. Of the 20% of patients with a nonanatomic reduction, 70% reported significant pain. There was no loss of reduction in patients in this series, and sacroiliac plate fixation anteriorly was determined to be a good form of fixation. There were, however, two patients with L5 neurapraxia.

Although most recent series demonstrate that modern internal fixation techniques that rely primarily on fixation with iliosacral screws for sacroiliac dislocations and sacral fractures and plate fixation of fracture-dislocations result in stable fixation that can be maintained to union, there is one important report to the contrary. Keating and associates[26] reported on a series of 38 patients with vertically unstable fractures, all of whom were treated with reduction and posterior iliosacral fixation. Thirty-two of the 38 patients had fixation of the anterior pelvic ring in addition to posterior fixation. This group reported 13% errant screw placement, 44% malunion, and an 85% rate of significant pain in follow-up, with only 46% of the patients returning to work. Of note, these authors used more stringent criteria for malunion than other series. This report from a group of experienced surgeons points out the risks of iliosacral screw placement and the potential problems for patients in whom posterior pelvic ring fixation is required.

Most recent series demonstrate that modern internal fixation techniques can maintain the reduction to union if the fracture is well reduced. This may not be the case if the fractures are not well reduced. In patients in whom the reduction is anatomic or near anatomic and maintained to union, the expected rate of successful outcomes for type III injuries is between 60% and 70% for most areas of evaluation, including having minimal pain, being able to walk without assistive devices, and returning to activities of daily living. Return to work is more dependent on job functional requirements than other areas of evaluation. Those who do strenuous labor have a much more difficult time returning to work than do sedentary workers. All of the series corroborate that maintaining a good reduction through union will diminish or eliminate any complaints related to limb-length discrepancy, sitting imbalance, and pelvic stability. In patients with type II injuries, in particular anterior-posterior compression type II injuries, good outcomes can be expected in 80% to 90% of patients as well as a high rate of return to work and near-normal function.

Outcomes Scores and General Health

Recently, more emphasis has been placed on general health measures and scoring systems in evaluating patient outcomes. This strategy is most effective for patients who are undergoing elective surgery because in such instances both preoperative and postoperative outcome scores can be obtained. In patients with traumatic injury, outcomes scoring can be useful only to identify or compare outcome with age-matched controls or to compare methods of treatment. Several investigators have looked at general health measures in patients with pelvic injuries. Oliver and associates[15] followed 55 multiply injured patients with pelvic injuries that required fixation. A Medical Outcomes Study 36-Item Short Form General Health Survey (SF-36) score was obtained for 46 of these patients 2 years

after surgery. These authors reported a 14% diminution in physical outcome and a 5.5% diminution in mental outcome compared with control subjects. These scores were not correlated with any injury-specific score. Brenneman and associates[27] obtained the SF-36 scores of 27 patients with open pelvic injuries at an average of 4 years and reported low scores in the areas of bodily pain, general health, and physical functioning. Cole and associates[16] followed 64 patients with unstable posterior pelvic ring injuries for an average of 36 months. Of the 52 patients available for complete follow-up, they reported that there was one sacral nonunion and all other fractures healed with acceptable reductions. The authors evaluated patients using a 40-point pelvic injury specific survey and the SF-36, and the results demonstrated a good correlation between the two scores. Forty percent of the patients had posterior tenderness, 37% had urinary dysfunction, and 29% had sexual dysfunction. Work status was affected in 35% of patients. Fracture location did not correlate with outcome in patients who went on to achieve union.

Miranda and associates[28] followed 80 patients with pelvic injuries for more than 5 years, 61% of whom were treated with only an external fixator. They evaluated the patients using the SF-36, the Iowa pelvic scores, and a questionnaire. The SF-36 evaluation demonstrated that the patients were more than two standard deviations below the norm in three of the eight measured categories. Seventy-five percent returned to normal sexual function, and 80% returned to work. These authors found no difference by class of instability (as classified by Tile[29]) and no difference in outcome based on displacement. These results demonstrate one of the problems in using summed scored outcome measurements. Although there was no apparent difference in outcome by Tile classification, there was no assessment of associated injuries. Thus, the

results of this study may have been subject to a floor effect. For example, a patient in whom the SF-36 scores were diminished because of an open ankle injury may have had a pelvic fracture that was fixed in good position and was not specifically the cause of any problem. Therefore, when evaluating the outcomes of patients with pelvic fractures, it is important to take associated injuries into account and subcategorize them during any reporting of general health.

Summary

Pelvic fractures are relatively common problems and are often associated with motor vehicle accidents and falls. Many level 1 trauma centers will treat more than 200 pelvic injuries each year. Most of these patients have stable injuries that can be treated with limited weight bearing or even weight bearing as tolerated and can be expected to go on to have a good result. Patients with rotational instability, particularly those with anterior-posterior compression type II fractures, benefit from surgical intervention to stabilize the pelvis in an anatomic position that allows it to heal appropriately. Good to excellent results can be expected in most of these patients. Patients with completely unstable posterior injuries in which the posterior pelvic ring is unstable rotationally and vertically comprise a different treatment class. Although modern treatment has been shown to diminish mortality, nonunion, limb-length discrepancy, sitting imbalance, gait impairment, and pelvic outlet obstruction, many of the sequelae of the initial injury, such as neurologic, urologic, and other skeletal injuries, will preclude the patient from having a good or excellent outcome. Even though much attention is initially given to treating the pelvic ring injury with regard to restoring the anatomy and gaining union, the long-term outcome will likely be affected more by the associated injuries than by a properly treated pelvic injury. It is, therefore, important to review this information with patients who have these injuries.

References

1. Holdsworth F: Dislocation and fracture-dislocation of the pelvis. *J Bone Joint Surg Br* 1948;30:461-466.

2. Huittinen VM: Lumbosacral nerve injury in fracture of the pelvis. *Acta Chir Scand* 1972;138(suppl):1-44.

3. Kellam J: The role of external fixation in pelvic disruptions. *Clin Orthop* 1989;241:66-82.

4. Raf L: Double vertical fractures of the pelvis. *Acta Chir Scand* 1966;131:298-305.

5. Slatis P, Huittinen VM: Double vertical fractures of the pelvis. *Acta Chir Scand* 1972;138:799-807.

6. Semba R, Yasukawa K, Gustilo R: Critical analysis of results of 53 Malgaigne fractures of the pelvic. *J Trauma* 1983;23:535-537.

7. Matta JM: Indications for anterior fixation of pelvic fractures. *Clin Orthop* 1996;329:88-96.

8. Matta JM, Tornetta P III: Internal fixation of unstable pelvic ring injuries. *Clin Orthop* 1996;329:129-140.

9. Bucholz R: The pathologic anatomy of Malgaigne fracture-dislocations of the pelvis. *J Bone Joint Surg Am* 1981;63:400-404.

10. Fell M, Meissner A, Rahmanzadeh R: Long-term outcome after conservative treatment of pelvic ring injuries and conclusions for current management. *Zentralbl Chir* 1995;120:899-904.

11. Templeman D, Goulet J, Duwelius PJ, Olson S, Davidson M: Internal fixation of displaced fractures of the sacrum. *Clin Orthop* 1996;329:180-185.

12. Pohlemann T, Gansslen A, Schellwald O, Culemann U, Tscherne H: Outcome after pelvic ring injuries. *Injury* 1996;27(suppl 2): 31-38.

13. Tornetta P III, Dickson K, Matta JM: Outcome of rotationally unstable pelvic ring injuries treated operatively. *Clin Orthop* 1996;329:147-151.

14. Tornetta P III, Matta JM: Outcome of operatively treated unstable posterior pelvic ring disruptions. *Clin Orthop* 1996;329:186-193.

15. Oliver CW, Twaddle B, Agel J, Routt ML Jr: Outcome after pelvic ring fractures: Evaluation using the medical outcomes short form SF-36. *Injury* 1996;27:635-641.

16. Cole JD, Blum DA, Ansel LJ: Outcome after fixation of unstable posterior pelvic ring injuries. *Clin Orthop* 1996;329:160-179.

17. Routt ML, Simonian PT, Defalco AJ, Miller J, Clarke T: Internal fixation in pelvic fractures and primary repairs of associated genitourinary disruptions: A team approach. *J Trauma* 1996;40:784-790.

18. Copeland CE, Bosse MJ, McCarthy ML, et al: Effect of trauma and pelvic fracture on female genitourinary, sexual, and reproductive function. *J Orthop Trauma* 1997;11:73-81.

19. Reilly MC, Zinar DM, Matta JM: Neurologic injuries in pelvic ring fractures. *Clin Orthop* 1996;329:28-36.

20. Van den Bosch EW, Van der Kleyn R, Hogervorst M, Van Vugt AB: Functional outcome of internal fixation for pelvic ring fractures. *J Trauma* 1999;47:365-371.

21. Dujardin FH, Hossenbaccus M, Duparc F, Biga N, Thomine JM: Long-term functional prognosis of posterior injuries in high-energy

pelvic disruptions. *J Orthop Trauma* 1998;12:145-151.

22. Kellam J, McMurtry R, Paley D, et al: The unstable pelvic fracture: Operative treatment. *Orthop Clin North Am* 1987;18:25-41.

23. Browner B, Cole D, Graham M, et al: Delayed posterior internal fixation of unstable pelvic fractures. *J Trauma* 1987;27:998-1006.

24. Draijer F, Egbers HJ, Havemann D: Quality of life after pelvic ring injuries: Follow-up results of a prospective study. *Arch Orthop Trauma Surg* 1997;116:22-26.

25. Leighton RK, Waddell JP: Techniques for reduction and posterior fixation through the anterior approach. *Clin Orthop* 1996;329:115-120.

26. Keating JF, Werier J, Blachut P, Broekhuyse H, Meek RN, O'Brien PJ: Early fixation of the vertically unstable pelvis: The role of iliosacral screw fixation of the posterior lesion. *J Orthop Trauma* 1999;13:107-113.

27. Brenneman FD, Katyal D, Boulanger BR, et al: Long-term outcomes in open pelvic fractures. *J Trauma* 1997;42:773-777.

28. Miranda MA, Riemer BL, Butterfield SL, Burke CJ III: Pelvic ring injuries: A long term functional outcome study. *Clin Orthop* 1996;329:152-159.

29. Tile M: Pelvic ring fractures: Should they be fixed? *J Bone Joint Surg Br* 1988;70:1-12.

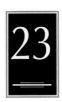

Primary Total Hip Arthroplasty After Acetabular Fracture

Dana C. Mears, MD, PhD
John H. Velyvis, MD

After a displaced acetabular fracture, a patient may be predisposed to the development of symptomatic posttraumatic degenerative arthritis of the hip joint or osteonecrosis of the femoral head. In selected patients, a total hip arthroplasty (THA) may eventually be necessary irrespective of the method of initial management.[1-3] On the basis of a review of the results described by Letournel and Judet[2] and Matta[4] and on the basis of our experience, we determined that the likelihood that treatment will culminate in an arthroplasty is related to the initial type of fracture; the magnitude of the provocative force; the age and weight of the patient; and, when the initial management of the fracture was open reduction and internal fixation, the duration of the delay from the injury to the surgical procedure. When the initial acetabular deformity is relatively minor and when the acetabulum unites, especially following nonsurgical treatment, a conventional arthroplasty is likely to lead to an uncomplicated recovery and a satisfactory outcome. Nevertheless, in selected cases, one or more complicating factors may be encountered. Following nonsurgical treatment of an acetabular fracture, residual displacement may hamper a subsequent arthroplasty because of an occult or frank nonunion of the acetabulum or possibly because of a malunion or a malaligned nonunion.[5] When the initial management of an acetabular fracture was surgical, a belated arthroplasty performed to manage posttraumatic arthritis may be impeded by dense scar tissue, heterotopic bone, avascularity of the hip muscles or the acetabulum, obstructive hardware, or occult infection.[6] On the basis of a review of the few prior studies in the literature,[7-10] we found that the overall prognosis for a patient managed with a THA after an acetabular fracture is less favorable than that for one managed with an arthroplasty performed because of primary degenerative arthritis. In the present study, we address the principal concerns regarding management with THA after initial treatment of an acetabular fracture with closed or open reduction.

In view of the principal shortcoming of acute management with THA following an acetabular fracture, namely, the vulnerability to premature failure and the subsequent need for one or more surgical revisions, the potential therapeutic alternatives merit serious consideration. For example, young male laborers or other young, exceptionally active individuals are highly susceptible to premature failure of an arthroplasty.[11] In such patients, one therapeutic alternative is arthrodesis of the hip, which is mainly indicated if there is relative preservation of the osseous architecture of the hip joint. The other criteria for an arthrodesis, namely, a normal contralateral hip, normal knees, and an asymptomatic lower back, also must be met.[12] Currently, most individuals in North America are reluctant to consider arthrodesis. When a patient has osteonecrosis of the femoral head, loss of acetabular bone stock, marked osteoporosis, or a persistent acetabular nonunion that impairs the mechanical stability of a hip fusion and hampers the healing of the bone, the likelihood of achieving a solid fusion is considerably compromised. In such complex cases, the main practical alternative is a resection arthroplasty, with or without the use of a cement spacer.[13]

Certain other symptomatic acetabular fractures may be associated with secondary problems that can be addressed by reconstruction of the hip, thus preserving the hip as a functional joint. Examples of the problems include heterotopic bone leading to hip stiffness; symptoms related to the hardware; a symptomatic nonunion or malunion of the acetabulum and/or hemipelvis; and, occasionally, a localized and indolent infection. In each of these situations, all relevant diagnostic clinical and radiographic methods are used in an attempt to determine whether the hip joint has intact and congruent bearing surfaces. Whenever it is technically possible, and especially in a younger patient, every attempt should be made to salvage a functional hip joint.[14]

Clinical Assessment

The typical presenting symptoms of posttraumatic arthritis or osteonecrosis of the femoral head include local or referred pain, a limp, and a decreased level of activity. If the acetabulum, or another site in the pelvic ring, has a persistent nonunion, the patient may complain of pelvic instability with gross motion of the nonunion site or sites. A marked deformity of the pelvic ring can be an associated complicating factor, but this is rare. After an open reduction of the acetabulum, particularly when an extensile exposure has been used, stiffness may develop secondary to extensive heterotopic bone. Young obese men who sustain a closed head injury in addition to the acetabular fracture are notoriously susceptible to this problem.

During the physical examination, a shortened leg or an antalgic or stiff-hipped gait may be evident. Tenderness about the hip and the presence of a surgical scar, along with a flexion or other type of contracture and stiffness, are commonly observed. The ipsilateral lower extremity is examined carefully for subtle findings of a sciatic nerve palsy, such as hypoesthesia of the foot or motor weakness. When a patient has these findings, even a slight intraoperative injury to the sciatic nerve creates a substantial risk for the development of a postoperative complete footdrop because of the extraordinary susceptibility of a peripheral nerve to a second injury, or "double crush syndrome" as described by Osterman.[15]

When open reduction of the acetabulum culminates in a chronically painful hip, the potential for a deep wound infection needs to be considered. Most such infections are occult, with such subtle clinical findings that hematologic, bacteriologic, and radiographic studies, and even an aspiration arthrogram, may not confirm the diagnosis. In an exceptional case, a frank wound infection with an open sinus tract may complicate the presentation of grossly infected bone. From the time of presentation, the patient should be managed with suitable antibiotic therapy, and surgical planning should include multiple débridements, techniques for plastic coverage of the wound, and consideration of a belated arthroplasty.

Radiographic Assessment

When a minimally displaced acetabular fracture progresses to posttraumatic arthritis, the preparation for a THA may be adequately accomplished by scrutiny of standard anteroposterior pelvic and frog-leg lateral radiographs. In more complex cases, additional pelvic radiographs may be helpful.[2,3] The 45° inlet and outlet radiographs reveal pelvic ring deformities, including central protrusion and vertical or posterior displacement of a hemipelvis. The 45° obturator oblique radiograph highlights deformities of the anterior column and the posterior wall, while the corresponding iliac oblique radiograph depicts the posterior column and the anterior wall. A CT scan may provide the optimal view of an occult nonunion and of incarcerated hardware such as a screw. When a patient has an exceptional deformity that involves the entire pelvic ring, a three-dimensional CT scan may help the surgeon to identify the sites and vectors of the deformity.[16] When there is extensive heterotopic bone formation, a combination of imaging modalities merits consideration in order to fully characterize the magnitude of the problem. A CT scan along with Judet oblique radiographs are crucial to fully ascertain the extent of the anterior and posterior heterotopic ossification.[17]

When an occult deep wound infection is suspected after a prior open acetabular reduction, either an aspiration arthrogram or a technetium Tc 99m bone scan may be helpful. An infection is a causative factor for heterotopic bone formation.[18] Ironically, when a patient has florid heterotopic bone, an aspiration arthrogram may be impossible and a technetium Tc 99m bone scan may lose much of its sensitivity in the detection of infection. In addition to a complete blood cell count with differential and a determination of the erythrocyte sedimentation rate and C-reactive protein level, a gallium Ga 67 citrate scan or an indium white blood cell scan may be valuable, but only in rare cases.[19,20]

Preoperative Planning

When the clinical and radiographic assessments are complete, the specific focal problems of the patient are carefully analyzed to plan the arthroplasty. A discrete acetabular defect may arise from the site of a displaced acetabular fragment following surgical removal of a loose fragment or from an area of marginal or central impaction. The defect may vary widely in size, from minute to structurally important. As a general rule, a defect with a diameter of less than 10 mm is not structurally important, a defect with a diameter of 10 to 25 mm is moderately important, and a defect with a diameter of greater than 25 mm is very important (Fig. 1). Such defects can be characterized by one of the available classification schemes, such as that of D'Antonio and associates[21] and that of Gross and associates[22] (Tables 1 and 2). Most of the available classification schemes distinguish isolated cavitary lesions from segmental defects. The more structurally important segmental group can be subdivided into defects involving a wall or a rim as opposed to a column or, ultimately, the most sinister form, a transverse dissociation or nonunion. These types of defects represent progressively more challenging reconstructive problems. Irrespective of its size, such a defect may possess a well-circumscribed boundary or a highly irregular one, and its borders may have well-vascularized or avascular bone. All of these factors have profound implications for the therapeutic plan.

A wide variety of deformities of the acetabulum and the pelvic ring may be encountered. When a late deformity is present, it may involve a limited portion of the acetabulum, such as the anterior or posterior column or the medial wall. This type of deformity may be evident as a linear step-off. Alternatively, after an unreduced fracture of both columns, a

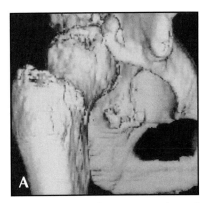 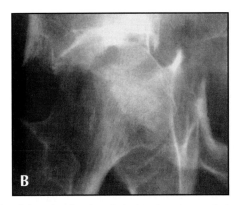 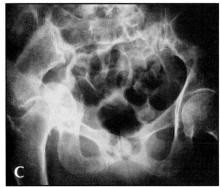

Fig. 1 The structural importance of acetabular defects is related to their size, location, and characterization as a cavitary or segmental lesion. **A,** Oblique three-dimensional CT scan, obtained 1 year after a fracture-dislocation of the posterior wall, showing a large segmental defect of the posterior wall secondary to failed fixation. **B,** Anteroposterior (AP) radiograph of a hip, obtained 2 years after a transtectal transverse fracture that was treated nonsurgically, showing a central segmental defect of moderate size, with a principal axis of more than 10 mm but less than 25 mm. **C,** AP radiograph of a pelvis, obtained 2 years after a transtectal T-type fracture that was treated nonsurgically, showing progression to a large central segmental defect with a principal axis of approximately 50 mm.

"secondary incongruity" may represent a malrotation of each portion of the acetabulum, manifesting as a protrusion of the fragments around the imploded femoral head.[2] Nevertheless, in this situation, while the center of rotation of the femoral head is somewhat altered biomechanically, there is no true focal acetabular defect. This deformity, therefore, is readily addressed with use of a standard cementless cup of a somewhat enlarged size, or a so-called jumbo cup[23] (Fig. 2).

At the time of a THA for posttraumatic arthritis following an acetabular fracture, a nonunion is particularly likely to be encountered after a posterior wall or column injury. However, after an injury pattern such as a transverse fracture or a fracture of both columns, a nonunion is an uncommon problem that occurs primarily when florid displacement is uncorrected. Preoperative multiplanar imaging of the acetabulum is particularly helpful to characterize the magnitude, site, and vector of displacement of the nonunion. The degree of malalignment of an acetabular nonunion has considerable therapeutic implications and can be broadly subdivided into three categories that correspond to the magnitude of the acetabular defect. When the

Table 1
Classification of acetabular deficiencies in THA according to the system of D'Antonio and associates[21]

Type	Deficiency
I	Segmental deficiencies
IA	Peripheral
IB	Central (medial wall absent)
II	Cavitary deficiencies
IIA	Peripheral
IIB	Central (medial wall intact)
III	Combined deficiencies
IV	Pelvic discontinuity
V	Arthrodesis

Table 2
Classification of acetabular deficiencies in THA according to the system of Gross and associates[22]

Type	Deficiency
I	Contained cavitary defect (protrusio)
II	Uncontained (structural rim defect)
IIA	Minor column (shelf defect) with > 50% of cup coverage
IIB	Major column (acetabular defect) with > 50% loss of cup contact and loss of one or both columns

nonunion gap is less than 10 mm, it can be readily obliterated by packing it with autograft harvested from the femoral head. Alternatively, the fracture fragments may be sufficiently mobile to approximate the fracture surfaces with use of suitable bone-holding forceps. The fixation of the fragments can be achieved with use of lag screws, a plate, a cup with multiple screws, or a ring. When a nonunion defect is 10 to 25 mm, scar tissue, heterotopic bone, or fracture callus may considerably impede an attempted open reduction. The gap can be obliterated with morcellized or bulk autograft. For structural augmentation, one of several strategies may be considered. Fine

stainless-steel or titanium mesh can be used to buttress the acetabulum to facilitate impaction grafting.[24] Alternatively, a cup inserted with multiple screws can be used as a form of a hemispherical plate. For defects that are larger than 25 mm, one of several specialized devices may be used. A cage or ring combined with a cemented cup can be used to immobilize multiple acetabular bone fragments and to obliterate the acetabular defect.[25,26] To fill a superior acetabular defect, a bilobed cup can be used. As an alternative strategy, when the nonunion gap exceeds 25 mm, serious consideration should be given to realignment and reapproximation of the acetabulum.[5] Otherwise, a

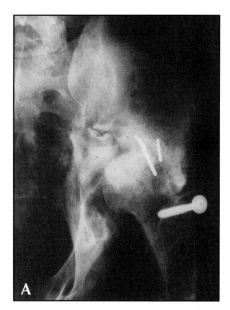
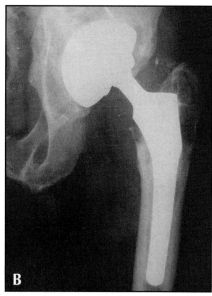

Fig. 2 A 48-year-old man sustained a T-type acetabular fracture, which was managed with limited internal fixation. Subsequent symptomatic posttraumatic arthritis was complicated by an excessively large superocentral acetabular defect and necrotic bone in the roof. Three years after the injury, as part of a THA, the necrotic bone was removed and a structural autograft from the femoral head was used to obliterate the acetabular defect. **A,** AP radiograph of the right hip, obtained 3 years after the injury, showing the large acetabular defect. **B,** AP radiograph obtained after the THA, showing the large defect obliterated by a jumbo cup.

technical failure with a persistent non-union, premature loosening of the cup, or other complication is likely to ensue. During preoperative preparation for such a case, a three-dimensional CT scan is helpful to optimally characterize the pelvic deformity.

Optimal Timing of the Arthroplasty

After initial management of an acetabular fracture, THA is typically considered when a patient is seen with evidence of secondary degenerative change 1 year or more after the initial injury. By that time, the acetabulum is usually united, even though there may be a defect or a deformity. Occasionally, a serious problem with the hip (for example, an early secondary displacement of the fracture, possibly with failed internal fixation) is recognized within a few days or weeks after the initial injury and following either nonsurgical or surgical treatment.

An unacceptable deformity often is not adequately appreciated radiographically. For instance, when a patient has a displaced transverse or posterior fracture-dislocation and osteopenia, the femoral head typically undergoes rapid abrasive wear that may culminate in the loss of 50% or more of its surface area. Likewise, late recognition of marginal or central acetabular impaction may not be consistent with a realistic capability to achieve a satisfactory belated surgical correction. Unfortunately, both conventional radiography and CT may fail to provide a realistic representation of a hip with an extraordinary amount of loss of surface area of the femoral head or extensive acetabular impaction.

When a THA is indicated, a question may arise about the need to delay the procedure until the acetabular fracture has fully united so that the cup can be inserted into a stable osseous bed. The best solution depends on the severity of

the particular acetabular deformity and the experience of the surgeon. There are potential advantages to undertaking a THA as soon as the hip has been shown radiographically to have incongruent articular surfaces and thus an overwhelming potential for a rapid onset of pain. The foremost advantage is minimization of the delay between the acute fracture and the recovery from the arthroplasty. Also, when an unacceptable deformity of the acetabulum is recognized soon after the injury, either as a failure to achieve an acceptable reduction or as a delayed displacement, the defect can typically be adequately minimized or even fully corrected at the time of a promptly executed arthroplasty.

For some hips with a displaced fracture, open reduction and internal fixation needs to be considered when an incongruity has been recognized early.[14] In the absence of marked impaction or abrasion of the articular surfaces, and especially in a young adult who has a simple fracture pattern, delayed open reduction is preferred. In an inactive elderly or otherwise infirm patient in whom comminution and impaction secondary to osteoporosis can be anticipated, acute management with an arthroplasty may be a more realistic endeavor. When it is difficult to predict the extent of irreversible damage radiographically, consent for open reduction with a possible THA is obtained and the appropriate resources are organized for both procedures.

Surgical Approaches

Depending on the focal anatomic and pathologic problem, such as heterotopic ossification, one of several standard surgical approaches may be preferred[26-31] (Fig. 3). Typically, when posttraumatic arthritis develops after an acetabular fracture has healed with minimal deformity, either a conventional anterior Hardinge approach[31] or a posterior approach is highly suitable. When there is a substantial acetabular deformity or heterotopic bone, a modified or alternative exposure may be preferred. If a fractured posterior wall or column requires an extensive surgical field, then a full Kocher-Langenbeck incision[2] is used. For adequate visualization of both the anterior and the posterior aspect of the acetabulum and the adjacent hip joint, a triradiate incision with preservation of the greater trochanter is highly appropriate. When the entire hemipelvis is involved in the deformity and needs a corrective osteotomy as part of the arthroplasty, then an extended iliofemoral approach may be used. In this situation, we prefer a modified or limited extended iliofemoral approach whereby the gluteal tendons and adjacent greater trochanter as well as the piriformis tendons are preserved intact. If the ipsilateral sacroiliac joint is displaced, typically in external rotation, open reduction can be achieved by means of a variety of exposures. With the extended iliofemoral or triradiate approach, a release of the insertions of the external oblique muscle from the iliac crest and the iliacus muscle from the internal iliac fossa provides a suitable access. Alternatively, if the arthroplasty is performed with a conventional anterior or posterior approach to the hip, a second incision along the anterior iliac crest can be used to approach the sacroiliac joint. Whenever a secondary deformity of the pelvic ring culminates in malalignment of the acetabulum by more than 25° in a single plane, initial correction of the pelvic ring is usually indicated prior to the THA. Otherwise, after insertion of the cup, an iatrogenic deformity would ensue as the pelvic ring deformity was corrected. For deformities that involve both hemipelves, the multiple corrective osteotomies and the arthroplasty may be undertaken as a combined sequential procedure (Fig. 4) or as separate procedures at two different times. The relevant determinants include the experience of the surgeon, the magnitude and complexity of the

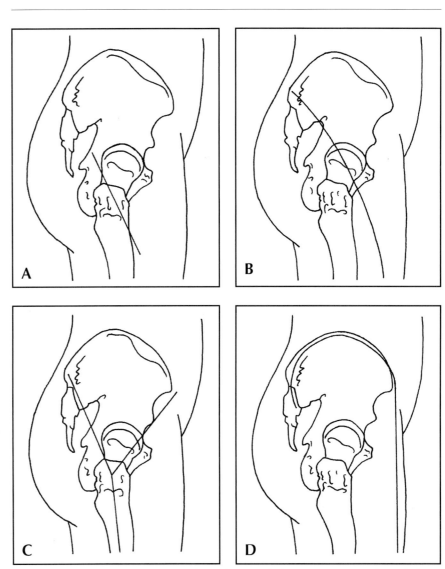

Fig. 3 The surgical approaches commonly used in THA for late reconstruction of acetabula with various defects and accompanying deformities. **A,** The modified Hardinge (anterolateral) incision. Our preferred modification of the approach includes an orientation of 30° from the long axis of the limb so that more direct visualization of the acetabulum is achieved with a shorter incision. **B,** The Kocher-Langenbeck incision. **C,** The modified triradiate incision, with preservation of the greater trochanter. **D,** The limited extended iliofemoral incision.

deformities, the presence of heterotopic bone, and the potential comorbidities of the patient. Some of the principal determinants and the corresponding therapeutic strategies are outlined in Table 3.

Preparation of the Acetabulum

After routine resection of the femoral neck and head, the acetabulum is débrided of residual fibrocartilage and granulation tissue. The acetabulum is carefully examined for a defect, deformity, or nonunion. If such a site is identified, its osseous surfaces are meticulously denuded so that the structural problem can be carefully assessed. The subsequent stages depend on the nature of the problem. If the acetabulum displays necrotic bone, then the dead bone is removed until a uniformly bleeding bed is achieved.

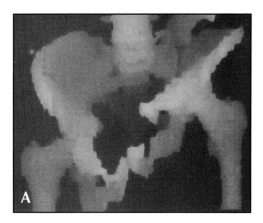 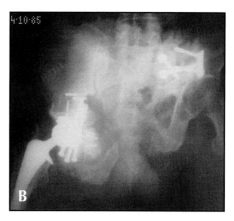 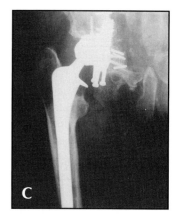

Fig. 4 CT scan and radiographs showing a displaced iliac-wing, or so-called crescent, fracture of the left hip and a T-type acetabular fracture of the right hip. **A,** A three-dimensional CT scan, obtained at the time of presentation, showing a persistent vertical and rotational deformity of the left hemipelvis and a displaced nonunion of the right T-type acetabular fracture with distal displacement of the inferior half of the acetabulum. **B,** Postoperative AP radiograph showing a partial correction of the left pelvic deformity and a right cementless total hip replacement with immobilization of the acetabulum. **C,** AP radiograph of the right hip, obtained 11 years after arthroplasty, showing a successful long-term result. The patient had no pain.

Subsequently, the acetabulum is reamed to restore a hemispherical concavity that is suitable for the insertion of a cementless cup. A large jumbo cup may be needed to obliterate a residual acetabular recess (Fig. 2).

Contained Defects

For a small contained defect, impaction grafting with morcellized bone from the femoral head is preferred.[24,32-35] When a defect is 25 mm or more in its largest dimension, a structural autograft should be considered. In some instances, a femoral head-and-neck autograft can be shaped to fit precisely into the defect (Fig. 5). If it is slightly oversized, it may be impacted to achieve a stable fit. In other instances, fixation with supplementary lag screws or a plate may be necessary. When the cup is placed on a bed of autograft, a cementless cup is the most appropriate choice. When the bed consists of allograft, and especially when it involves the weight-bearing surface, use of a cemented cup is preferred.[36] If the defect greatly exceeds 25 mm in its largest dimension, another useful option is a ring or cage.

Use of a Ring or Cage

Historically, a ring or cage was used in conjunction with a cemented polyethylene cup (Fig. 6). The more recent designs include the availability of a metal-backed polyethylene liner that is mechanically secured to the cage so that the use of bone cement is unnecessary. A wide variety of cages with diverse extension plates are available for special problems[25,26,28] (Fig. 7). The principal advantage of the cage is the potential to use a device with a predictable shape to obliterate a highly irregular defect. Frequently, supplementary bone graft is needed to fill any gaps that remain between the outer surface of the cage and the intact pelvis. The cage may function as a type of fixation plate that immobilizes the site of a transverse nonunion. Nevertheless, despite its current popularity, a cage has certain shortcomings. The foremost problem is a potential for loosening when its anchoring screws are inserted in osteopenic bone. Where there is a nonunion and osteopenic bone, failure to achieve a rapid union of the acetabulum contributes greatly to premature loosening of the cage. A shortcoming that pertains to pre-

vious designs in which the cup was attached to the cage with bone cement is late deterioration of this interface, with subsequent loss of fixation of the cup. This problem is not uncommon after a period of 5 to 10 years. An additional shortcoming of the various cages with a superior or inferior flange or hook is the anatomic configuration of such devices. Typically, such a cup does not fit properly in a highly deformed acetabulum. Most cages are too thick to permit realistic contouring with standard bending instrumentation. A review of the indications for the use of a variety of these devices is summarized in Table 4.

Intermediate or Uncontained Defects

The most common site of an intermediate or uncontained defect is the posterior wall (Fig. 8). In this situation, the displaced and ununited fragment of wall typically is maintained, by scar tissue, in a highly displaced location with superior and posterior malalignment. To achieve a nearly anatomic reduction, the surfaces attached by scar tissue must be fully mobilized, which inevitably provokes extensive avascularity. As an alternative technique, we prefer to denude the deep, former articular surface of the displaced fragment so that it contacts the structural graft and provides a potential source of blood supply.

After curettage, whenever feasible, the defect is prepared with conventional acetabular reamers. Likewise, the true acetabulum is reamed in a conventional manner. The resected femoral head is denuded of residual cartilage with use of cup arthroplasty reamers or so-called reverse acetabular reamers and is used as a structural autograft. A v-shaped notch is made in the femoral head so that the notch interlocks into the damaged section of the posterior wall. The autograft is anchored with use of three 3.5- or 4.0-mm fully threaded screws. Then, the acetabulum is reamed again to the optimal diameter. Any persistent small defect at the junction between the graft and the residual acetabulum is filled with morcellized cancellous bone. Then, a metal backing for a cementless cup in an appropriate size is impacted into the acetabular recess and is anchored with two or three cancellous screws.

Large Uncontained Defects

Large uncontained defects present a principal structural problem in the posterior, superior, or central aspect of the acetabulum. Some reconstructive recommendations are described for each type of defect.

When a patient has a large defect in the posterior part of the acetabulum that involves the wall and the adjacent column, perhaps the most formidable mechanical challenge is the transfer of the patient from the bed to a chair. Thus, a highly stable configuration of the reconstruction is essential. Historically, the most popular form of reconstruction has been the application of a posterior plate with the use of a structural autograft (Figs. 5 and 8). Alternative potential solutions include the use of a cage or a mesh, which is anchored

Table 3
Guidelines for surgical strategies to address pelvic and acetabular deformities as part of a THA

Type of Defect	Treatment
Intrinsic acetabular defects	
Small superior acetabular defect	Morcellized impaction grafting if contained defect, supplementary mesh if uncontained defect, cementless cup
Large superior acetabular defect	Structural or morcellized grafting, cementless cup, jumbo cup, bilobed cup, protrusio cage
Medial acetabular defect	Central mesh, morcellized impaction grafting, cage
Posterior acetabular defect	Structural or morcellized grafting, posterior plate, mesh, standard cup, cage
Associated deformities of pelvic ring	
Iliac defect, nonunion, malalignment	Open reduction and internal fixation of ilium, standard cup
External rotational deformity of ipsilateral or contralateral sacroiliac joint	Open reduction and internal fixation of sacroiliac joint, standard cup
Unstable, windswept pelvis	Open reduction and internal fixation of both sacroiliac joints, standard cup
Vertical defect	
Ipsilateral	Reduction of hemipelvis, long-stemmed component
Contralateral	Reduction of hemipelvis, standard cup

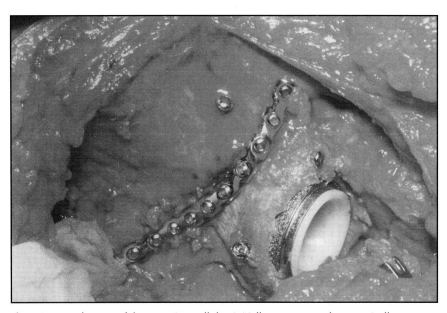

Fig. 5 A T-type fracture of the posterior wall that initially was managed nonsurgically progressed to a nonunion with deformity and degenerative change. Two years later, the posterior column was stabilized through a Kocher-Langenbeck approach with a reconstruction plate, while the defective wall was replaced with a precisely fitting structural autograft and lag screws. This intraoperative photograph was obtained after a metal-backed cup was secured to the pelvis while the autograft was secured with multiple screws.

around the rim of the defect with screws. Then, impaction grafting of the defect is performed with autologous bone in order to create a suitable bed for the cup.

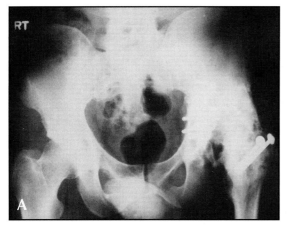
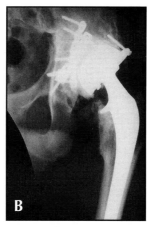

Fig. 6 Radiographs of a 28-year-old man who sustained a transverse fracture of the posterior wall of the left acetabulum. Open reduction and internal fixation was performed with use of a triradiate incision. Within 2 weeks, the posterior wall fragment had displaced; subsequently, the hip progressed to posttraumatic arthritis with grade IV heterotopic bone formation. Two years later, a THA was performed and augmented with a Müller ring to stabilize the wall defect. **A,** AP radiograph, obtained 2 years after the open reduction and internal fixation, showing grade IV heterotopic bone formation and a fusion of the hip. **B,** AP radiograph, obtained 5 years after THA, showing stable fixation of the ring along with a cemented polyethylene cup and a cementless stem.

Table 4	
Devices to manage a large defect and indications for their use	
Device	**Indication**
Mesh	Superior or middle central defect or superior posterior wall defect (remaining acetabulum must be intact)
Bilobed cup	Superior wall and dome defect
Müller ring	Central, superior defect
Ganz ring with hook inobturator foramen	Nonunion of transverse fracture

Another option is the fabrication of a custom implant that is designed on the basis of a three-dimensional CT scan or a corresponding model of the hip (Fig. 9). While this method permits the use of an unlimited variety of shapes to address truly unique structural problems, it possesses several shortcomings. Not only is this technique costly, but only a single implant design can be available during the procedure. If an unanticipated defect within an avascular bed is identified during the surgery, so that additional bone has to be excised, then the custom implant no longer fits precisely into the defect. In this situation, structural autograft or, suboptimally, allograft is needed to restore the structural stability of the reconstruction.

A viable solution for a defect in the superior aspect of the acetabulum that includes a corresponding segment of wall is a bilobed or oblong cup.[37] One newer modular model permits the application of a lobe of three different sizes for obliteration of the corresponding defects (Fig. 10). The principal shortcoming of a bilobed cup is the need to orient it so that the lobe is directed superiorly. If a defect is posterosuperior, the lobe cannot be redirected or the articular portion of the cup will be malaligned and provoke instability of the total hip prosthesis.

For repair of a defect in the central aspect of the acetabulum, use of a structural autograft, a cage, or a central mesh should be considered[38] (Fig. 11). For the latter two methods, morcellized autograft initially is placed into the base of the defect prior to insertion of the hardware. If a central mesh is used, a 5- to 10-mm-thick layer of morcellized cancellous bone graft is impacted in place after insertion of the mesh.

If the defect is exceedingly large, a bed of morcellized cancellous bone graft is inserted into the acetabulum to a thickness of approximately 5 mm. A layer of mesh that obliterates the entire defect is placed inside the bone graft and is supported by the adjacent intact acetabulum. Extra-articular screws may be inserted to anchor the periphery of the mesh to the lateral wall of the acetabular rim. Additional bone graft is impacted into the mesh until a continuous layer that is 5 to 10 mm thick has been established. A second layer of mesh is inserted into the acetabulum with two additional extra-articular anchoring screws. An additional layer of impacted bone graft is used to cover the second mesh. Then, a cup is cemented into the bone graft. In this construct, the secondary layer of mesh serves to compartmentalize the bone graft and thereby to inhibit late subsidence.

Nonunion

When a partial union of a displaced acetabular fracture creates a gap of as much as 25 mm, the fracture gap is usually managed with débridement and obliteration with autograft. If a mobile nonunion is encountered, the opposing surfaces are approximated and immobilized with appropriate fixation. Any residual fracture gaps are obliterated with bone graft. The preferred strategies for fixation of a nonunion site include the use of lag screws or the insertion of a cup as a hemispherical plate, both of which avoid exposure of the posterior column, which is the most suitable site for plate fixation. The application of a plate to the posterior column in the setting of a nonunion is likely to result in osteo-

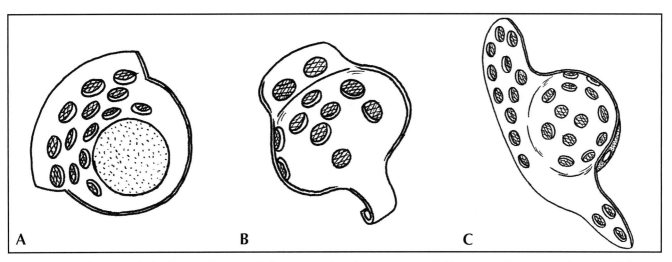

Fig. 7 Drawings showing multiple designs of cages with diverse extension plates that are available for use with a cemented cup. **A,** Müller ring with a smaller posterosuperior flange. **B,** Ganz ring with a superior flange and an inferior hook for anchorage in the obturator foramen. **C,** Burch-Schneider cage with large superior and inferior flanges for anchoring screws.

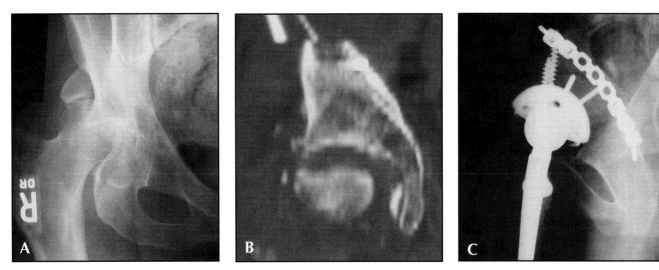

Fig. 8 Radiographs and CT scan from a 53-year-old man who had a fracture of the posterior wall that was managed with an acute open reduction and internal fixation with use of a plate. **A,** AP radiograph of the right hip, obtained at the time of the injury, showing the fracture-dislocation of the posterior wall. **B,** Transaxial CT scan, obtained 4 weeks after the injury, showing erosive damage to more than 30% of the femoral head. This finding was not visualized on plain radiographs made at that time. **C,** Iliac oblique radiograph, obtained after THA, showing the structural autograft secured with two cancellous screws.

necrosis of the acetabulum as the periosteal blood supply is compromised by the elevation of soft tissues and revascularization is impeded by the plate.

Another technique of fixation is the use of cables around the acetabulum[39] (Fig. 12). This method is particularly suitable for a transverse fracture pattern. The cable is passed around the inner

pelvic wall with a standard or modified Statinski vascular clamp. We have procured custom-made modified clamps that are stiffer and have jaws designed to rigorously grip the end of a 2-mm cable. The advantages of this method include minimal denuding and devascularizing of the hemipelvis and prolonged integrity of the fixation in osteopenic bone, where

screws are vulnerable to a rapid onset of loosening. The principal liability of the cabling technique is the potential for a neurovascular injury during the passage of the cable along the inner pelvic table.

Insertion of the Femoral Stem
Currently, the optimal design of a cemented or cementless femoral stem

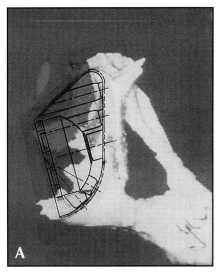

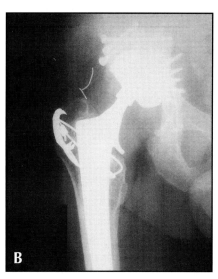

Fig. 9 CT scan and radiograph from a 35-year-old man who sustained a fracture of the posterior wall and posterior column of the right acetabulum and was managed initially with limited internal fixation. **A,** Transaxial three-dimensional CT reconstruction with a template of the custom cup. **B,** AP radiograph of the right hip, obtained 6 years after THA, showing continued stable fixation of the cup in a superior position.

Fig. 10 Photograph showing the modular bilobed cup (Mars, Biomet, Warsaw, IN), which allows application of a lobe of three different sizes to obliterate corresponding acetabular defects. The polyethylene liner is secured mechanically to the bilobed cup, in contrast to the conventional cage.

remains highly controversial.[40] As a general rule, in the United States, a cementless design is favored for use in younger adults. In the few previous reports in the literature on THA performed after an acetabular fracture, some investigators acknowledged an exceptionally high prevalence of premature loosening of cementless stems.[6,7,41,42] They described the development of a relative osteopenia of the proximal part of the femur even in young men. This observation has been interpreted to mean that the period of inactivity and limited weight bearing that immediately follows the acute injury, combined with the additional period of limited weight bearing that accompanies the onset of posttraumatic arthritis of the hip before the THA, culminates in disuse osteoporosis. In such a patient, the application of a cemented stem merits consideration.

Strategies to Address Anticipated Problems

When a THA is performed after an acetabular fracture, problems may arise that need special consideration and an appropriate alteration of the technique. Infrequently, a concomitant fracture of the proximal part of the femoral shaft or an intertrochanteric fracture is an additional problem that may lead to a secondary malunion, retained metal, the development of heterotopic bone, or a nonunion in rare cases.[43-47] The principal factors that are most likely to influence acetabular reconstruction are sciatic nerve injury, obstructive hardware, heterotopic ossification, occult infection, and osteonecrosis.

Sciatic Nerve Injury

After initial surgical management of a posterior fracture-dislocation of the acetabulum, the sciatic nerve usually becomes attached to the site of the posterior fixation with scar tissue. The extent of the scar tissue varies considerably and may progress to its most sinister form, in which supplementary heterotopic bone is encountered. When a THA is performed after a posterior fracture-dislocation has been initially managed with

surgery, we prefer to use an anterolateral or a modified Hardinge approach[31] (Fig. 3, A). In this way, the need for posterior dissection is minimized. In many cases, some degree of contusion of the sciatic nerve accompanies the initial traumatic injury. At the time of the arthroplasty, the sciatic nerve is particularly vulnerable to a clinically important secondary injury as a manifestation of the "double crush syndrome," which may result from a seemingly trivial retraction.[15] Whenever possible, the principal posterior fixation is left in situ, although not infrequently one or two obstructive screws may need to be entirely or partly removed. In certain cases in which a persistent nonunion or malunion of the posterior column or a retained plate needs to be exposed, a complete exposure of the relevant segment of the sciatic nerve should precede the osseous reconstruction or metal removal. In order to minimize the tension on the nerve, the knee is maintained in a position of more than 90° of flexion during the remainder of the arthroplasty except for the brief period when the hip is being reduced.

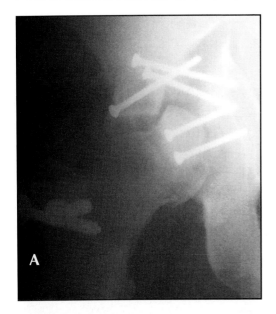

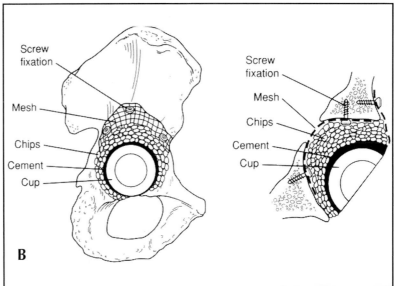

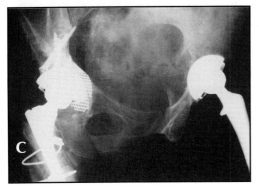

Fig. 11 Radiographs and schematic of the hip of a 56-year-old man who had failure of fixation of a transverse acetabular fracture of the right hip and was managed with a THA with use of central mesh, morcellized bone graft, and lag screws. **A,** AP radiograph, obtained before THA, showing failure of internal fixation solely with lag screws and marked abrasive destruction of the femoral head. **B,** Schematic drawing of the central mesh and morcellized impacted bone chip. **C,** Obturator oblique radiograph, obtained after hybrid THA, showing a central mesh and a metal-backed cup secured with three screws.

In an attempt to monitor the function of the sciatic nerve during a surgical procedure, somatosensory evoked potentials and continuous electromyographic measurements both have been used. Some early reports expressing enthusiasm for measurements of somatosensory evoked potentials have been published.[48-50] Nevertheless, a disturbing trend, which has been documented, has been a prevalence, albeit a low one, of false-positive and false-negative results.[48,51,52] The latter is a particular problem that undermines the confidence of the surgeon in the reliability of this method. Other problems include a substantial latent period, which may be exacerbated by the complexities in the interpretation of the results. Recent evaluations of continuous elec-tromyographic monitoring have indicated that this method has more advantages than the former one.[53,54] Unlike recordings of somatosensory evoked potentials, electromyographic measurements represent virtually instantaneous changes in nerve function. Also, electromyographic measurements are technically less demanding to obtain and require less sophisticated and less costly instrumentation. While the methods can be used in combination, it appears that isolated use of motor-nerve monitoring is the most practical option.

Intraoperative spontaneous electromyographic recordings are obtained with use of sterile needle electrodes from the muscles innervated by the common peroneal nerve (tibialis anterior and per-oneus longus muscles) and the posterior tibial nerve (abductor hallucis and flexor hallucis longus muscles). Unlike the situation with somatosensory evoked potential monitoring, a neurotechnologist is not needed to evoke electromyographic activity. The data are continuously recorded from the muscles; any mechanical or thermal irritation of the sciatic nerve results in a burst or train of neuromuscular discharges, which usually persists until the offending stimulus is removed.[54]

Obstructive Hardware
In many patients who have a THA after open reduction and internal fixation of an acetabular fracture, some of the hardware is directly visualized once the

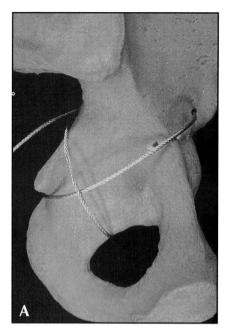 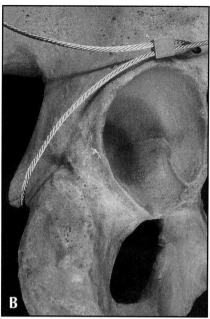 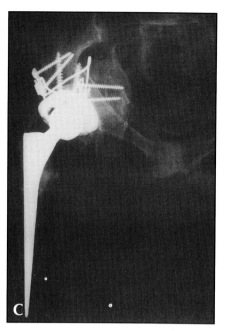

Fig. 12 The use of cables for reconstruction of the inner pelvic table in a so-called geriatric acetabular fracture pattern in which the quadrilateral plate is displaced medially. **A,** Photograph of an intact anatomic pelvic model, showing the position of the cables on the inner pelvic table. **B,** Photograph of an intact anatomic pelvic model, showing the position of a cable on the outer pelvic table. **C,** AP radiograph made after THA with two cables that buttress the crucial quadrilateral surface; the patient is a 62-year-old woman with osteopenic bone who sustained a T-type acetabular fracture with marked displacement of the posterior column, including most of the quadrilateral surface.

articular surface of the acetabulum is exposed. This problem may be indicative of loose or broken hardware that has migrated, or it may be a sequela to an eroded osseous surface or a malpositioned implant. Generally, appropriate preoperative imaging allows this problem to be recognized or at least suspected so that a suitable preoperative plan can be made. When a plate on the posterior column is directly visualized within the acetabulum, or when the plate or its associated screw is struck by an acetabular reamer, the feasibility of leaving the plate in situ needs to be considered. The potential problems that may be encountered during an attempt to remove the entire plate include the risk of an iatrogenically induced injury to the sciatic nerve, the inevitable blood loss, and the extensive surgical time needed to remove the plate. Occasionally, with certain patterns of acetabular malunion in the presence of a thick layer of heterotopic bone,

most of the structural integrity of the posterior column is provided by the heterotopic bone. On removal of the heterotopic bone and the underlying plate, the residual acetabulum may be weakened to a substantial degree, even to the point where a fracture occurs through the remaining defective bone.[6] Once this problem arises, a successful arthroplasty necessitates structural replacement of the posterior column, which is a formidable technical challenge. We recommend that, whenever feasible, impaction grafting of the acetabulum with morcellized femoral-head autograft be performed to cover the exposed bottom surface of the plate and to restore a 5- to 10-mm thick osseous supportive layer for the cup. If a segment of a protruding screw or another nonstructural portion of hardware intrudes into the acetabulum, it may be trimmed with a diamond burr without compromising the structural integrity of the posterior column.

Heterotopic Ossification

When a lateral exposure (especially an extended lateral approach) was used for the fixation of an acetabular fracture, some degree of heterotopic bone is typically seen.[5] Occasionally, clinically important heterotopic ossification develops after a Kocher-Langenbeck approach, whereas it rarely develops after an ilioinguinal exposure. While the amount of heterotopic ossification may be limited, an extensive region of dense scar tissue usually surrounds the radiographically demonstrable area. This area may be impregnated with multiple small deposits of bone that are radiographically invisible. Such tissue must be excised to permit dislocation of the hip and subsequent completion of the THA. If the preoperative radiographs display extensive grade III or IV heterotopic bone according to the system of Brooker and associates,[55] a rigorous characterization of the extent of the problem is essential. Both supplementary iliac and obturator oblique radiographs are needed to determine the magnitude of the anterior and posterior extent of the heterotopic ossification.[17] A CT scan is useful to document that the hip capsule and adjacent muscles are intact, which indicates that excision of the heterotopic ossification is feasible. Prior to the removal of the heterotopic ossification, the precise distribution of the bone, the optimal approaches to the sites, and the potential anatomic hazards are reviewed. One typical pattern involves heterotopic ossification that is limited to the site of the hip capsule and does not extend into the adjacent hip muscles or femoral head. In this situation, removal of the heterotopic ossification during the THA may be highly successful (Fig. 6). The opposite extreme involves circumferential heterotopic bone that infiltrates radially from the femoral head and neck to pervade the capsule and the adjacent muscles, with associated osseous bars that anchor the entire proximal part of the femur to the pelvis. Almost all of these more florid cases are encountered in patients who have had a closed head injury, particularly young obese men. Despite the use of postoperative radiation therapy, the likelihood for recurrent formation of massive heterotopic ossification is great.[51] With the loss of the normal tissue planes and mobile interfaces, resection of heterotopic ossification when there is such extensive involvement is a formidable undertaking. Considerable blood loss can be anticipated, and arrangements for transfusion and intraoperative salvage of blood are needed.

Following such an extensive procedure, the risk of a serious deep wound infection is considerable. If such an infection does develop, it has been our experience that, despite the use of multiple surgical débridements, formation of scar tissue usually progresses to a virtual fusion of the hip. Alternatively, a resection arthroplasty may become necessary to

control the infection. This measure is reserved solely for infections that culminate in extensive necrosis of the involved bone and neighboring soft tissues. After adequate débridements of bone and soft tissue, a cement spacer is inserted to obliterate the dead space and to provide a temporary reservoir of a suitable antibiotic. It has been our experience that, when the residual viable tissues have been extensively covered with scar tissue in the aftermath of the infection, the late functional outcome of a resection arthroplasty with a cement spacer often is functionally equivalent to that of a secondarily performed THA with regard to pain relief, stability, and mobility. In fact, after a resection arthroplasty with a cement spacer, many patients refuse to consider additional surgery even if a surgeon recommends conversion to a total hip replacement.

Once the amount and the site of distribution of the heterotopic ossification have been characterized, the optimal surgical approach can be selected. Although grade I or II heterotopic ossification does not materially influence the approach, grade III or IV heterotopic ossification has an impact on the surgical plan. If heterotopic ossification is localized solely to the posterior aspect of the hip joint, the use of a Kocher-Langenbeck approach is recommended (Fig. 3, B). If heterotopic ossification is both anterior and posterior to the hip joint, we prefer to use a triradiate incision with preservation of the greater trochanter and the adjacent gluteal insertions.[30]

The excision of two patterns of heterotopic ossification is especially challenging. In some patients with mature heterotopic ossification, the extra bone is virtually indistinguishable from the intact pelvis. Furthermore, the soft-tissue boundaries, such as the capsule, may be wholly or substantially lost because they have been replaced by bone. In contrast, progressive removal of heterotopic ossification in a patient who has preservation of

the soft-tissue intervals can be documented by visualization of conspicuous osseous landmarks, such as the anterior inferior iliac spine and the junction between the femoral neck and the greater trochanter. The other challenging pattern of heterotopic ossification is ossification that infiltrates deeply into the adjacent soft tissues such as the gluteus minimus. At the time of the initial cutaneous incision, the first hint of this pattern is typified by evidence of bone in the deep fascia. To dislocate the hip, resection of the involved portion of the gluteus minimus may be necessary. Other local muscles that are likely to contain ossified portions include the indirect head of the rectus femoris, the iliopsoas, and the short external rotators.

During resection of heterotopic ossification around the superior portion of the hip joint, the insertions of the gluteal muscles into the trochanteric region must be carefully preserved. The exposure of a fixation plate on the posterior column or an isolated screw is a valuable landmark for identifying the surface of the intact pelvis. As a rule, such hardware is left in situ. In this way, if another approach to the hip subsequently becomes necessary, possibly for a revision arthroplasty, the hardware continues to serve as a marker of the normal pelvic surface, so that overenthusiastic removal of recurrent heterotopic bone does not progress to a catastrophic resection of the acetabulum. In cases with the most extensive heterotopic ossification, the anterior inferior iliac spine is an additional useful anterior landmark. Supplementary image intensification can be used to delineate the position of the acetabular rim. During THA, the femoral neck is provisionally divided in its midportion with a power saw. Sufficient heterotopic ossification is removed so that the proximal part of the femoral shaft can be placed in approximately 90° of external rotation. Afterward, the standard cut at the base of the femoral neck is made with the use of an alignment guide. Once the heterotopic ossification has been completely removed, the remainder of the arthroplasty continues in a conventional fashion.

Often, the most extensive cases of heterotopic bone around the hip are encountered in patients with an acetabular fracture and an associated fracture of the proximal or midpart of the femur who had combined internal fixation performed through contiguous surgical fields. In the most florid cases, the heterotopic bone can extend from the iliac crest to the distal femoral metaphysis so that both the hip and the ipsilateral knee are ankylosed. A suitable release of the hip and knee involves both a resection of the massive amount of bone and a complete quadricepsplasty. Despite the use of postoperative radiation therapy and/or treatment with indomethacin, recurrent heterotopic ossification is almost a certainty.[51,56] Nevertheless, the patient may be grateful for a moderate functional improvement in gait and the ability to transfer.

In some cases of massive heterotopic ossification, the findings on preoperative radiographs are consistent with some degree of posttraumatic degenerative arthritis of the hip. Even with an adequate CT scan, the surgeon may be unable to determine whether complete removal of the heterotopic ossification will permit a functional restoration of a mobile and painless hip joint. The patient's preoperative consent and the corresponding discussion may be directed toward surgical resection of the heterotopic ossification, with a possible supplementary THA, if features of severe degenerative changes in the hip joint are observed during the procedure.

Following a THA that is accompanied by the removal of extensive heterotopic ossification, the use of one or more postoperative prophylactic measures is recommended.[51] Radiation therapy with a dose of 700 cGy on the first postoperative day is a standard recommendation.[57] Alternatively, the use of indomethacin

for a period of at least 6 weeks has been advised. In a recent randomized, prospective study to assess the formation of heterotopic ossification after open reduction of acute acetabular fractures, Matta and Siebenrock[56] reported that indomethacin had no therapeutic beneficial effect as prophylaxis against heterotopic ossification. Other surgeons have used a combination of radiation therapy and indomethacin.[58] Despite the use of prophylactic regimens, the formation of clinically important heterotopic ossification or a complete recurrence of it after resection is not unlikely in hips with florid heterotopic ossification following a closed head injury. It has been our experience that this sobering event may transpire even though years of "maturation" of the heterotopic ossification may ensue after the acetabular fracture and prior to the THA.

Occult Infection

An occult infection may be a source of chronic pain in the hip after open reduction and internal fixation of the acetabulum, and it may be the cause of deterioration of the joint surfaces. Certain circumstances should heighten suspicion of an occult infection. The use of an extended lateral approach for the initial treatment of an acetabular fracture is a risk factor, particularly when the dissection is undertaken along both the inner and the outer pelvic table. Another factor is heterotopic ossification, which may be provoked in part by the infection itself. Additional factors include morbid obesity, an immunocompromised patient, and previous radiation therapy to the pelvis.

While clinical, hematologic, radiographic, or other findings may indicate an infection, clear evidence of an infection is typically not available until the arthroplasty is performed. When dense scar tissue or heterotopic bone is anticipated, a preoperative aspiration or even a trephine biopsy of the hip may fail to confirm the

infection. At the time of the arthroplasty, specimens of joint fluid should be sent to the laboratory for analysis, including a Gram stain and a histologic scrutiny for white blood cells. A highly reliable method is intraoperative examination of a frozen section obtained from membrane or pericapsular granulation tissue. The presence of 10 white blood cells per high-power field is presumptive evidence of an infection.[59] If the hip is infected, our preferred method is to perform a thorough débridement, including resection of the femoral head and neck and any necrotic acetabular bone. Following pulsatile jet lavage and antibiotic irrigation, a cement spacer that has been impregnated with an antibiotic, typically gentamicin, is inserted into the acetabulum.[60,61] The wound is closed in layers over a suction drain. Postoperatively, after the identification of the pathogen, appropriate intravenous antibiotics are given for at least 6 weeks. Upon the cessation of antibiotic therapy, a trephine biopsy of the hip is performed under image intensification. If the specimen is sterile, insertion of the total hip prosthesis is considered. If the specimen reveals a persistent infection, multiple surgical débridements with replacement of the cement spacer and continued intravenous antibiotic therapy are undertaken until the infection is eradicated.

Osteonecrosis of the Acetabulum

Another potential complicating factor is osteonecrosis of the acetabulum.[62] Following a single extensile approach or two simple approaches for acute reconstruction of an acetabular fracture, the blood supply to the acetabular bone may be heavily compromised for a prolonged period of years. At the time of a belated arthroplasty, necrotic acetabular bone may thwart the insertion of the cup and may predispose the patient to premature acetabular loosening. When a THA is being considered for a patient with posttraumatic arthritis after an extended lateral approach or a two-incision approach, the surgeon is advised to review the prior surgical report to determine whether an extensive intra-operative dissection on the inner and outer pelvic tables was performed. A helpful, although subtle, radiographic sign of acetabular necrosis is an increased radiodensity, especially in the region of the dome (Fig. 13). If the cup is inserted into an avascular bed, a serious potential complication is an insidious protrusion of the cup through the medial acetabular wall. In the most florid case, a transverse dissociation may occur (Fig. 14).

The optimal method of addressing acetabular osteonecrosis is to reduce its potential for development at the time of the initial open reduction; for instance, use of the extended lateral approach should be minimized, and the blood supply to all of the major acetabular fragments should be maintained. At the time of the arthroplasty, if a cementless cup is used, it must be placed on viable bone. Even if a cemented cup is selected, a viable osseous bed markedly improves the longevity of the fixation. When the preoperative radiographs indicate an extensive area of periacetabular osteonecrosis, the feasibility of successfully anchoring the cup on viable bleeding and structurally sound bone must be carefully reviewed. In exceptional cases, a resection arthroplasty may provide a superior and more predictable outcome than a THA.

After a thorough inspection of the preoperative images, the feasibility of reconstructing a stable acetabulum needs to be determined. For a particularly large acetabular defect that is further complicated by a suspicion of extensive avascular bone, a frank discussion with the patient about the magnitude of the problem and the potential need for resection arthroplasty may be advisable before embarking on the procedure. If the potential for acetabular

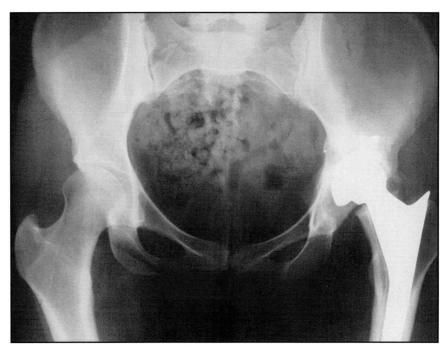

Fig. 13 Increased radiodensity of the acetabular roof on the left side is a subtle but important finding of acetabular osteonecrosis. The radiograph is that of a 28-year-old woman who sustained a transverse fracture that was managed acutely with open reduction and was managed 1 year later with removal of the metal. Three years after the injury, a THA was performed to manage posttraumatic arthritis. Within another 2-year period, the patient complained of recurrent hip pain, and an aspiration arthrogram confirmed an aseptically loose cup. This AP radiograph shows superior migration of the failed cup into the necrotic acetabular roof.

reconstruction remains unclear to the surgeon, a review of the clinical and radiographic features with an orthopaedist who is highly experienced with this problem may be beneficial.

Salvage of Complex Late Cases
A limited spectrum of acetabular fractures, after failure of the initial open reduction and internal fixation, have a heterogeneous mixture of complicating factors. A patient may have a serious deep wound infection, possibly with persistent drainage through a sinus tract. The gluteus medius and minimus muscles may have been damaged by an injury to the superior gluteal nerve, heterotopic bone formation, or osteonecrosis, or they may even have been injured secondary to a life-saving embolic occlusion of a traumatic laceration of the internal iliac ar-

tery. Substantial acetabular bone loss may have occurred as a result of avascularity or infection or occasionally other factors. In some of these situations, a THA may be feasible, even if a multistaged reconstruction is necessary. Nevertheless, in certain situations, such as complete loss of the posterior column (Fig. 15), a THA may be technically unrealistic. Furthermore, the functional outcome of a THA with respect to pain relief and durability may not be any better than that of the principal surgical alternative, a resection arthroplasty with or without the insertion of a cement spacer.[63-66]

Acute Management With THA After Acetabular Fracture in Highly Selected Patients
Fractures in elderly individuals represent the most rapidly growing spectrum of

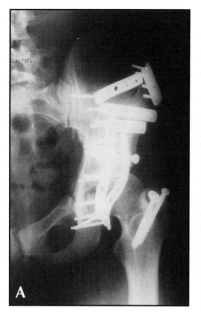 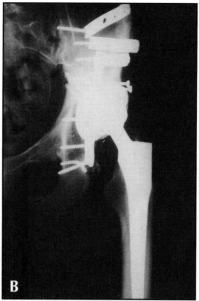 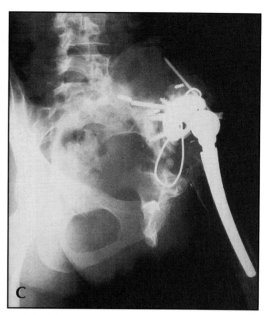

Fig. 14 Radiographs from a 24-year-old woman who sustained a fracture of both columns of the left acetabulum, which was initially treated with open reduction through a triradiate approach and dissection on the outer and inner pelvic tables. **A,** AP radiograph obtained 10 months after open reduction and internal fixation. **B,** AP radiograph made soon after THA and 6 years after the initial injury. **C,** Iliac oblique radiograph, obtained 2 years after THA, showing a completely loose cup and a transverse dissociation secondary to marked osteolysis of the anterior and posterior columns.

acetabular trauma.[67-69] The specific indications for acute management with THA after a displaced acetabular fracture have yet to be clearly defined but may include marked impaction, extensive abrasion or fracture of the femoral head, a completely displaced femoral neck fracture, marginal or central impaction of the acetabulum involving more than 30% of its surface area, and extensive acetabular comminution in the presence of osteopenic bone. Other relative indications include delayed presentation, substantial medical comorbidities, morbid obesity, and advanced age. We have been encouraged by our early experience with THA in the treatment of selected acute fractures.[39]

Postoperative Management

After the THA, a patient is managed with an abduction bolster or split Russell traction for 24 hours to minimize the risk of postoperative dislocation. In general, bed-to-chair transfers are initiated on the first postoperative day, with touch-down or light partial weight bearing beginning on the second day. Substantial partial weight bearing is begun at 4 to 6 weeks after the arthroplasty, with full weight bearing at 6 to 8 weeks. When an elderly patient who has compromised strength, agility, and balance compared with a younger adult is managed with a THA, partial weight bearing or weight bearing as tolerated is almost essential or the risk of a fall becomes excessive. Therefore, the acetabular repair requires sufficient structural integrity so that some degree of immediate weight bearing is feasible.

Whenever practical, vigorous progressive resistance exercises of the hip abductors, quadriceps, and hamstrings, as well as active range-of-motion exercises, including flexion, extension, and abduction of the hip joint, are encouraged.[6,70] A program of continuous passive motion may be used at the discretion of the surgeon. Prophylactic intravenous antibiotics with a second-generation cephalosporin are used routinely for 48 hours. Prophylaxis against thromboembolism includes the application of elastic stockings, sequential compression devices, and an appropriate course of anticoagulation with warfarin or low-molecular-weight heparin.

Patients who have previously had open reduction and internal fixation of an acetabular fracture and who had grade I or II heterotopic ossification and/or an extended lateral approach prior to the belated THA are managed with low-dose radiation (a single dose of 700 cGy). Alternatively, indomethacin can be used in younger female patients in whom radiation exposure should be avoided. When indomethacin and anticoagulation with low-molecular-weight heparin or warfarin are used concomitantly, appropriate medical supervision is needed to minimize the risk of a coagulopathy.

Clinical Outcome of THA After Acetabular Fracture

According to a few prior studies on the late outcome of a belated total hip replacement after closed or open treatment of an acetabular fracture,[7,8,42,71] the clinical outcome is generally less favorable than that after THA performed to manage degenerative arthritis. Undoubtedly, the outcome of belated THA after acetabular fracture is best when the fracture pattern is one of minor displacement with union, especially following nonoperative treatment. In earlier published reports, such as one by Boardman and Charnley,[72] even when open reduction of the acute acetabular fracture had been performed, the indication for the late THA typically was a posterior fracture-dislocation, such as a posterior wall fracture, for which an isolated posterior surgical approach was used to achieve fixation with lag screws or a single plate. In contrast to the simple pattern fractures of the posterior column, posterior wall, and transverse fractures, few of the more complex patterns, such as a fracture of both columns, a T-type fracture, or an anterior column-posterior hemitransverse fracture, were managed surgically until recently. For example, Boardman and Charnley,[72] in a study of the outcomes of 68 Charnley low-friction arthroplasties, reported that 55 of the acute acetabular fractures were managed nonsurgically and the remaining 13 were treated with primary open reduction and internal fixation. After a relatively short period of follow-up (an average of 3.5 years), the patients had good results with respect to pain and function. Waddell and Morton (unpublished data, 1994), in a study of 34 patients, reported that 29 were managed initially with open reduction. Satisfactory rates of success were noted after an average follow-up period of 2 years. Earlier studies by multiple authors have described comparable rates of success over similarly brief follow-up periods, regardless of whether the initial management of the diverse patterns of the acetabular fractures was open or closed.[8,10,73-75]

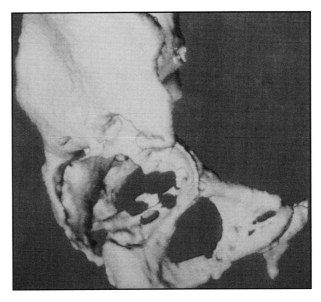

Fig. 15 Three-dimensional CT scan of the hip of a 73-year-old woman who had complete, traumatic loss of the posterior acetabular column. This acetabular defect presents one of the most challenging reconstruction problems because it can be very difficult to achieve a stable acetabular component that will resist the forces that are imposed by sitting and sitting transfers, as well as standing and walking.

Romness and Lewallen,[7] in a longer-term evaluation of 55 belated arthroplasties performed after an acetabular fracture, observed that the rate of radiographic acetabular loosening at an average of 7.5 years postoperatively was 52.9%; the loosening was symptomatic in 27.5%, and it progressed to a revision in 13.7%. In contrast, Stauffer,[9] in a 10-year follow-up study of 231 hips in which a Charnley arthroplasty had been performed for degenerative arthritis, reported that 36.8% had features of radiographic loosening and the rate of revision was 8.2%. The rates of radiographic loosening of the femoral component (29%), symptomatic loosening (16%), and revision (8%) were remarkably similar in the two series. When the two series were compared with respect to the results in patients who were older than age 60 years, the rates of loosening of the femoral component were similar; however, the rate of loosening of the acetabular component was 38.5% in the series described by Romness and Lewallen compared with approximately 4.8% in the series reported by Stauffer. Romness and Lewallen concluded that the fourfold to fivefold increase in the rate of failure of THA after an acetabu-

lar fracture was primarily attributable to damage or loss of acetabular bone stock. They recommended an initial open reduction as a way to reconstruct the osseous anatomy, even if that procedure fails to prevent posttraumatic degeneration. In contrast, Carnesale and associates,[71] in a study of 56 hips with an acetabular fracture, including 11 that were treated surgically, discouraged open reduction as the initial choice of treatment for an acetabular fracture because of the corresponding deterioration of the outcome after belated arthroplasty.

More recently, Mears and Ward (unpublished data, 1996) evaluated a series of 36 patients who underwent a THA after previous open reduction and internal fixation of the acetabulum. Most patients (83%) had had a triradiate extended lateral surgical exposure with dissection along the inner and outer pelvic walls. The rate of radiographic loosening was 58%, and the rate of surgical revision was 36% within 2 years after the primary arthroplasty. The high rate of premature technical failure was, in part, a reflection of the use of an unsatisfactory design of a cementless femoral stem. Nevertheless, at the time of the revision arthroplasties, multiple acetabular biopsies confirmed the high likelihood of widespread osteonecrosis in the central aspect of the acetabulum that correlated with the initial dissections along the inner and outer pelvic walls.

Weber and associates[42] reported on 63 patients who were followed for an average of 9.6 years after a primary THA following failed open reduction of an acetabular fracture. The 10-year rate of survival of the components was 78%, and the rate of revision, which was performed mainly because of aseptic loosening of one or both components, was 51%. Notable risk factors for revision included age younger than 50 years, weight greater than 80 kg, and large residual combined segmental and cavitary deficiencies in the osseous acetabulum. Mont and associates[11] also observed a poorer outcome after THAs performed in younger patients, who generally are more active and have an increased body weight compared with older individuals.

For many reasons, the use of extensile or multiple pelvic incisions has diminished greatly during the past decade. Nevertheless, there is currently no convincing documented evidence that acute management with open reduction and internal fixation improves the success of a subsequent THA performed for posttraumatic arthritis. Ironically, it has been our experience that the best late results of THA after acetabular fracture have been documented when the arthroplasties were performed acutely. In a series of 57 patients managed with an acute THA after acetabular fracture, the principal problems were postoperative dislocation in two hips (3.5%), one of which progressed to a revision of the cup, and a symptomatic loose cup in one hip (1.6%), which was revised at 3 years.[76] In one other hip, grade IV heterotopic bone developed after the acute THA. The heterotopic ossification was resected, and there was no recurrence at 20 months

after the arthroplasty. There were no deep wound infections and no cases of radiographic or symptomatic femoral loosening. The discussion of these results is not meant to be a recommendation for THA for more than an exceptional acetabular fracture, especially in elderly patients. Nevertheless, an analysis of the results of open reduction and internal fixation of acute acetabular fractures highlights a therapeutic dilemma. Even in the most experienced hands, as Letournel and Judet[2] meticulously documented, certain patterns of acetabular fracture have an abysmal prognosis.

A small group of patterns of displaced acetabular fractures and clinical scenarios have a low likelihood for a favorable outcome after open reduction and internal fixation, and an open reduction of such fractures may compromise the outlook for a successful subsequent THA. These fracture patterns include abrasion, impaction, or fracture of the femoral head; a displaced fracture of the femoral neck; acetabular impaction; certain comminuted fractures; multiple associated fractures; and osteopenic bone. The clinical scenarios include advanced patient age, morbid obesity, substantial medical comorbidities, and a delay between the injury and the surgery. In certain patients who have several of these complicating factors, some alternative method of primary management seems to be preferable. When the primary factor is comminution and impaction with relatively minor displacement, most surgeons may lean toward nonsurgical treatment. When a patient has substantial displacement, especially an elderly patient with osteopenic bone, acute THA merits more careful consideration.

Summary

In most cases, when THA is performed after an acetabular fracture, it is done to manage secondary degenerative change or, possibly, osteonecrosis of the femoral

head. Secondary complicating factors may be encountered during the THA. After initial nonsurgical treatment of an acetabular fracture, an occult or frank acetabular nonunion and malunion are not uncommon and may extend to the residual pelvic ring. After surgical treatment, intrusive hardware, heterotopic bone, dense scar tissue, ischemic muscle or bone, and occult infection are additional hazards that may be encountered. When acute sciatic nerve palsy, whether induced traumatically or iatrogenically, accompanies the initial acetabular injury, the palsy is likely to be exacerbated during a subsequent THA. A careful clinical and radiographic evaluation is needed, along with the formulation of a detailed surgical strategy. The need for specialized arthroplasty instruments, fixation devices, and autograft or, occasionally, allograft has to be identified.

When heterotopic bone is evident, an extensile approach may be needed to allow adequate exposure for its complete removal. After a bone defect and/or a nonunion with displacement has been characterized, one or more strategies for obliteration of the defect are considered; these include the use of impaction grafting, a structural graft, a cup inserted with multiple screws, mesh, or a suitable ring or other fixation device.

Evaluation of results has shown that, overall, the late outcome of THA after acetabular fracture is inferior to that of arthroplasty performed because of degenerative arthritis. Although open reduction and internal fixation of an acute acetabular fracture was previously hypothesized as an effective way to improve the anticipated late outcome of THA by the elimination of a large fracture gap or the prevention of a potential nonunion, current observations do not support that hypothesis. An initial open reduction may compromise the outcome of a subsequent THA by compromising the blood supply of the acetabulum and by initiating the formation of scar tissue, heterotopic bone, or an occult or frank infection.

For a highly selected group of especially severe acetabular fractures, particularly those in elderly patients, THA appears to be a promising therapeutic alternative.

References

1. Vail TP, McCollum DE: Complex primary acetabular replacement, in Callaghan JJ, Rosenberg AG, Rubash HE (eds): *The Adult Hip.* Philadelphia, PA, Lippincott-Raven, 1998, vol 2, pp 1183-1200.

2. Letournel E, Judet R: *Fractures of the Acetabulum,* ed 2. Berlin, Germany, Springer-Verlag, 1993, pp 359-386.

3. Tile M (ed): *Fractures of the Pelvis and Acetabulum,* ed 2. Baltimore, MD, Williams & Wilkins, 1995, pp 176-184.

4. Matta JM: Fractures of the acetabulum: Accuracy of reduction and clinical results in patients managed operatively within three weeks after the injury. *J Bone Joint Surg Am* 1996;78:1632-1645.

5. Mears DC, Rubash HE (eds): *Pelvic and Acetabular Fractures.* Thorofare, NJ, Slack, 1986, pp 422-439.

6. Jimenez ML, Tile M, Schenk RS: Total hip replacement after acetabular fracture. *Orthop Clin North Am* 1997;28:435-446.

7. Romness DW, Lewallen DG: Total hip arthroplasty after fracture of the acetabulum: Long-term results. *J Bone Joint Surg Br* 1990;72(suppl 5):761-764.

8. Pritchett JW, Bortel DT: Total hip replacement after central fracture dislocation of the acetabulum. *Orthop Rev* 1991;20:607-610.

9. Stauffer RN: Ten-year follow-up study of total hip replacement. *J Bone Joint Surg Am* 1982;64:983-990.

10. Rogan IM, Weber FA, Solomon L: Abstract: Total hip replacement following fracture dislocation of the acetabulum. *J Bone Joint Surg Br* 1979;61(suppl 2):252.

11. Mont MA, Maar DC, Krackow KA, Jacobs MA, Jones LC, Hungerford DS: Total hip replacement without cement for non-inflammatory osteoarthrosis in patients who are less than forty-five years old. *J Bone Joint Surg Am* 1993;75:740-751.

12. Callaghan JJ, McBeath AA: Arthrodesis in, Callaghan JJ, Rosenberg AG, Rubash HE (eds): *The Adult Hip.* Philadelphia, PA, Lippincott-Raven, 1998, pp 749-759.

13. Carangelo RJ, Schutzer SF: Resection arthroplasty in, Callaghan JJ, Rosenberg AG, Rubash HE (eds): *The Adult Hip.* Philadelphia, PA, Lippincott-Raven, 1998, pp 737-747.

14. Johnson EE, Matta JM, Mast JW, Letournel E: Delayed reconstruction of acetabular fractures 21-120 days following injury. *Clin Orthop* 1994;305:20-30.

15. Osterman AL: The double crush syndrome. *Orthop Clin North Am* 1988;19:147-155.

16. Mears DC, Ward AJ, Wright MS: The radiological assessment of pelvic and acetabular fractures using three-dimensional computed tomography. *Intern J Orthop Trauma* 1992;2:196-209.

17. Moed BR, Smith ST: Three-view radiographic assessment of heterotopic ossification after acetabular fracture surgery. *J Orthop Trauma* 1996;10:93-98.

18. Evans BG: Late complications and their management, in Callaghan JJ, Rosenberg AG, Rubash HE (eds): *The Adult Hip.* Philadelphia, PA, Lippincott-Raven, 1998, pp 1149-1161.

19. Fitzgerald RH Jr, Davis LP, Rajan DK: Radionuclide imaging, in Callaghan JJ, Rosenberg AG, Rubash HE (eds): *The Adult Hip.* Philadelphia, PA, Lippincott-Raven, 1998, pp 373-391.

20. Schauwecker DS: The scintigraphic diagnosis of osteomyelitis. *AJR Am J Roentgenol* 1992;158:9-18.

21. D'Antonio JA, Capello WN, Borden LS, et al: Classification and management of acetabular abnormalities in total hip arthroplasty. *Clin Orthop* 1989;243:126-137.

22. Gross AE, Allan DG, Catre M, Garbuz DS, Stockley I: Bone grafts in hip replacement surgery: The pelvic side. *Orthop Clin North Am* 1993;24:679-695.

23. Emerson RH Jr, Head WC: Dealing with the deficient acetabulum in revision hip arthroplasty: The importance of implant migration and use of the jumbo cup. *Sem Arthroplasty* 1993;4:2-8.

24. Slooff JH, Schreurs BW, Buma P, Gardeniers JWM: Impaction morcellized allografting and cement. *Instr Course Lect* 1999;48:79-89.

25. Müller ME: Acetabular revision, in Salvati EA (ed): *The Hip: Proceedings of the Ninth Open Scientific Meeting of the Hip Society.* St Louis, MO, CV Mosby, 1981, pp 46-56.

26. Peters CL, Curtain M, Samuelson KM: Acetabular revision with the Burch-Schneider antiprotrusio cage and cancellous allograft bone. *J Arthroplasty* 1995;10:307-312.

27. Moed BR: Acetabular fractures: The Kocher-Langenbeck approach, in Wiss DA (ed): *Fractures: Master Techniques in Orthopaedic Surgery.* Philadelphia, PA, Lippincott-Raven, 1998, pp 631-655.

28. Matta JM, Reilly MC: Acetabular fractures: The ilioinguinal approach, in Wiss DA (ed): *Fractures: Master Techniques in Orthopaedic Surgery.* Philadelphia, PA, Lippincott-Raven, 1998, pp 657-673.

29. Helfet DL, Bartlett CS, Malkani AL: Acetabular fractures: The extended iliofemoral approach, in Wiss DA (ed): *Fractures: Master Techniques in Orthopaedic Surgery.* Philadelphia, PA, Lippincott-Raven, 1998, pp 675-695.

30. Mears DC, MacLeod MD: Acetabular fractures: The triradiate and modified triradiate approaches, in Wiss DA (ed): *Fractures: Master Techniques in Orthopaedic Surgery.* Philadelphia, PA, Lippincott-Raven, 1998, pp 697-724.

31. Hardinge K: The direct lateral approach to the hip. *J Bone Joint Surg Br* 1982;64:17-19.

32. Gie GA, Linder L, Ling RS, Simon JP, Slooff TJ, Timperley AJ: Impacted cancellous allografts and cement for revision total hip arthroplasty. *J Bone Joint Surg Br* 1993;75:14-21.

33. Ling RS: Femoral component revision using impacted morsellised cancellous graft. *J Bone Joint Surg Br* 1997;79:874-875.

34. Paprosky WG, Magnus RE: Principles of bone grafting in revision total hip arthroplasty: Acetabular technique. *Clin Orthop* 1994;298:147-155.

35. Slooff TJ, Huiskes R, van Horn J, Lemmens AJ: Bone grafting in total hip replacement for acetabular protrusion. *Acta Orthop Scand* 1984;55:593-596.

36. Capello WN, Hellman EJ, Feinberg JR: Revision of the acetabular component: Use of cement, in Callaghan JJ, Rosenberg AG, Rubash HE (eds): *The Adult Hip.* Philadelphia, PA, Lippincott-Raven, 1998, vol 2, pp 1439-1448.

37. DeBoer DK, Christie MJ: Revision of the acetabular component: Oblong cup, in Callaghan JJ, Rosenberg AG, Rubash HE (eds): *The Adult Hip.* Philadelphia, PA, Lippincott-Raven, 1998, vol 2, pp 1461-1468.

38. Slooff TJ JH, Buma P, Gardeniers JWM, Schreurs BW, Schimmel JW, Huiskes R: Revision of the acetabular component: Bone packing, in Callaghan JJ, Rosenberg AG, Rubash HE (eds): *The Adult Hip.* Philadelphia, PA, Lippincott-Raven, 1998, vol 2, pp 1449-1459.

39. Mears DC, Shirahama M: Stabilization of an acetabular fracture with cables for acute total hip arthroplasty. *J Arthroplasty* 1998;13:104-107.

40. Galante JO: Overview of total hip arthroplasty in, Callaghan JJ, Rosenberg AG, Rubash HE (eds): *The Adult Hip.* Philadelphia, PA, Lippincott-Raven, 1998, vol 2, pp 829-838.

41. Sim FH, Stauffer RN: Management of hip fractures by total hip arthroplasty. *Clin Orthop* 1980;152:191-197.

42. Weber M, Berry DJ, Harmsen WS: Total hip arthroplasty after operative treatment of an acetabular fracture. *J Bone Joint Surg Am* 1998;80:1295-1305.

43. Mehlhoff T, Landon GC, Tullos HS: Total hip arthroplasty following failed internal fixation of hip fractures. *Clin Orthop* 1991;269:32-37.

44. Soballe K, Boll KL, Kofod S, Severinsen B, Kristensen SS: Total hip replacement after medial-displacement osteotomy of the proximal part of the femur. *J Bone Joint Surg Am* 1989;71:692-697.

45. Tabsh I, Waddell JP, Morton J: Total hip arthroplasty for complications of proximal femoral fractures. *J Orthop Trauma* 1997;11:166-169.

46. Patterson BM, Salvati EA, Huo MH: Total hip arthroplasty for complications of inter-trochanteric fracture: A technical note. *J Bone Joint Surg Am* 1990;72:776-777.

47. Boos N, Krushell R, Ganz R, Müller ME: Total hip arthroplasty after previous proximal femoral osteotomy. *J Bone Joint Surg Br* 1997;79:247-253.

48. Vrahas M, Gordon RG, Mears DC, Krieger D, Sclabassi RJ: Intraoperative somatosensory evoked potential monitoring of pelvic and acetabular fractures. *J Orthop Trauma* 1992;6:50-58.

49. Helfet DL, Koval KJ, Hissa EA, Patterson S, DiPasquale T, Sanders R: Intraoperative somatosensory evoked potential monitoring during acute pelvic fracture surgery. *J Orthop Trauma* 1995;9:28-34.

50. Helfet DL, Schmeling GJ: Somatosensory evoked potential monitoring in the surgical treatment of acute, displaced acetabular fractures: Results of a prospective study. *Clin Orthop* 1994;301:213-220.

51. Templeman DC, Olson S, Moed BR, Duwelius P, Matta JM: Surgical treatment of acetabular fractures. *Instr Course Lect* 1999;48:481-496.

52. Middlebrooks ES, Sims SH, Kellam JF, Bosse MJ: Incidence of sciatic nerve injury in opera-tively treated acetabular fractures without somatosensory evoked potential monitoring. *J Orthop Trauma* 1997;11:327-329.

53. Helfet DL, Anand N, Malkani AL, et al: Intraoperative monitoring of motor pathways during operative fixation of acute acetabular fractures. *J Orthop Trauma* 1997;11:2-6.

54. Moed BR, Ahmad BK, Craig JG, Jacobson GP, Anders MJ: Intraoperative monitoring with stimulus-evoked electromyography during placement of iliosacral screws: An initial clini-cal study. *J Bone Joint Surg Am* 1998;80:537-546.

55. Brooker AF, Bowerman JW, Robinson RA, Riley LH Jr: Ectopic ossification following total hip replacement: Incidence and a method of classification. *J Bone Joint Surg Am* 1973;55:1629-1632.

56. Matta JM, Siebenrock KA: Does indomethacin reduce heterotopic bone formation after opera-tions for acetabular fractures? A prospective randomised study. *J Bone Joint Surg Br* 1997;79:959-963.

57. Lo TC, Healy WL, Covall DJ, et al: Heterotopic bone formation after hip surgery: Prevention with single-dose postoperative hip irradiation. *Radiology* 1988;168:851-854.

58. Moed BR, Letournel E: Low-dose irradiation and indomethacin prevent heterotopic ossifica-tion after acetabular fracture surgery. *J Bone Joint Surg Br* 1994;76:895-900.

59. Della Valle CJ, Bogner E, Desai P, et al: Analysis of frozen sections of intraoperative specimens obtained at the time of reoperation after hip or knee resection arthroplasty for the treatment of infection. *J Bone Joint Surg Am* 1999;81:684-689.

60. Spangehl MJ, Masri BA, O'Connell JX, Duncan CP: Prospective analysis of preopera-tive and intraoperative investigations for the diagnosis of infection at the sites of two hun-dred and two revision total hip arthroplasties. *J Bone Joint Surg Am* 1999;81:672-683.

61. Hanssen AD, Rand JA: Evaluation and treat-ment of infection at the site of a total hip or knee arthroplasty. *Instr Course Lect* 1999;48:111-122.

62. Mears DC: Avascular necrosis of the acetabu-lum. *Op Tech Orthop* 1997;7:241-249.

63. Younger AS, Duncan CP, Masri BA, McGraw RW: The outcome of two-stage arthroplasty using a custom-made interval spacer to treat the infected hip. *J Arthroplasty* 1997;12:615-623.

64. Haddad FS, Masri BA, Garbuz DS, Duncan CP: The treatment of the infected hip replace-ment: The complex case. *Clin Orthop* 1999;369:144-156.

65. Pagnano MW, Trousdale RT, Hanssen AD: Outcome after reinfection following reimplan-tation hip arthroplasty. *Clin Orthop* 1997;338:192-204.

66. Nestor BJ, Hanssen AD, Ferrer-Gonzalez R, Fitzgerald RH Jr: The use of porous prosthe-ses in delayed reconstruction of total hip replacements that have failed because of infection. *J Bone Joint Surg Am* 1994;76:349-359.

67. Lonner JH, Koval KJ: Polytrauma in the elder-ly. *Clin Orthop* 1995;318:136-143.

68. DeMaria EJ, Kenney PR, Merriam MA, Casanova LA, Gann DS: Survival after trauma in geriatric patients. *Ann Surg* 1987;206:738-743.

69. McCoy GF, Johnston RA, Duthie RB: Injury to the elderly in road traffic accidents. *J Trauma* 1989;29:494-497.

70. Joly JM, Mears DC: The role of total hip arthroplasty in acetabular fracture management. *Op Tech Orthop* 1993;3:80-102.

71. Carnesale PG, Stewart MJ, Barnes SN: Acetabular disruption and central fracture-dislocation of the hip: A long-term study. *J Bone Joint Surg Am* 1975;57:1054-1059.

72. Boardman KP, Charnley J: Low-friction arthro-plasty after fracture-dislocations of the hip. *J Bone Joint Surg Br* 1978;60:495-497.

73. Coventry MB: The treatment of fracture-dislo-cation of the hip by total hip arthroplasty. *J Bone Joint Surg Am* 1974;56:1128-1134.

74. Harris WH: Traumatic arthritis of the hip after dislocation and acetabular fractures: Treatment by mold arthroplasty: An end-result study using a new method of result evaluation. *J Bone Joint Surg Am* 1969;51:737-755.

75. Westerborn A: Central dislocation of the femoral head treated with mold arthroplasty. *J Bone Joint Surg Am* 1954;36:307-314.

76. Mears DC: Surgical treatment of acetabular fractures in elderly patients with osteoporotic bone. *J Am Acad Orthop Surgeons* 1999;7:128-141.

Periprosthetic Fractures of the Acetabulum

David L. Helfet, MD
Arif Ali, MD

Abstract

Periprosthetic fractures of the acetabulum after total hip arthroplasty are uncommon, but are increasing in number and severity. These fractures may occur intraoperatively, during the perioperative period, or many years after the total hip arthroplasty. Periprosthetic fractures of the acetabulum vary in severity and may involve stress fractures of the pubis or medial wall, significant bone loss secondary to osteolysis and subsequent loss of column integrity, or complete pelvic discontinuity.

Treatment differs depending on the complexity of the fracture and the stability of the acetabular prosthesis. Surgical treatment for an unstable acetabulum should stabilize the bony columns of the acetabulum, provide bone grafting of defects, and should maintain adequate bone stock for replacement of a stable acetabular implant. Strict adherence to the principles of fracture surgery is required to achieve bony union of the acetabular columns and provide a stable environment for reimplantation of an acetabular component.

Periprosthetic fractures of the acetabulum after total hip arthroplasty (THA) are relatively uncommon and few reports in the literature describe the occurrence or treatment of this significant complication. It is expected that the number of primary joint arthroplasties will continue to increase and that the joint replacements will be in use longer as the population ages, thus leading to an increase in the number of periprosthetic fractures.[1] This situation along with an increased incidence of osteolysis and high molecular-weight polyethylene wear in hip prostheses will require the orthopaedic surgeon to understand the principles needed to diagnose and treat these injuries.

The treatment goals for acetabular fractures in native hips significantly differ from those in patients with arthroplasties. Rather than attempting to achieve a perfect articular reduction, surgery for periprosthetic fractures involves stabilizing the bony columns of the acetabulum, bone grafting of defects, and maintaining adequate bone stock for replacement of a stable acetabular implant.

Historical Review

In 1972, Miller[2] reported on nine patients with ischiopubic fractures occurring 14 to 48 months after THA. The fractures failed to unite with nonsurgical treatment and resection arthroplasty was performed in all patients. In 1974, McElfresh and Coventry[3] reported on 5,400 THAs performed at the Mayo Clinic and reported 1 acetabular fracture and 3 stress fractures of the pubis. The pubic stress fractures were treated with protected weight bearing, and the acetabular fracture was treated with a resection arthroplasty because the patient had a deep infection.

More recently, Peterson and Lewallen[4] reported on a study of 11 patients with a periprosthetic acetabular fracture. Patients were divided into two groups. Those in the type 1 group (eight patients) had fractures in which the acetabular component was clinically and radiographically stable and those in the type 2 group (three patients) had fractures in which the component was unstable. Eight patients (including both type 1 and type 2 patients) ultimately underwent a revision of the acetabular component.

As the longevity of THAs increases, more cases of periprosthetic acetabular fractures associated with extensive pelvis osteolysis are being documented.[1,5,6] Pelvic osteolysis predisposes patients to fractures secondary to loss of the structural integ-

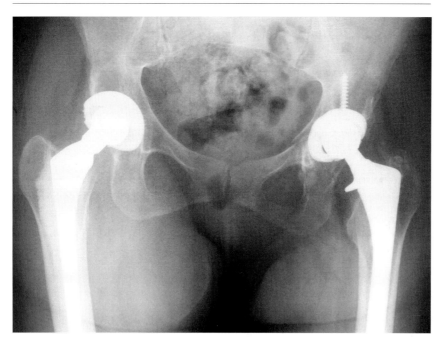

Figure 1 A 65-year-old woman underwent a staged bilateral THA for treatment of severe osteoarthritis. The postoperative AP radiograph shows an incomplete transverse type periprosthetic acetabular fracture.

rity of the acetabulum and should be treated with techniques that allow replacement of the bony defects with bone grafting as necessary, and revision of the acetabular prosthesis.

Treatment

Periprosthetic acetabular fractures may occur at the time of intraoperative placement of the acetabular implant, during the perioperative pe-

riod, or may occur many years after the THA.[7,8]

Intraoperative Fractures

Callaghan and associates[8] have identified underreaming of the acetabulum for placement of a press-fit component as an important risk factor that may predispose patients to intraoperative periprosthetic acetabular fractures (Figure 1). Kim and associates[9] showed that underreaming by 2 mm or more significantly increases the risk of an acetabular fracture. Care must also be taken when preparing an acetabulum in osteopenic bone.[8,10]

If an intraoperative fracture is suspected, judicious exposure of the fracture should be undertaken to determine if the fracture involves simply the acetabular wall or is a component of a transverse fracture (Figure 2). Wall fractures require assessment of the stability of the implant; if there is any instability, augmentation of the fixation is required with screws or buttress plating. If the fracture pattern is more extensive, with a trans-

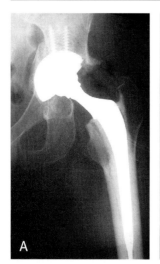
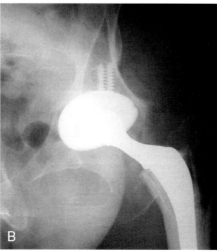
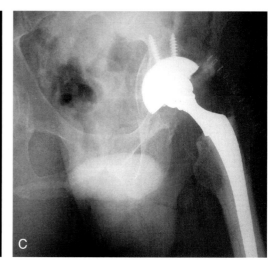

Figure 2 Postoperative AP (**A**) and Judet (**B** and **C**) views showing a left-sided anterior wall type periprosthetic acetabular fracture of a 50-year-old man who underwent hybrid THA. The fracture was noted during impaction of the cup on the left acetabulum and was evaluated and determined to be stable. The cup was upsized by 2 mm, two stabilizing screws were placed, and bone grafting of the medial defect was performed. The patient was progressed from toe-touch weight bearing to weight bearing as tolerated at 6 weeks after THA. At last follow-up, a good result was noted and the patient reported a return to preinjury functional status.

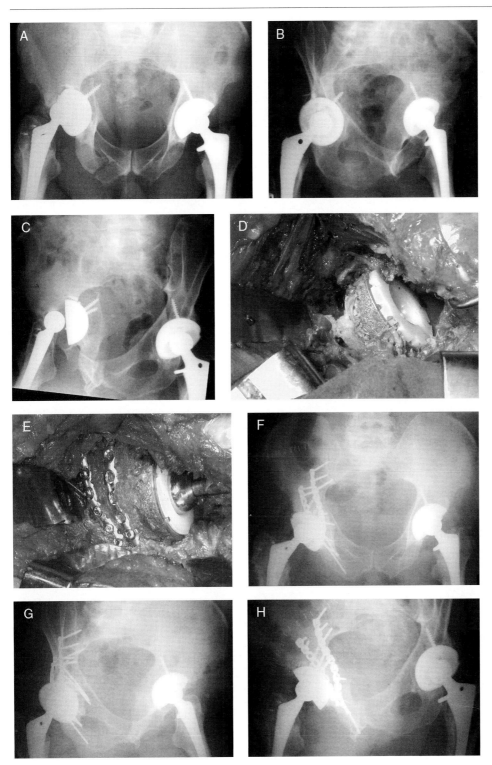

Figure 3 AP (**A**) and Judet (**B** and **C**) views of a 64-year-old man who fell and sustained a right-sided posterior column type periprosthetic acetabular fracture. The cup remained attached to the acetabulum and was intraoperatively confirmed as stable. **D,** The intraoperative image shows displacement of the acetabular component and posterior column and superior osteolysis. **E,** Open reduction and internal fixation was done through a Kocher-Langenbeck approach with placement of two pelvic reconstruction plates along the posterior wall and posterior column. The intraoperative image is shown after reduction of the posterior column with placement of plates and bone graft. Postoperative AP (**F**), Judet AP (**G**), and Judet (**H**) views of the patient are shown.

verse component, or if displacement is present, formal stabilization is done with posterior column plating and additional lag screw fixation anterior-ly as indicated, with bone grafting. The goal of fixation of the acetabular fracture is to provide structurally sound bony columns to support an acetabular component; the acetabular component should not be compromised to provide stability for an unstable acetabular column.

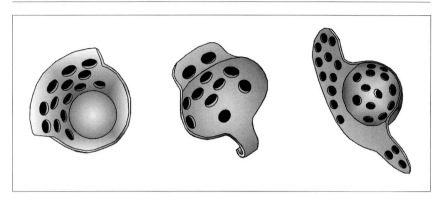

Figure 4 Several types of antiprotrusio cages are shown.

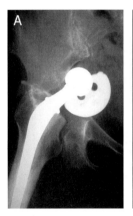
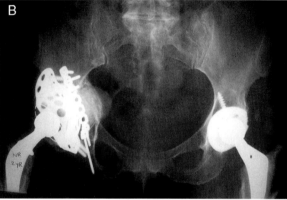

Figure 5 A, A preoperative AP radiograph is shown of a 74-year-old woman who previously had a bilateral THA and presented with right-sided periprosthetic insufficiency fractures with pelvic discontinuity and medial migration of the acetabular component into the pelvis. **B,** A postoperative AP radiograph is shown after open reduction and internal fixation was performed with a posterior reconstruction plate and screws for the posterior column. An antiprotrusio cage was used for additional medial support with bone graft to treat the defect.

Postoperative Fractures

Acute groin pain in patients after THA should be monitored and an acetabular fracture should be included in the differential diagnosis. These patients usually have experienced some form of blunt trauma; however, some patients may have no antecedent trauma, especially if there is significant osteoporosis or osteolysis.[6] Because standard radiographs may not show subtle acetabular fractures for these patients, standard and Judet views of the pelvis, along with a CT scan for accurate delineation of the fracture and extent of bone loss,

should be done.[6,11]

Elderly osteoporotic patients may report groin pain caused by stress fractures of the pubis that often are undiagnosed and may lead to lengthy and exhaustive testing for infection and other possible causes.[12,13] Launder and Hungerford[13] also attributed these stress fractures to repetitive trauma to a pubis that had been weakened by osteoporosis; it was theorized that the disease was exacerbated by the less active lifestyle adopted by elderly patients who had experienced pain from degenerative joint disease.

Patients with a periprosthetic acetabular fracture are assessed to determine the stability of the acetabular component because this finding affects the initial treatment plan. Fractures with clinically and radiographically stable implants may be treated with 6 to 8 weeks of toe-touch weight bearing. Conservative treatment may allow the fracture to heal; however, a study by Peterson and Lewallen[4] found that six of eight patients with radiographically stable implants required revision surgery despite healing of the fracture. The fracture may heal with delayed treatment, thus limiting the extent of subsequent surgery to only revision of the acetabular component, if the patient remains symptomatic.

Patients with clinically unstable acetabular components and/or periprosthetic acetabular fractures are best treated with fixation of the acetabulum and revision of the component. The patient's existing bone stock, degree of osteopenia, and pattern of acetabular fracture are treatment considerations.

The principles for treating periprosthetic acetabular fractures generally remain the same irrespective of etiology. The goal is to restore the structural integrity of the columns and restore bone stock with bone graft, allowing for stable reimplantation of the acetabular prosthesis. Acute fractures after blunt trauma require assessment of the fracture pattern and choice of a surgical approach that will allow the best access for fixation of the fracture and revision of the component as needed.

Fractures associated with pelvic dissociation usually are seen at the time of acetabular reconstruction of cemented and cementless components that have been in vivo for many years.[8,14,15] Pelvic discontinuity usually occurs as a result of severe

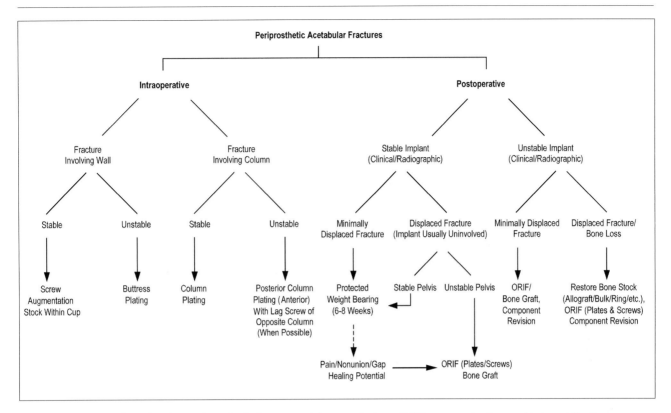

Figure 6 Treatment algorithm for periprosthetic fractures of the acetabulum. ORIF, open reduction and internal fixation.

and progressive osteolysis with loss of bone.[5,12,15] Reduction and fixation of at least one column with a pelvic reconstruction plate is done and followed by appropriate bone grafting (occasionally bulk allograft) to treat any bony defect, and reimplantation of an acetabular component. Isolated anterior column defects can be treated with an iliac crest or femoral head allograft with lag screws. However, posterior column defects, even when isolated, should be treated with the addition of a posterior column buttress plate because of the high stress forces that occur on the posterior column during activities of daily living.[16] Occasionally, patients with osteolysis and subsequent trauma have a fractured column with an acetabular component that remains fixed to the displaced column. Open reduction and internal fixation of the column and a change of the polyeth-

ylene is all that is required for treatment (Figure 3).

Acetabular fractures of the medial wall are a complication in patients who have undergone THA. Bone loss secondary to osteolysis causes weakening of the medial wall and continued weight bearing can cause protrusio acetabuli. These patients often have significant bone loss secondary to osteolysis and require treatment with a bulk structural allograft and acetabular reconstructive cages. A wide variety of cages with diverse extension plates are available for special problems[17,18] (Figure 4). The cage may also function as a type of fixation plate that immobilizes the site of a transverse nonunion.[18]

The antiprotrusio cage (APC) was originally designed by Burch in 1974 and modified by Schneider in 1975 to treat pelvic discontinuities and massive bone loss.[17] The cage can

bridge areas of bone loss, allowing grafting and bone augmentation in areas of protected stress, and can provide support for the socket. The APC provides a large contact area between the implant and eroded pelvic bone, transferring resultant forces across the hip under the acetabular roof while providing a metal backing for the polyethylene cup.[17] Although the selection of bone graft for use with the APC must be individualized, solid graft is reserved for segmental defects in the weight-bearing dome.[16,17,19] Medial support is provided by resting the superior flange against the ilium and sinking the inferior flange into the ischium. Implant stability is obtained by placing multiple screws in the superior flange, preferably with at least two screws placed at right angles to each other, to lock the implant proximally[17] (Figure 5).

Summary

Periprosthetic fractures of the acetabulum vary in significance, complexity, and time of occurrence in relationship to the THA. Unlike standard hip arthroplasties, successful outcome requires adherence to the principles of fracture surgery. Assessment of the fracture and the stability of the implant after the fracture is important. Radiographic analysis is more difficult and must clearly delineate the acetabular fracture pattern. A treatment algorithm for periprosthetic fractures of the acetabulum is shown in Figure 6. All periprosthetic acetabular fractures with an unstable component should undergo fixation of the bony acetabulum with standard techniques using reconstruction plates/screws and lag screws and with bone grafting (including bulk allograft for extensive bony loss). The goal of surgery is to provide a stable construct to allow successful reimplantation of an acetabular prosthetic component; an APC should be used when needed.

References

1. Younger ASE, Dunwoody J, Duncan CP: Periprosthetic hip and knee fractures: The scope of the problem. *Instr Course Lect* 1998;47:251-256.

2. Miller AJ: Late fracture of the acetabulum after total hip replacement. *J Bone Joint Surg Br* 1972;54:600-606.

3. McElfresh EC, Coventry MB: Femoral and pelvic fractures after total hip arthroplasty. *J Bone Joint Surg Am* 1974;56:483-492.

4. Peterson CA, Lewallen DG: Periprosthetic fractures of the acetabulum after total hip arthroplasty. *J Bone Joint Surg Am* 1996;78:1206-1213.

5. Chatoo M, Parfitt J, Pearse MF: Periprosthetic acetabular fracture associated with extensive osteolysis. *J Arthroplasty* 1998;13:843-845.

6. Sanchez-Sotelo J, McGrory BJ, Berry DJ: Acute periprosthetic fracture of the acetabulum associated with osteolytic pelvic lesions. *J Arthroplasty* 2000;15:126-130.

7. Berry DJ: Management of periprosthetic fractures: The hip. *J Arthroplasty* 2002;17:11-13.

8. Callaghan JJ: Periprosthetic fractures of the acetabulum during and following total hip arthroplasty. *Instr Course Lect* 1998;47:231-235.

9. Kim YS, Callaghan JJ, Ahn PB, et al: Fracture of the acetabulum during insertion of an oversized hemispherical component. *J Bone Joint Surg Am* 1995;77:111-117.

10. Kyle RF, Crickard GE: Periprosthetic fractures associated with total hip arthroplasty. *Orthopedics* 1998;21:982-984.

11. Haddad FS, Masri BA, Garbuz DS, et al: The prevention of periprosthetic fractures in total hip and knee arthroplasty. *Orthop Clin North Am* 1999;30:191-207.

12. Andrews P, Barrack RL, Harris WH: Stress fracture of the medial wall of the acetabulum adjacent to a cementless acetabular component. *J Arthroplasty* 2002;17:117-120.

13. Launder WL, Hungerford DS: Stress fracture of the pubis after total hip arthroplasty. *Clin Orthop* 1981;159:183-185.

14. Callaghan JJ, Kim YS, Pederson DR, et al: Periprosthetic fractures of the acetabulum. *Orthop Clin North Am* 1999;30:221-234.

15. Mahoney CR, Garvin KL: Periprosthetic acetabular stress fracture causing pelvic discontinuity. *Orthopedics* 2002;25:83-85.

16. D'Antonio JA: Periprosthetic bone loss of the acetabulum. *Orthop Clin North Am* 1992;23:279-290.

17. Gill TJ, Sledge JB, Müller ME: The Burch-Schneider anti-protrusio cage in revision total hip arthroplasty. *J Bone Joint Surg Br* 1998;80:946-953.

18. Mears DC, Velyvis JH: Primary total hip arthroplasty after acetabular fracture. *Instr Course Lect* 2001;50:335-354.

19. Maloney WJ, Peters P, Engh CA, et al: Severe osteolysis of the pelvis in association with acetabular replacement without cement. *J Bone Joint Surg Am* 1993;75:1627-1635.

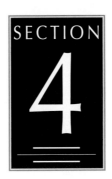

SECTION 4

Care of the Trauma Patient

Care of the Trauma Patient

Care of the trauma patient presents a wide variety of problems, ranging from identification of specific, numerous injuries to challenges associated with patient factors such as age, comorbidities, social challenges, and personal goals. The perioperative care of patients with musculoskeletal injuries includes correctly timing fracture fixation and implementing strategies to avoid postoperative complications. This section of *Instructional Course Lectures Trauma* focuses on patient management. New concepts in the appropriate timing of fracture fixation, pain control, and prevention of deep venous thrombosis are addressed. An excellent article by Vern Tolo describes the care of pediatric trauma patients, distinguishing the differences in management of our young trauma patients.

The most appropriate timing of fracture care in the multiply injured patient is the subject of much controversy. As with many other aspects of medicine, and with musculoskeletal trauma in particular, we have come full circle in our philosophy for treatment of these severely injured patients. Only several decades ago, immediate fracture care in multiply injured patients was considered contraindicated. The adage that these patients were "too sick to operate on" has been replaced with the adage that they are "too sick not to operate on." Hence, the concept of early total fracture care evolved during the 1980s. More recently, the tide has turned again to the thought that a certain subset of multiply injured patients may be too sick to tolerate the physiologic burden of total fracture care.

Many patients with fractures, including multiple fractures, are best treated by early total fracture care. However, in some subsets of multiply injured patients, major orthopaedic surgery may have a deleterious effect. Patients with severe chest and/or head injuries, along with those who have not been adequately resuscitated are the focus of this debate. The recognition that major orthopaedic procedures, when performed during the early phases of care, may increase the inflammatory response of the initial injury and lead to organ system failure is an evolving concept in the care of multiply injured patients.

Craig Roberts and associates describe the evolving concept of damage control orthopaedics (DCO). Because much is still being debated, indications for the use of provisional external fixation are not yet firmly established. However, this article provides an excellent framework for approaching multiply injured patients and developing guidelines to help decide when early total fracture care is appropriate or when following DCO principles may be best.

The management of acute and chronic pain has received greater attention, which has extended to notoriety in the lay press. Because this is an issue of concern to the orthopaedist, the review of postoperative pain management strategies by Evan Ekman and Andrew Koman is a timely and important addition to this volume. Strategies are outlined based on the molecular basis of pain. Because postoperative pain is one of the greatest concerns to patients, understanding pain mechanisms and methods for managing postoperative pain remains a critical part of patient care.

The next article by Daniel Berry does not specifically focus on the treatment of trauma patients, but it outlines the modalities for the prevention and treatment of deep venous thrombosis, which is a concern in this patient population. Since Geerts and associates documented that patients who sustain blunt trauma have a high incidence of deep venous thrombosis, prevention and management of this problem has been of interest to physicians caring for multiply injured patients. This problem is well recognized as a cause of morbidity and mortality after hip fractures, and now there is greater appreciation that many patients with pelvic and lower extremity fractures also are at risk for deep venous thrombosis.

David C. Templeman, MD
Associate Professor
Department of Orthopaedic Surgery
University of Minnesota
Hennepin County Medical Center
Minneapolis, Minnesota

William M. Ricci, MD
Associate Professor
Department of Orthopaedic Surgery
Washington University School of
   Medicine at Barnes-Jewish Hospital
St. Louis, Missouri

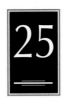

Damage Control Orthopaedics: Evolving Concepts in the Treatment of Patients Who Have Sustained Orthopaedic Trauma

Craig S. Roberts, MD
Hans-Christoph Pape, MD
Alan L. Jones, MD
Arthur L. Malkani, MD
Jorge L. Rodriguez, MD
Peter V. Giannoudis, MD

Abstract

In some groups of polytrauma patients, particularly those with chest injuries, head injuries, and those with mangled extremities, early total care of major bone fractures may be potentially harmful. Delaying all orthopaedic surgery, however, is also not always the best approach. In these situations, damage control orthopaedics, which emphasizes the stabilization and control of the injury rather than repair, will add little additional physiologic insult to the patient and is a treatment option that should be considered.

Many orthopaedic patients who have sustained multiple injuries benefit from the early total care of major bone fractures. However, the strategy is not the best option, and indeed might be harmful, for some multiply injured patients. Because foregoing all early surgery is not the optimal approach for those patients, the concept of damage control orthopaedics has evolved. Damage control orthopaedics emphasizes the stabilization and control of the injury, often with use of spanning external fixation, rather than immediate fracture repair. The concept of damage control orthopaedics is not new; it has evolved out of the rich history of fracture care and abdominal surgery. This chapter traces the roots of damage control orthopaedics, reviews the physiologic basis for it, describes the subgroups of patients and injury complexes that are best treated with damage control orthopaedics, reports the early clinical results, and provides a rationale for modern fracture care for the multiply injured patient.

Definition of Damage Control Orthopaedics

Damage control orthopaedics is an approach that contains and stabilizes orthopaedic injuries so that the patient's overall physiology can improve. Its purpose is to avoid worsening of the patient's condition by the "second hit" of a major orthopaedic procedure and to delay definitive fracture repair until a time when the overall condition of the patient is optimized. Minimally invasive surgical techniques such as external fixation are used initially. Damage control focuses on control of hemorrhage, management of soft-tissue injury, and achievement of provisional fracture stability, while avoiding additional insults to the patient.

History of Fracture Surgery and Birth of Damage Control Orthopaedics

It has been stated that: "Information illustrating the benefits of fracture stabilization after multiple trauma has been gathering for almost a century."[1] It also has been noted that during this time "fears of the 'fat embolism syndrome' also dominated the philosophy in managing polytrauma patients." Early manipulation of long-bone fractures was considered unsafe.[2]

External fixation, an essential component of damage control orthopaedics, developed slowly and was outpaced by the development of internal fixation. In Switzerland, in 1938, Räoul Hoffmann produced an external fixator frame that allowed the fracture to be mechanically manipulated and reduced.[3] In 1942, Roger Anderson advocated castless ambulatory treatment of fractures with use of a versatile linkage system, but the device was banned in World War II for being too elaborate.[3] In 1950, a survey by the Committee on Fractures and Traumatic Surgery of the American Academy of Orthopaedic Surgeons concluded that the complications of external fixation frequently exceed any advantages of the procedure.[3] Also in 1950, Gavril Abramovich Ilizarov developed the ring system for fractures and deformities, but his device did not reach the West until the late 1970s. On March 15, 1958, Maurice Müller, Hans Willenegger, and Martin Allgöwer convened a group of interested Swiss general and orthopaedic surgeons, including Robert Schneider and Walter Bandi at the Kantonsspital, Chur, Switzerland, to discuss the status of fracture treatment, which usually included traction and prolonged bed rest and led to poor functional results in a high percentage of patients.[4] On November 6, 1958, these pioneering surgeons established the Arbeitsgemeinschaft für Osteosynthesefragen (the Association for the Study of Internal Fixation, or ASIF), or AO, in Biel, Switzerland.[4] The key objective of the AO was the early restoration of function, whether a patient was being treated for an isolated fracture or for multiple injuries.[4] Matter noted that this strategy led to "aggressive traumatology involving early total care of the trauma victim, culminating in the statement: This patient is too sick not to be treated surgically."[4]

By the 1980s, the accepted care of a major fracture was early or immediate fixation.[5] Substantiating this approach were 11 studies (10 retrospective and one prospective), with the one by Bone and associates[6] being most frequently cited. Bone and associates reported that the incidence of pulmonary complications (adult respiratory distress syndrome, pneumonia, and fat embolism) was higher and stays in the hospital and the intensive care unit were increased when femoral fixation was delayed.

In 1990, Border[7] reported on a comprehensive study of patients with blunt trauma that challenged the accepted practice of immediate definitive fixation. This changed practice in the early 1990s, and a more selective approach to fracture fixation was used; however, early fixation was still performed in most cases. During the 1990s, more was learned about the parameters associated with adverse outcomes in multiply injured patients and about the systemic inflammatory response to trauma.[8] It became clear that fracture surgery, especially intramedullary nailing, has systemic physiologic effects. These effects became known as the "second-hit" phenomenon.

The era of damage control orthopaedics started around 1993. Two reports from one institution[9,10] described temporary external fixation of femoral shaft fractures in severely injured patients. From 1989 to 1990, the frequency of using temporary external fixation increased from less than 5% to more than 10%. The mean duration of external fixation until intramedullary nailing was less than one week. Compared with patients treated with immediate definitive fixation, those treated initially with external fixation had more severe injuries, with higher injury severity scores and transfusion requirements in the initial 24 hours. The term "damage control" began to be used in the orthopaedic literature over the past 6 to 7 years.[1,9-12]

History of Abdominal Damage Control Surgery

The concept of damage control surgery was developed first in the field of abdominal surgery. The benefits of controlling hemorrhage and contamination and leaving the abdomen open, in lieu of definite repair of injuries and closure of the abdomen, improved the survival of patients with the lethal triad of hypothermia, acidosis, and coagulopathy. Abdominal damage control surgery was described as the sum total of all maneuvers required

to ensure survival of a multiply injured patient who was exsanguinating; its purpose was to control rather than definitely repair injuries.[13]

In the 1940s and 1950s, Arnold Griswold of Kentucky used a damage control approach to penetrating injuries of the abdominal cavity.[14] In 1981, Feliciano and associates[15] reported that 9 of 10 patients who had undergone hepatic packing for the treatment of exsanguinating hemorrhage survived. Stone and associates,[16] in 1983, described a stepwise approach involving intra-abdominal packing and a laparotomy that was terminated rapidly. In 1992, Burch and associates[17] reported a 33% survival rate in a group of 200 patients treated with abbreviated laparotomy and a planned reoperation. Rotondo and Zonies,[18] in 1993, coined the term "damage control" and reported a 58% rate of survival of patients treated with a standardized protocol. In short, the concept of damage control was first used in abdominal surgery to describe a systematic three-phase approach designed to disrupt a lethal cascade of events leading to death by exsanguination.[13] Phase one involved an immediate laparotomy to control hemorrhage and contamination.[18] Phase two was resuscitation in the intensive care unit with improvement of hemodynamics, rewarming, correction of coagulopathy, ventilatory support, and continued identification of injuries. Phase three consisted of a reoperation for removal of intra-abdominal packing, definitive repair of abdominal injuries, and closure and possible repair of extra-abdominal injuries. Damage control surgery in the abdomen has gained widespread acceptance throughout North America and Israel.[18,19]

Physiology of Damage Control Orthopaedics

The physiologic basis of damage control orthopaedics is beginning to be understood. Traumatic injury leads to systemic inflammation (systemic inflammatory response syndrome) followed by a period of recovery mediated by a counterregulatory anti-inflammatory response[20] (Figure 1). Severe inflammation may lead to acute organ failure and early death after an injury. A lesser inflammatory response followed by an excessive compensatory anti-inflammatory response syndrome may induce a prolonged immunosuppressed state that can be deleterious to the host. This conceptual framework may explain why multiple organ dysfunction syndrome develops early after trauma in some patients and much later in others.

Within this inflammatory process, there is a fine balance between the beneficial effects of inflammation and the potential for the process to cause and aggravate tissue injury leading to adult respiratory distress syndrome and multiple organ dysfunction syndrome. The key players in the host response appear to be the cytokines, the leukocytes, the endothelium, and subsequent leukocyte-endothelial cell interactions.[21] Reactive oxygen species, eicosanoids, and microcirculatory disturbances also play pivotal roles.[22] The development of this inflammatory response and its subsequent, often fatal consequences are part of the normal response to injury.

When the initial massive injury and shock give rise to an intense systemic inflammatory syndrome with the potential to cause remote organ injury, this "one hit" can cause an excessive inflammatory response that activates the innate immune system, including macrophages, leukocytes, natural killer cells, and inflammatory cell migration enhanced by interleukin (IL)-8 production and complement components (C5a and C3a). When the stimulus is less intense and would normally resolve without consequence, the patient is vulnerable to secondary inflammatory insults that can reactivate the systemic inflammatory response syndrome and precipitate late

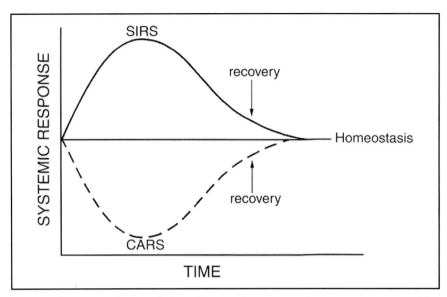

Figure 1 After trauma, there is a balance between the systemic inflammatory response and the counterregulatory anti-inflammatory response. Severe inflammation can lead to acute organ failure and early death. A lesser inflammatory response coupled with an excessive counterregulatory antiinflammatory response may also induce a prolonged immunosuppressed state that can be deleterious to the host. SIRS = systemic inflammatory response syndrome, and CARS = counterregulatory anti-inflammatory response syndrome.

multiple organ dysfunction syndrome. The second insult may take many forms as a result of a variety of circumstances, such as sepsis and surgical procedures, and is the basis for the decision-making process regarding when and how much to do for a "borderline" multiply injured patient (defined later). Hyperstimulation of the inflammatory system, by either single or multiple hits, is considered by many to be the key element in the pathogenesis of adult respiratory distress syndrome and multiple organ dysfunction syndrome.[23]

The First- and Second-Hit Phenomena
Numerous studies have demonstrated that stimulation of a variety of inflammatory mediators takes place in the immediate aftermath of trauma.[24-27] This response initially corresponds to the first-hit phenomenon.[25] Hoch and associates[28] reported elevation in plasma concentrations of IL-6 and IL-8 in patients

with an injury severity score of 25 points. An immediate increase in expression of neutrophil L-selectin was reported in patients with an injury severity score of 16 points.[29] Similarly, a significant ($P < 0.05$) increase in the expression of the integrin CD11b was noted in more severely injured patients.[29] The development of multiple organ dysfunction syndrome has also been associated with a persistent elevation of CD11b expression on both neutrophils and lymphocytes for 120 hours, a finding that is suggestive of neutrophil activation in the early development of leukocyte-mediated end-organ injury. Several other studies have clearly demonstrated the effect of injury severity on the degree of stimulation of the inflammatory markers.[8,30]

Although selective immunostimulation may play a critical role in the development of severe complications after injuries, it is also clear that the governing effect of surgical or accidental trauma on immune function is immunosuppres-

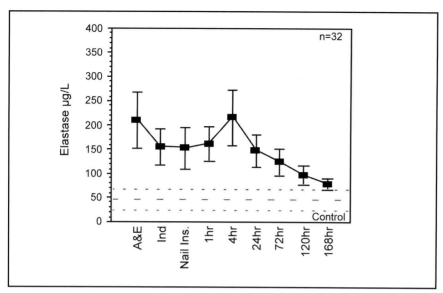

Figure 2 Mean plasma elastase concentrations (and 95% confidence intervals) before and after intramedullary nailing of the femur from the time of admission to the emergency room (A&E) to 168 hours after surgery.[8] The control group is shown by the dotted line. Ind = induction of anesthesia, and Nail Ins. = nail insertion. (Reproduced with permission from Giannoudis PV, Smith RM, Bellamy MC, Morrison JF, Dickson RA, Guillou PJ. Stimulation of the inflammatory system by reamed and unreamed nailing of femoral fractures: An analysis of the second hit. *J Bone Joint Surg Br* 1999;81:359.)

sion. Several authors have demonstrated the immunosuppressive effect of trauma.[31,32] Following trauma, the production of immunoglobulins and interferon decreases and many patients become anergic, as assessed with delayed hypersensitivity skin testing, and are thus exposed to an increased risk of posttraumatic sepsis.[33] Defects in neutrophil chemotaxis, phagocytosis, lysosomal enzyme content, and respiratory burst have also been reported. Immunosuppression contributes to the etiology of infection and sepsis after trauma.[34]

The biologic profile of the first hit in trauma patients is being defined. Obertacke and associates[35] demonstrated the importance of the first hit by using bronchopulmonary lavage to assess changes in pulmonary microvascular permeability in patients who had sustained multiple trauma. The permeability of the pulmonary capillaries increased following multiple trauma, and patients in whom adult respiratory distress syn-

drome later developed had a high correlation (r = 0.81) with increased permeability within just 6 hours after admission than did those who had experienced an uneventful recovery. The development of a massive immune reaction in a patient with bilateral femoral fracture who showed a massive inflammatory reaction, which was subsequently hyperstimulated by the surgical procedure itself (bilateral reamed femoral nailing), further supports the importance of the first-hit phenomenon.[36] Although there was no obvious additional risk factor present (such as no chest injury), the patient died from full-blown adult respiratory distress syndrome 3 days after the injury. This case not only clearly illustrates the existence of biologic variation in the inflammatory response to injury, but also confirms the importance of the degree of the response to the first hit and the response to the second (surgical) hit that created the final fatal event. The above studies suggest that the degree of the initial injury is impor-

tant in determining a patient's susceptibility to posttraumatic complications.

The concept that a secondary surgical procedure creates an additional inflammatory insult (a second hit) was specifically addressed in a prospective study of 106 patients with an average injury severity score of 40.6 points.[37] Forty patients in whom respiratory, renal, or hepatic failure developed, alone or in combination, following a secondary surgical procedure, were compared with patients in whom no such complications developed. There was a significant ($P < 0.05$) elevation of the neutrophil elastase and C-reactive protein levels and a reduction in the platelet counts in the 40 patients with systemic complications. Abnormality of those three parameters predicted postoperative organ failure with an accuracy of 79%.[37]

The first- and second-hit phenomena in trauma patients were demonstrated in a study in which femoral nailing was considered to be the second hit[8] (Figure 2). That study demonstrated similar responses to reamed and unreamed nailing in terms of neutrophil activation, elastase release, and expression of adhesion molecules. These concepts of biologic responses to different stimuli (first and second hits) have now become the basis of our treatment plans and illustrate the impact of the surgical procedure on trauma patients at risk for exhaustion of their biologic reserve (Figure 3).

Markers of Immune Reactivity
Inflammatory markers may hold the key to identifying patients at risk for the development of posttraumatic complications such as multiple organ dysfunction syndrome (Table 1). Common serum markers can be divided into markers of mediator activity such as C-reactive protein, tumor necrosis factor-α (TNF-α), IL-1, IL-6, IL-8, IL-10, and procalcitonin and markers of cellular activity such as CD11b surface receptor on leukocytes, endothelial adhesion molecules (intercel-

lular adhesion molecule-1 [ICAM-1] and e-selectin), and HLA-DR class II molecules on peripheral mononuclear cells.

C-reactive protein, procalcitonin, TNF-α, IL-1, and IL-8 have not been shown to be reliable markers.[38-43] However, IL-6 correlates well with the degree of injury, appears to be a reliable index of the magnitude of systemic inflammation, and correlates with the outcome.[12] IL-10 inhibits the activity of TNF-α and IL-1, and the levels detectable in the circulation correlate with the initial degree of injury. Persistently high levels of IL-10 also correlate with sepsis. However, its role in predicting outcome is still debatable.[44]

Regarding the markers of cellular activity, mixed results have been reported in the literature about the efficacy of endothelial adhesion molecules (ICAM-1 and e-selectin) and the CD11b receptor of leukocytes.[45] HLA-DR class II molecules mediate the processing of antigen to allow for cellular immunity. They are considered to be reliable markers of immune reactivity and a predictor of outcome following trauma.[46,47]

Napolitano and associates[48] reported that the severity of the systemic inflammatory response syndrome at admission might be an accurate predictor of mortality and the length of stay in the hospital by trauma patients. In another study, the ratio of IL-6 to IL-10 was found to correlate with injury severity after major trauma, and this ratio was recommended as a useful marker to predict the degree of injury following trauma.[49] The level of plasma DNA has been found to increase after major trauma and has also been suggested as a potentially valuable prognostic marker for patients at risk.[50]

It appears that, at present, only two markers, IL-6 and HLA-DR class II molecules, accurately predict the clinical course and outcome after trauma. IL-6 measurement has already been implemented as a routine laboratory test in sev-

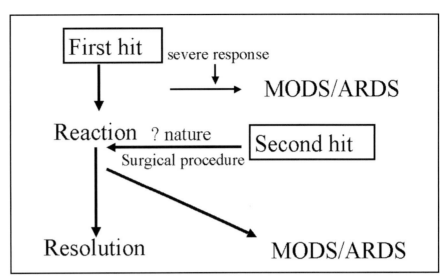

Figure 3 The two-hit theory is shown schematically. The first hit is the initial traumatic event, and the second hit is the definitive orthopaedic procedure, usually femoral nailing. MODS = multiple organ dysfunction syndrome, and ARDS = adult respiratory distress syndrome.

Table 1
Cytokines That Are Important Inflammatory Mediators

Group	Examples
Interleukins (IL)	IL-1, IL-2, IL-3, IL-4, IL-5, IL-6, IL-7, IL-8, IL-10, IL-11, IL-12, IL-13, IL-18
Tumor necrosis factors (TNF)	TNF, lymphotoxin (LT)
Interferons (IFN)	IFN-alpha, IFN-beta, IFN-gamma
Colony stimulating factors (CSF)	G-CSF, M-CSF, GM-CSF

eral trauma centers. Because of the additional laboratory processing required for tests of HLA-DR class II molecules (antibody staining of cells and flow cytometric analysis), the use of these tests has not found great clinical acceptance.

Genetic Predisposition and Adverse Outcomes

Biologic variation and genetic predisposition are increasingly mentioned as explanations of why serious posttraumatic complications develop in some patients and not in others.[51] Some individuals may be "preprogrammed" to have a hyperreaction to a given traumatic insult. Genetic polymorphism of the neutrophil receptor for immunoglobulin G, CD16, has been reported and is associated with

functional differences in neutrophil phagocytosis.[52] An inherited predisposition toward high or low levels of HLA-DR expression is further evidence of a genetic component in the immune response to injury.[46]

Additional evidence of genetic predisposition is found in the cytokine genes. The single base pair polymorphism at position –308 in the *TNF* gene was associated with an increased incidence of sepsis and with a worse outcome after major trauma, postoperative sepsis, and sepsis in a medical intensive care unit.[53-55] This association depends on the presence of the TNF2 allele. Homozygosity for the TNFB2 allele is associated with an increased incidence of severe sepsis and a worse outcome. The risk of

Table 2
Clinical Parameters Used in Hanover, Germany, to Define the "Borderline" Patient for Whom Damage Control Orthopaedics is Often Preferred

Polytrauma + injury severity score of > 20 points and additional thoracic trauma (abbreviated injury score > 2 points)

Polytrauma with abdominal/pelvic trauma (Moore score[75] > 3 points) and hemorrhagic shock (initial blood pressure < 90 mm Hg)

Injury severity score of ≥ 40 points in the absence of additional thoracic injury

Radiographic findings of bilateral lung contusion

Initial mean pulmonary arterial pressure of > 24 mm Hg

Increase of > 6 mm Hg in pulmonary arterial pressure during intramedullary nailing

posttraumatic sepsis developing is 5.22 times higher in patients who are homozygous for TNFB2.[56] Homozygous patients also have higher circulating TNF-α concentrations and higher multiple organ dysfunction syndrome scores compared with heterozygotes.[57]

IL-6 polymorphisms have been reported and were detected in both the 3' and the 5' flanking regions and exon.[58,59] The *Sfa*NI polymorphism is located at position 174. A homozygotic constellation of this polymorphism coincided with decreased IL-6 serum levels during inflammation.[60,61] Polymorphisms in the *IL-10* gene have also been demonstrated.[62] Eskdale and associates[63] reported that stimulation of human blood cultures with bacterial lipopolysaccharide showed large interindividual variation in IL-10 secretion. They concluded that the ability to secrete IL-10 can vary in humans according to the genetic composition of the IL-10 locus.

Recently, isolated case reports of germline defects in the cellular receptor for interferon-gamma were described, and the mutations were characterized.[64,65] Davis and associates[66] conducted a pilot study of 38 patients who had sustained blunt trauma and found that the microsatellite polymorphism AA correlated strongly with infection. These findings portend polymorphism in the receptor itself and thus represent a genetic basis for the development of the infection.

Early identification of patients at risk for adverse outcomes and complications may allow directed intervention with biologic response modifiers in order to improve morbidity and mortality rates. Use of biochemical and genetic markers to identify patients "at risk" after orthopaedic trauma may facilitate clinical decision making regarding when to switch from early total care to damage control orthopaedics.

Patient Selection for Damage Control Orthopaedics

Because biomechanical and genetic testing is currently not practical, it remains a clinical decision when to shift from early total care to damage control orthopaedics. Which patient should be treated with damage control orthopaedics instead of early total care after orthopaedic trauma should be decided on the basis of the patient's overall physiologic status and injury complexes. Many trauma scoring systems (for example, the abbreviated injury scale,[67] injury severity score,[68,69] revised trauma score,[70] anatomic profile,[71] and Glasgow coma scale[72]) have been developed in an attempt to describe the overall condition of the trauma patient. However, Bosse and associates[73] noted that, "there is no score that assists in decision making during the acute resuscitation phase." Therefore, it may be that one cannot rely exclusively on a scoring system.

Additional data must be synthesized, and the overall status of the patient should be stratified into one of four categories. Patients who have sustained orthopaedic trauma have been divided into four groups: stable, borderline, unstable, and in extremis.[74] Stable patients, unstable patients, and patients in extremis are fairly easy to define. Stable patients should be treated with the local preferred method for managing their orthopaedic injuries. Unstable patients and patients in extremis should be treated with damage control orthopaedics for their orthopaedic injuries. Borderline patients are more difficult to define. One of the authors (HCP) and other colleagues defined them as patients with polytrauma and an injury severity score of more than 40 points in the absence of thoracic injury, or an injury severity score of less than 20 points with thoracic injury (an abbreviated injury score of > 2 points); polytrauma with abdominal trauma (a Moore score[75] of > 3 points); a chest radiograph showing bilateral lung contusions; an initial mean pulmonary artery pressure of more than 24 mm Hg; or an increase in pulmonary artery pressure of more than 6 mm Hg during nailing[74] (Table 2). Borderline orthopaedic trauma patients are probably best treated with damage control orthopaedics.

The term "borderline patient" describes a predisposition for deterioration.[74] Among other factors, thoracic trauma appears to play a crucial role in this predisposition. However, whether femoral fractures in patients with chest trauma should be treated with definitive stabilization or should be stabilized with a temporary external fixator remains a subject of debate. The clinical situation, including the presence or absence of a criterion indicating borderline status (Table 2) and factors associated with a high risk of adverse outcomes (Table 3), should determine how the patient is treated. In Louisville, some of the additional clinical criteria that we have used as a basis for shifting to damage control orthopaedics include a pH of less than 7.24, a temperature of less than 35°C, surgical times of more than 90 minutes, coagulopathy, and transfusion of more than 10 units of packed red blood cells. Furthermore, certain specific orthopaedic injury complexes appear to be more amenable to damage control orthopaedics; these include, for example, femoral fractures in a multiply injured patient, pelvic ring injuries with exsanguinating hemorrhage, and polytrauma in a geriatric patient.

Femoral Fractures

Femoral fractures in a multiply injured patient are not automatically treated with intramedullary nailing because of concerns about the second hit of such a procedure. In addition to the second hit, which results in an additional systemic inflammatory response, embolic fat from use of instrumentation in the medullary canal will worsen the pulmonary status. Patients with a chest injury (an abbreviated injury score of > 2 points) are most prone to deterioration after an intramedullary nailing procedure.[76]

Bilateral femoral fracture is a unique scenario in polytrauma that is associated with a higher mortality rate and incidence of adult respiratory distress syndrome than is a unilateral femoral fracture.[77] Copeland and associates[77] noted that the increase in mortality may be more closely related to associated injuries and physiologic parameters than to the bilateral femoral fracture itself. Wu and Shih[78] noted that bilateral femoral fracture indicates severe systemic and local injuries. Thus, such injuries are ideal for damage control orthopaedics.

Pelvic Ring Injuries

Exsanguinating hemorrhage associated with pelvic fracture is another injury complex suitable for damage control orthopaedics. Hemorrhage can result from a combination of osseous, venous,

---

Table 3

Clinical Parameters Associated With Adverse Outcomes in Multiply Injured Patients as Reported in Hannover, Germany

Unstable condition or resuscitation difficult (borderline patient)

Coagulopathy (platelet count < 90,000)

Hypothermia (< 32°C)

Shock and > 25 units of blood needed

Bilateral lung contusion on first plain radiograph

Multiple long-bone injuries and truncal injury; abbreviated injury score of ≥ 2 points

Presumed surgery time > 6 hr

Arterial injury and hemodynamic instability (blood pressure < 90 mm Hg)

Exaggerated inflammatory response (eg, IL-6 > 800 pg/mL)

---

and arterial bleeding. Although the most common arterial injuries involve the internal iliac artery or its branches (for example, the superior gluteal artery), injuries to the common and external iliac arteries have been reported and are associated with a poor outcome.[79] The specific radiographic pattern of the pelvic ring injury and the mechanism of the injury can help one to anticipate the amount of bleeding, but there is no precise injury pattern that predicts hemorrhage consistently. An additional complicating factor can be the presence of a pelvic binder put in place by emergency medical responders, as it may decrease the pelvic volume, realign the pelvic ring, and contribute to a benign-looking pelvic radiograph.

There are nonetheless some consistent findings associated with a higher likelihood of hemorrhage. Posterior pelvic ring injuries are associated with a twofold to threefold increase in blood replacement requirements compared with anterior injuries.[80,81] Anterior-posterior compression type III injuries and lateral compression injuries are associated with a high prevalence of vascular injury (22% and 23%, respectively).[82] Finally, pelvic fractures in patients older than 55 years of age are more likely to produce hemorrhage and require angiography.[83]

The main controversy regarding the treatment of patients with profuse, exsan-

guinating hemorrhage relates to the role of angiography and embolization. In North America, both are most commonly used in the initial treatment of pelvic fractures with associated hypotension that have not responded to the placement of a pelvic binder, external fixator, pelvic c-clamp, or pelvic stabilizer and transfusion of four units or more of blood. Additional indications for angiography are an expanding retroperitoneal hematoma, a vascular blush seen on CT, and a massive retroperitoneal hematoma observed on CT. The timing of embolization is also important. Agolini and associates[84] reported that embolization later than 3 hours after injury increased the risk of mortality fivefold and that the average procedure time for embolization was 90 minutes.

Alternatively, pelvic packing for the control of hemorrhage has been advocated at some centers in Europe.[85] This technique appears to be used for patients with severe hypotension and a pelvic fracture that is unresponsive to other initial treatment measures, and that is associated with the imminent risk of death and thus a high likelihood that the patient will not survive the trip to the angiography suite. However, there are limited data to support the use of pelvic packing.

Damage control orthopaedics for a pelvic ring injury with exsanguinating hemorrhage involves rapid clinical deci-

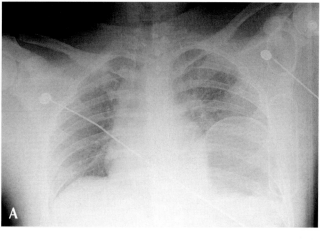
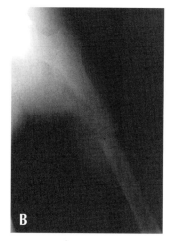
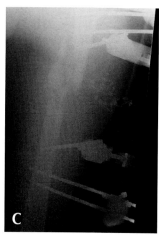
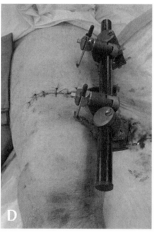
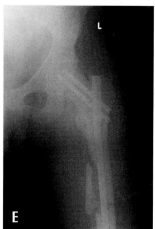

Figure 4 Chest radiograph demonstrating a ruptured left hemidiaphragm (**A**) and radiograph showing a grade II open femoral fracture (**B**) in a multiply injured patient. **C** and **D,** Initial external fixation was performed at the time of the diaphragmatic repair. **E,** Staged intramedullary nailing was performed on postinjury day 2.

sion making and multiple teams for resuscitation and minimally invasive pelvic stabilization (for example, with a pelvic binder, external fixator, pelvic c-clamp, or pelvic stabilizer). Patients who do not respond to these measures should be considered for angiography and embolization if they are likely to survive the trip to the angiography suite; otherwise, they should be considered for pelvic packing once any underlying coagulopathy has been corrected.

Geriatric Trauma

Elderly trauma patients require special evaluation and treatment because of their higher mortality rate following trauma, even minor trauma. Greenspan and associates[86] reported that the average Lethal Dose (LD) 50 injury severity score was 20 points for individuals older than 65 years of age. This value is essentially half of the LD 50 injury severity score for individuals between 24 and 44 years of age. In addition, pelvic ring fractures in patients older than 55 years of age are associated with an increased chance of arterial injuries and higher transfusion requirements.[83] In a study of patients who were older than 60 years of age, Tornetta and associates[87] noted that increased mortality was associated with a lower Glasgow coma score (11.5 points for the patients who died compared with 13.9 points for the patients who survived), greater transfusion requirements (10.9 units for the patients who died compared with 2.9 units for those who survived), and greater fluid infusion (12.4 L for the patients who died com-

pared with 4.9 L for those who survived). These differences highlight the importance of considering damage control orthopaedics for elderly patients. In addition, treatment should be directed toward measures that enhance immediate mobilization and the avoidance of prolonged bed rest in this patient population.

Special Situations in Damage Control Orthopaedics
Chest Injuries

Traditionally, there have been two divergent schools of thought related to the treatment of multiply injured patients with long-bone fractures and a chest injury (Figure 4), with some believing that early fracture stabilization is safe and possibly beneficial[6,88-91] and others believing that early fracture stabilization is not safe and may be harmful.[76] The classic article by Bone and associates[6] has probably had the most influence on the care and treatment of orthopaedic trauma patients in the United States. More recently, Boulanger and associates[92] reported no increase in morbidity or mortality in association with early intramedullary nailing (within 24 hours) of femoral fractures in patients who had sustained blunt thoracic trauma.

The Eastern Association for the Surgery of Trauma Practice Management Guidelines Work Group reviewed the current literature and found no randomized clinical trials of the treatment of patients with chest injuries with immediate long bone stabilization (within 48 hours).[93] They noted that available prospective studies or retrospective analyses comparing long bone stabilization within 48 hours with later stabilization in patients with a chest injury showed that the two groups had similar rates of mortality and adult respiratory distress syndrome, mechanical ventilation requirements, lengths of stay in the intensive care unit, and total lengths of stay in the hospital. The authors indicated that five clinical parameters might be helpful in determining the appropriateness of early long bone stabilization: severity of pulmonary dysfunction, hemodynamic status, estimated operative time, estimated blood loss, and fracture status (open or closed).

A selective approach should be used for patients with long bone fractures and a chest injury. Defining the subgroup of patients for whom early nailing would increase the risk of early complications is the goal of damage control orthopaedics. Treatment should be individualized. When early intramedullary nailing is not deemed to be the best alternative, damage control orthopaedics, with short-term external fixation of the femur followed by staged conversion to an intramedullary nail in the first week after injury, can be used.

Head Injuries

The Eastern Association for the Surgery of Trauma Practice Management Guidelines Work Group also searched the literature for studies regarding the timing of long-bone fracture stabilization in a multiply injured patient with a head injury.[93] The group found no level I studies (randomized clinical trials). On the basis of level II studies (prospective, noncomparative clinical studies or retrospective analyses of reliable data) and level III studies (retrospective case series or database reviews), it was concluded that patients with mild, moderate, or severe brain injury who underwent long bone stabilization within 48 hours were similar to those treated with later stabilization with regard to mortality rate, length of stay in the intensive care unit, need for mechanical ventilation, and total length of stay in the hospital. The overall conclusion was that there was no compelling evidence that early long bone stabilization either enhances or worsens the outcome in patients with a mild, moderate, or severe head injury.

Many clinical issues arise during an examination of the available literature on patients with a head injury and long bone fractures. Early definitive fracture stabilization is potentially beneficial in this situation because it reduces persistent pain at the fracture site by minimizing involuntary movements by an unconscious or not yet cooperative patient. Fracture stabilization also has a positive effect on the patient's metabolism, muscle tone, and body temperature, and, as a result, cerebral function.[94] Furthermore, unstabilized fractures may cause physiologic deterioration in these patients as a result of increased soft-tissue damage, fat embolism, and respiratory insufficiency.[95-99]

In recent years, some authors have reported a worse outcome in patients with secondary brain injury resulting from hypotension, hypoxia, and increased intraoperative administration of fluid related to early surgical fracture fixa-

tion.[100,101] In a study of multiply injured patients with fractures of the femur, tibia, and pelvis, Martens and Ectors[102] reported a 38% prevalence of early neurologic deterioration in a group treated with early fixation but no early neurologic deterioration in a group treated with late fixation. McKee and associates[103] reported that neurologic complications developed in the postoperative period in three patients treated with early fixation, but they did not attribute any of these complications to the femoral fracture or its fixation. Also, they found no difference in the long-term neurologic outcome between the patients treated with early fixation and those treated with delayed fixation.

In contrast, in a study of patients with a head injury and a fracture of the neck or shaft of the femur or the shaft of the tibia, Poole and associates[104] found that those who had undergone early definitive fracture fixation had a significantly ($P < 0.0001$) lower prevalence of perioperative neurologic complications compared with those who had been treated with late fixation. Brundage and associates[105] reported that, in a series of multiply injured patients with head injuries, femoral shaft fractures, and an injury severity score of more than 15 points, those treated with fixation within 24 hours after the injury had the highest Glasgow coma scale scores at the time of discharge. However, because only the mean head abbreviated injury scale score, and not the Glasgow coma scale score on admission, was reported, these results are very difficult to interpret accurately. Hofman and Goris[106] found that the Glasgow coma scale score was better in a group treated with early fixation than it was in a group treated with late fixation, but the difference did not reach significance.

The initial management of a patient with a head injury should be similar to that of other trauma patients, with a focus on the rapid control of hemorrhage and restoration of vital signs and tissue perfusion. A brain injury can be made worse if resuscitation is inadequate or if surgical intervention such as long-bone fixation decreases mean arterial pressure or increases intracranial pressure. The treatment protocol for unstable patients should be based on the individual clinical assessment and treatment requirements rather than on mandatory policies with respect to the timing of fixation of long-bone fractures. In such cases, damage control orthopaedics can provide temporary osseous stability to an injured extremity, functioning as a temporary bridge to staged definitive osteosynthesis, without worsening the patient's head injury or overall condition. Intracranial pressure monitoring should be used in the intensive care unit as well as during surgical procedures in the operating room. Aggressive management of intracranial pressure appears to be related to an improved outcome. Maintenance of cerebral perfusion pressure at more than 70 mm Hg and intracranial pressure at less than 20 mm Hg should be mandatory before, during, and after surgical procedures. Orthopaedic injuries should be managed aggressively with the assumption that full neurologic recovery will occur.

Mangled Extremities

Prior to the Lower Extremity Assessment Project (LEAP) study, there were limited data on the contemporary treatment of severely injured or mangled lower extremities.[107-109] Lange[110] performed a retrospective study of 23 Gustilo and Anderson type IIIC tibial fractures (severe open fractures with limb-threatening vascular compromise requiring repair), 14 of which eventually led to amputation (5 of the amputations were primary and 9, delayed). The absolute indications for amputation in that study included anatomic disruption of the tibial nerve and a crush injury with a warm ischemia time of more than 6 hours, or

the presence of two of three relative indications (serious polytrauma, severe injury of the ipsilateral foot, and anticipation of a protracted course to obtain soft-tissue coverage and tibial reconstruction). Caudle and Stern[111] reported that seven of nine type III open tibial fractures required secondary amputation.

Hansen[112] called for a multicenter study to develop guidelines to "avoid prolonged, costly, and fruitless salvage procedures when such a course is not indicated." Helfet and associates[113] reported that a mangled extremity severity score of 7 points was associated with a 100% rate of amputation. Georgiadis and associates[114] reported that, of 45 patients with a severe open tibial fracture requiring free tissue transfer for soft-tissue coverage, 27 were treated with limb salvage and 18 were treated with early amputation. The patients in the limb salvage group had an average of three complications, whereas there was a total of 17 complications in the early amputation group.

Renewed interest in treatment of the mangled lower extremity has been generated by the dissemination of the results from the LEAP study, a prospective, longitudinal, observational, outcomes study at eight level I American trauma centers.[107-109] In this study, the attending surgeons directed all evaluations, decisions, and extremity treatment. There were 656 eligible patients ranging in age from 16 to 69 years. Fifty-five patients were excluded from the study: 36 refused to participate, 13 died in the hospital, and 6 were not enrolled because of administrative failure, which left a study group of 601 patients. In that group, 32 patients had bilateral injuries, which were analyzed separately, and 569 had a unilateral injury.

The main hypothesis of the study was that after the investigators controlled for the severity of the limb injury, the presence and severity of other injuries, and patient characteristics, amputation would prove to have a better functional outcome

than reconstruction for the treatment of traumatic amputations, type IIIB and IIIC open tibial fractures, selected type IIIA open tibial fractures, vascular injuries, major soft-tissue injuries, and severe foot injuries.

The LEAP study patients differed from the general population with regard to many characteristics. They were more likely to be male; they were less educated; they were more often blue collar workers; they were less insured (38% had no insurance); they were more likely to be healthy, heavy drinkers, smokers, neurotic, and extroverted; they were less agreeable; and they had a lower income.

Patients with a severe injury of the lower extremity and absent plantar sensation at the time of admission had substantial impairment at 20 and 24 months. Patients treated with limb salvage did not have poorer outcomes than those treated with amputation. Absent plantar sensation did not even predict the state of plantar sensation at 24 months. Neither the injury characteristics nor the presence and severity of ipsilateral or contralateral limb injuries significantly correlated with the outcomes as assessed with the Sickness Impact Profile (SIP). Patients with a through-the-knee amputation had worse regression-adjusted SIP scores ($P = 0.05$) and slower self-selected walking speeds ($P = 0.004$) than did patients with either a below-the-knee or an above-the-knee amputation.[109] Patients who had been rehospitalized for a major complication also had poorer outcomes. Significant ($P = 0.05$) predictors of a poor outcome were a high-school education or less, a household income below the federal poverty line, being nonwhite, a lack of insurance, receiving Medicaid benefits, a poor social support network, low self-efficacy, smoking, and involvement in the legal system for injury compensation. A proportion of the patients who had undergone limb reconstruction had not fully recovered by 2 years; 10.8% of those patients had nonunion, 4.7% did

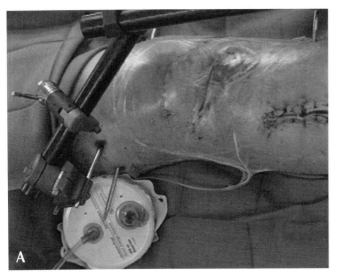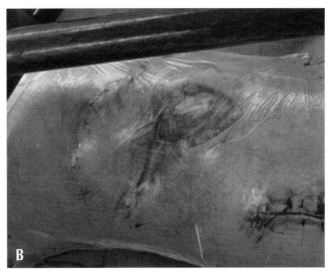

Figure 5 Antibiotic bead pouch for treatment of an open proximal tibial fracture (**A**), with a close-up view (**B**). Adjacent to the bead pouch are traumatic arthrotomy and fasciotomy wounds that have been closed. Spanning external fixation across the knee for management of the tibial fracture and a femoral traction pin for management of an ipsilateral acetabular fracture were also used in this patient.

not have soft-tissue healing, and 15% needed additional surgery.

The SIP scores in the LEAP study were significantly higher ($P < 0.01$) than published population scores.[115] Significant ($P < 0.05$) improvement was observed over time for all dimensions of the SIP except for psychosocial functioning. The percentage of patients with a slower walking speed was higher in the amputation group than in the reconstruction group ($P < 0.05$). There was no difference between the two groups in terms of SIP scores for disability or the percentage who returned to work. The patients who had undergone reconstruction took longer to achieve full weight bearing, and they had more rehospitalizations and hospital days ($P < 0.01$). Contrary to the study's hypothesis, the 2-year outcomes following the reconstructions were not significantly worse, or better, than those following the amputations. However, reconstruction involves a higher complication risk, additional surgical procedures, and more hospital readmissions. Also, the risk of late amputation was 6.4%. As a result of this study, it cannot be assumed that either an amputation or

a successful reconstruction will provide a superior result.

It was reported (LX Webb, MD, and associates, Salt Lake City, UT, unpublished data, 2003) that patients with a limb-threatening type III open tibial shaft fracture managed with limb salvage had outcomes that were similar to those of patients who had undergone an amputation. Several surgeon-controlled variables that appeared to influence the course of the fracture and the patient outcome. Wound coverage with simple methods provided better results than flap coverage, external fixation and flap coverage provided worse results than amputations, and bone grafting performed within 3 months after the injury had a trend for a better outcome than did bone grafting that was accomplished later. In addition, it was found (LX Webb, MD, and associates, Salt Lake City, UT, unpublished data, 2003) that the timing of débridement and of soft-tissue coverage did not influence the outcome, and the most common complications warranting readmission were nonunion and infection.

It was reported (DG Smith, MD, and associates, Salt Lake City, UT, unpub-

lished data, 2003) that patients treated with late amputation after a complex lower extremity injury reported significantly ($P < 0.05$) higher levels of disability than did those who previously had an amputation either during the first hospitalization or within the first 3 months after the injury. These investigators noted a high number of hospitalizations for complications ($P < 0.0001$), a high number of infections ($P < 0.001$), and a high number of surgical procedures in the late-amputation group ($P < 0.0001$). They stated that "when severe lower limb trauma places an individual at risk of amputation there is value in making that difficult decision in a timely fashion."

The LEAP data suggest an increasing trend toward limb salvage rather than immediate amputation for complex open lower extremity injuries. A damage control orthopaedics approach to saving the limb may make it possible to improve surgeon-controlled variables that appear to be related to better outcomes. The use of spanning external fixation, antibiotic bead pouches[116-118] (Figure 5), and the vacuum-assisted wound closure technique may provide a bridge to staged

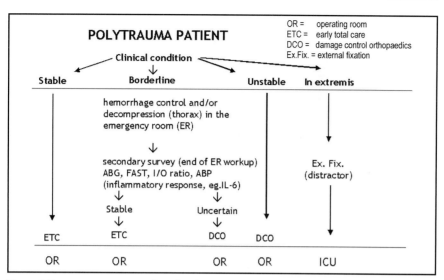

Figure 6 The current treatment algorithm from Hanover, Germany, for the use of damage control orthopaedics is based on a prompt and accurate determination of whether the patient is stable, borderline, unstable, or in extremis. ER = emergency room, ABG = arterial blood gases, FAST = focused assessment sonography for trauma, I/O ratio = intake/output ratio, ABP = arterial blood pressure, IL-6 = interleukin-6, ETC = early total care, OR = operating room, DCO = damage control orthopaedics, and ICU = intensive care unit.

osseous reconstruction and soft-tissue coverage procedures.[119] Vacuum-assisted wound closure subjects the wound bed to negative pressure by way of a closed system and thereby removes edema from the extravascular space.[119]

Isolated Complex Lower Extremity Trauma

An isolated complex extremity injury (other than a mangled limb) is a possible indication for a limited form of damage control orthopaedics that has been termed "limb damage control orthopaedics." Specific injuries that are amenable to this approach include complex proximal tibial articular and metaphyseal fractures and distal tibial pilon fractures. These clinical situations usually combine a complex fracture pattern, either open or closed, with a substantial soft-tissue injury. Limb damage control orthopaedics is useful for preventing soft-tissue complications by spanning the articular segment with an external fixator and avoiding areas of future incisions.

Then minimally invasive plate osteosynthesis can be performed at a stage when the condition of the soft-tissue envelope is optimized.

When Can Secondary Orthopaedic Procedures Be Performed?

One of the most important issues in damage control orthopaedics is the timing of the secondary surgical procedures (definitive osteosynthesis). Days 2, 3, and 4 are not safe for performing definitive surgery. During this period, marked immune reactions are ongoing and increased generalized edema is observed. A recent prospective study demonstrated that multiply injured patients subjected to secondary definitive surgery between days 2 and 4 had a significantly ($P < 0.0001$) increased inflammatory response compared with that in patients operated on between days 6 and 8.[12,120] It was concluded that, in different posttraumatic periods, variable inflammatory responses to comparable stimuli are

observed. This variation may contribute to the differences in clinical outcome (for example, a higher incidence of multiple organ failure) that have been reported.[12]

In Hannover, Germany, all high-risk patients have been managed with a treatment plan that involves a reevaluation of clinical and laboratory parameters in the emergency department after the primary diagnostic workup.[1] On the basis of this reevaluation, specific recommendations can be made for specific groups of patients in the form of an algorithm (Figure 6).

Clinical Outcomes of Damage Control Orthopaedics

In the early 1990s, the approach in Hannover changed from performing definitive surgery in all patients to using an external fixator as a temporary measure to stabilize the fracture and subsequently carrying out secondary definitive internal fixation.[1] In a retrospective evaluation, three different periods were identified. In the early total care period, between January 1, 1981, and December 31, 1989, the protocol for the treatment of a femoral shaft fracture was early definitive stabilization (within 24 hours). In the intermediate period, between January 1, 1990, and December 31, 1992, the usual protocol for treating a femoral shaft fracture in a multiply injured patient at risk for posttraumatic complications changed from early definitive stabilization to early temporary fixation. In the damage control orthopaedics period, beginning in 1993, the protocol for such an injury in such a patient was early temporary stabilization (within 24 hours) followed by secondary conversion to intramedullary nailing. The rates of multisystem organ failure and adult respiratory distress syndrome were found to be significantly higher ($P < 0.05$) in the earlier periods (Table 4). In addition, during the latest period, patients who were treated with damage control orthopaedics demonstrated a lower risk of adult respiratory distress syndrome than those treated with initial intramedullary nailing.

Risk of Local Infection with Damage Control Orthopaedics

The use of spanning external fixation carries the risk of pin track infection. In the series in Hannover, the risk of infection following definitive intramedullary nailing (Table 5) was not greater than that in other studies of patients who had undergone intramedullary stabilization after external fixation.[121-123] Contemporary rates of pin track infection are still substantial, but they are minimized when the duration of external fixation is brief.[124]

Practical Considerations for Damage Control Orthopaedics

Practical considerations for spanning external fixation include the use of an external fixation system that is user-friendly and can be applied rapidly. Self-drilling pins, which can be manually inserted, can be applied quickly with a limited need for fluoroscopy. Operating time can be decreased by multiple operating teams working on opposite ends of the same limb or on different extremities. External fixation systems that use snap-and-click clamps can be assembled rapidly. In addition, a system that allows flexibility in pin placement is preferable so that areas of future incisions can be avoided.

Summary

Damage control orthopaedics is ideal for an unstable patient or a patient in extremis, and it has some utility for the borderline patient as well. Specific injury complexes for which damage control orthopaedics should be considered are femoral fractures (especially bilateral fractures), pelvic ring injuries with profound hemorrhage, and multiple injuries in elderly patients. Specific subgroups of multiply injured orthopaedic patients who may benefit from damage control orthopaedics are those with a head injury,

Table 4
Prevalence of Adult Respiratory Distress Syndrome, According to Type of Femoral Fixation, Associated With Three Different Approaches to Treatment of a Multiply Injured Patient in Hannover, Germany

	Patients With Adult Respiratory Distress Syndrome*			
	Early Total Care Period	Intermediate Period	Damage Control Orthopaedics Period	P Value[†]
Primary intramedullary nailing	77 (32.7)‡	20 (22.7)‡	29 (15.1)‡	0.003
Primary external fixation, secondary intramedullary nailing	38 (16.2)	10 (11.4)	15 (7.8)	0.002
Primary plate fixation	45 (19.1)	14 (15.9)	42 (21.9)	0.001

*The values are given as the number of patients with the percentage in parentheses
[†] P values indicate significant differences between Early Total Care and Damage Control Orthopaedics; the prevalence of Adult Respiratory Distress Syndrome was significantly lower with the Damage Control Orthopaedics approach
‡ Indicates a significant difference (P < 0.05) between primary intramedullary nailing and primary external fixation with secondary intramedullary nailing

Table 5
Comparative Data on Postoperative Local Complications During the Three Periods of Fracture Care in Hannover, Germany

	Patients With Complications*			
	Early Total Care Period	Intermediate Period	Damage Control Orthopaedics Period	P Value[†]
Pin track infection	2/39	3/21	4/68	NS
Wound infection	5/235	2/88	3/191	NS
Osteomyelitis	2/235	0/88	1/191	NS

*Number of patients with a complication/total number of patients.
† NS = not significant

chest trauma, or a mangled limb. A limited form of damage control orthopaedics (limb damage control orthopaedics) is a rational alternative for the treatment of isolated, complex limb injuries.

Clinical data and emerging discoveries in molecular medicine may continue to provide answers to the question of when orthopaedic surgeons should use a damage control orthopaedics approach. Prospective, multicenter studies similar to LEAP may ultimately be necessary to better understand the role of damage control orthopaedics in the treatment of patients who have sustained orthopaedic

trauma, especially those with concomitant injuries to the chest and head. Despite the lack of prospective clinical studies, many trauma centers have already modified their approach to the treatment of orthopaedic patients with multiple injuries by incorporating the principles of damage control orthopaedics.[1]

Acknowledgments
The authors thank Paul Tornetta III, MD, for his encouragement and enthusiasm, which contributed greatly to this instructional course lecture. They also express their appreciation to Timothy E.

Hewett, PhD, for his thoughtful review of this manuscript.

References

1. Pape HC, Giannoudis P, Krettek C: The timing of fracture treatment in poly-trauma patients: Relevance of damage control orthopedic surgery. *Am J Surg* 2002;183:622-629.

2. Bradford DS, Foster RR, Nossel HL: Coagulation alterations, hypoxemia, and fat embolism in fracture patients. *J Trauma* 1970;10:307-321.

3. Rang M: *The Story of Orthopaedics*. Philadelphia, PA, WB Saunders, 2000.

4. Matter P: History of the AO and its global effect on operative fracture treatment. *Clin Orthop* 1998;347:11-18.

5. Pape HC, Schmidt RE, Rice J, et al: Biochemical changes after trauma and skeletal surgery of the lower extremity: Quantification of the operative burden. *Crit Care Med* 2000;28:3441-3448.

6. Bone LB, Johnson KD, Weigelt J, Scheinberg R: Early versus delayed stabilization of femoral fractures: A prospective randomized study. *J Bone Joint Surg Am* 1989;71:336-340.

7. Border JR: *Blunt Multiple Trauma: Comprehensive Pathophysiology and Care*. New York, NY, Marcel Dekker, 1990.

8. Giannoudis PV, Smith RM, Bellamy MC, Morrison JF, Dickson RA, Guillou PJ: Stimulation of the inflammatory system by reamed and unreamed nailing of femoral fractures: An analysis of the second hit. *J Bone Joint Surg Br* 1999;81:356-361.

9. Nowotarski PJ, Turen CH, Brumback RJ, Scarboro JM: Conversion of external fixation to intramedullary nailing for fractures of the shaft of the femur in multiply injured patients. *J Bone Joint Surg Am* 2000;82:781-788.

10. Scalea TM, Boswell SA, Scott JD, Mitchell KA, Kramer ME, Pollak AN: External fixation as a bridge to intramedullary nailing for patients with multiple injuries and with femur fractures: Damage control orthopedics. *J Trauma* 2000;48:613-623.

11. Townsend RN, Lheureau T, Protech J, Riemer B, Simon D: Timing fracture repair in patients with severe brain injury (Glasgow Coma Scale score < 9). *J Trauma* 1998;44:977-983.

12. Pape HC, van Griensven M, Rice J, et al: Major secondary surgery in blunt trauma patients and perioperative cytokine liberation: Determination of the clinical relevance of biochemical markers. *J Trauma* 2001;50:989-1000.

13. Rotondo MF, Schwab CW, McGonigal MD, et al: 'Damage control': An approach for improved survival in exsanguinating penetrating abdominal injury. *J Trauma* 1993;35:375-383.

14. Richardson D, Seligson D: Dudley and Griswold: The development of fracture treatment in Kentucky. *J Ky Med Assoc* 1993;91:226-230.

15. Feliciano DV, Mattox KL, Jordan GL Jr: Intra-abdominal packing for control of hepatic hemorrhage: A reappraisal. *J Trauma* 1981;21:285-290.

16. Stone HH, Strom PR, Mullins RJ: Management of the major coagulopathy with onset during laparotomy. *Am Surg* 1983;197:532-535.

17. Burch JM, Ortiz VB, Richardson RJ, Martin RR, Mattox KL, Jordan GL Jr: Abbreviated laparotomy and planned reoperation for critically injured patients. *Am Surg* 1992;215:476-484.

18. Rotondo MF, Zonies DH: The damage control sequence and underlying logic. *Surg Clin North Am* 1997;77:761-777.

19. Mattox KL: Introduction, background, and future projections of damage control surgery. *Surg Clin North Am* 1997;77:753-759.

20. Smith RM, Giannoudis PV: Trauma and the immune response. *J R Soc Med* 1998;91:417-420.

21. Granger DN, Kubes P: The microcirculation and inflammation: Modulation of leukocyte-endothelial cell adhesion. *J Leukoc Biol* 1994;55:662-675.

22. Cipolle MD, Pasquale MD, Cerra FB: Secondary organ dysfunction: From clinical perspectives to molecular mediators. *Crit Care Clin* 1993;9:261-298.

23. Anderson BO, Harken AH: Multiple organ failure: Inflammatory priming and activation sequences promote autologous tissue injury. *J Trauma* 1990;30(suppl 12):S44-S49.

24. Giannoudis PV, Smith RM, Ramsden CW, Sharples D, Dickson RA, Guillou PJ: Molecular mediators and trauma: Effects of accidental trauma on the production of plasma elastase, IL-6, sICAM-1, and sE-selectin. *Injury* 1996;27:372.

25. Giannoudis PV, Smith RM, Banks RE, Windsor AC, Dickson RA, Guillou PJ: Stimulation of inflammatory markers after blunt trauma. *Br J Surg* 1998;85:986-990.

26. Giannoudis PV, Smith RM, Windsor AC, Bellamy MC, Guillou PJ: Monocyte human leukocyte antigen-DR expression correlates with intrapulmonary shunting after major trauma. *Am J Surg* 1999;177:454-459.

27. Pape HC, Grimme K, Van Griensven M, et al: Impact of intramedullary instrumentation versus damage control for femoral fractures on immunoinflammatory parameters: Prospective randomized analysis by the EPOFF Study Group. *J Trauma* 2003;55:7-13.

28. Hoch RC, Rodriguez R, Manning T, et al: Effects of accidental trauma on cytokine and endotoxin production. *Crit Care Med* 1993;21:839-845.

29. Maekawa K, Futami S, Nishida M, et al: Effects of trauma and sepsis on soluble L-selectin and cell surface expression of L-selectin and CD11b. *J Trauma* 1998;44:460-468.

30. Smith RM, Giannoudis PV, Bellamy MC, Perry SL, Dickson RA, Guillou PJ: Interleukin-10 release and monocyte human leukocyte antigen-DR expression during femoral nailing. *Clin Orthop* 2000;373:233-240.

31. Ertel W, Keel M, Bonaccio M, et al: Release of anti-inflammatory mediators after mechanical trauma correlates with severity of injury and clinical outcome. *J Trauma* 1995;39:879-887.

32. Tan LR, Waxman K, Scannell G, Ioli G, Granger GA: Trauma causes early release of soluble receptors for tumor necrosis factor. *J Trauma* 1993;34:634-638.

33. Meakins JL, Pietsch JB, Bubenick O, et al: Delayed hypersensitivity: Indicator of acquired failure of host defenses in sepsis and trauma. *Ann Surg* 1977;186:241-250.

34. Polk HC Jr: Non-specific host defence stimulation in the reduction of surgical infection in man. *Br J Surg* 1987;74:969-970.

35. Obertacke U, Kleinschmidt C, Dresing K, Bardenheuer M, Bruch J: Repeated routine determination of pulmonary microvascular permeability after polytrauma. *Unfallchirurg* 1993;96:142-149.

36. Giannoudis PV, Abbott C, Stone M, Bellamy MC, Smith RM: Fatal systemic inflammatory response syndrome following early bilateral femoral nailing. *Intensive Care Med* 1998;24:641-642.

37. Waydhas C, Nast-Kolb D, Trupka A, et al: Posttraumatic inflammatory response, secondary operations, and late multiple organ failure. *J Trauma* 1996;40:624-631.

38. Giannoudis PV, Smith MR, Evans RT, Bellamy MC, Guillou PJ: Serum CRP and IL-6 levels after trauma: Not predictive of septic complications in 31 patients. *Acta Orthop Scand* 1998;69:184-188.

39. Mimoz O, Benoist JF, Edouard AR, Assicot M, Bohuon C, Samii K: Procalcitonin and C-reactive protein during the early posttraumatic systemic inflammatory response syndrome. *Intensive Care Med* 1998;24:185-188.

40. Andermahr J, Greb A, Hensler T, et al: Pneumonia in multiple injured patients: A prospective controlled trial on early prediction using clinical and immunological parameters. *Inflamm Res* 2002;51:265-272.

41. Wanner GA, Keel M, Steckholzer U, Beier W, Stocker R, Ertel W: Relationship between procalcitonin plasma levels and severity of injury, sepsis, organ failure, and mortality in injured patients. *Crit Care Med* 2000;28:950-957.

42. Oberhoffer M, Karzai W, Meier-Hellmann A, Bogel D, Fassbinder J, Reinhart K: Sensitivity and specificity of various markers of inflammation for the prediction of tumor necrosis factor-alpha and interleukin-6 in patients with sepsis. *Crit Care Med* 1999;27:1814-1818.

43. Abraham E: Why immunomodulatory therapies have not worked in sepsis. *Intensive Care Med* 1999;25:556-566.

44. Giannoudis PV, Smith RM, Perry SL, Windsor AJ, Dickson RA, Bellamy MC: Immediate IL-10 expression following major orthopaedic trauma: Relationship to anti-inflammatory response and subsequent development of sepsis. *Intensive Care Med* 2000;26:1076-1081.

45. Weigand MA, Schmidt H, Pourmahmoud M, Zhao Q, Martin E, Bardenheuer HJ: Circulating intracellular adhesion molecule-1 as an early predictor of hepatic failure in patients with septic shock. *Crit Care Med* 1999;27:2656-2661.

46. Cheadle WG, Hershman MJ, Wellhausen SR, Polk HC Jr: HLA-DR antigen expression on peripheral blood monocytes correlates with surgical infection. *Am J Surg* 1991;161:639-645.

47. Giannoudis PV, Smith RM, Windsor AC, Bellamy MC, Guillou PJ: Monocyte human leukocyte antigen-DR expression correlates with intrapulmonary shunting after major trauma. *Am J Surg* 1999;177:454-459.

48. Napolitano LM, Ferrer T, McCarter RJ Jr, Scalea TM: Systemic inflammatory response syndrome score at admission independently predicts mortality and length of stay in trauma patients. *J Trauma* 2000;49:647-653.

49. Taniguchi T, Koido Y, Aiboshi J, Yamashita T, Suzaki S, Kurokawa A: The ratio of interleukin-6 to interleukin-10 correlates with severity in patients with chest and abdominal trauma. *Am J Emerg Med* 1999;17:548-551.

50. Lo YM, Rainer TH, Chan LY, Hjelm NM, Cocks RA: Plasma DNA as a prognostic marker in trauma patients. *Clin Chem* 2000;46:319-323.

51. Guillou PJ: Biological variation in the development of sepsis after surgery or trauma. *Lancet* 1993;342:217-220.

52. Salmon JE, Edberg JC, Brogle NL, Kimberly RP: Allelic polymorphisms of human Fc gamma receptor IIA and Fc gamma receptor IIIB: Independent mechanisms for differences in human phagocyte function. *J Clin Invest* 1992;89:1274-1281.

53. O'Keefe GE, Hybki DL, Munford RS: The G—>A single nucleotide polymorphism at the -308 position in the tumor necrosis factor-alpha promoter increases the risk for severe sepsis after trauma. *J Trauma* 2002;52:817-826.

54. Tang GJ, Huang SL, Yien HW, et al: Tumor necrosis factor gene polymorphism and septic shock in surgical infection. *Crit Care Med* 2000;28:2733-2736.

55. Mira JP, Cariou A, Grall F, et al: Association of TNF2, a TNF-alpha promoter polymorphism, with septic shock susceptibility and mortality: A multicenter study. *JAMA* 1999;282:561-568.

56. Majetschak M, Flohe S, Obertacke U, et al: Relation of a TNF gene polymorphism to severe sepsis in trauma patients. *Ann Surg* 1999;230:207-214.

57. Stüber F, Petersen M, Bokelmann F, Schade U: A genomic polymorphism within the tumor necrosis factor locus influences plasma tumor necrosis factor-alpha concentrations and outcome of patients with severe sepsis. *Crit Care Med* 1996;24:381-384.

58. Bowcock AM, Ray A, Erlich H, Sehgal PB: Rapid detection and sequencing of alleles in the 3' flanking region of the interleukin-6 gene. *Nucleic Acids Res* 1989;17:6855-6864.

59. Fishman D, Faulds G, Jeffery R, et al: The effect of novel polymorphisms in the interleukin-6 (IL-6) gene on IL-6 transcription and plasma IL-6 levels, and an association with systemic-onset juvenile chronic arthritis. *J Clin Invest* 1998;102:1369-1376.

60. Osiri M, McNicholl J, Moreland LW, Bridges SL Jr: A novel single nucleotide polymorphism and five probable haplotypes in the 5' flanking region of the IL-6 gene in African-Americans. *Genes Immun* 1999;1:166-167.

61. Fernandez-Real JM, Broch M, Vendrell J, et al: Interleukin-6 gene polymorphism and insulin sensitivity. *Diabetes* 2000;49:517-520.

62. Turner DM, Williams DM, Sankaran D, Lazarus M, Sinnott PJ, Hutchinson IV: An investigation of polymorphism in the interleukin-10 gene promoter. *Eur J Immunogenet* 1997;24:1-8.

63. Eskdale J, Gallagher G, Verweij CL, Keijsers V, Westendorp RG, Huizinga TW: Interleukin 10 secretion in relation to human IL-10 locus haplotypes. *Proc Natl Acad Sci USA* 1998;95:9465-9470.

64. Newport MJ, Huxley CM, Huston S, et al: A mutation in the interferon-gamma-receptor gene and susceptibility to mycobacterial infection. *N Engl J Med* 1996;335:1941-1949.

65. Jouanguy E, Altare F, Lamhamedi S, et al: Interferon-gamma-receptor deficiency in an infant with fatal bacille Calmette-Guerin infection. *N Engl J Med* 1996;335:1956-1961.

66. Davis EG, Eichenberger MR, Grant BS, Polk HC Jr: Microsatellite marker of interferon-gamma receptor 1 gene correlates with infection following major trauma. *Surgery* 2000;128:301-305.

67. Association for the Advancement of Automotive Medicine: *The Abbreviated Injury Scale: 1990 Revision.* Des Plaines, IL, Association for the Advancement of Automotive Medicine, 1990.

68. Baker SP, O'Neill B, Haddon W Jr, Long WB: The Injury Severity Score: A method for describing patients with multiple injuries and evaluating emergency care. *J Trauma* 1974;14:187-196.

69. Copes WS, Champion HR, Sacco WJ, Lawnick MM, Keast SL, Bain LW: The Injury Severity Score revisited. *J Trauma* 1988;28:69-77.

70. Champion HR, Sacco WJ, Copes WS, Gann DS, Gennarelli TA, Flanagan ME: A revision of the Trauma Score. *J Trauma* 1989;29:623-629.

71. Copes WS, Champion HR, Sacco WJ, et al: Progress in characterizing anatomic injury. *J Trauma* 1990;30:1200-1207.

72. Teasdale G, Jennett B: Assessment of coma and impaired consciousness: A practical scale. *Lancet* 1974;2:81-84.

73. Bosse MJ, MacKenzie EJ, Riemer BL, et al: Adult respiratory distress syndrome, pneumonia, and mortality following thoracic injury and a femoral fracture treated either with intramedullary nailing with reaming or with a plate: A comparative study. *J Bone Joint Surg Am* 1997;79:799-809.

74. Pape HC, Hildebrand F, Pertschy S, et al: Changes in the management of femoral shaft fractures in polytrauma patients: From early total care to damage control orthopedic surgery. *J Trauma* 2002;53:452-462.

75. Moore EE, Cogbill TH, Malangoni MA, et al: Organ injury scaling. *Surg Clin North Am* 1995;75:293-303.

76. Pape HC, Auf'm'Kolk M, Paffrath T, Regel G, Sturm JA, Tscherne H: Primary intramedullary femur fixation in multiple trauma patients with associated lung contusion: A cause of posttraumatic ARDS? *J Trauma* 1993;34:540-548.

77. Copeland CE, Mitchell KA, Brumback RJ, Gens DR, Burgess AR: Mortality in patients with bilateral femoral fractures. *J Orthop Trauma* 1998;12:315-319.

78. Wu CC, Shih CH: Simultaneous bilateral femoral shaft fractures. *J Trauma* 1992;32:289-293.

79. Carrillo EH, Wohltmann CD, Spain DA, Schmieg RE Jr, Miller FB, Richardson JD: Common and external iliac artery injuries associated with pelvic fractures. *J Orthop Trauma* 1999;13:351-355.

80. McMurtry R, Walton D, Dickinson D, Kellam J, Tile M: Pelvic disruption in the polytraumatized patient: A management protocol. *Clin Orthop* 1980;151:22-30.

81. Gilliland MD, Ward RE, Barton RM, Miller PW, Duke JH: Factors affecting mortality in pelvic fractures. *J Trauma* 1982;22:691-693.

82. Hak DJ: Pelvic ring injuries, in Brinker MR (ed): *Review of Orthopaedic Trauma.* Philadelphia, PA, WB Saunders, 2001, p 188.

83. Henry SM, Pollak AN, Jones AL, Boswell S, Scalea TM: Pelvic fracture in geriatric patients: A distinct clinical entity. *J Trauma* 2002;53:15-20.

84. Agolini SF, Shah K, Jaffe J, Newcomb J, Rhodes M, Reed JF III: Arterial embolization is a rapid and effective technique for controlling pelvic fracture hemorrhage. *J Trauma* 1997;43:395-399.

85. Pohlemann T, Gänsslen A, Bosch U, Tscherne H: The technique of packing for control of hemorrhage in complex pelvic fractures. *Tech Orthop* 1995;9:267-270.

86. Greenspan L, McLellan BA, Greig H: Abbreviated Injury Scale and Injury Severity Score: A scoring chart. *J Trauma* 1985;25:60-64.

87. Tornetta P III, Mostafavi H, Riina J, et al: Morbidity and mortality in elderly trauma patients. *J Trauma* 1999;46:702-706.

88. Meek RN, Vivoda EE, Pirani S: Comparison of mortality of patients with multiple injuries according to type of fracture treatment: A retrospective age-and injury-matched series. *Injury* 1986;17:2-4.

89. Goris RJ, Gimbrére JS, van Niekerk JL, Schoots FJ, Booy LH: Early osteosynthesis and prophylactic mechanical ventilation in the multitrauma patient. *J Trauma* 1982;22:895-903.

90. Johnson KD, Cadambi A, Seibert GB: Incidence of adult respiratory distress syndrome in patients with multiple musculoskeletal injuries: Effect of early operative stabilization of fractures. *J Trauma* 1985;25:375-384.

91. Riska EB, von Bonsdorff H, Hakkinen S, Jaroma H, Kiviluoto O, Paavilainen T: Prevention of fat embolism by early internal fixation of fractures in patients with multiple injuries. *Injury* 1976;8:110-116.

92. Boulanger BR, Stephen D, Brenneman FD: Thoracic trauma and early intramedullary nailing of femur fractures: Are we doing harm? *J Trauma* 1997;43:24-28.

93. Dunham CM, Bosse MJ, Clancy TV, et al: Practice guidelines for the optimal timing of long-bone fracture stabilization in polytrauma patients: The EAST Practice Management Guidelines Work Group. *J Trauma* 2001;50:958-967.

94. Giannoudis PV, Veysi VT, Pape HC, Krettek C, Smith MR: When should we operate on major fractures in patients with severe head injuries? *Am J Surg* 2002;183:261-267.

95. Seibel R, LaDuca J, Hassett JM, et al: Blunt multiple trauma (ISS 36), femur traction, and the pulmonary failure-septic state. *Ann Surg* 1985;202:283-295.

96. Rüedi T, Wolff G: Prevention of post-traumatic complications through immediate therapy in patients with multiple injuries and fractures. *Helv Chir Acta* 1975;42:507-512.

97. Wilber MC, Evans EB: Fractures of the femoral shaft treated surgically: Comparative results of early and delayed operative stabilization. *J Bone Joint Surg Am* 1978;60:489-491.

98. Beck JP, Collins JA: Theoretical and clinical aspects of posttraumatic fat embolism syndrome. *Instr Course Lect* 1973;22:38-87.

99. Wald SL, Shackford SR, Fenwick J: The effect of secondary insults on mortality and long-term disability after severe head injury in a rural region without a trauma system. *J Trauma* 1993;34:377-382.

100. Bhandari M, Guyatt GH, Khera V, Kulkarni AV, Sprague S, Schemitsch EH: Operative management of lower extremity fractures in patients with head injuries. *Clin Orthop* 2003;407:187-198.

101. Jaicks RR, Cohn SM, Moller BA: Early fracture fixation may be deleterious after head injury. *J Trauma* 1997;42:1-6.

102. Martens F, Ectors P: Priorities in the management of polytraumatised patients with head injury: Partially resolved problems. *Acta Neurochir (Wien)* 1988;94:70-73.

103. McKee MD, Schemitsch EH, Vincent LO, Sullivan I, Yoo D: The effect of a femoral fracture on concomitant closed head injury in patients with multiple injuries. *J Trauma* 1997;42:1041-1045.

104. Poole GV, Miller JD, Agnew SG, Griswold JA: Lower extremity fracture fixation in head-injured patients. *J Trauma* 1992;32:654-659.

105. Brundage SI, McGhan R, Jurkovich GJ, Mack CD, Maier RV: Timing of femur fracture fixation: Effect on outcome in patients with thoracic and head injuries. *J Trauma* 2002;52:299-307.

106. Hofman PA, Goris RJ: Timing of osteosynthesis of major fractures in patients with severe brain injury. *J Trauma* 1991;31:261-263.

107. MacKenzie EJ, Bosse MJ, Kellam JF, et al: LEAP Study Group: Factors influencing the decision to amputate or reconstruct after high-energy lower extremity trauma. *J Trauma* 2002;52:641-649.

108. McCarthy ML, MacKenzie EJ, Edwin D, Bosse MJ, Castillo RC, Starr A: LEAP study group: Psychological distress associated with severe lower-limb injury. *J Bone Joint Surg Am* 2003;85:1689-1697.

109. MacKenzie EJ, Bosse MJ, Castillo RC, et al: Functional outcomes following trauma-related lower-extremity amputation. *J Bone Joint Surg Am* 2004;86:1636-1645.

110. Lange RH: Limb reconstruction versus amputation decision making in massive lower extremity trauma. *Clin Orthop* 1989;243:92-99.

111. Caudle RJ, Stern PJ: Severe open fractures of the tibia. *J Bone Joint Surg Am* 1987;69:801-807.

112. Hansen ST Jr: The type-IIIC tibial fracture: Salvage or amputation. *J Bone Joint Surg Am* 1987;69:799-800.

113. Helfet DL, Howey T, Sanders R, Johansen K: Limb salvage versus amputation: Preliminary results of the Mangled Extremity Severity Score. *Clin Orthop* 1990;256:80-86.

114. Georgiadis GM, Behrens FF, Joyce MJ, Earle AS, Simmons AL: Open tibial fractures with severe soft-tissue loss: Limb salvage compared with below-the-knee amputation. *J Bone Joint Surg Am* 1993;75:1431-1441.

115. Gilson BS, Bergner M, Bobbitt RA, Carter WB: *The Sickness Impact Profile: Final Development and Testing*. Seattle, WA, Department of Health Services, University of Washington School of Public Health and Community Medicine, 1979.

116. Goodell JA, Flick AB, Hebert JC, Howe JG: Preparation and release characteristics of tobramycin-impregnated polymethylmethacrylate beads. *Am J Hosp Pharm* 1986;43:1454-1461.

117. Flick AB, Herbert JC, Goodell J, Kristiansen T: Noncommercial fabrication of antibiotic-impregnated polymethylmethacrylate beads: Technical note. *Clin Orthop* 1987;223:282-286.

118. Seligson D: Antibiotic-impregnated beads in orthopedic infectious problems. *J Ky Med Assoc* 1984;82:25-29.

119. Webb LX: New techniques in wound management: Vacuum-assisted wound closure. *J Am Acad Orthop Surg* 2002;10:303-311.

120. Pape H, Stalp M, v Griensven M, Weinberg A, Dahlweit M, Tscherne H: Optimal timing for secondary surgery in polytrauma patients: An evaluation of 4,314 serious-injury cases. *Chirurg* 1999;70:1287-1293.

121. Tornetta P III, DeMarco C: Intramedullary nailing after external fixation of the tibia. *Bull Hosp Jt Dis* 1995;54:5-13.

122. Blachut PA, Meek RN, O'Brien PJ: External fixation and delayed intramedullary nailing of open fractures of the tibial shaft: A sequential protocol. *J Bone Joint Surg Am* 1990;72:729-735.

123. Winkler H, Hochstein P, Pfrengle S, Wentzensen A: Change in procedure to reamed intramedullary nail in diaphyseal femoral fractures after stabilization with external fixator. *Zentralbl Chir* 1998;123:1239-1246.

124. Parameswaran AD, Roberts CS, Seligson D, Voor M: Pin tract infection with contemporary external fixation: How much of a problem? *J Orthop Trauma* 2003;17:503-507.

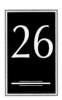

Controversies in Intramedullary Nailing of Femoral Shaft Fractures

Philip Wolinsky, MD
Nirmal Tejwani, MD
Jeffrey H. Richmond, MD
Kenneth J. Koval, MD
Kenneth Egol, MD
David J.G. Stephen, MD, FRCSC

Intramedullary fixation with reaming is an excellent surgical procedure that has revolutionized the treatment of fractures of the femoral shaft. Instead of being confined to bed in traction, patients can be mobilized on the first postoperative day. The expected union rate is between 95% and 99%, with infrequent malunion and infection, at least for closed fractures and for grade 1 and grade 2 open fractures. Stabilization of a femoral fracture within the first 24 hours after the injury has been shown to reduce morbidity and mortality in multiply injured patients. However, there are still controversial issues related to intramedullary femoral fixation. This chapter addresses several of these, including the effect of intramedullary reaming on pulmonary complications and the rate of fracture union, whether a fracture table or a flat radiolucent table should be used for nail insertion, and whether the presence

of a head injury alters the treatment selection.

Fracture Table Compared With Flat Radiolucent Table

Classically, intramedullary nailing is done with use of a fracture table. The table assists with fracture reduction by applying sustained longitudinal traction. A perineal post provides a fulcrum against which traction is applied. The design of most fracture tables allows circumferential access to the extremity for manipulation, surgical exposure, and imaging. When surgery is delayed and length has not been maintained, the mechanical advantage of a fracture table or a femoral distractor is needed to regain length.

Alternatively, intramedullary nailing can be done on a radiolucent table[1-3] (Stephen DJG, et al, San Antonio, TX, unpublished data presented at the Orthopaedic Trauma Association annual meeting, 2000). Traction can be applied manually or with the use of a femoral distractor, although it takes almost as long to apply the distractor as it does to perform the entire nailing procedure, and manual traction is usually sufficient to regain length. Manual traction works best when nailing is done within 24 hours after the

injury; otherwise, muscle-shortening can not be overcome with manual traction alone. If surgery is to be delayed, the patient should be placed in skeletal traction to maintain the normal length or even slight distraction of the fracture fragments. Radiographic documentation is suggested. The use of a flat radiolucent table keeps setup time to a minimum, and access to the piriformis fossa is improved by adduction of the limb. Disadvantages include difficulty in visualizing the hip and the proximal part of the femur in the lateral projection; difficulty in reducing and holding fracture alignment; and, if a distractor is used, risk to the femoral neurovascular structures and blockage of the surgical field.

With either method, the patient can be placed in the lateral decubitus or supine position. An advantage of the lateral decubitus position is the improved access to the piriformis fossa, especially in obese patients or in those with ipsilateral hip disease associated with a decreased range of motion of the hip. The disadvantages of the lateral position include respiratory compromise in patients with pulmonary injuries, valgus angulation of the fracture, difficulty in determining proper rotation, and greater difficulty inserting distal locking screws.

Although femoral nailing with use of a fracture table has been associated with excellent results, there are problems with the technique. Obese patients are difficult to fit on a fracture table, and it can be extremely difficult to establish the correct starting hole. It is cumbersome to treat patients with multiple injuries on a fracture table because access to the chest, abdomen, contralateral limb, and the distal part of the ipsilateral limb is limited. These patients require table changes as well as multiple preparation and draping procedures, all of which add to the complexity of the operation and increase surgical time. Unstable pelvic and spinal injuries make it difficult to use a fracture table as well. There are also several unique complications associated with the use of a fracture table, including compartment syndrome in the contralateral leg, perineal slough, and pudendal nerve palsy.[4-6]

More recently, surgeons have begun to use flat radiolucent tables to treat femoral shaft fractures. There are several advantages to placement of the patient in the supine position, including ease of setup, less respiratory compromise, better fracture alignment, and easier insertion of distal screws. Because the injured leg is draped free and can be adducted, it is easier to find the starting point, particularly in larger patients. Moreover, because the entire involved extremity as well as the contralateral lower extremity can be prepared and draped at the same time and because it is not necessary to reposition the patient and repeat the preparation and draping at the conclusion of femoral nailing, it is easier to address multiple fractures. The intramedullary nailing can be performed on the same table used for a laparotomy, eliminating the need for a table change. Two studies have shown that use of a radiolucent table rather than a fracture table results in a significant reduction ($P < 0.05$) in the time needed

for preparation and draping; in the surgical and anesthesia times; and, if multiple injuries are present, in the number of table changes and times that the patient needs to be prepared and draped in order to address all of the injuries.[1] (Stephen DJG, et al, San Antonio, TX, unpublished data presented at the Orthopaedic Trauma Association annual meeting, 2000).

When a fracture table is used, a closed reduction is performed with use of traction applied through the fracture table combined with external manipulation of the leg by the surgeon. To minimize the risk of pudendal nerve palsy,[4] traction is decreased during the preparation and draping of the patient and during proximal exposure. A small-diameter intramedullary nail can be placed in the proximal fragment and used as a joystick to manipulate the proximal fragment and reduce the fracture. This can be particularly useful for fractures of the proximal third of the femur. Many implant manufacturers include a device in the nailing sets for this purpose.

When a radiolucent table is used, the fracture is reduced with use of in-line manual traction combined with sterile bumps placed posteriorly to correct angulation in the sagittal plane. Percutaneously placed Schantz pins in the proximal or distal fragments may aid in the reduction of fracture fragments. A small-diameter nail can be used to correct angulation of short proximal segments. The most difficult fractures to reduce with this method are noncomminuted fractures of the isthmus in young patients with large thigh muscles. A small incision to allow direct reduction of the fracture with use of a bone-hook may be necessary.

A proper entry point is critical to ensure proper nail placement and fracture reduction. A 2-cm longitudinal incision is made one handbreadth proximal to the greater trochanter in line with the femoral shaft. The fascia of the gluteus maximus is incised, and the muscle is split bluntly in line with its fibers down

to the piriformis fossa. A clamp is placed in the piriformis fossa, its position is confirmed with fluoroscopy, and then it is spread open upon withdrawal. A guide-pin is then placed into the piriformis fossa and checked on AP and lateral fluoroscopic views. Next, the guide-pin is overreamed. Medial portal placement should be avoided, because it may cause a femoral neck fracture. Lateral portal placement may lead to comminution and varus alignment in fractures of the proximal part of the femur. Alternatively, an awl may be placed in the piriformis fossa and the proximal part of the femur may be opened by creating a pilot hole. If this technique is chosen, a larger skin incision is required.

When a radiolucent table is used, judging the length of the femur can be problematic. The typical error when such a table is used is to fail to restore length fully, whereas the typical error when a fracture table is used is to overlengthen the limb. If the fracture is minimally comminuted, radiographic landmarks can be used to judge the proper length of the femur. If the fracture is so comminuted that radiographic landmarks cannot be used, it is critical to know the proper length before beginning the operation. Several methods can be used. A radiograph of the intact femur can be made with a radiopaque ruler placed along the thigh, and the distance between two reproducible landmarks, such as the tip of the greater trochanter and the adductor tubercle, can be used to determine length. In the operating room, the C-arm can be used to image nails of different lengths held over the intact femur until the proper length of nail is found. If both femora are fractured and comminuted, the length should be determined by measuring the less comminuted fracture and then making both femora the same length.

Radiographs of the contralateral limb also may be used to assess the diameter of the medullary canal and the degree of curvature of the intact femur. Patients with an extremely small medullary canal may require a special-size implant, which should be determined preoperatively to ensure implant availability.

The proper rotation is also difficult to judge. We find that it is easier to judge rotation when a radiolucent table is used, as it allows the use of several methods. External and internal rotation of the contralateral hip can be assessed prior to preparation and draping, and hip rotation on the injured side can be checked after proximal locking and placement of a drill-bit through a distal locking hole have been performed. Nearly symmetrical hip rotation indicates that proper rotation has been restored. Confirmation of proper rotation is performed by first making a perfect lateral fluoroscopic view of the knee with the image intensifier. Next, the image intensifier is slid proximally to the hip and the machine is rotated 15° to account for femoral anteversion. If the rotation at the fracture site is correct, this maneuver should produce a true lateral fluoroscopic view of the hip.

In conclusion, reaming and femoral intramedullary nailing can be performed safely and effectively on a flat radiolucent table. Surgical and anesthesia times have been shown to be reduced, and the care of a multiply injured patient is facilitated.

Antegrade Compared With Retrograde Nailing

Antegrade femoral nailing (passing the intramedullary nail from proximal to distal) is the gold standard for surgical treatment of diaphyseal femoral shaft fractures. It has a high rate of union (99%) and a low rate of infection and malunion (< 1%).[7,8] However, antegrade nailing is associated with a number of complications (including heterotopic ossification around the hip, abductor weakness resulting in a limp, and limited ability to walk or climb stairs), and its use is limited in certain situations.[9] If a fracture table is used, additional problems arise, including prolonged setup time, possible pudendal nerve palsy, and the inability to address other injuries simultaneously.[10-11] Recent clinical studies have shown that the results of retrograde nailing (passing the intramedullary nail from distal to proximal) are currently comparable with those of antegrade nailing.[12-14]

Indications for Retrograde Nailing

Retrograde nailing may be the treatment of choice for certain femoral fractures.[15] Distal femoral fractures with or without articular involvement are easier to reduce and stabilize with use of an implant that is inserted closer to the fracture site. For patients with fractures of the ipsilateral femoral neck and shaft, use of a retrograde nail allows the fracture of the shaft to be fixed with one implant and the fracture of the neck to be fixed with a separate implant, thus allowing each fracture to be treated optimally. Retrograde nailing is useful for the treatment of obese patients because the femoral intercondylar notch is easier to access than the piriformis fossa, and it is advantageous for pregnant patients because the radiation exposure to the fetus is reduced. Antegrade nailing can be problematic in patients who need surgical fixation of an acetabular or pelvic fracture, as the incision for antegrade nailing is usually inappropriate for the fixation of these injuries. With use of an incision around the knee, it is possible to avoid a second approach in patients with an open knee joint, knee disarticulation, or a fracture of the ipsilateral tibia (a floating knee). Retrograde nails can also be used to stabilize femoral shaft fractures proximal to a knee replacement or distal to a total hip replacement. However, not all femoral components used for total knee replacement allow the passage of a nail and, if this is the case, a retrograde nail cannot be used.

Retrograde Nailing Technique

Retrograde nailing is performed with the patient placed in the supine position on a flat radiolucent table, with a bolster under the knee to allow approximately 60° of flexion. A medial parapatellar approach, either open or percutaneous, is used. The starting point is in the intercondylar notch, just anterior to the posterior cruciate ligament attachment and in line with the axis of the femoral shaft. Once the starting point is identified, a starting hole is made with a threaded guide-wire. This hole is then enlarged with use of a cannulated drill, followed by passage of the ball-tipped guide-wire. The fracture can be reduced with use of bolsters and manual traction. The femoral distractor can be used, if necessary, to achieve and maintain length and alignment. The ideal nail diameter is 1.5 to 2 mm less than the largest reamer used. The nail should be driven proximal to the level of the lesser trochanter and distally should be flush with or buried 1 to 2 mm deep to the articular cartilage to avoid impingement on the patella.[16]

Distal locking of the nail is done with use of the jig, and the length of the screws is carefully judged to avoid medial prominence, which can cause subsequent symptoms. In elderly patients with osteoporotic bones and poor screw purchase, washers are recommended. Proximal locking is done freehand in the anterior-posterior direction. The mass of the quadriceps muscle and the curved anterior femoral surface make this difficult. The proximal screw should be placed at or proximal to the level of the lesser trochanter to avoid damage to the neurovascular structures.[17]

It is essential that the fracture be reduced before the nail is inserted so that the correct length and rotation can be ascertained. The determination of appropriate length and rotation can be difficult, especially when indirect reduction techniques are used. The correct nail length should be determined preoperatively, particularly when the fracture is comminuted and radiographic markers cannot be used to judge length. Scanograms of the intact femur, fluoroscopic imaging of the actual implants over the intact femur, or an intraoperative modified scanogram measuring with a sterile electrocautery cord and C-arm are all methods that can be used to determine the proper length of the femur. Rotation is more difficult to judge. Comparing the cortical diameter of the femur proximal and distal to the fracture on the fluoroscopic image can help. Palpating the greater trochanter and comparing its position to that of the intact femur also can help obtain the correct rotation.

Complications

Malunion is more frequent after retrograde nailing than it is after antegrade nailing. Malunion is a problem after the retrograde nailing of very proximal fractures because the capacious canal makes it difficult to judge and control length and rotation. It is important to reduce the distal femoral fracture prior to insertion of the nail. The nail holds the reduction but will not reduce the fracture. Retrograde nails are not the implant of choice for fractures of the proximal third of the femur. Early series[18] demonstrated a higher prevalence of delayed union and nonunion after retrograde nailing; however, with improved technique and the use of canal-matched implants, the rate of union after retrograde nailing is currently comparable with that after antegrade nailing.

Clinical Studies

The early reports on the use of retrograde nails were retrospective, and the results were compared with those of historical controls. Swiontkowski and associates[19] were the first, as far as we know, to report on the use of retrograde nails. They used a cloverleaf femoral nail in seven patients who had an ipsilateral fracture of the femoral neck and shaft. The nail was inserted by means of an extra-articular portal through the medial femoral condyle. Sanders and associates[20] expanded the indications for retrograde

nailing to include ipsilateral acetabular, pelvic, or femoral neck fractures; polytrauma requiring multiple simultaneous procedures; and pregnancy. Initial difficulties with insertion of the femoral nail necessitated a change to a tibial nail. The authors reported a healing rate of 92% (23 of 25 fractures), with no instances of infection or nail failure. Patterson and associates,[21] in a study of 17 fractures (11 of which were open), were the first to report on the use of the intercondylar portal as a starting point. They attributed the poor results in their study to the severity of the initial injury and the high proportion of open fractures. Herscovici and Whiteman[22] also reported on a series in which this approach was used.

Ostrum and associates[18] recommended caution when retrograde nailing is used to treat type IIIB open fractures. They reported a healing rate of 95% (58 of 61 fractures) but noted that for seven fractures a secondary procedure was needed to obtain union. They recommended the use of canal-diameter-matched implants to increase rates of union and to decrease the need for secondary procedures.

In a follow-up to their earlier study,[23] Moed and associates[24] reported that 94% (33) of 35 fractures united after retrograde nailing, with a shorter time to union and with excellent knee scores.

Laboratory Studies

ElMaraghy and associates,[25] in a laboratory study, showed that retrograde femoral nailing after reaming led to a 52% de-crease in anterior cruciate ligament perfusion and a 49% decrease in posterior cruciate ligament perfusion in adult dogs. It is not known whether this decrease in perfusion occurs in humans or is clinically important for long-term knee function. Stubbs and associates[26] examined rabbit knees at 2, 6, and 12 months after insertion of a stainless-steel implant and found that the insertion site was completely covered with fibrous tis-

sue. No histologic difference was seen in the cartilage or synovial tissue compared with that on the contralateral side, and there was no evidence of metallosis.

Koval and associates[27] found no significant difference during axial loading when the two nailing techniques were compared with regard to strength.

Randomized Trials

The results of a number of randomized trials comparing antegrade and retrograde nailing have been published during the last several years. Tornetta and Tiburzi[12] prospectively compared 38 fractures treated with antegrade nailing and 31 fractures treated with retrograde nailing and found no difference in surgical time, blood loss, or union rate. They found that it was more difficult to judge rotation and length with use of the retrograde technique. In the most recent prospective, randomized trial of which we are aware, Ostrum and associates[14] found no difference between antegrade nailing (46 fractures) and retrograde nailing (54 fractures) with respect to the rate of union or the range of motion of the knee. Knee motion improved more quickly and knee effusion resolved earlier in the group that had antegrade nailing. However, the group that had retrograde nailing had an increased need for distal hardware removal and conversion from a static to a dynamic construct as well as a longer time to union. These findings were attributed to undersizing of the nail diameter. Antegrade nailing was associated with an increased prevalence of hip and thigh pain. The prevalence of knee pain was similar in both groups.

Overview

The results of retrograde nailing of femoral shaft fractures are comparable with those of antegrade nailing. Retrograde nails are useful for fractures of the distal part of the femur with intra-articular involvement. Intra-articular fractures can be managed with compression lag screws before the nail is inserted. Fractures of the distal third of the femoral shaft may be better suited for retrograde nailing, and they have a lower rate of malalignment.[19]

Retrograde fixation may be better than antegrade fixation for the treatment of femoral shaft fractures associated with (1) fracture of the ipsilateral femoral neck, (2) obesity, (3) pregnancy, (4) knee disarticulation, (5) ipsilateral acetabular or pelvic fracture, (6) periprosthetic fracture, (7) a floating knee, or (8) an open knee joint. It is also better for the treatment of a femoral shaft fracture in a paraplegic patient with decubitus ulcers. The use of intercondylar portal nails designed for retrograde insertion and of larger-diameter nails has decreased the prevalence of complications, including malunion, nonunion, and implant failure. Retrograde nailing requires the creation of an intra-articular entry hole. There is concern about the long-term effect of such an entry hole in young patients as well as the potential for infection of the joint in patients with an open fracture, as the knee joint then communicates with the open fracture site. The long-term effects are still unknown, although the prevalence of knee pain and the limitation of range of motion in the short to medium term seem to be no higher than those associated with antegrade nailing. At present, antegrade nailing remains the gold standard for the treatment of isolated fractures of the proximal third of the femur and the femoral diaphysis. Studies with larger numbers and long-term follow-up are needed before the current recommendations for the use of retrograde nails can be extended.

Nailing With or Without Reaming: Effect on Fracture Union

Early-generation intramedullary nails were open-section devices designed to achieve a tight intramedullary fit in order to control rotation. Reaming was necessary to enlarge the canal sufficiently to maximize implant contact with the endosteum. Since the advent of locked intramedullary devices, a tight endosteal fit is less necessary because rotational control, as well as axial control, is achieved by means of proximal and distal locking bolts. These intramedullary devices behave more as rods than as nails.[28]

Reaming of the femoral canal prior to intramedullary nailing has a multitude of local and systemic effects. Some of the systemic effects are described in subsequent sections. Local effects have been classified as biologic or mechanical[29] and are discussed in this section.

Biologic Factors

Rhinelander[30] described the blood supply of the normal femoral diaphysis as coming from one or more nutrient arteries supplying the inner two thirds of the cortex, with the outer third supplied by means of periosteal vessels derived from the abundant soft tissue surrounding the femoral shaft. The cortical circulation is defined as centrifugal, with the predominant flow directed from the medullary canal toward the outer cortex. The medullary blood supply is disrupted by fracture, leading to necrosis of approximately 50% to 70% of the cortical bone near the fracture.[28] Fracture-healing is dependent on the reestablishment of blood flow to the disrupted cortical bone. This revascularization may be periosteal, endosteal, intracortical, or, additionally, by a transient extraosseous flow derived from the soft tissue surrounding the fracture. This extraosseous flow is particularly important in providing nutrients to callus as well as to detached fracture fragments.[31]

Trueta[32] suggested that the overall direction of cortical blood flow after a fracture is reversed from centrifugal to centripetal. This was confirmed by Strachan and associates,[33] who showed that ligation of the nutrient artery did not reduce blood flow to callus following diaphyseal osteotomy. This reversal of flow takes place over approximately 2 weeks, demonstrating that the intramedullary and extramedullary circulations supplement each other through revascularization across the cortex of the bone.[34] Several animal studies have confirmed these findings.[35,36]

Placement of any intramedullary device, either with or without reaming, damages the endosteal blood supply. However, reaming of the medullary canal causes more substantial destruction of the endosteal circulation and may lead to necrosis of the inner one half to two thirds of the cortical bone.[37] This was well demonstrated in a fractured sheep tibia model with use of Doppler flowmetry.[38] Cortical perfusion was significantly decreased in the group that had nailing with reaming ($P < 0.0009$). Revascularization was established by 6 weeks in the group that had nailing without reaming compared with 12 weeks in the group that had nailing with reaming. Hupel and associates[39] studied the effects of limited reaming on cortical blood flow in a canine model. They demonstrated that minimal reaming, to allow easy passage of a small-diameter nail, had significantly less impact on the immediate postoperative cortical blood flow than did standard reaming ($P = 0.009$).

In addition to the destruction of endosteal blood flow, reaming causes a hyperemic response in the periosteum and the surrounding soft tissues. Reichert and associates[35] demonstrated, with use of radiolabeled microspheres, a substantial increase in periosteal blood flow after reaming in sheep tibiae. Schemitsch and associates[40] showed that muscle perfusion is markedly increased following long-bone reaming. Despite the reduced cortical blood flow that has been demonstrated after reaming, an experimental model demonstrated no difference between long bones treated with reaming and those treated without reaming with respect to the perfusion of callus and the early strength of union.[41]

Intramedullary nailing with reaming clearly disrupts endosteal blood circulation to a greater degree than nailing without reaming does. However, given the change in cortical circulation from centrifugal to centripetal following fracture, periosteal and extraosseous flow seems to be the dominant method of revascularization and healing after fracture fixation with intramedullary nails. This circulation is stimulated by reaming and is dependent on a more-or-less intact soft-tissue envelope surrounding the fracture. The excellent soft-tissue coverage of the femur likely provides a means for this revascularization, which may not be available after fractures of the tibia, particularly those associated with open injuries. Reaming of the femur in and of itself does not seem to have a deleterious effect on the revascularization necessary for the healing of a fracture treated with intramedullary nailing.

In addition to the circulatory effects, reaming is also thought to improve fracture-healing by means of autogenous bone-grafting through the deposition of bone from the reaming at the fracture site.

Mechanical Factors

Nails used without reaming of the femoral canal are typically of smaller diameter than are nails used with reaming. The moment of inertia of a nail is a component of its overall strength, increasing with the fourth power of the nail diameter. Reaming permits the insertion of a larger-diameter, hence stronger, intramedullary nail, and a larger nail can accept larger locking bolts. A larger nail with larger locking bolts also may allow earlier or immediate weight bearing,[42] even in the presence of a comminuted fracture. Reaming also increases the contact area between the nail and the endosteal bone, resulting in a stiffer fracture construct. However, reaming results in the removal of bone, theoretically decreasing the overall bone strength. Even

so, the outer diameter of the cortex is the primary contributor of strength of the bone; thus, reaming removes the bone that contributes least to the overall strength yet allows a substantially stronger nail to be inserted.[43] Finite element analysis has demonstrated that, within clinical limits, it is not possible to ream a bone enough to substantially reduce its strength.[44]

Clinical Outcomes

Numerous studies have demonstrated that use of a locked intramedullary femoral nail after reaming leads to a union rate of 97% to 100%.[7,8,45,46] Kröpfl and associates[47] reported a union rate of 100% in a study of 81 femoral fractures treated with an intramedullary device inserted without reaming. However, several studies have demonstrated lower union rates[24] and an increased need for secondary procedures[48,49] after nailing without reaming.

Clatworthy and associates[50] performed a prospective, randomized study comparing femoral nailing with and without reaming. They demonstrated that the group treated with reaming had a faster time to union (28.5 weeks compared with 39.4 weeks) and that the group treated without reaming required substantially more secondary procedures (conversion to a dynamic construct or bone-grafting) to achieve union. Tornetta and Tiburzi[51,52] also demonstrated faster union with reaming (80 days) than without reaming (109 days.) Distal fractures had a more dramatic difference in time to union with reaming (80 days) than without reaming (158 days). No significant difference was found between the groups with respect to surgical time or transfusion requirements. The group treated with reaming had fewer technical complications. A meta-analysis of randomized trials showed similar findings.[53]

The use of reaming in the treatment of open tibial fractures is controversial

because of concerns about the destruction of the endosteal blood supply in a bone with already compromised circulation. However, the femur has a more substantial soft-tissue envelope than the tibia does, so periosteal and extraosseous blood supply is better. Clinical studies of open femoral fractures treated with nailing after reaming have demonstrated excellent rates of union with a low risk of infection.[54,55]

Overview

Reaming of the medullary canal has been shown to disrupt the endosteal circulation. However, fracture-healing involves a reversal of the normal centrifugal blood flow across the cortex to a circulation dominated by periosteal and extraosseous flow. Reaming stimulates this flow. Despite the disruption of the nutrient vessel circulation, reaming seems actually to lead to increased circulation around a femoral shaft fracture in the presence of an adequate soft-tissue envelope. Reaming also permits the insertion of a larger, more stable nail, which is advantageous for fracture-healing. Numerous clinical studies have demonstrated that intramedullary nailing with reaming provides more reliable and faster healing with fewer complications than does nailing without reaming. Fixation with a femoral nail after reaming is the treatment of choice for most femoral fractures that are managed surgically.

Pulmonary Effects of Intramedullary Nailing of the Femur After Reaming: Is the Risk of Pulmonary Complications Increased?

The fat embolism syndrome is a multisystem disorder that results from fat embolization. Clinically, it causes dysfunction of the pulmonary and central nervous systems as well as fever and rash.[56] Almost all patients who sustain blunt trauma have some degree of pulmonary fat embolization as a result of the soft-tissue injury. The clinical severity of fat embolism syndrome ranges from subclinical symptoms to the adult respiratory distress syndrome (ARDS).[57-62]

No consistent factors other than the number of long-bone fractures can be used to identify patients who are at risk. Pulmonary fat embolization apparently alters pulmonary hemodynamics, increases pulmonary vascular permeability, activates the fibrinolytic and coagulation systems, and causes pulmonary leukostasis.[56,57,63-65]

The clinical pulmonary effects are thought to occur as a result of an increase in pulmonary vascular resistance secondary to widespread vascular occlusion due to multiple small emboli. Larger fat emboli may obstruct the pulmonary circulation, causing a ventilation-perfusion mismatch and hypoxia. Death occurs as a result of right ventricular failure.[56,66,67]

Prevention of Pulmonary Complications

The best treatment of fat embolism syndrome and ARDS is prevention. Prior to the work of Riska and associates[58,59] and Goris and associates,[68] fracture fixation was usually performed on a delayed basis. One reason given for the delay was to allow the peak dose of fat emboli to pass before fracture fixation was undertaken.[69] Riska and associates[59] demonstrated that early stabilization of long-bone fractures in multiply injured patients decreased the prevalence of fat embolism syndrome. They thought that fat embolization was an ongoing process that began at the time of injury. Early fracture stabilization stopped this process and prevented the development of related symptoms.[58,59] Goris and associates[68] then showed that early fracture stabilization in combination with mechanical ventilation not only decreased the prevalence of ARDS but also decreased the mortality rate in patients with an Injury Severity Score of greater than 50 points. Death was most often due to sepsis and multiple organ failure.

Bone and associates,[70] in a prospective, randomized trial, demonstrated that patients with femoral shaft fractures and an Injury Severity Score of greater than 18 points benefited from fracture stabilization within 24 hours after injury. Early stabilization led to a decrease in the rates of ARDS, fat embolism syndrome, and pneumonia and to a shorter length of stay in the intensive care unit. The authors hypothesized that the decreased fat embolization and the reduced need for narcotics associated with early stabilization, as well as the ability to position the patient with the torso upright, may explain these findings.

Femoral Intramedullary Nailing After Reaming: The Present Controversy

The results of these and other studies have led to the consensus that early stabilization of long-bone fractures is beneficial to the multiply injured patient. The current treatment of choice for fractures of the femoral shaft in adults is insertion of a statically locked intramedullary nail after reaming. When the nail is inserted with use of a closed technique, union rates of 95% to 99%, with low rates of infection and malunion, can be expected.[8,71] Several clinical studies have shown that early fixation with an intramedullary nail after reaming has a beneficial effect in this group of patients, leading to a decrease in pulmonary complications without an increase in other complications.[70,72,73] On the basis of the studies reported to date, it appears that trauma patients without thoracic injuries benefit from early nailing of a femoral shaft fracture, with a reduction in the prevalence of pulmonary complications. The potential downside of using a nail after reaming is the possibility that fat emboli generated during nail insertion are harmful. This issue was first raised, to our knowledge, by Pape and associates,[74] who analyzed a group of patients with thoracic injuries and femoral shaft frac-

tures. Those authors noted a trend toward an increase in pulmonary complications among patients in whom the fracture was stabilized with intramedullary nailing with reaming within 24 hours after the injury compared with those in whom the fracture was stabilized more than 24 hours after the injury. Although this finding was not significant, the authors concluded that nailing after reaming in the presence of thoracic trauma led to additional pulmonary damage.

There is no doubt that intramedullary nailing after reaming causes fat embolization. Numerous clinical and animal studies have demonstrated that pressurizing the medullary canal results in fat embolization that can be visualized with use of echocardiography.[56,75] The questions are whether this fat embolization has a clinically important effect and whether particular subgroups of patients are at risk. The study by Pape and associates[74] suggested that patients with thoracic injuries are at an increased risk for postoperative complications when early intramedullary nailing with reaming is done.

Since the cause of pulmonary dysfunction is multifactorial, it is hypothesized that an otherwise trivial pulmonary insult such as fat embolization may potentiate another noxious stimulus, leading to respiratory impairment. Evidence for this "second hit" phenomenon has been presented in animal studies.[64] In addition to the study by Pape and associates,[74] two other clinical studies have been performed to examine this issue. Charash and associates[76] performed a study quite similar to that of Pape and associates and came to different conclusions. They found that delayed femoral shaft stabilization in patients with thoracic trauma led to an increase in pulmonary complications. In fact, the more severely injured the patient, the more pronounced the difference. Bosse and associates,[77] in a report on femoral shaft fractures that were treated at two institutions, divided patients into groups on the basis of whether a thoracic injury was also present. The fractures at one institution were stabilized with a plate, and those at the other institution were stabilized with an intramedullary nail after reaming. Presumably, the patients treated with a plate would have had no pulmonary fat embolization as a result of the femoral stabilization procedure, whereas those treated with intramedullary nailing after reaming would have had fat embolization. If fat embolization were harmful, the group treated with intramedullary nailing after reaming would have a higher prevalence of pulmonary complications. However, Bosse and associates found no difference between the two groups with respect to the prevalence of pulmonary complications.

In a study of sheep, Pape and associates[78] subjected the animals to a lung crush injury and systemic hypotension on day 1. On day 3, the animals underwent nailing either with or without reaming. Pulmonary permeability increased in both groups, but only the group that had reaming had an increase in pulmonary arterial pressures. The authors concluded that nails inserted after reaming cause more pulmonary damage than do nails inserted without reaming. In contrast, Wozasek and associates[79] found that intramedullary nailing after reaming alone did not cause an increase in pulmonary permeability, whereas nailing combined with systemic hypotension caused a transient increase. This raises the question of whether the nailing with reaming or the hypotension altered the pulmonary permeability in the study by Pape and associates.[78]

Since it is unclear what pulmonary permeability means clinically, one of us (P.W.) and colleagues used a sheep model to investigate the effects of intramedullary nailing after reaming on clinically applicable hemodynamic and oxymetric parameters.[80,81] Two groups of animals were used. The first had a lung crush injury, and the second had a chemically induced "ARDS-like" state. No alteration in pulmonary function was noted in either group after nailing with reaming was performed.

Current investigations are centered on the role of the inflammatory response in the development of ARDS. Trauma can cause the systemic inflammatory response syndrome (SIRS) early after injury. Hemorrhagic shock and the reperfusion injury can overstimulate the immune system and lead to complications, such as acute lung injury, ARDS, SIRS, and multiple organ dysfunction syndromes. Oxygen free radicals released by activated neutrophils are thought to play a key role in this process by damaging endothelial tissues.[61,82-84] The SIRS score has been developed, and studies have shown that patients with blunt trauma and higher SIRS scores have an increased mortality rate and length of stay.[85] Presumably, these findings are related to the extent of the inflammatory reaction.[85]

The association between shock and the development of ARDS is well known. In fact, the likelihood of development of ARDS and the mortality rate have been found to be related to the initial base deficit, presumably reflecting the depth of the initial hypoxic event.[86,87] In a recent study, no relationship was found between the injury pattern (that is, chest injury, abdominal injury, fracture, and so on), patient age, Injury Severity Score on admission, Glasgow Coma Scale score, hypotension on admission, or time spent in the operating room and the development of ARDS.[86] However, the transfusion requirements in the initial 24 hours were substantially higher in the patients in whom ARDS developed. Those patients also had a lower base deficit in the initial 24 hours after the injury, and the deficit normalized more slowly than did the base deficit in those in whom ARDS did not develop. In addition, the magnitude of the lowest base deficit was found to correlate with the increase in cytokines on days 1 through 4, presumably reflecting an increased stimulation of the inflammatory cascade. It appears that the depth of the initial hypoperfusion correlates with the development of an early inflammatory response. The findings in that study suggest that the most effective prevention of ARDS is the early aggressive treatment of shock.[86]

It is hypothesized that the initial shock and resuscitation serve to prime the immune system so that a second, trivial stimulus can lead to an exaggerated inflammatory response. There are experimental and clinical data to support this hypothesis.[79,84,88,89] Wozasek and associates,[79] in a sheep model, demonstrated that only nailing with reaming and hypotension led to an increase in pulmonary permeability. Other studies have shown that animals in shock can tolerate less of a fat load.[83,90]

The neutrophils of trauma patients have been found to be more responsive to stimuli to the release of superoxides than are the neutrophils of healthy donors.[88] Since neutrophils are thought to play a central role in the development of lung injury, this finding suggests that trauma patients who have had an initial stimulus of the inflammatory cascade as a result of hypoperfusion may be extremely sensitive to the stimulus of fat embolization that results from intramedullary nailing after reaming. Without the initial stimulus, this fat embolization may have had no significant detectable effect.[88]

In a recent clinical study, Crowl and associates[89] investigated the effect of occult hypoperfusion on complications following intramedullary fixation of the femoral shaft within 24 hours after admission in patients with an Injury Severity Score of more than 18 points. Patients were retrospectively divided into two groups on the basis of lactate levels. No patient had overt clinical signs of shock. The group with occult hypoperfusion had a higher complication rate and higher hospital costs. The authors hypothesized that all trauma patients have activation of the inflammatory process and that patients who have persistent occult end-organ hypoperfusion may be more susceptible to a second-hit injury. This suggests that the patients who may be harmed by early intramedullary nailing after reaming are those with inadequate resuscitation.

Overview

There is controversy with regard to whether intramedullary nailing after reaming can cause clinically important additional pulmonary damage in trauma patients. The studies to date have indicated that this is not an issue in trauma patients without chest injuries who have been well resuscitated. The bulk of the literature has indicated that intramedullary nailing after reaming does not seem to have a detrimental effect on patients with only a thoracic injury. The current controversy centers on the systemic inflammatory response syndrome in underresuscitated patients. It appears that the depth of initial hypoperfusion is an indicator of the extent of stimulation of the inflammatory cascade. This factor is thought to play a role in the development of endothelial injury, one aspect of which is the development of pulmonary dysfunction including ARDS. The already stimulated inflammatory reaction may exhibit inappropriate exuberance if stimulated again by factors such as the fat embolization generated during intramedullary nailing after reaming. Therefore, prior to intramedullary nailing with reaming, the patient must be fully resuscitated according to laboratory data (such as base deficit or lactate) to make sure that occult hypoperfusion is not present. If a patient is hemodynamically unstable or is not fully resuscitated, femoral fixation should be delayed or an alternative, less invasive procedure for stabilization, such as external fixation, should be

used.[91,93] It seems that the extent of resuscitation rather than the presence or absence of a thoracic injury is the critical risk factor for further pulmonary damage as a result of intramedullary nailing after reaming.

Management of Femoral Fractures Associated With Head Injury

The management of patients with a femoral fracture associated with a severe head injury is controversial.[92-99] A head injury is usually considered severe if the patient presents with a Glasgow Coma Scale score of 8 points or less or an Abbreviated Injury Scale score of 3 points or more.[100] It is postulated that patients undergoing early stabilization of a long-bone fracture in the presence of a severe head injury may be at risk for a secondary brain injury as a result of reduced cerebral perfusion pressure, hypoxemia, hypotension, and fat embolization.[57,93,97,101] This raises the question of whether the risk of secondary brain injury outweighs the benefits of early stabilization of a long-bone fracture in a patient with a severe head injury and a femoral fracture. If so, can traumatologists decide who should and who should not undergo early stabilization of a femoral fracture in the presence of a severe head injury?

After a severe head injury, numerous factors can lead to secondary ischemic brain injury, and ischemic brain injury has been shown to be the major determinant of long-term neurologic disability.[102] Hypotension on or before admission substantially increases the rate of poor neurologic outcomes.[102-104] Immediately after a severe head injury, the normal autoregulation that maintains a stable cerebral perfusion pressure (and thus cerebral blood flow and oxygen) is altered. This effect is most pronounced in the first 24 to 48 hours after injury.[105,106] During this time, cerebral perfusion pressure is directly propor-

tional to mean arterial pressure. Thus, any hypotension during this period can lead to cerebral hypoperfusion and hypoxemia—that is, the so-called secondary brain injury.[102] The complicating issues are that the duration of altered autoregulation varies and that there can be regional cerebral ischemia up to 48 hours following the injury.[107]

Cerebral perfusion pressure reflects cerebral blood flow, and the current method of assessment is to monitor the intracranial pressure. In this way, once the mean arterial pressure is determined (by means of arterial line monitoring), the cerebral perfusion pressure is determined by subtracting the intracranial pressure from the mean arterial pressure. The generally accepted normal values are less than 20 to 25 mm Hg for intracranial pressure and greater than 70 mm Hg for cerebral perfusion pressure.[108] This means that the mean arterial pressure should stay in the range of 90 mm Hg to avoid cerebral hypoperfusion and thus cerebral hypoxemia. Additional information concerning cerebral oxygenation can be obtained by sampling the central venous oxygen tension through a central venous catheter.[109] Thus, during the initial period following a severe head injury, protection against secondary brain injury requires aggressive resuscitation with crystalloid, blood products, and, if necessary, inotropic support as well as invasive monitoring of arterial, central venous, and intracerebral pressures to avoid systemic hypotension and cerebral hypoperfusion and ischemia.

Despite the known benefit of early stabilization of long-bone fractures and increased knowledge with regard to the treatment of patients with head injuries, there is no consensus on how best to manage a patient with both injuries. There are no large, prospective, randomized studies comparing early and delayed stabilization of long-bone fractures in the setting of a severe head injury. The advocates of each approach base their decision on small retrospective studies.

The advocates for delaying long-bone stabilization in patients with a head injury cite published reports indicating that hypotension leads to worse neurologic outcomes in patients undergoing an early operation (within the first 24 hours after injury).[93,97,101] Jaicks and associates[93] reported on a cohort of 33 patients who had blunt trauma associated with severe head injury (an Abbreviated Injury Scale score of $\geq$ 2 points) and femoral fracture. Nineteen patients underwent early fracture fixation (within 24 hours after injury), and 14 patients underwent late fixation (more than 24 hours after injury). The two groups were matched for age, Glasgow Coma Scale score, Injury Severity Score, and neurologic and orthopaedic Abbreviated Injury Scale scores. The early fixation group required significantly more fluids ($P < 0.05$) in the first 48 hours and tended toward a higher rate of intraoperative hypotension (observed in three patients who had early fixation and one who had late fixation) and intraoperative hypoxia (observed in two patients who had early fixation and one who had late fixation). Despite these findings, the neurologic complication rate was similar in the two groups. Although the mean Glasgow Coma Scale score on discharge was lower in the early-fixation group (13.5 ± 3.7 points) than in the late-fixation group (15 ± 0.0 points), the mean hospital stay was 5 days longer in the late-fixation group (27 ± 13 days) than in the early-fixation group (22 ± 20 days). No confidence intervals were given for these data. The authors concluded that early fracture fixation leads to greater fluid administration in patients with head injuries. They thought that prospective studies were required to evaluate the impact of the timing of fracture fixation on head injury.

The advocates of early stabilization cite an equal (if not greater) number of reports indicating that the severity of the initial head injury—not the timing of long-bone stabilization—determines the ultimate neurologic function.[94-96,98,99] McKee and associates[96] reported on a group of 46 patients with a femoral fracture and a severe head injury (mean Glasgow Coma Scale score, < 8 points) who had early fracture stabilization (85% had stabilization within 24 hours after injury) and compared them with a cohort of 99 patients with a severe head injury alone (mean Glasgow Coma Scale Score, 8 points; range, 3 to 13 points). There were no differences between the two groups with respect to demographic data or other injury patterns. No significant differences between the two groups were found in terms of early mortality, length of hospitalization, length of stay in the intensive-care unit, level of neurologic disability, or results of cognitive testing. The authors concluded that (1) femoral fractures in patients with head injuries should be aggressively managed with early fixation; (2) adequate oxygenation and cerebral perfusion pressure must be maintained during surgical procedures, including femoral nailing after reaming; and (3) early femoral nailing after reaming did not negatively affect neurologic outcome in this subset of trauma patients.[96] Thus, each side of the argument is supported in the literature— albeit by small retrospective cohort studies—and the only solution may be to perform a large, multicenter, prospective, randomized study.

When faced with a patient with a severe head injury and a femoral fracture, it is imperative to adopt a multidisciplinary approach that includes the trauma service, the orthopaedic surgeon, the neurosurgeon, and the anesthesiologist. This approach will allow optimal resuscitation of the patient, establishment of the diagnosis and prognosis of the head injury, and placement of invasive monitors prior to orthopaedic intervention. The aggressive correction of hypothermia and coagulopathy, as well as timely use of inotropes to maintain optimal mean arterial pressure (and thus cerebral perfusion pressure), must be undertaken. The exact timing of long-bone stabilization is determined on the basis of the status of the patient, the results of the CT scan of the head, and the parameters made available by invasive monitoring. Prolonged orthopaedic interventions should be avoided, with timely fracture stabilization being the goal. A mass lesion, such as a subdural or epidural hematoma, seen on the CT scan of the head requires urgent neurosurgical intervention. A constellation of bad prognostic signs on the CT scan, such as extensive amounts of subarachnoid blood, a ventricular shift, and/or cerebellar herniation, may preclude any surgical intervention. Certainly, if the intracranial pressure or the cerebral perfusion pressure remains abnormal or labile, a delay in definitive stabilization of long-bone fractures is recommended. In these patients, external fixation for temporary fracture stabilization may be of benefit. This would be especially important in the presence of an open femoral fracture, in which case there is an urgency to get to the operating room. External fixation would then be followed by definitive stabilization with an intramedullary nail. The external fixator is usually applied as an anterior half-frame, with two pins in each fracture segment. In one series, this approach, called "damage control orthopaedics," was required for 13% of 327 patients with a femoral fracture and multiple injuries who were treated at a level-I trauma center. This approach mirrors the experience with devastating abdominal injuries[110] and is appropriate for patients who cannot tolerate additional blood loss, including those with head injuries and those who are not yet fully resuscitated. External fixation has been associated with a shorter operating-room time and less blood loss than has intramedullary nailing after reaming.[91] In rare cases, when the patient is in extremis, temporary skeletal traction may be required.

The timing of definitive stabilization with an intramedullary nail is determined by the status of the patient, but because of the risk of contamination of the external fixator pin site it is desirable to perform the procedure within 5 to 7 days. In some cases, when the patient's general or neurologic parameters do not stabilize, the external fixator can be used for definitive fixation.[91]

In summary, there is no evidence in the literature that early fixation of femoral fractures is deleterious in the presence of a severe head injury. However, aggressive resuscitation and invasive monitoring are required to achieve and maintain stable intracranial and systemic parameters. If these parameters remain unstable, temporization with external fixation or, rarely, skeletal traction may be required. A multidisciplinary approach must be adopted to allow an optimal outcome in this subset of trauma patients.

References

1. Wolinsky PR, McCarty EC, Shyr Y, Johnson KD: Length of operative procedures: Reamed femoral intramedullary nailing performed with and without a fracture table. *J Orthop Trauma* 1998;12:485-495.

2. Karpos PA, McFerran MA, Johnson KD: Intramedullary nailing of acute femoral shaft fractures using manual traction without a fracture table. *J Orthop Trauma* 1995;9:57-62.

3. Sirkin MS, Behrens F, McCracken K, Aurori K, Aurori B, Schenk R: Femoral nailing without a fracture table. *Clin Orthop* 1996;332:119-125.

4. Brumback RJ, Ellison TS, Molligan H, Molligan DJ, Mahaffey S, Schmidhauser C: Pudendal nerve palsy complicating intramedullary nailing of the femur. *J Bone Joint Surg Am* 1992;74:1450-1455.

5. Callanan I, Choudhry V, Smith H: Perineal sloughing as a result of pressure necrosis from the traction post during prolonged bilateral femoral nailing. *Injury* 1994;25:472.

6. Anglen J, Banovetz J: Compartment syndrome in the well leg resulting from fracture-table positioning. *Clin Orthop* 1994;301:239-242.

7. Wolinsky PR, McCarty E, Shyr Y, Johnson K: Reamed intramedullary nailing of the femur: 551 cases. *J Trauma* 1999;46:392-399.

8. Winquist RA, Hansen ST Jr, Clawson DK: Closed intramedullary nailing of femoral fractures: A report of five hundred and twenty cases. *J Bone Joint Surg Am* 1984;66:529-539.

9. Bain GI, Zacest AC, Paterson DC, Middleton J, Pohl AP: Abduction strength following intramedullary nailing of the femur. *J Orthop Trauma* 1997;11:93-97.

10. Benirschke SK, Melder I, Henley MB, et al: Closed interlocking nailing of femoral shaft fractures: Assessment of technical complications and functional outcomes by comparison of a prospective database with retrospective review. *J Orthop Trauma* 1993;7:118-122.

11. Johnson EE, Marroquin CE, Kossovsky N: Synovial metallosis resulting from intraarticular intramedullary nailing of a distal femoral nonunion. *J Orthop Trauma* 1993;7:320-326.

12. Tornetta P III, Tiburzi D: Antegrade or retrograde reamed femoral nailing: A prospective, randomised trial. *J Bone Joint Surg Br* 2000;82:652-654.

13. Ricci WM, Bellabarba C, Evanoff B, Herscovici D, DiPasquale T, Sanders R: Retrograde versus antegrade nailing of femoral shaft fractures. *J Orthop Trauma* 2001;15:161-169.

14. Ostrum RF, Agarwal A, Lakatos R, Poka A: Prospective comparison of retrograde and antegrade femoral intramedullary nailing. *J Orthop Trauma* 2000;14:496-501.

15. Gellman RE, Paiement GD, Green HD, Coughlin RR: Treatment of supracondylar femoral fractures with a retrograde intramedullary nail. *Clin Orthop* 1996;332:90-97.

16. Morgan E, Ostrum RF, DiCicco J, McElroy J, Poka A: Effects of retrograde femoral intramedullary nailing on patellofemoral articulation. *J Orthop Trauma* 1999;13:13-16.

17. Riina J, Tornetta P III, Ritter C, Geller J: Neurologic and vascular structures at risk during anterior-posterior locking of retrograde femoral nails. *J Orthop Trauma* 1998;12:379-381.

18. Ostrum RF, DiCicco J, Lakatos R, Poka A: Retrograde intramedullary nailing of femoral diaphyseal fractures. *J Orthop Trauma* 1998;12:464-468.

19. Swiontkowski MF, Hansen ST Jr, Kellam J: Ipsilateral fractures of the femoral neck and shaft: A treatment protocol. *J Bone Joint Surg Am* 1984;66:260-268.

20. Sanders R, Koval KJ, DiPasquale T, Helfet DL, Frankle M: Retrograde reamed femoral nailing *J Orthop Trauma* 1993;7:293-302.

21. Patterson BM, Routt ML Jr, Benirschke SK, Hansen ST: Retrograde nailing of femoral shaft fractures. *J Trauma* 1995;38:38-43.

22. Herscovici D, Whiteman KW: Retrograde nailing of the femur using an intercondylar approach. *Clin Orthop* 1996;332:98-104.

23. Moed BR, Watson JT: Retrograde intramedullary nailing, without reaming, of fractures of the femoral shaft in multiply injured patients. *J Bone Joint Surg Am* 1995;77:1520-1527.

24. Moed BR, Watson JT, Cramer KE, Karges DE, Teefey JS: Unreamed retrograde intramedullary nailing of fractures of the femoral shaft. *J Orthop Trauma* 1998;12:334-342.

25. ElMaraghy AW, Schemitsch EH, Richards RR: Femoral and cruciate blood flow after retrograde femoral reaming: A canine study using laser Doppler flowmetry. *J Orthop Trauma* 1998;12:253-258.

26. Stubbs M, Zhang H, Vrahas MS, Baratta RV, Zieske A: Effect of intraarticular stainless steel implants on the health of the rabbit knee joint: An experimental study. *J Orthop Trauma* 2000;14:567-570.

27. Koval KJ, Kummer FJ, Bharam S, Chen D, Halder S: Distal femoral fixation: A laboratory comparison of the 95 degrees plate, antegrade and retrograde inserted reamed intramedullary nails. *J Orthop Trauma* 1996;10:378-382.

28. Brumback RJ, Virkus WW: Intramedullary nailing of the femur: Reamed versus non-reamed. *J Am Acad Orthop Surg* 2000;8:83-90.

29. Chapman MW: The effect of reamed and nonreamed intramedullary nailing on fracture healing. *Clin Orthop* 1998;355(suppl):S230-S238.

30. Rhinelander FW: Effects of medullary nailing on the normal blood supply of diaphyseal cortex. *Instr Course Lect* 1973;22:161-187.

31. Rhinelander FW: The vascular response of bone to internal fixation, in Browner BD, Edwards CC (eds): *The Science and Practice of Intramedullary Nailing*. Philadelphia, PA, Lea and Febiger, 1987, pp 25-60.

32. Trueta J: Blood supply and the rate of healing of tibial fractures. *Clin Orthop* 1974;105:11-26.

33. Strachan RK, McCarthy I, Fleming R, Hughes SP: The role of the tibial nutrient artery: Microsphere estimation of blood flow in the osteotomised canine tibia. *J Bone Joint Surg Br* 1990;72:391-394.

34. Whiteside LA, Lesker PA: The effects of extraperiosteal and subperiosteal dissection: II. On fracture healing. *J Bone Joint Surg Am* 1978;60:26-30.

35. Reichert IL, McCarthy ID, Hughes SP: The acute vascular response to intramedullary reaming: Microsphere estimation of blood flow in the intact ovine tibia. *J Bone Joint Surg Br* 1995;77:490-493.

36. Cole JD: The vascular response of bone to internal fixation, in Browner BD (ed): *The Science and Practice of Intramedullary Nailing*, ed 2. Baltimore, MD, Williams & Wilkins, 1996, pp 43-70.

37. Klein MP, Rahn BA, Frigg R, Kessler S, Perren SM: Reaming versus non-reaming in medullary nailing: Interference with cortical circulation of the canine tibia. *Arch Orthop Trauma Surg* 1990;109:314-316.

38. Schemitsch EH, Kowalski MJ, Swiontkowski MF, Senft D: Cortical bone blood flow in reamed and unreamed locked intramedullary nailing: A fractured tibia model in sheep. *J Orthop Trauma* 1994;8:373-382.

39. Hupel TM, Aksenov SA, Schemitsch EH: Effect of limited and standard reaming on cortical bone blood flow and early strength of union following segmental fracture. *J Orthop Trauma* 1998;12:400-406.

40. Schemitsch EH, Kowalski MJ, Swiontkowski MF: Soft-tissue blood flow following reamed versus unreamed locked intramedullary nailing: A fractured sheep tibia model. *Ann Plast Surg* 1996;36:70-75.

41. Schemitsch EH, Kowalski MJ, Swiontkowski MF, Harrington RM Comparison of the effect of reamed and unreamed locked intramedullary nailing on blood flow in the callus and strength of union following fracture of the sheep tibia. *J Orthop Res* 1995;13:382-389.

42. Brumback RJ, Toal TR Jr, Murphy-Zane MS, Novak VP, Belkoff SM: Immediate weight-bearing after treatment of a comminuted fracture of the femoral shaft with a statically locked intramedullary nail. *J Bone Joint Surg Am* 1999; 81:1538-1544.

43. Bechtold JE, Kyle RF, Perren SM: Biomechanics of intramedullary nailing, in Browner BD (ed): *The Science and Practice of Intramedullary Nailing*, ed 2. Baltimore, MD, Williams & Wilkins, 1996, pp 89-101.

44. Sandvig S: Effect of reaming on the torsional strength of femora. Masters' thesis, University of Minnesota, 1995.

45. Brumback RJ, Uwagie-Ero S, Lakatos RP, Poka A, Bathon GH, Burgess AR: Intramedullary nailing of femoral shaft fractures: Part II. Fracture-healing with static interlocking fixation. *J Bone Joint Surg Am* 1988;70:1453-1462.

46. Wiss DA, Fleming CH, Matta JM, Clark D: Comminuted and rotationally unstable fractures of the femur treated with an interlocking nail. *Clin Orthop* 1986;212:35-47.

47. Kröpfl A, Naglik H, Primavesi C, Hertz H: Unreamed intramedullary nailing of femoral fractures. *J Trauma* 1995;38:717-726.

48. Bone L, Kowalski J, Rohrbacher B, Stegemann P: Reamed versus unreamed femoral nailing: A prospective randomized study. *Orthop Trans* 1997;21:603.

49. Le TT, Wilber JH, Patterson BM, Sontich JK, Ziran BH: Early results of femur fractures treated with reamed vs unreamed intramedullary nailing: A prospective study. *Orthop Trans* 1997;21:604.

50. Clatworthy MG, Clark DI, Gray DH, Hardy AE: Reamed versus unreamed femoral nails: A randomized, prospective trial. *J Bone Joint Surg Br* 1998;80:485-489.

51. Tornetta P III, Tiburzi D: The treatment of femoral shaft fractures using intramedullary interlocked nails with and without intramedullary reaming: A preliminary report. *J Orthop Trauma* 1997;11:89-92.

52. Tornetta P III, Tiburzi D: Reamed versus nonreamed anterograde femoral nailing. *J Orthop Trauma* 2000;14:15-19.

53. Bhandari M, Guyatt GH, Tong D, Adili A, Shaughnessy SG: Reamed versus nonreamed intramedullary nailing of lower extremity long bone fractures: A systematic overview and meta-analysis. *J Orthop Trauma* 2000;14:2-9.

54. Brumback RJ, Ellison PS Jr, Poka A, Lakatos R, Bathon GH, Burgess AR: Intramedullary nailing of open fractures of the femoral shaft. *J Bone Joint Surg Am* 1989;71:1324-1331.

55. Lhowe DW, Hansen ST: Immediate nailing of open fractures of the femoral shaft. *J Bone Joint Surg Am* 1988;70:812-820.

56. Pell AC, Christie J, Keating JF, Sutherland GR: The detection of fat embolism by transoesophageal echocardiography during reamed intramedullary nailing: A study of 24 patients with femoral and tibial fractures. *J Bone Joint Surg Br* 1993;75:921-925.

57. Levy D: The fat embolism syndrome: A review. *Clin Orthop* 1990;261:281-286.

58. Riska EB, von Bonsdorff H, Hakkinen S, Jaroma H, Kiviluoto O, Paavilainen T: Prevention of fat embolism by early internal fixation of fractures in patients with multiple injuries. *Injury* 1976;8:110-116.

59. Riska EB, von Bonsdorff H, Hakkinen S, Jaroma H, Kiviluoto O, Paavilainen T: Primary operative fixation of long bone fractures in patients with multiple injuries. *J Trauma* 1977; 17:111-121.

60. Riska EB, Myllynen P: Fat embolism in patients with multiple injuries. *J Trauma* 1982;22:891-894.

61. Flick MR: Pulmonary edema and acute lung injury, in Murray JF, Nadel JA (eds): *Textbook of Respiratory Medicine*, ed 2. Philadelphia, PA, WB Saunders, 1994, vol 2, pp 1725-1777.

62. Gurd AR: Fat embolism: An aid to diagnosis. *J Bone Joint Surg Br* 1970;52:732-737.

63. Barie PS, Minnear FL, Malik AB: Increased pulmonary vascular permeability after bone marrow injection in sheep. *Am Rev Respir Dis* 1981;123:648-653.

64. Regel G, Nerlich ML, Dwenger A, Siedel J, Schmidt C, Sturm JA: Induction of pulmonary injury by polymorphonuclear leucocytes after bone marrow fat injection and endotoxemia: A sheep model. *Theoret Surg* 1989;4:22-30.

65. Nakata Y, Dahms TE: Triolein increases microvascular permeability in isolated perfused rabbit lungs: Role of neutrophils. *J Trauma* 2000;49:320-326.

66. Peltier LF: Fat embolism: An appraisal of the problem. *Clin Orthop* 1984;187:3-17.

67. Peltier LF: Fat embolism: A perspective. *Clin Orthop* 1988;232:263-270.

68. Goris RJ, Gimbrere JS, van Niekerk JL, Schoots FJ, Booy LH: Early osteosynthesis and prophylactic mechanical ventilation in the multitrauma patient. *J Trauma* 1982;22:895-903.

69. Wickstrom J, Corban MS: Intramedullary fixation for fractures of the femoral shaft: A study of complications in 298 operations. *J Trauma* 1967;7:551-583.

70. Bone LB, Johnson KD, Weigelt J, Scheinberg R: Early versus delayed stabilization of femoral fractures: A prospective randomized study. *J Bone Joint Surg Am* 1989;71:336-340.

71. Wolinsky PR, McCarty E, Shyr Y, Johnson K: Reamed intramedullary nailing of the femur: 551 cases. *J Trauma* 1999;46:392-399.

72. Behrman SW, Fabian TC, Kudsk KA, Taylor JC: Improved outcome with femur fractures: Early vs. delayed fixation. *J Trauma* 1990;30: 792-798.

73. Talucci RC, Manning J, Lampard S, Bach A, Carrico CJ: Early intramedullary nailing of femoral shaft fractures: A cause of fat embolism syndrome. *Am J Surg* 1983;146:107-111.

74. Pape HC, Auf'm'Kolk M, Paffrath T, Regel G, Sturm JA, Tscherne H: Primary intramedullary femur fixation in multiple trauma patients with associated lung contusion: A cause of posttraumatic ARDS? *J Trauma* 1993;34:540-548.

75. Wenda K, Runkel M, Degreif J, Ritter G: Pathogenesis and clinical relevance of bone marrow embolism in medullary nailing: Demonstrated by intraoperative echocardiography. *Injury* 1993;24(suppl 3):S73-S81.

76. Charash WE, Fabian TC, Croce MA: Delayed surgical fixation of femur fractures is a risk factor for pulmonary failure independent of thoracic trauma. *J Trauma* 1994;37:667-672.

77. Bosse MJ, MacKenzie EJ, Riemer BL, Brumback RJ, McCarthy ML, Burgess AR: Adult respiratory distress syndrome, pneumonia, and mortality following thoracic injury and a femoral fracture treated either with intramedullary nailing with reaming or with a plate: A comparative study. *J Bone Joint Surg Am* 1997;79:799-809.

78. Pape HC, Dwenger A, Regel G, et al: Pulmonary damage after intramedullary femoral nailing in traumatized sheep: Is there an effect from different nailing methods. *J Trauma* 1992;33:574-581.

79. Wozasek GE, Thurnher M, Redl H, Schlag G: Pulmonary reaction during intramedullary fracture management in traumatic shock: An experimental study. *J Trauma* 1994;37:249-254.

80. Wolinsky PR, Sciadini MF, Parker RE: Effects on pulmonary physiology of reamed femoral intramedullary nailing in an open-chest sheep model. *J Orthop Trauma* 1996;10:75-80.

81. Wolinsky PR, Banit D, Parker RE, et al: Reamed intramedullary femoral nailing after induction of an "ARDS-like" state in sheep: Effect on clinically applicable markers of pulmonary function. *J Orthop Trauma* 1998;12: 169-176.

82. Marrhay MA, Matthay RA: Pulmonary edema: Cardiogenic and noncardiogenic, in George RB (ed): *Chest Medicine: Essentials of Pulmonary and Critical Care Medicine*, ed 2. Baltimore, MD, Williams & Wilkins, 1990, p 439.

83. Bulger EM, Jurkovich GJ, Gentilello LM, Maier RV: Current clinical options for the treatment and management of acute respiratory distress syndrome. *J Trauma* 2000;48:562-572.

84. Rhee P, Morris J, Durham R, et al: Recombinant humanized monoclonal antibody against CD18 (rhuMAb CD18) in traumatic hemorrhagic shock: Results of a phase II clinical trial: Traumatic Shock Group. *J Trauma* 2000;49:611-620.

85. Napolitano LM, Ferrer T, McCarter RJ, Scalea TM: Systemic inflammatory response syndrome score at admission independently predicts mortality and length of stay in trauma patients. *J Trauma* 2000;49:647-653.

86. Rixen D, Siegel JH: Metabolic correlates of oxygen debt predict posttrauma early acute respiratory distress syndrome and the related cytokine response. *J Trauma* 2000;49:392-403.

87. Davis JW, Parks SN, Kaups KL, Gladen HE, O'Donnell-Nicol S: Admission base deficit predicts transfusion requirements and risk of complications. *J Trauma* 1996;41:769-774.

88. Rotstein OD: Novel strategies for immunomodulation after trauma: Revisiting hypertonic saline as a resuscitation strategy for hemorrhagic shock. *J Trauma* 2000;49:580-583.

89. Crowl AC, Young JS, Kahler DM, Claridge JA, Chrzanowski DS, Pomphrey M: Occult hypoperfusion is associated with increased morbidity in patients undergoing early femur fracture fixation. *J Trauma* 2000;48:260-267.

90. Harman JW, Ragatz FJ: Abstract: The pathogenesis of experimental fat embolism. *Am J Pathol* 1949;25:809-810.

91. Scalea TM, Boswell SA, Scott JD, Mitchell KA, Kramer ME, Pollak AN: External fixation as a bridge to intramedullary nailing for patients with multiple injuries and with femur fractures: Damage control orthopedics. *J Trauma* 2000;48:613-623.

92. Garland DE, Rothi B, Waters RL: Femoral fractures in head-injured adults. *Clin Orthop* 1982;166:219-225.

93. Jaicks RR, Cohn SM, Moller BA: Early fracture fixation may be deleterious after head injury. *J Trauma* 1997;42:1-6.

94. Poole GV, Miller JD, Agnew SG, Griswold JA: Lower extremity fracture fixation in head-injured patients. *J Trauma* 1992;32:654-659.

95. Malisano LP, Stevens D, Hunter GA: The management of long bone fractures in the head-injured polytrauma patient. *J Orthop Trauma* 1994;8:1-5.

96. McKee MD, Schemitsch EH, Vincent LO, Sullivan I, Yoo D: The effect of a femoral fracture on concomitant closed head injury in patients with multiple injuries. *J Trauma* 1997; 42:1041-1045.

97. Townsend RN, Lheureau T, Protetch J, Riemer B, Simon D: Timing fracture repair in patients with severe brain injury (Glasgow Coma Scale score < 9). *J Trauma* 1998;44:977-983.

98. Starr AJ, Hunt JL, Chason DP, Reinert CM, Walker J: Treatment of femur fracture with associated head injury. *J Orthop Trauma* 1998; 12:38-45.

99. Scalea TM, Scott JD, Brumback RJ, et al: Early fracture fixation may be "just fine" after head injury: No difference in central nervous system outcomes. *J Trauma* 1999;46:839-846.

100. Greenspan L, McLellan BA, Greig H: Abbreviated Injury Scale and Injury Severity Score: A scoring chart. *J Trauma* 1985;25:60-64.

101. Pietropaoli JA, Rogers FB, Shackford SR, Wald SL, Schmoker JD, Zhuang J: The deleterious effects of intraoperative hypotension on outcome in patients with severe head injuries. *J Trauma* 1992;33:403-407.

102. Chesnut RM, Marshall LF, Klauber MR, et al: The role of secondary brain injury in determining outcome from severe head injury. *J Trauma* 1993;34:216-222.

103. Shackford SR, Mackersie RC, Davis JW, Wolf PL, Hoyt DB: Epidemiology and pathology of traumatic deaths occurring at a Level I Trauma Center in a regionalized system: The importance of secondary brain injury. *J Trauma* 1989; 29:1392-1397.

104. Wald SL, Shackford SR, Fenwick J: The effect of secondary insults on mortality and long-term disability after severe head injury in a rural region without a trauma system. *J Trauma* 1993;34:377-382.

105. Go KG: The fluid environment of the central nervous system, in Go KG (ed): *Cerebral pathophysiology: An Integral Approach with Some Emphasis on Clinical Implications.* Amsterdam, Netherlands, Elsevier Science Publishers, 1991, pp 66-172.

106. Bouma GJ, Muizelaar JP, Bandoh K, Marmarou A: Blood pressure and intracranial pressure: Volume dynamics in severe head injury. Relationship with cerebral blood flow. *J Neurosurg* 1992;77:15-19.

107. Marion DW, Darby J, Yonas H: Acute regional cerebral blood flow changes caused by severe head injuries. *J Neurosurg* 1991;74:407-414.

108. Shackford SR, Zhuang J, Schmoker J: Intravenous fluid tonicity: Effect on intracranial pressure, cerebral blood flow, and cerebral oxygen delivery in focal brain injury. *J Neurosurg* 1992;76:91-98.

109. Fortune JB, Feustel PJ, Weigle CG, Popp AJ: Continuous measurement of jugular venous oxygen saturation in response to transient elevations of blood pressure in head-injured patients. *J Neurosurg* 1994;80:461-468.

110. Rotondo MF, Schwab CW, McGonigal MD, et al: "Damage control": An approach for improved survival in exsanguinating penetrating abdominal injury. *J Trauma* 1993;35: 375-383.

Orthopaedic Treatment of Fractures of the Long Bones and Pelvis in Children Who Have Multiple Injuries

Vernon T. Tolo, MD

A large number of children who are admitted to the hospital after trauma have multiple injuries. Although most of the fractures associated with polytrauma are obvious, with deformity and swelling of the injured extremity, it is essential to examine all extremities and axial areas carefully in this setting. It has been suggested that technetium bone scans be used for young patients who have multiple injuries in order to diagnose all skeletal injuries,[1] but careful physical examination will usually suffice. The orthopaedic treatment of fractures in children who have multiple injuries is clearly affected by what other injuries the child has sustained. These injuries of other systems not only may change the timing of the orthopaedic care but also often alter the type of treatment chosen for the fracture.

Special Factors in Children Who Have a Head Injury

Injury to the brain needs immediate attention and has a higher priority than fractures of the extremities of patients who have multiple injuries. The extent of injury to the brain and coma resulting from the head injury can be quantified, with use of the Glasgow Coma Scale or a similar grading system,[2] to follow the course of the child after he or she arrives at the hospital. Commonly, intracranial pressure is monitored to evaluate the need for neurosurgical intervention.

The orthopaedist can help to control the intracranial pressure by initially providing effective immobilization of the fractures. The stimulus from the manipulation of fractures or the movement of unsplinted fractures of the extremities can lead to an increase in the intracranial pressure. Although this immobilization may be limited to application of a splint or cast in the first few hours, if the child is brought to the operating room for the treatment of another system injury displaced fractures of the long bones should be stabilized operatively at the same time.

When treating fractures in a comatose child, the orthopaedist should assume that full neurologic recovery will take place. It has been clearly demonstrated that a child's recovery from a head injury is substantially better than an adult's recovery from the same type of injury.[3] This means that orthopaedic care needs to be extensive and complete. If a fracture would be treated surgically in an alert child, it should be treated surgically in a comatose child. General anesthesia should not be avoided if it is thought to be necessary, as it will not adversely affect the neurologic status of a comatose child.[4]

Invasive measurements of compartment pressure should be used readily if there is any chance of a compartment syndrome. The decision to measure compartment pressure should be based on the mechanism and location of the fracture and the swelling of the soft tissues. The compartment pressure that would lead me to recommend fasciotomy for a child who is comatose and who cannot cooperate with a clinical examination is lower than the pressure that would lead me to make such a recommendation for a conscious child. I recommend fasciotomy for a comatose child if the pressure readings for the compartments in the leg exceed 30 mm/Hg (4.00 kPa).

Treatment of Fractures of the Long Bones in Children Who Have Multiple Injuries

The orthopaedic care given to fractures of the long bones in patients who have trauma to multiple organ systems often differs in some way from the care recommended for a solitary fracture of a long bone. Generally, solitary fractures of the long bones in children are treated with closed reduction and immobilization with a cast, but casts can cause problems for some patients with multiple injuries. The creation of windows in the cast, which are needed to change dressings on wounds in the extremities, can lead to displacement of previously reduced fractures. Involuntary movement due to spasticity from a head injury can lead to pressure sores within the cast. A hip spica cast makes it more difficult to examine the abdomen clinically and to perform imaging studies in the abdominal and pelvic areas.

As a result, well-padded casts and splints are used for primary treatment of closed, nondisplaced fractures in children with multiple injuries. The preferred treatment for open, nondisplaced fractures, once irrigation and debridement in the operating room has been completed, often is fixation with pins and an external frame, particularly if the cutaneous wound is large. Consideration should be given to operative treatment of all displaced fractures in this setting, even though many can be adequately and safely treated closed. The decision to use nonsurgical or surgical treatment depends on many factors and needs to be made on the basis of the individual needs of each child with multiple injuries.

Treatment of Open Fractures

The ideal time for stabilization of closed fractures is a bit unclear, but there is no doubt that open fractures need to be treated on an emergency basis. Although only a relatively small number of fractures in children who have multiple injuries are open, it is these fractures that need immediate care.[5]

An open fracture is generally classified with use of the criteria of Gustilo and Anderson[6] when the patient arrives in the emergency room. When used for adults, this classification is associated with the number and extent of sequelae from the open fracture, including risks of infection, delayed union, nonunion, amputation, and residual functional impairment. The 3 major classifications of open fractures are based on the size of the wound, extent of the injury of the soft tissues, contamination of the wound, and associated vascular injury.

A fracture is classified as type I when the wound is less than 1 cm in size and there is minimum contamination or injury of the soft tissues. Most of these wounds are inside-to-outside punctures, caused when the sharp end of the fractured bone punctures the skin. Even open fractures associated with a small puncture wound should be treated with irrigation and debridement in the operating room. The fracture is considered to be type II when the wound is larger than 1 cm with moderate soft-tissue injury, and it is classified as type III when there is extensive soft-tissue injury and crushing as well as a large, open, contaminated wound. Fractures are classified as subtypes IIIB and IIIC when there is exposed bone and as subtype IIIC when there is associated vascular injury. The Gustilo-Anderson system can be used as a guide to classify open fractures in children, but the treatment, particularly that of type III fractures, in children may differ from that in adults, given that wounds and fractures heal more quickly in young children than they do in adults. Subtype IIIC injuries that may be considered an indication for primary amputation in adults should be considered treatable with a limb-salvage operation in most children.

In the emergency room, a sterile gauze dressing containing povidone-iodine solution should be applied to the open wound, and the fracture should be immobilized for transport to the radiology unit. It is not necessary to take samples for culture in the emergency room, but it may be helpful to obtain them in the operating room at the time of debridement. A broad-spectrum antibiotic, usually cefazolin at a dose of 25 mg/kg of body weight, is administered intravenously in the emergency room to all patients who have an open fracture. An aminoglycoside antibiotic is added for primary coverage for all patients who have a type III fracture. It is also added for some patients who have a type II fracture, such as those who have had a delay in treatment of longer than 12 hours or those who have contamination from a farmyard accident.

The open fracture should be irrigated and debrided in the operating room as soon as possible after the injury. Although an attempt should be made to perform irrigation and debridement within 6 hours after the injury, as has been recommended by some authors to decrease the risk of later infection,[7] debridement in patients with multiple injuries may be delayed for a few more hours to allow time for stabilization of the patient and for the imaging of other organ systems. If there is a delay in operative irrigation and debridement, early intravenous administration of cefazolin (25 mg/kg of body weight) in the emergency room may help to keep the risk of infection acceptably low.

In the operating room, a systematic approach to irrigation and debridement is helpful. A sample for culture is usually obtained, but there is controversy about the importance of the result of this culture with regard to determining the later treatment of the wound. The edges of the wound are excised, and the wound is extended to allow for a more complete exploration. The hematoma is evacuated, and any necrotic soft tissue is excised. The ends of the proximal and distal fracture fragments are inspected. During this exploration of the wound, a pulsatile irrigation system is used to gently debride both the soft tissues and the ends of the bone. It is customary to use 10 liters of fluid for irrigation of each open fracture. Reduction of the fracture is then completed under direct vision, and the fracture is assessed to determine the reconstruction options for stabilization. After the fracture is stabilized, the portion of the wound that was incised in the operating room is closed and the wound associated with the open fracture is left open. When the fracture is type I, a small drain is left in the wound for 2 days. Cefazolin, administered intravenously at a dosage of 25 mg/kg of body weight every 8 hours, is generally used for a total of 3 days. A longer course of appropriate antibiotics, based on the results of culture and sensitivity studies, is used if additional problems with the wound occur.

Timing of Treatment of Multiple Closed Fractures

It is standard practice in adult trauma centers to stabilize fractures of the long bones within 24 hours after the injury in order to decrease the risk of pulmonary and other medical complications. There is much less concern about pulmonary disease developing in children after multiple injuries, unless the child has sustained severe trauma to the chest or multiple fractures of the ribs. In addition, children who have multiple injuries were typically active and healthy before the trauma.

Generally, closed fractures of the long bones should be treated expeditiously. Treatment of fractures within 72 hours after the time of the multiple injuries, as opposed to more than 72 hours after the injuries, usually results in a shorter stay in the hospital, a shorter stay in the intensive care unit, and a shorter period of ventilatory assistance. Children who have earlier surgical management have fewer complications.[8] General anesthesia does not have a negative effect on the brain of a comatose child, and early fixation of fractures facilitates evaluation and care of the other injured organ systems.[4]

Indications for External or Internal Fixation of Fractures

Indications for surgical treatment of long-bone fractures have to be examined individually in each child with multiple injuries, as the combination of organ-system injuries is seldom fully predictable. Nonetheless, there are some relatively frequent clinical situations in which it is best to treat fractures by either external or internal fixation. These situations include a displaced and shortened fracture of a long bone in a comatose child, an open or closed fracture associated with a large wound or loss of skin, a fracture associated with vascular injury, a fracture associated with compartment syndrome necessitating fasciotomy, a so-called floating joint (long-bone fractures on both sides of the joint), and a displaced pelvic fracture in a preteenager or teenager.

Internal Fixation of Fractures

The techniques used for internal fixation of fractures in children differ somewhat from those used in adults. The main types of internal fixation in children are Kirschner wires or Steinmann pins, flexible intramedullary rods, and AO plates. The primary purposes of internal fixation in children are to align the fracture fragments enough to allow healing, to facilitate the care of other injured organ systems, and to prevent complications that may be associated with immobilization of the extremity. Since nonunion of fractures is unusual in children, the fixation does not need to be as rigid as it needs to be in adults. As stiffness of adjacent joints caused by immobilization is not an important risk in most children, casts or splints can be used to supplement the internal fixation while healing rapidly occurs. In addition, intramedullary fixation with reaming should be avoided in order to prevent iatrogenic injury to the open growth plates.

Radial or Ulnar Fractures Most closed fractures of the forearms of children who are less than ten years of age should be treated with closed reduction and the application of a cast. In certain situations—such as when the fracture is open or irreducible or is unstable after closed reduction—intramedullary rod fixation, currently the most common form of internal fixation used for the treatment of fractures of the forearm, is indicated.[9] In these children and young adolescents, flexible intramedullary implants are useful for providing sufficient stability to allow healing. These implants have included Steinmann pins, Rush rods, and, more recently, the new flexible titanium implants of 2 to 4 mm in diameter. The type of device that is used for fixation depends on the surgeon's experience and on the size of the child's bone. Steinmann pins are used in the ulna to

provide stabilization of this straight bone, but they are less applicable to the radius. Rush rods can be used in both the ulna and the radius, with the implant contoured to accommodate the bow of the radius when it is inserted in that bone. Flexible titanium nails have a slightly hooked end that facilitates passage across the site of the fracture, and they can be inserted either straight into the ulna or with a contoured bow into the radius.

When intramedullary implants are used for fractures of the forearm, the ulna is stabilized first. The point of entry into the ulna is at the olecranon or in the proximal ulnar metaphysis. Once entry into the medullary canal is achieved, the implant should be inserted by hand, not with a power drill, particularly if the end of the implant is sharp. The implant is advanced with fluoroscopic control while the fracture is held in the reduced position. After the ulna is stabilized, fluoroscopic examination is done to assess the adequacy of the reduction of the radial fracture. If the stability provided by the ulnar implant has allowed satisfactory reduction of the radius, a cast is applied without additional surgical stabilization of the radius. If the radius is not adequately reduced after the ulna is stabilized, an intramedullary rod is placed in the radius as well.

The standard point of entry of the intramedullary implant into the radius is the distal metaphysis, just proximal to the distal physis. Patients who have a closed fracture of the middle or proximal part of the radius are good candidates for intramedullary fixation, as these fractures are more difficult to control with closed reduction and a cast. Here again, the implant is manually advanced across the site of the fracture under fluoroscopic guidance. In the proximal aspect of the radius, limited surgical exposure of the fracture may be necessary to align the fracture fragments, particularly if the pinning is being done several days after the initial fracture.

A surgical alternative to the use of an intramedullary rod in the forearm is the use of an AO plate.[10] Generally, AO plates used in preteenagers can be shorter and can have a smaller number of sites of cortical fixation than those needed in teenagers or adults, as a splint or cast is applied postoperatively for preteenagers. A second operative procedure is needed to remove the plate, and, even in children and teenagers, there is a risk of refracture through the empty screw holes for approximately 6 weeks after the plate and the screws are removed.

Humeral Fractures Nonoperative treatment is preferred for most fractures of the proximal aspect of the humerus; substantial angulation and displacement can be accepted because the bone remodels excellently after this fracture, even in teenagers. If open reduction is needed because of the presence of interposed soft tissue, fixation with Steinmann pins is sufficient to provide stability for healing. Fixation with an AO plate is usually used for diaphyseal fractures in a teenager or when there is a special circumstance, such as a floating elbow with associated fracture of the forearm. Recently available flexible intramedullary nails can also be used in this setting, without the risk of injuring the radial nerve during either insertion of the plate or its subsequent removal. Fixation with smooth pins is generally sufficient for distal fractures in preteenagers. In adolescents, as in adults, T condylar fractures need to be treated with open reduction and the insertion of a contoured AO reconstruction plate.

Tibial Fractures Internal fixation is not often used for diaphyseal fractures of the tibia; it is more common for this bone to be treated operatively with pins and an external fixation device when surgical stabilization is needed. The primary use of internal fixation is for stabilization after reduction of physeal fractures. A Salter-Harris type I fracture in the proximal aspect of the tibia can be stabilized with the percutaneous insertion of smooth Steinmann pins in a crossed fashion between the epiphysis and metaphysis. Fixation of fractures in this manner usually negates the need for an extreme reduction position in a cast and allows for care of arterial injury, which is often associated with this type of fracture. An above-the-knee cast is used to protect the fracture reduction for 4 weeks, after which time the pins are removed.

A Salter-Harris type III fracture is temporarily stabilized with 2 Kirschner wires inserted into the epiphysis, parallel to the joint surface, under fluoroscopic imaging. Two parallel cannulated screws are then inserted over the Kirschner wires for permanent stabilization, and the Kirschner wires are removed. A washer is frequently used to prevent the screw from being buried into the epiphysis as it is tightened. A similar technique of temporary stabilization with a Kirschner wire followed by permanent fixation with cannulated screws is used for Salter-Harris type II and type IV fractures with a sizable metaphyseal fragment. The cannulated screws used in this setting must avoid crossing the physis and are inserted parallel to the joint line and to the physis. When either Steinmann pins or cannulated screws are used for fixation of a physeal fracture, it is necessary to use an above-the-knee cast as well until the fracture has healed.

Reaming to insert an intramedullary fixation device, an approach often used to treat a tibial fracture in an adult, is avoided in skeletally immature patients because of the possibility of a recurvatum deformity developing as a result of iatrogenic injury to the anterior part of the proximal tibial physis. Flexible intramedullary nails, entering the proximal metaphysis, will likely be used more in the future, but currently their use is more popular in other long bones.

Femoral Fractures Femoral fractures commonly are treated with surgical stabilization in children with multiple injuries. As in the tibia, distal physeal fractures in the femur can be stabilized with smooth Steinmann pins or cannulated screws, depending on the amount of displacement and the type of fracture.

Physeal growth arrest is rather common after any distal femoral physeal fracture. Nonetheless, with Salter-Harris type I fractures, percutaneous smooth Steinmann pins can be inserted in a crossed fashion to hold the fracture fragments securely enough to allow for placement of a cast or splint with slight flexion of the knee. With Salter-Harris type II fractures, the insertion of cannulated screws through the metaphyseal fragment, parallel to the physis, provides adequate stability of the fracture reduction to allow placement of a cast or splint. Supracondylar distal femoral fractures are usually best reduced with the knee flexed to relax the pull of the gastrocnemius muscle. However, with the knee in this position it is not possible to easily recognize varus or valgus malalignment of the fracture reduction. Percutaneous crossed Steinmann pins are useful to hold the reduction in a position to allow full extension of the knee and to provide the opportunity to accurately assess for varus or valgus malalignment.

There may be a small risk of physeal injury from the use of Steinmann pins, but it is better to achieve excellent alignment of the fracture here than to avoid the insertion of smooth pins across the physis because of this risk. These pins are left protruding through the skin and are removed on an outpatient basis 3 to 4 weeks after insertion. Cannulated screws are used commonly for Salter-Harris type III fractures of the distal epiphysis and for Salter-Harris type II and type IV fractures with a large enough metaphyseal fragment to allow for internal fixation without physeal damage. All patients who have treatment of a distal femoral physeal fracture must be followed carefully to look for subsequent longitudinal or angulatory growth disturbance.

It is the surgical treatment of the

femoral diaphyseal fracture that remains controversial.[11] Intramedullary rods inserted in any fashion after reaming are used in teenagers and adults. In children between 5 and 12 years of age, the primary choice of operative stabilization is external fixation, retrograde flexible intramedullary fixation, or fixation with AO plates.

Open reduction with AO plate fixation has been shown to be successful in treating femoral fractures in children who have multiple injuries.[12] This is a particularly effective technique when there is an injury of the femoral artery needing repair adjacent to the fracture. Prompt stabilization of the fracture is achieved through the same wound that is used for exploration of the artery; with the internal fixation, an external fixation frame, which can make the arterial repair more cumbersome, is unnecessary. A disadvantage of fixation with a plate is that a second surgical procedure is needed in order to remove the plate. Also, there is possibly more subsequent femoral overgrowth than occurs with other treatment methods, although a recent study demonstrated a mean of only 9 mm of overgrowth after fixation with an AO plate in children.[12]

An increasingly popular method of internal fixation of femoral fractures in children is the use of flexible retrograde intramedullary nails that range in diameter from 2 to 4 mm.[13,14] I prefer this method for stabilization of femoral fractures in children who are 6 to 12 years of age. Two intramedullary implants are inserted at the medial and lateral metaphyseal areas just proximal to the distal femoral physis. The implant is bent into a gentle C-shape and is inserted through a drill hole. The implant is then manually advanced proximally across the site of the fracture under fluoroscopic imaging. The second implant that is used is generally 5 mm smaller than the first to facilitate passage across the fracture site. The curved tip of one nail should end in the femoral neck and that of the other should end in the region of the greater trochanter to improve the rotational stability. The distal ends of the nails are cut off 1 to 2 cm from the surface of the bone to facilitate later removal of the implants. Although general anesthesia is needed for a brief time, the implants are removed easily through the distal insertion wounds once fracture healing is complete.

The use of standard techniques of antegrade femoral intramedullary nailing in children who are younger than 12 years of age remains controversial.[11] Interference with the appositional growth of the proximal aspect of the femoral neck leads to narrowing of the femoral neck in some preteenagers. The appearance of avascular necrosis of the femoral head following treatment of fractures of the femoral shaft with antegrade nails has suggested that injury to the circumflex artery near the piriformis fossa is the most likely cause of the necrosis. Implants recently have been designed to enter from the tip of the greater trochanter to avoid this problem of osteonecrosis, but follow-up information regarding these new implants is incomplete to date.

External Fixation of Fractures

As is the case with internal fixation, external fixation of fractures of the long bones can greatly facilitate the overall care of children with multiple injuries.[15-22] Although the technique is applicable to any fracture of a long bone, external fixation is used primarily to treat fractures of the lower extremities in children. The main reason to use external fixation in the upper extremity of a comatose child may be to lengthen a bone that has shortened excessively. The placement of pins for external fixation has more potential for causing iatrogenic injury to the peripheral nerves in the arm and forearm than it has in the lower extremity. In some patients, it may be safer to place certain pins (for example, those in the distal aspect of the humerus) under direct vision through a limited incision in order to avoid nerve injury. Familiarity with the cross-sectional anatomy of the forearm is essential if external fixation is used there.

In contrast, external fixation is a widely used, valuable method for the stabilization of fractures of the lower extremities of children. Most orthopaedists can apply the pins and the external fixator frame relatively quickly. Unlike the use of pins for external fixation in the upper extremity, placement of the pins in the lower extremity is associated with a low risk of iatrogenic neurovascular problems. External fixation is the preferred method for treatment of open fractures of the femur and tibia. The external fixator can be used to bridge the knee or ankle joint to achieve stability of metaphyseal fractures as well as to avoid the use of pins inside large wounds. It is my preferred technique of surgical stabilization for fractures of the tibial shaft and for spiral or oblique femoral fractures in preteenagers.

Usually a unilateral frame provides sufficient stabilization of tibial and femoral fractures. A number of fixators are commercially available, and each has its relative merits. All require that at least 2 pins be placed in the proximal and distal fragments of the fracture. When pins are to be placed in a skeletally immature patient, the sites of insertion should be predrilled. Half-pins, inserted through a stab wound and engaging both bone cortices but not exiting the skin on the opposite side of the thigh or leg, are used routinely. These half-pins are inserted laterally in the femur and either anteriorly or medially in the tibia. The size of the pin that should be used varies with the size of the bone and the age of the child, but the diameter of the pin should be less than 30% of the diameter of the bone in order to minimize the risk of fracture through the site of the pin. The most distal and proximal pins should be placed at least 1 to 2 cm away from the physis to avoid physeal injury from insertion of the pin and later from infections at the sites of the pins. Weight bearing is encouraged after the child has recovered from the other injuries and walking is permitted. If a rigid frame is used, some of the connectors of the pins to the frame are loosened a few weeks before removal of the pins and the frame to allow weightbearing forces to pass through the bone rather than through the external fixator. This process, which has been termed dynamization, appears to strengthen the bone at the site of the fracture and to decrease the prevalence of refracture after removal of the pins and the frame.

There are several potential problems with the use of pins and an external fixator in children. The most commonly encountered problem is pin-track infection. The risk of such an infection can be decreased by ensuring that there is no skin tension at the sites of entry of the pins and by meticulous care of the pin sites; hydrogen-peroxide-soaked swabs should be used twice daily to remove any crusted material. This home care may be augmented at times with whirlpool cleansing. If local erythema and seropurulent drainage occurs, the oral administration of broad-spectrum antibiotics, usually cephalexin at a dosage of 50 mg/kg of body weight per day in 4 divided doses, will suffice to control the local infection and allow for continued use of the external fixator. If radiographs demonstrate progressive lucency around a pin with drainage, the pin needs to be removed and the pin track must be debrided with curettage and irrigation in the operating room and the patient under general anesthesia. In the case of established osteomyelitis, intravenous antibiotic therapy is generally used initially in conjunction with the operative curettage and irrigation to control the infection. At first, cefazolin at a dosage of 25 mg/kg of body weight is given every 8 hours, but other antibiotics may be used if the cultures indicate that the bacteria are more

susceptible to them. Although many patients have some wound drainage during the course of treatment, the prevalence of deep bone infection is very low in children.

The use of external fixation can lead to delayed healing of a fracture, particularly a transverse fracture in a teenager. Use of a rigid frame and a lack of dynamization of a frame also lead to a delay in fracture-healing. Early weightbearing should be encouraged. In preteenagers in whom femoral overgrowth is expected after a fracture heals, bayonet apposition with 0.5 to 1.0 cm overriding allows faster healing of a transverse fracture than if it is reduced anatomically. In reports on external fixation of fractures of the lower extremity, rates of refracture have ranged from 0 of 27[20] to 3 of 14,[21] with refractures occurring either through the site of the old fracture or through the pin track. The use of a flexible frame, the loosening of the connectors of the pins to the rods to allow weightbearing through the fractured bone before removal of the pin and rod, bayonet apposition of the fracture ends, and the use of pins of appropriate size all minimize the rate of refracture after removal of the fixator.

Overgrowth of a limb usually amounts to a few millimeters after treatment of a solitary closed fracture of the femoral shaft. It is primarily a concern in a preteenager who has had anatomic reduction of the femoral fracture and who has also had associated extensive soft-tissue injury in the ipsilateral extremity. Use of bayonet apposition for preteenagers who have a femoral fracture helps to eliminate this problem with limb length and possibly decreases the time to healing. Joint stiffness is unusual, even if the external fixator is used to bridge a joint, unless there is marked soft-tissue injury adjacent to the joint. Malalignment of the fracture in the frontal plane should be preventable, as the frame can be adjusted to correct malalignment quite readily. Rotational alignment of the

femur is more difficult to judge at the time of placement of the fixator pins. The use of an anteroposterior radiograph to view both ends of the bone helps to ensure correct alignment when pins are placed, thus avoiding malalignment, which most often results from internal rotation of the distal femoral fragment.

Treatment of Floating Joints
A floating joint, an injury involving a fracture of a long bone on each side of a joint, is a special injury that requires surgical stabilization of at least one of the fractures.[23,24] This injury most commonly involves the long bones adjacent to the knee and the elbow. Although floating joints are sometimes treated nonoperatively in children who are younger than 10 years of age,[23] I prefer some surgical stabilization even in young children. Treatment of floating joints in teenagers and of those involving fractures in the juxta-articular position has poorer results than treatment of fractures of the midpart of the shaft and those in children who are less than 10 years of age.[23] If there is swelling of the involved joint, I prefer to stabilize both fractures in order to evaluate the joint for ligamentous instability or another injury of bone or cartilage and in order to institute joint motion earlier. The primary difference between treatment of a floating joint in children and treatment of this injury in adults is that the fixation usually can be less rigid in children and skeletally immature adolescents; AO plates are used less often, and external fixation or fixation with an intramedullary rod is generally employed.

Treatment of Pelvic Fractures in Children Who Have Multiple Injuries
High-energy trauma often leads to pelvic fractures as a part of the multiple-system injury. Injuries to the pelvis and spine are associated with the longest hospital stays, the most admissions to the intensive care

unit, and the highest rates of mortality among patients with multiple injuries.[25] It has been demonstrated that associated head and abdominal injuries should be strongly suspected when a pelvic fracture and at least one other fracture are present, so careful examination of other systems is essential.[26] Trauma to viscera and soft-tissue structures adjacent to the osseous pelvis can cause life-threatening injuries, so resuscitation of the child initially takes precedence over stabilization of the pelvic fracture. Although at times a pelvic fracture may need to be stabilized immediately to help to control hemorrhage, it appears that the death of children who have a pelvic fracture usually results from a head injury, not the visceral or vascular injuries associated with the pelvic fracture.[27] However, while soft-tissue and visceral injuries are of high priority, incompletely treated orthopaedic injuries of the pelvis may lead to more permanent disability. Thus, these displaced fractures, like those of the long bones, need to be treated definitively and expeditiously, with the assumption that the child will eventually recover fully from any head injury that has occurred.

Pubic and Ischial Injuries
A fracture of the pubic or ischial ramus needs little orthopaedic treatment if it is the only osseous injury present in the pelvis. However, care needs to be taken to assess two primary areas: the posterior aspect of the pelvic ring and the genitourinary system. If the child is awake, examination for tenderness at the sacroiliac joints is indicated, and, if tenderness is present, a computed axial tomography scan of this area is needed. As most genitourinary injuries that occur with pelvic fractures are associated with those of the anterior aspect of the pelvic ring,[28] it is necessary to ensure that a urethral injury is not missed in a patient who has this type of fracture. If this is the only fracture of the pelvis, the patient should be managed with analgesics and bed rest until the pain is sufficiently relieved to allow weightbearing. Full weightbearing after a fracture of the pubic or ischial ramus will not displace the fracture, but the patient usually walks with crutches until the pain resolves, after which time full weightbearing is resumed.

Bilateral fracture of the pubic and ischial rami is a more severe injury, with more potential for injury to the adjacent soft-tissue structures, especially the urethra. Urologic consultation should be arranged in the emergency room soon after admission to assess the patient for a possible urethral injury. Although a bilateral fracture of the rami is relatively stable, there is often an associated injury of the posterior aspect of the pelvic ring or of the sacroiliac joint (a Malgaigne fracture). Because of this possibility, a computed axial tomography examination of the pelvis is needed to assess for injuries of the posterior sacroiliac joint or the ilium and to provide more information for the formulation of treatment plans. External fixation has been used,[19] but surgical stabilization is usually not needed in children and preteenagers, as healing is expected to occur quickly in these patients. Guidelines for internal stabilization of an injury of the posterior aspect of the pelvis in a teenager are similar to those for stabilization of this injury in adults. An injury of the posterior aspect of the pelvis in a child or a preteenager usually can be treated adequately with 4 weeks of bed rest to allow enough bone-healing for the commencement of weightbearing. If there is no posterior injury, weightbearing can begin when the pain subsides and the other injuries have healed sufficiently.

Diastasis of the pubic symphysis involves injury to the sacroiliac joints or the adjacent posterior part of the pelvic ring. Again, urologic consultation should be obtained in the emergency room or shortly after admission to the hospital to assess the patient for a possible urethral injury. The degree of injury of the poste- rior aspect of the pelvic ring is related to the degree of spread of the pubis anteriorly. Bed rest, with the patient lying either supine or on the side, is used for mild diastasis until the pain is gone, at which point walking is begun. In more severe cases, an external fixator placed anteriorly can be used to close the diastasis.[29] If a wide diastasis is left unreduced, the child will walk with increased external rotation of the lower limbs but should not have other functional problems.

Acetabular Injuries
An acetabular injury in a child usually occurs from the extension of an adjacent fracture into the acetabular region and usually is stable. Fractures of the pubic and ischial rami can extend into the triradiate cartilage and may lead to premature closure with cessation of the centrifugal growth of the triradiate cartilage. A fracture of the iliac wing may extend into the superior aspect of the acetabulum. If plain radiographs suggest extension of a fracture into the acetabulum or the triradiate cartilage, computed axial tomography scans should be made to define the injury more completely. If the acetabular fracture is displaced, open reduction and internal fixation is recommended to restore joint congruity.

Vertical Shear Fractures
A vertical shear fracture is the most serious type of pelvic injury in children. These fractures are unstable and are associated with visceral and other soft-tissue injuries.[30] The immediate problem associated with these fractures is bleeding, which can be either retroperitoneal from the fracture or intraperitoneal from injured abdominal organs.[31] Of the different types of pelvic fracture, bilateral anterior and posterior fractures are the most likely to cause severe hemorrhage.[32] The initial treatment usually involves replacement of blood volume and stabilization of the child's overall condition. While adults often die from the loss of

blood associated with severe pelvic fracture, it is much less common for a child to do so.[27] There may be instances in which a child needs external fixation of the pelvis to control hemorrhage, but children need such treatment far less often than adults do.[19] Although an anterior external fixation frame that is attached with pins to the iliac wings does not anatomically reduce a vertical shear fracture, the stability provided by the fixator appears to help to limit motion of the posterior aspect of the pelvis and, in this way, aid in controlling retroperitoneal hemorrhage.

Once lost blood has been replaced and blood loss has been controlled, imaging studies of the abdomen and pelvis should be performed to define the degree of injury. Plain radiography is used first, but it is nearly always necessary to perform a computed axial tomography scan of the abdomen and pelvis. At times, a 3-dimensional reconstruction of the computed axial tomography scan of the osseous pelvis is helpful to better visualize the extent of the injuries.[33] Stabilization with internal fixation is not usually needed in a young child with a vertical shear pelvic fracture, as these fractures heal even if they are moderately displaced. All children and preteenagers who do not have internal or external fixation of the pelvic fracture should be managed with skeletal traction, with use of a Steinmann pin in the distal aspect of the femur, to prevent further cephalad migration of the hemipelvis. If there is a concomitant femoral fracture, either external fixation or traction is used to reduce the femoral fracture to full length or the femur is slightly overlengthened to compensate for the approximately 1 cm of shortening of the lower extremity that occurs with cephalad displacement of the hemipelvis. In teenagers who have a vertical shear fracture, posterior reduction and plate-and-screw internal fixation is used in the same way as it is used in adults.

Nonorthopaedic Injuries Associated With Pelvic Fractures

Nonorthopaedic injuries associated with pelvic fractures are common; in one series, they occurred in 24 of 36 patients (67%) and 11 of these 36 patients (30%) had long-term morbidity or died.[34]

Neurologic Injuries Displacement of the hemipelvis or the iliac wing posteriorly can result in local neurologic deficits, either from injury to the sciatic nerve at the sciatic notch or from nerve-root avulsion at the lumbosacral level. The level of injury can be partially determined with a clinical examination, but it may be necessary to perform other imaging studies to assess the feasibility of treating this injury operatively. Myelography with computed axial tomography can be used to diagnose nerve-root avulsions by visualizing small meningoceles at the level of the injured nerve roots. If no nerve-root avulsion is noted and there is no clinical or electromyographic evidence of recovery in 6 to 9 months after the injury, exploration of the sciatic nerve is probably indicated in children before adolescence. The younger the child is, the better the outlook is for success of nerve-grafting for an injury of the sciatic nerve, if such a repair is possible. Surgical repair of nerve-root avulsion or of injury of the proximal aspect of the sciatic nerve generally is not recommended for teenagers because the distance between the injured area and the motor end plate in the muscles ennervated by these neural elements is too great to expect functional return.

Vascular Injuries Retroperitoneal hemorrhage may be a severe problem in children who have a pelvic fracture, but, as a rule, it is less of a problem in children than in adults. I do not recommend exploration of the retroperitoneal area. Blood replacement, external compression devices, and, at times, external fixation of the pelvis should allow control of the bleeding. If there is marked cephalad displacement of the hemipelvis, the superior

and inferior gluteal arteries at the sciatic notch can be injured, which may lead to local soft-tissue necrosis. Unless there is an open fracture involving the anterior aspect of the pelvic ring, injury of the iliac artery or femoral artery is uncommon.

Urologic Injuries Most urologic injuries occur from fractures of the anterior aspect of the pelvic ring. The injury is most common at the bulb of the urethra, but the bladder, the prostate, and other portions of the urethra also can be injured. When the trauma is severe, injury to a kidney is also possible, but most urologic injuries associated with pelvic fractures occur in the lower genitourinary tract distal to the ureters.[35]

Gynecologic Injuries Vaginal tears and fistulae between the vagina and the bladder may occur from severe injuries of the anterior aspect of the pelvic ring. Other fractures that displace the ilia or change the shape of the pelvic ring can lead to later problems associated with narrowing of the birth canal. The rate of cesarean section is substantially higher for young women who have had a pelvic fracture than in those who have not.[36] In children and adolescents, pelvic fractures heal in a predictable way, and nonunions are unusual, so it is very important that, in girls, the fracture be reduced at least to the degree needed to allow freedom from later complications during pregnancy and delivery.

Late Orthopaedic Sequelae of Pelvic Fractures

There are few late orthopaedic effects of pelvic fractures that have been appropriately treated initially. Limb-length discrepancy may result from vertical shear-type fractures, with cephalad migration of one hemipelvis. This discrepancy is usually mild, but if it is more than 2 cm consideration can be given to contralateral epiphyseodesis at the appropriate time to allow for equality of the limb lengths at maturity. Premature closure of the triradiate cartilage may result from a fracture that extended into this area, usually from the region of the pubic ramus. If the child is young when this occurs, the acetabulum will not develop its normal depth and hip dysplasia will occur in early adolescence. Surgical procedures to increase acetabular coverage of the femoral head may be needed at a later date.

References

1. Heinrich SD, Gallagher D, Harris M, Nadell JM: Undiagnosed fractures in severely injured children and young adults: Identification with technetium imaging. *J Bone Joint Surg* 1994;76A:561–572.

2. Cramer KE: The pediatric polytrauma patient. *Clin Orthop* 1995;318:125–135.

3. Colombani PM, Buck JR, Dudgeon DL, Miller D, Haller JA Jr: One-year experience in a regional pediatric trauma center. *J Pediatr Surg* 1985;20:8–13.

4. Poole GV, Miller JD, Agnew SG, Griswold JA: Lower extremity fracture fixation in head-injured patients. *J Trauma* 1992;32:654–659.

5. Tolo VT: Management of the multiply injured child, in Rockwaood CA Jr, Wilkins KE, Beaty JH (eds): *Fractures in Children*, ed 4. Philadelphia, PA, Lippincott-Raven, 1996, pp 83–95.

6. Gustilo RB, Anderson JT: Prevention of infection in the treatment of one thousand and twenty-five open fractures of long bones: Retrospective and prospective analyses. *J Bone Joint Surg* 1976;58A:453–458.

7. Kreder HJ, Armstrong P: A review of open tibia fractures in children. *J Pediatr Orthop* 1995;15:482–488.

8. Loder RT: Pediatric polytrauma: Orthopaedic care and hospital course. *J Orthop Trauma* 1987;1:48–54.

9. Lascombes P, Prevot J, Ligier JN, Metaizeau JP, Poncelet T: Elastic stable intramedullary nailing in forearm shaft fractures in children: 85 cases. *J Pediatr Orthop* 1990;10:167–171.

10. Wyrsch B, Mencio GA, Green NE: Open reduction and internal fixation of pediatric forearm fractures. *J Pediatr Orthop* 1996;16:644–650.

11. Canale ST, Tolo VT: Fractures of the femur in children. *J Bone Joint Surg* 1995;77A:294–315.

12. Kregor PJ, Song KM, Routt MLC Jr, Sangeorzan BJ, Liddell RM, Hansen ST Jr: Plate fixation of femoral shaft fractures in multiply injured children. *J Bone Joint Surg* 1993;75A: 1774–1780.

13. Heinrich SD, Drvaric DM, Darr K, MacEwen GD: The operative stabilization of pediatric diaphyseal femur fractures with flexible intramedullary nails: A prospective analysis. *J Pediatr Orthop* 1994;14:501–507.

14. Huber RI, Keller HW, Huber PM, Rehm KE: Flexible intramedullary nailing as fracture treatment in children. *J Pediatr Orthop* 1996;16: 602–605.

15. Aronson J, Tursky EA: External fixation of femur fractures in children. *J Pediatr Orthop* 1992;12:157–163.

16. Blasier RD, Aronson J, Tursky EA: External fixation of pediatric femur fractures. *J Pediatr Orthop* 1997;17:342–346.

17. Evanoff M, Strong ML, MacIntosh R: External fixation maintained until fracture consolidation in the skeletally immature. *J Pediatr Orthop* 1993;13:98–101.

18. Kirschenbaum D, Albert MC, Robertson WW Jr, Davidson RS: Complex femur fractures in children: Treatment with external fixation. *J Pediatr Orthop* 1990;10:588–591.

19. Reff RB: The use of external fixation devices in the management of severe lower-extremity trauma and pelvic injuries in children. *Clin Orthop* 1984;188:21–33.

20. Schranz PJ, Gultekin C, Colton CL: External fixation of fractures in children. *Injury* 1992;23:80–82.

21. Tolo VT: External skeletal fixation in children's fractures. *J Pediatr Orthop* 1983;3:435–442.

22. Tolo VT: External fixation in multiply injured children. *Orthop Clin North Am* 1990;21: 393–400.

23. Bohn WW, Durbin RA: Ipsilateral fractures of the femur and tibia in children and adolescents. *J Bone Joint Surg* 199173A:429–439.

24. Letts M, Vincent N, Gouw G: The "floating knee" in children. *J Bone Joint Surg* 1986;68B: 442–446.

25. Buckley SL, Gotshall C, Robertson W Jr, Sturm P, Tosi L, Thomas M, Eichelberger M: The relationships of skeletal injuries with trauma score, injury severity score, length of hospital stay, hospital charges, and mortality in children admitted to a regional pediatric trauma center. *J Pediatr Orthop* 1994;14:449–453.

26. Vazquez WD, Garcia VF: Pediatric pelvic fractures combined with an additional skeletal injury as an indicator of significant injury. *Surg Gynecol Obstet* 1993;177:468–472.

27. Musemeche CA, Fischer RP, Cotler HB, Andrassy RJ: Selective management of pediatric pelvic fractures: A conservative approach. *J Pediatr Surg* 1987;22:538–540.

28. Batislam E, Ates Y, Germiyanoglu C, Karabulut A, Gulerkaya B, Erol D: Role of tile classification in predicting urethral injuries in pediatric pelvic fractures. *J Trauma* 1997;42:285–287.

29. Torode I, Zieg D: Pelvic fractures in children. *J Pediatr Orthop* 1985;5:76–84.

30. Bond SJ, Gotshall CS, Eichelberger MR: Predictors of abdominal injury in children with pelvic fracture. *J Trauma* 1991;31:1169–1173.

31. Ismail N, Bellemare JF, Mollitt DL, DiScala C, Koeppel B, Tepas JJ III: Death from pelvic fracture: Children are different. *J Pediatr Surg* 1996;31:82–85.

32. McIntyre RC Jr, Bensard DD, Moore EE, Chambers J, Moore FA: Pelvic fracture geometry predicts risk of life-threatening hemorrhage in children. *J Trauma* 1993;35:423–429.

33. Magid D, Fishman EK, Ney DR, Kuhlman JE, Frantz KM, Sponseller PD: Acetabular and pelvic fractures in the pediatric patient: Value of two- and three-dimensional imaging. *J Pediatr Orthop* 1992;12:621–625.

34. Garvin KL, McCarthy RE, Barnes CL, Dodge BM: Pediatric pelvic ring fractures. *J Pediatr Orthop* 1990;10:577–582.

35. Abou-Jaoude WA, Sugarman JM, Fallat ME, Casale AJ: Indicators of genitourinary tract injury or anomaly in cases of pediatric blunt trauma. *J Pediatr Surg* 1996;31:86–89.

36. Copeland CE, Bosse MJ, McCarthy ML, MacKenzie EJ, Guzinski GM, Hash CS, Burgess AR: Effect of trauma and pelvic fracture on female genitourinary, sexual, and reproductive function. *J Orthop Trauma* 1997;11:73–81.

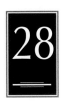

Acute Pain Following Musculoskeletal Injuries and Orthopaedic Surgery: Mechanisms and Management

Evan F. Ekman, MD

L. Andrew Koman, MD

Abstract

The undertreatment of acute pain associated with musculoskeletal conditions and surgical procedures is a focus of growing concern to orthopaedic surgeons. Fortunately, the armamentarium now includes recent advances in the understanding of how undertreated acute pain can lead to chronic pain, the development of new therapeutic agents, and new approaches to pain management. The concept of neuronal plasticity (the ability of neurons to profoundly alter their structure, function, or biochemical profile in response to repeated afferent sensory input) is now central to the understanding of the development of chronic pain from acute pain. Local inflammation in injured tissue increases the sensitization of specialized peripheral sensory neurons (nociceptors), leading to repeated afferent input into the central nervous system. Resolving inflammation before these events occur may prevent modifications in the central nervous system that lead to chronic pain. Therefore, it is important to reduce pain and inflammation at both the central and peripheral level. In addition to traditional agents (aspirin, nonspecific nonsteroidal anti-inflammatory drugs, opioids, local anesthetics, and regional blocks), more recently developed agents, such as cyclooxygenase-2 specific inhibitors, are now available. Combinations of these agents, as well as combinations of pharmacologic and nonpharmacologic approaches, are being used as multimodal therapy to treat the multiple sources of acute pain. Clinical practice guidelines for the management of acute pain now emphasize the incorporation of new knowledge into solid, evidence-based practice. This knowledge, combined with further understanding of the anatomic, physiologic, cellular, and molecular basis of pain, will provide the basis for future approaches to the management of acute pain in orthopaedic practice.

With the advent of new pain assessment standards and guidelines and advances in the development of analgesic agents, it is timely to discuss current and future approaches to the management of acute pain in orthopaedic practice. With the percentage of elderly patients increasing in the general population, orthopaedic specialists will see an unprecedented number of patients who not only report pain from acute musculoskeletal conditions but who also expect to stay active longer than previous generations.

It is increasingly acknowledged that acute postoperative pain from ambulatory surgery is undertreated and that the consequences of this add to the already huge burden of pain management on patients and society.[1-3] Recent advances in the elucidation of the biologic mechanisms underlying the development of both acute and chronic pain suggest that inadequately treated acute pain can result in the sensitization of the peripheral and central nervous system, which may ultimately lead to the development of chronic pain.[4-6]

The most common musculoskeletal injuries are those involving the back or spine, followed by sprains, dislocations, and fractures—the sum of which account for almost half of all musculoskeletal injuries.[7] Ankle injuries are the most common sports and recreational injuries, accounting for 38% to 45% of those injuries.[8,9] In 2001, 2.6 million people in North America were treated for foot and ankle injuries.[10] More than 40% of ankle sprains can progress to chronic problems.[11] Knee injuries also burden a considerable portion of the general population.

Arthroscopy of the knee is the second most common type of ambulatory surgical procedure in individuals between the ages of 15 and 44 years, with 357,000 such procedures performed in the United States in 1995.[12] Approximately 95,000 new instances of acute rupture of the anterior cruciate ligament occur annually in the United States, and approximately 50,000 of those are reconstructed each year.[13]

Orthopaedic procedures may induce more intense pain than other surgical procedures because bone injury is more painful than soft-tissue injury. This is because the periosteum has the lowest pain threshold of the deep somatic structures.[14] In two separate studies involving more than 10,000 patients in Canada and Sweden, patients who had undergone orthopaedic surgery had the most intense pain of all patients who had undergone ambulatory surgery.[1,15]

On the basis of these trends and statistics, orthopaedic surgeons should be adept at addressing acute pain associated with a variety of musculoskeletal conditions, including ankle sprains, back pain, and outpatient procedures. However, studies have suggested that the pain associated with these problems is often undertreated, particularly after ambulatory surgery. One study implied that orthopaedic surgeons undertreat pain, especially after shoulder surgery, surgery for hardware removal, and elbow arthroscopy.[1]

In addition, health care professionals may lack formal education in pain management or may have mistaken beliefs regarding potential opioid addiction and drug tolerance. Additional factors may be inadequate pain assessment, misinterpretation of orders, and the traditional emphasis on pro re nata dosing.[16,17]

Clinicians have primarily considered the undertreatment of pain to be a humanitarian concern. However, consequences can include adverse clinical outcomes and additional economic costs to the patient and provider.[18-20] Acute pain results in various physiologic changes that have important effects on the patient's clinical course. Unrelieved pain is likely to cause adverse effects on more than one body system, particularly in high-risk surgical patients, and the development of chronic pain.[21-23] For example, severe postoperative pain and increased levels of sympathetic activity may cause reductions in arterial inflow and venous emptying. In a patient who is relatively immobilized because of pain, a hypercoagulable state can lead to venous thrombosis and pulmonary embolism.[17,24] It is also generally believed that joint splinting and relative immobilization lead to joint

stiffness (such as arthrofibrosis in the knee and adhesive capsulitis in the shoulder). Reduced mobility of high-risk patients may also lead to pneumonia.[25]

Moreover, severe postoperative pain is a common reason for delays in hospital discharge and unanticipated hospital admissions.[26] Effective pain relief after surgery or acute injury can increase mobility and expedite a patient's return to normal function.[22] Furthermore, effective pain relief can lead to an earlier return to work and to psychologic benefits.

Over the past 30 years, great strides have been made in understanding the anatomic, physiologic, and molecular basis of pain mechanisms as well as in developing new therapeutic agents to manage pain. There have been major initiatives to refine and standardize guidelines for the assessment and treatment of acute pain. It is important for orthopaedic surgeons to be aware of these developments because they are relevant to current and future orthopaedic practice.

Anatomic, Physiologic, Cellular, and Molecular Considerations in Acute and Postoperative Pain Management

Pain Transmission in the Peripheral and Central Nervous Systems

To determine the most effective methods of treating acute pain and to avoid the subsequent development of chronic pain, it is important to understand the biologic mechanisms by which perception of acute pain develops and how acute pain can progress to chronic pain. Acute pain results from mechanically, chemically, or thermally induced damage to tissue integrity. Nociceptors, which are specialized peripheral sensory neurons, are activated in response to noxious stimuli and lead to neurotransmitter release in dorsal horn neurons in the spinal cord. Neurotransmitters, in turn, relay sensory information to the cerebral cortex by means of the thalamus and elicit acute pain as well as the withdrawal reflex and a variety of

heightened physiologic and emotional responses.[5]

A variety of chemicals released by damaged cells in response to tissue injury and local inflammation, including histamine, bradykinin, prostaglandins, serotonin, substance P, acetylcholine, and leukotrienes, further sensitizes nociceptors to other noxious stimuli.[4,27,28] Sensitization lowers the nociceptive threshold to painful stimuli and can result in repeated afferent input into the nervous system that leads to activation-dependent neuronal plasticity (the ability of neurons to profoundly alter their structure, function, or biochemical profile). Plasticity has been described as proceeding in three dynamically overlapping stages: activation, modulation, and modification[5] (Figure 1).

If inflammation from an injury is treated appropriately, the hypersensitivity that normally develops in damaged tissue resolves without causing major biochemical or cellular changes in the neurons. If inflammation persists, modulation of the pain perception system by inflammatory mediators induces biochemical alterations in receptors and ion channels on the cell surface of peripheral nociceptors. This results in increased sensitization of peripheral sensory neurons (peripheral sensitization).[5,29-31]

Increased and persistent afferent input to the dorsal horn leads to increased neurotransmitter release, activating signaling cascades in postsynaptic neurons. This increased signaling causes posttranslational changes (modulation) in secondary sensory neurons, such as phosphorylation of neuropeptide receptors (such as N-methyl-D-aspartate and α-amino-3-hydroxy-5-methyl-isoxazole-4-proprionic acid ion channels), which result in increased sensitivity to neurotransmitter activity, an influx of calcium and potassium ions, and depolarization of the neuronal membrane. These changes in neuronal sensitivity enhance activity in pain transmission neurons (central sensitization). These processes lead to amplified responses to all sensory input and result in allodynia (pain evoked by a normally innocuous stimulus) and hyperalgesia (an exaggerated, prolonged pain response). Disinhibition of spinal inhibitory mechanisms also occurs. Modification occurs in both peripheral and central neurons and involves induced expression of normally dormant genes that encode ion channels, receptors, and neurotransmitters.[31-36]

Cyclooxygenase-2 (COX-2) is also induced in dorsal horn neurons, with a concomitant increase in production of inflammatory prostaglandins such as prostaglandin E_2 (PGE$_2$). Additionally, there is widespread induction of COX-2 throughout the central nervous system, including the thalamus, ventral midbrain, and pons. Administration of nerve blocks in animal models of inflammation has resulted in partial, but not complete, inhibition of central COX-2 expression, suggesting that factors other than afferent input from the periphery are responsible for COX-2 induction in the central nervous system.[6] The inflammatory cytokine interleukin-1 (IL-1) also induces COX-2 expression and subsequent PGE$_2$ production in the central nervous system.[6] Administration of a COX-2–specific inhibitor or IL-1 receptor antagonist in these animal models reduced mechanical hyperalgesia, suggesting a role for COX-2 in the development of central sensitization.[6]

Sensitization of the peripheral and central nervous systems, if improperly treated, can result in neuronal plasticity such that hypersensitive pain responses persist even after the initial injury has resolved. It is believed that such modification of the central nervous system may ultimately lead to the development of chronic pain in some patients. Additionally, there is evidence of a neuropathic component in some chronic conditions arising from acute pain syndromes when nerve damage may have been sustained during the initial trauma.[5]

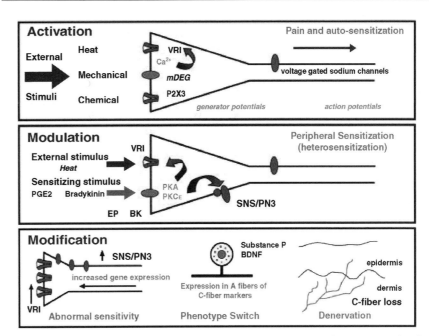

Figure 1 Illustration showing that the activation of nociceptive pathways begins at peripheral terminals of primary sensory neurons and that neuronal plasticity (activation, modulation, and modification) contributes to alteration of the nociceptor terminal threshold. (Reproduced with permission from Woolf CJ, Salter MW: Neuronal plasticity: Increasing the gain in pain. *Science* 2000;288:1765-1769.)

The complexity of the pain pathways involved in the perception and transmission of pain and in the development of peripheral and central sensitization suggests that no single analgesic agent will manage pain adequately. Multimodal therapy (such as the use of two or more analgesic agents with different modes of action) is becoming increasingly common.

Cognitive and Metabolic Modifiers of the Physiologic Pain Process

Pain is recognized not only as a sensory experience but also as a phenomenon with affective and cognitive components.[28,37] Factors such as age, gender, culture, communication skills, and previous pain experiences may play a role in determining an individual's perception of pain.[38,39] Physiologic and behavioral studies have shown that perception of pain is altered by previously conditioned cues in the environment or by the expectation of pain and suffering. In addition to pain,

tissue injury produces stress, which leads to the release of chemical mediators from the injury site, the adrenal cortex, and the immune system, all of which, in turn, interact with mediators of pain.[40]

The general stress response to surgical and other trauma results in endocrine and metabolic changes that affect respiratory, cardiovascular, gastrointestinal, genitourinary, and musculoskeletal systems. These changes can cause nausea, intestinal stasis, alterations in blood flow, coagulation, and fibrinolysis; increase demands on the cardiovascular and respiratory systems; and affect water and electrolyte flux.[23,41] The general stress response may be caused by nociceptive impulses and by factors including anxiety, hemorrhage, and infection as well as local tissue factors.[22,42]

Unrelieved pain can produce physiologic and psychologic effects, including delayed wound repair, muscle spasm, sensitization, limited mobility, and impaired immunocompetence. Anxiety and fear resulting from unrelieved severe acute pain can exacerbate the perception of pain and lead to behavioral changes, including depression. Pain also can cause sleeplessness, which can compound a vicious cycle of acute pain, anxiety, and additional sleep deprivation.[22,43] Acute pain has been associated with decreased peripheral blood flow, which can have deleterious effects on wound repair. Reflex responses, such as vasoconstriction, may be partly reversed by effective pain relief.[16,17]

Segmental and suprasegmental motor activity in response to pain results in muscle spasm, which can compound the pain. This cycle also may activate sharp increases in sympathetic activity and further increase the sensitivity of peripheral nociceptors.[22] Persistent postoperative pain and limited mobility may be associated with impaired muscle metabolism, muscular atrophy, and marked delays in the return to normal muscular function. In addition, changes in immunocompetence and acute-phase proteins after surgical trauma have been documented.[22]

The profound effects of pain transmission on the nervous system as well as the cognitive, metabolic, and physiologic responses to pain greatly emphasize the need for further development of effective therapeutic agents. After decades without fundamental advances in pain management options, discoveries in the past 30 years have led to the development of a variety of new modalities and the refinement of old ones.[44,45] Inflammatory mediators that sensitize nociceptors (such as prostaglandins and neurotransmitters) are major targets of both old and new drugs.

Pain Assessment Guidelines and Standards

Over the past 20 years, new pain management guidelines and standards have been proposed. In 1986, the World Health Organization proposed guidelines for the selection of appropriate drug regimens for pain.[46] Guidelines specifically for postoperative pain management were introduced in Australia in 1988 and in the United Kingdom in 1990.[47,48] The first Clinical Practice Guidelines for pain treatment were published in 1992 by the Agency for Health Care Policy and Research[49] (now called the Agency for Healthcare Research and Quality). The American Society of Anesthesiologists published Clinical Practice Guidelines for managing both acute and chronic pain.[50,51]

The National Pharmaceutical Council in collaboration with the Joint Commission on Accreditation of Healthcare Organizations recently published a comprehensive review of pain assessment and treatment guidelines.[52] These and other organizations have also developed clinical practice guidelines in specific disciplines and for management of pain resulting from specific conditions. The most current initiatives in postoperative pain management focus on providing comprehensive evidence-based research related to specific anatomic sites of surgery.[53,54] One such initiative is the Procedure Specific Postoperative Pain Management initiative, which can be found online (http://www.postoppain.org). The American Academy of Orthopaedic Surgeons has produced clinical guidelines, which are also available online (http://www.aaos.org/wordhtml/research/guidelin/guide.htm), for managing hip, knee, low back, wrist, and shoulder pain; ankle and knee injury; and knee osteoarthritis.

In 1995, the American Pain Society coined the phrase "Pain: The Fifth Vital Sign," with the intention that pain assessment should be considered to be as important as measurement of other vital signs.[55] The standards recommend that patients be assessed for pain every time pulse, blood pressure, core temperature, and respiration are measured. The Joint Commission on Accreditation of Healthcare Organizations adopted this idea and proposed that pain become a fifth vital sign for their 2000-2001 pain standards. An important concept in these standards is that patients have a right to have appropriate assessment and management of their pain. Organizations accredited by the Joint Commission on Accreditation of Healthcare Organizations are required not only to recognize each patient's right to pain assessment and treatment, but also to monitor responses to pain interventions and to provide pain management education to staff and patients.[56]

The development of a pain management plan should be a collaborative effort among the physician, nursing staff, anesthesiology team, patient, and patient's family.[57] A member of the anesthesiology department should obtain a pain history during the preoperative visit.[57]

According to the guidelines of the American Society of Anesthesiologists, pain assessment and reassessment should take place during the preoperative, intraoperative, and postoperative management of pain. The patient and family should be prepared preoperatively to understand their responsibilities in pain management, and pain management tools should be reviewed. The guidelines of the American Society of Anesthesiologists also recommend that the patient be involved in the determination of the pain score criteria that will result in a dose increment or another intervention and that the assessment of pain after surgery be frequent and simple.[58] Once the patient has recovered from anesthesia, the mainstay of pain assessment should be the patient's self-report, which should be used to assess pain perceptions and cognitive response, and the patient should be assessed for pain during routine activity such as movement.[57] It should be recognized that a patient's behavior and self-report of pain may show discrepancies as a result of excellent coping skills. Therefore, members of the health care team should emphasize the importance of a factual report from the patient.[57]

Pain Assessment Instruments

Pain measurement instruments are used to evaluate and document pain and are useful for studying pain mechanisms and for assessing methods for controlling pain. Clinicians also use pain end points as sensitive surrogates to demonstrate how a method of pain relief mediates postoperative responses, such as clinical course or recovery time. However, proving a correlation between a pain relief modality and postoperative responses requires very large sample populations because major outcomes, such as death or morbidity, are uncommon events among patients undergoing elective surgery. Other outcome variables, such as hypoxemia, return of bowel function, and pulmonary function, can be defined clearly and timed, but relationships between such variables and outcomes such as major morbidity are indirect.

Common pain assessment measures include pain intensity, pain relief, and function. When an appropriate measurement tool is being selected, the patient's age; developmental status; physical, emotional, or cognitive condition; and preference should be considered. Most pain instruments rely on verbal assessments of pain because the correlation between physical abnormalities and patients' reports of pain has been found to be poor and ambiguous. Intensity is considered to be the most salient dimension of pain, and many procedures for quantifying this dimension have been validated. However, because pain is a complex, multidimensional, subjective experience, the use of a single dimension, such as intensity, does not capture the other qualities and dimensions of the pain experience.

The visual analog scale is commonly used to measure pain intensity and pain relief.[59] It consists of a 10-cm horizontal line with the descriptors "no pain" and "pain as bad as it could possibly be" at the two ends. The patient places a mark at the point between the two ends that best represents the intensity of his or her pain. This scale has the advantage of being easy to administer and minimally obtrusive, but it does not take into account the subjective and multidimensional characteristics of pain, including affective qualities. It is, however, widely accepted and validated, and it is easily added to any existing medical record.

Another common tool for measuring pain intensity or pain relief is the Patient's Global Evaluation. Typically, the assessment uses a query such as "How would you rate the maximum pain relief after treatment?" or "How would you rate the study medication you received for pain?" Patients respond with a discrete number on a scale or select from among possible ratings such as excellent, very good, good, fair, or poor. The format of the Patient's Global Evaluation can also be used to measure a specific component, such as nausea.

In addition to the visual analog scale, the McGill Pain Questionnaire is the most frequently used self-rating instrument. It was designed to assess the multidimensional nature of the pain experience with use of sensory, affective, and evaluative words, and it has been demonstrated to be a reliable, valid, and consistent measurement tool. The McGill Pain Questionnaire evolved into components of the American Pain Society Patient Outcome Questionnaire.[60] It uses small groups of descriptive words to assess the sensory, subjective, and affective qualities of pain. The questionnaire is often used to assess chronic pain. Its purpose is to examine the level of disability and interference caused by pain.

Other ways to measure pain include assessing physical function, the behavioral manifestations of pain, and the psychologic contributions to the pain experience. Physical function can be evaluated with objective measures as well as with self-report of the ability to engage in a range of functional activities. Self-report devices measure components such as function, interference, and other affective qualities. Studies have shown high correlations among self-reports, disease characteristics, physicians' ratings of functional abilities, and objective functional performance. Although pain behaviors have not been found to be uniquely or invariably associated with the experience of pain, psychologic factors have been found to modulate pain responses. Therefore, instruments to assess psychologic factors associated with pain also have been developed and validated. Psychologic status, particularly anxiety, seems to influence pain and patient-controlled analgesia. Educating the patient about what to expect before, during, and after surgery can decrease anxiety and decrease postoperative pain. Anxiety can be measured by using a combination of qualitative components from the McGill Pain Questionnaire and the State-Trait Anxiety Inventory. Comprehensive approaches that address psychologic contributions to pain and suffering have been proposed for the measurement of pain.

Approaches to the Treatment of Acute Pain

Some of the oldest known analgesics are still used for the treatment of acute injury as well as pain after orthopaedic surgery. Use of opium as an analgesic dates back to before the first century BC. In the mid-nineteenth century, morphine and codeine were purified as alkaloids from opium. The bark of the willow tree, long known for its medicinal properties, was the predecessor to aspirin, which was first synthesized in 1860 for use as an antipyretic. Acetaminophen was first used medically in 1893.[61] In the late 1970s, ibuprofen was the first propionic acid derivative to be used in the United States. Naproxen, ketoprofen, and others followed in the 1980s.

In 1971, Vane[62] proposed inhibition of prostaglandin synthesis as the primary mechanism of action of nonsteroidal anti-inflammatory drugs. The enzyme responsible for the initial steps of prostaglandin synthesis from arachidonic acid, COX, was first isolated and purified in enzymatically active form in 1976.[63] The discovery in the early 1990s of two isoforms of COX (COX-1 and COX-2)[64,65] was followed by the development of a novel group of anti-inflammatory agents, the COX-2–specific inhibitors. A third COX enzyme, COX-3, was recently identified[66] and will be discussed in greater detail. In 1999, neuropeptides, including substance P, were discovered to have a role as the primary transmitters of nociceptive information; subsequently, a substance-P agonist was discovered.[67]

Although many targets for pain and analgesia have been discovered, no individual therapy targets them all, and it is unlikely that therapies under development will do so. Therefore, multimodal approaches to pain relief[41] and the potential for preemptive pain relief[68,69] have been studied.

Mechanisms and Actions of Therapies

The goals of pain management in orthopaedics are to meet the humanitarian need for pain relief and to facilitate rehabilitation and return to normal function. These goals are accomplished by reducing pain and inflammation at both the central and the peripheral levels.

Opioids Opioids include all endogenous and exogenous compounds that possess morphine-like analgesic properties. They are classified as agonists, agonist-antagonists, and antagonists and are characterized by their effects on individual or multiple opioid receptors. Categories of agonists commonly used for analgesia include the phenanthrene alkaloids (such as morphine and codeine), the semisynthetic opioids (such as hydrocodone and oxycodone), and the

synthetic opioids (such as meperidine, fentanyl, and sufentanil). Commonly used agonist-antagonists are the semisynthetic opioids (such as buprenorphine and nalbuphine).

In orthopaedic practice, opioids are commonly used to treat moderate-to-severe pain, usually acute in nature, such as that associated with fractures and soft-tissue injury. Opioids produce their analgesic effect by mimicking the actions of endogenous opioid peptides at specific receptors within the central nervous system. The three major classes of opioid receptors are mu (μ) (to which morphine binds), kappa (κ), and delta (δ); in addition, there are subtype receptors within each class. For example, μ_1 produces supraspinal analgesia, and μ_2 affects respiratory, cardiovascular, and gastrointestinal function. The κ and δ receptors also produce spinal analgesia, and sedation results from the activation of the κ receptors.[70]

Although μ agonists produce alterations in mood and sleep, unconsciousness cannot be guaranteed at anesthetic doses. The effects of μ agonists on bowel motility are the result of concomitant reduction in the propulsive peristaltic contractions of both the small and the large intestine and enhanced sphincteric tone. Also, by stimulating the vagal nucleus in the medulla, agonists produce dose-dependent bradycardia.[70,71]

Nonspecific Nonsteroidal Anti-Inflammatory Drugs The primary mechanism of action of nonsteroidal anti-inflammatory drugs is inhibition of prostaglandin production by the COX enzyme.[62] Analgesia and the anti-inflammatory activity of nonsteroidal anti-inflammatory drugs are produced by inhibition of the COX-2 isoenzyme.

Arachidonic acid metabolism produces prostanoids that regulate normal cell activity, notably in the gastric mucosa, kidney, and vascular endothelial cells. COX-1 is expressed constitutively in these and most other tissues, whereas COX-2 is inducibly expressed only in the

central nervous system, kidney, tracheal epithelium, and testicles.[72] PGE_2 is produced in the gastrointestinal tract; it acts as a vasodilator and plays a key role in defense and repair mechanisms designed to maintain gastrointestinal mucosal integrity. In the kidney, PGE_2 induces diuresis and natriuresis.[73] It also exerts an inhibitory action on lymphocytes and on other cells that participate in inflammatory and allergic responses.[74] In platelets, thromboxane A_2 is the primary metabolite of arachidonic acid.[73] Prostacyclin potently inhibits platelet aggregation and has vasodilatory effects.[73] Conventional nonsteroidal anti-inflammatory drugs such as ibuprofen, meloxicam, naproxen, and diclofenac have a relatively linear structure, which allows them to fit readily into the active site of both COX-1 and COX-2 and thus to nonspecifically inhibit both isoforms.[75,76] The anti-inflammatory and analgesic effects of nonspecific nonsteroidal anti-inflammatory drugs result from the inhibition of COX-2, whereas the inhibition of COX-1 adversely affects the production of prostanoids involved in normal homeostatic mechanisms such as protection of gastric mucosa.

COX-2–Specific Inhibitors In contrast to nonspecific nonsteroidal anti-inflammatory drugs, COX-2–specific agents, including celecoxib, rofecoxib (recently withdrawn from the market), and valdecoxib, were developed with a bulky side chain that binds to the catalytic binding site of COX-2 with substantially greater affinity than it binds to the binding site of COX-1, allowing selective inhibition.

A parenteral water-soluble prodrug of valdecoxib, parecoxib sodium (parecoxib), is available in the European Union for treatment of short-term postoperative pain[77] and is currently an investigational drug in the United States. Other COX-2–specific inhibitors, such as etoricoxib[78,79] and lumiracoxib,[80] are also being investigated.

COX-2–specific inhibitors are at least

as effective as nonspecific nonsteroidal anti-inflammatory drugs for managing pain associated with chronic conditions such as osteoarthritis[81-86] and rheumatoid arthritis[87-89] as well as pain resulting from acute soft-tissue injury. In a study of acute ankle sprains, the time to return to normal activity was reduced by 1 day for patients treated with celecoxib compared with those treated with a nonspecific nonsteroidal anti-inflammatory drug.[90] COX-2–specific inhibitors have also been shown to be as effective as hydrocodone or acetaminophen in relieving postoperative pain following various ambulatory orthopaedic procedures, including anterior cruciate ligament repair, laminectomy, open reduction and internal fixation of long bone fractures, and osteotomy.[91] They have also demonstrated efficacy in relieving postoperative pain from oral surgery,[92] hip arthroplasty,[93] and bunionectomy.[94]

COX-2–specific inhibitors not only have similar efficacy but also have greater gastrointestinal safety and tolerability compared with nonspecific nonsteroidal anti-inflammatory drugs. The results of multiple clinical trials have shown that treatment with COX-2–specific inhibitors is associated with significantly fewer ulcer-related complications than treatment with nonspecific nonsteroidal anti-inflammatory drugs ($P < 0.05$).[95] One example is the Vioxx Gastrointestinal Outcomes Research (VIGOR) trial,[96] which compared the safety and efficacy of rofecoxib (50 mg daily) and naproxen (500 mg daily) in 8,076 patients with rheumatoid arthritis who were treated over 9 months. The results of this trial indicated that rofecoxib caused significantly fewer upper gastrointestinal events than did naproxen ($P < 0.05$). On September 30, 2004, Merck withdrew rofecoxib worldwide because of cardiovascular safety concerns. Another example is the Celecoxib Long-Term Arthritis Safety Study (CLASS),[97] which was conducted over 6 months and involved 8,059

patients with osteoarthritis and rheumatoid arthritis. The results of this study showed that, even at supratherapeutic doses (400 mg twice daily), celecoxib was associated with a lower prevalence of gastrointestinal ulcers and ulcer-related complications than were therapeutic doses of ibuprofen (800 mg three times daily) or diclofenac (75 mg twice daily). Analysis of long-term (13- to 15-month) follow-up data from the CLASS study revealed that the combined prevalence of complicated and symptomatic gastrointestinal ulcers associated with nonspecific nonsteroidal anti-inflammatory drugs was greater than that associated with celecoxib.[98]

Other studies have shown that even short-term use of COX-2–specific inhibitors is significantly less toxic to the upper gastrointestinal mucosa than short-term use of nonspecific nonsteroidal anti-inflammatory drugs ($P < 0.05$). A preliminary endoscopic study of the upper gastrointestinal tract demonstrated gastric ulcers in 19% of patients who had taken naproxen for 1 week but in none who had taken celecoxib for the same duration.[99] Another study comparing the effects of valdecoxib (40 mg twice daily) and naproxen (500 mg twice daily) in healthy elderly subjects showed that, even after only 1 week of treatment, naproxen was associated with a significantly higher prevalence of gastroduodenal ulcers than was valdecoxib ($P < 0.05$).[100]

There is some evidence that use of rofecoxib is associated with an increased prevalence of adverse cardiovascular events. In the VIGOR trial, the rate of myocardial infarction with rofecoxib was threefold to fourfold higher than the rate with naproxen.[96] However, in the CLASS trial, there were no significant differences among celecoxib, diclofenac, and ibuprofen with regard to the prevalence of adverse cardiovascular events, even in patients who were not taking aspirin.[97] In a recent matched case-control study of 54,475 patients with osteoarthritis taking

either celecoxib or rofecoxib, use of rofecoxib was associated with an increased adjusted relative risk of acute myocardial infarction.[101] This risk was highest in patients taking more than 25 mg of rofecoxib. Although the most recent data have yet to be published, cardiovascular safety with COX-2–specific inhibitor use is an issue sparking enormous medical and public concern.

Platelet aggregation and hemostasis depend on the ability of platelets to generate thromboxane A_2, which is synthesized from arachidonic acid by COX. Platelets lack COX-2 and depend on COX-1 to indirectly produce thromboxane. Because nonspecific nonsteroidal anti-inflammatory drugs prevent the formation of prostaglandins through the inhibition of COX-1, the tendency toward bleeding is increased.[102] Aspirin exerts these effects irreversibly for the life of the circulating platelet, whereas other nonspecific nonsteroidal anti-inflammatory drugs have a reversible, dose-dependent effect. Normal platelet function is reflected by a normal bleeding time. For the orthopaedist, normal platelet function is clinically important in surgically treated patients in whom appropriate hemostasis decreases perioperative bleeding and the comorbidities associated with it (including hemarthrosis, wound problems, infection, poor visualization during arthroscopy, and an increased need for transfusion). In patients with acute injuries such as ankle sprain, bleeding causes volumetric changes in addition to pain and inflammation; thus, normal platelet aggregation is again important. Bleeding also has a bearing on rehabilitation because hemarthroses have a deleterious effect on motion and strength. In this area, COX-2–specific inhibitors are an attractive alternative to nonspecific nonsteroidal anti-inflammatory drugs because of their lack of clinically important effects on platelet aggregation and bleeding time. All COX-2–specific inhibitors, including celecoxib, valdecoxib, parecoxib, and rofecoxib—even at supratherapeutic doses—have been shown to not interfere with platelet function, even in elderly patients.[103-107]

The decision whether to use a nonspecific nonsteroidal anti-inflammatory drug or a COX-2–specific inhibitor depends on the individual situation. Although COX-2–specific inhibitors and nonspecific nonsteroidal anti-inflammatory drugs have similar efficacy, care must be taken to assess the risks, limitations, and benefits before selecting the appropriate treatment. When the risk of gastrointestinal complications and compromised platelet function is not a consideration, nonspecific nonsteroidal anti-inflammatory drugs may be the treatment of choice. On the other hand, if there is an elevated risk of gastrointestinal bleeding, ulceration, or ulcer-related complications, it would be preferable to use a COX-2–specific inhibitor—even if only short-term treatment is warranted. In situations in which normal platelet function is useful, as in any surgical procedure, or in cases of acute injury in which bleeding, hemarthrosis, and ecchymosis may be part of the pathology, a COX-2–specific inhibitor should be considered. At present, it is not clear how cardiovascular disease should affect clinical decision making in regard to COX-2–specific inhibitors.

Centrally Acting Nonopioids The antipyretic and analgesic effects of acetaminophen (paracetamol) are centrally mediated. Acetaminophen is believed to exert its analgesic effects by increasing the pain threshold, possibly by means of central inhibition of prostaglandin production. Its antipyretic properties have been attributed to its action on the hypothalamic heat center.[108] Acetaminophen has been shown to selectively inhibit COX-3, a COX-1 variant recently cloned from the canine cerebral cortex.[66] There is some biochemical evidence of the existence of a third human COX isoform, the human COX-3 isoform, which may play a role in the central analgesic and antipyretic effects of acetaminophen.[66,109-111]

Acetaminophen or aspirin, when compounded with narcotics, effectively relieves moderate-to-severe acute postoperative pain.[17] Oral preparations of opioids such as morphine and meperidine are not well absorbed alone. However, oxycodone is particularly effective as a result of its relatively high absorption rate, and it is often used in combination with acetaminophen.[17]

Tramadol, a synthetic analog of codeine,[112] has a dual mode of action, both as a centrally acting analgesic agent with a weak affinity for the μ, omega (ω), and opioid receptors and as an inhibitor of norepinephrine and serotonin uptake. Orally administered tramadol and nonsteroidal anti-inflammatory drugs are useful as supplements to treatment with regional neural blockade in patients with mild-to-moderate pain.

The combination of tramadol and acetaminophen has been used successfully to treat moderate to moderately severe acute and chronic pain. This combination has several advantages, including rapid onset of analgesia from the acetaminophen and a longer duration of analgesia from the tramadol. Adverse events associated with this combination are similar to those observed with tramadol monotherapy, such as dizziness or vertigo and seizure.[113,114] In studies of postoperative dental pain, the combination of tramadol and acetaminophen has been shown to be more effective than either agent alone and to provide efficacy similar to that of a hydrocodone-paracetamol combination.[115]

Local and Regional Anesthesia Local anesthetics are used primarily for surgery, as opposed to acute injury or nonsurgical pain. Local anesthesia and regional blocks are often used by themselves for anesthesia and as part of a multimodal approach to perioperative pain management.

Local anesthetics may block peripheral nerve function through several mechanisms, with their primary mode being through sodium channel and axonal conductive blockade. These agents may reduce sodium conductance by interacting with the surrounding lipid membrane or by altering membrane fluidity.[116] Local anesthetics have extensive effects on presynaptic calcium channels that function to stimulate the release of neurotransmitters. Interference with calcium channel conductance can potentiate spinal anesthesia.[117]

When administered as an epidural infusion, local anesthetics such as ropivacaine or bupivacaine are effective analgesics, particularly in patients who are highly susceptible to the adverse effects associated with opioids. Placement of the epidural tip at the dermatomal level relevant to the surgery, with continuous infusions of dilute anesthetic (approximately 0.1% at 5 to 12 mL/h) can minimize adverse events such as hypotension and impaired micturition and can maximize the analgesic effect.[17]

It is important to note that the analgesic effects of neuraxial blocks only partially inhibit pain responses and do not affect any humoral component such as the activity of inflammatory cytokines like IL-1.[6] Additionally, the analgesic effects are quickly reversed when the block is removed.[16] Therefore, these agents should be used in conjunction with other forms of pain control.

Neuraxial analgesia can be associated with adverse effects such as respiratory depression, nausea, and pruritus; patients should be monitored constantly to minimize these problems. Prophylactic naloxone infusions can relieve respiratory depression as well as other opioid-related adverse effects in elderly patients.[118] Prophylaxis against deep venous thrombosis with low-molecular-weight heparin in patients treated with spinal or epidural neuraxial analgesia is associated with a risk of epidural hematoma. Guidelines for preventing this problem were recently proposed by the American

Society of Regional Anesthesia and Pain Medicine.[119]

Novel Approaches to Treatment of Acute Pain

Multimodal Analgesia

There is a trend toward increasing utilization of multimodal analgesia in orthopaedic surgery and for the management of musculoskeletal injury. A combination of approaches, both pharmacologic and nonpharmacologic (such as the use of ice or cooling units), can address multiple mechanisms of pain, with the added benefit of reducing adverse effects through the use of lower doses of individual modalities.[120] There is increasing evidence that multimodal therapy can shorten the hospital stay, lessen the adverse effects of opioids by decreasing dosage, and improve patient outcomes.[41]

Several randomized trials have demonstrated the effectiveness and opioid-sparing properties of nonspecific nonsteroidal anti-inflammatory drugs such as ibuprofen, diclofenac,[121] and piroxicam[122] in the relief of acute postoperative pain.

Recently, several studies have shown that following hip or knee arthroplasty administration of the COX-2–specific inhibitors valdecoxib[93,123] (off-label use) and parecoxib[124,125] (investigational in the United States) significantly reduces the dose of opioid required for effective acute postoperative analgesia and provides better pain relief than does opioid analgesia alone ($P < 0.05$). A study of the efficacy of intravenous doses of parecoxib (20 and 40 mg), ketorolac (30 mg), and morphine (4 mg) in relieving postoperative pain following total knee replacement showed that parecoxib and ketorolac have a similar onset of action, duration of analgesia, and level of analgesia.[126] Morphine was similar to parecoxib and ketorolac with regard to onset of action but provided a significantly shorter duration and lower level of analgesia ($P < 0.01$).

Several studies have shown that parecoxib administered intravenously before laparoscopic cholecystectomy followed by postoperative treatment with oral valdecoxib (off-label use) reduces opioid use, with concomitant improvement in health outcomes and a reduction in opioid-related adverse effects.[127-129]

Preemptive Analgesia

The overall value of preemptive analgesia has been examined in several reviews and still remains controversial.[68,130] Until recently, the central question regarding preemptive analgesia was whether an intervention performed before pain starts has a greater analgesic effect than does the same intervention (with the same route and dose) performed after the onset of pain.[131] Using this strict definition of preemptive analgesia, McQuay and associates[131] concluded that there was no evidence that nonsteroidal anti-inflammatory drugs or acetaminophen had a preemptive effect. Their studies of opioid or local anesthetic infiltration showed mixed results, and they did not find spinal and nerve blocks to have any effect.

Few studies have provided unequivocal support for the concept of preemptive analgesia according to this conventional definition. However, Kissin[69] reviewed the studies on preemptive analgesia and recommended that the definition be extended to include the reduction of central sensitization. Using this definition, the author concluded that the evidence from positive clinical studies in combination with basic science sufficiently validates the phenomenon of preemptive analgesia.

Preemptive analgesia may have less of an effect in patients with preoperative pain who undergo orthopaedic procedures, as was demonstrated in a study showing a definitive preemptive effect on postoperative pain following hardware removal and mass excision, but less of an effect after fracture and arthritis-related surgery.[132,133] Although preemptive analgesia had been considered the domain of anesthesiologists, orthopaedic surgeons are now taking a more active role in developing preemptive analgesia protocols.

It has also been suggested that the timing of preemptive analgesia, coordinated so that the analgesic reaches peak levels in the peripheral and central nervous system as a surgical procedure begins, may influence the effectiveness of postoperative pain relief. It has been proposed that additional studies on the timing of aggressive protective perioperative multimodal therapy, rather than conventional perioperative doses, be performed to determine whether this is the case.[134]

The terms preoperative analgesia and preemptive analgesia have often been used interchangeably; however, they are not necessarily equivalent. Preemptive analgesia is preventive and does not simply imply administration before surgery. Therefore, not all preoperative analgesia is preemptive.[69,134]

Nonpharmacologic Management

Nonpharmacologic interventions include behavioral interventions and physical agents. Cognitive behavioral therapies can change patients' perceptions of pain, alter pain behavior, and provide patients with a greater sense of control over pain. Physical agents provide comfort, correct physical dysfunction, alter physiologic responses, and reduce fears associated with pain-related immobility or restriction of activity. Examples of physical modalities include application of superficial heat or cold, massage, exercise, immobility, and electroanalgesia, such as transcutaneous electrical nerve stimulation. Nonpharmacologic interventions are not intended to substitute for pharmacologic or other invasive techniques of pain management. However, they are sometimes used in the multimodal approach to analgesia by contributing to the effects of pharmacologic analgesia.[57]

Summary

In recent years, orthopaedic surgeons have become increasingly aware of the problems caused by undertreated acute pain following musculoskeletal injuries and orthopaedic surgery. As outlined in this chapter, many steps have been taken to improve awareness as well as treatment of acute pain. In addition, there are new approaches to anesthesia and analgesia, including preemptive analgesia and multimodal therapy. Potential future therapeutic targets include IL-1, which has been shown to induce expression of COX-2 in the central nervous system.[6] Inhibition of IL-1 possibly prevents not only production of COX-2 but also other mediators of inflammation such as PGE synthase.[45] The future of pain management requires further development of standards, guidelines, and pain assessment tools rooted in evidence-based practice. Advances in the understanding of the molecular mechanisms underlying neuronal plasticity should provide the basis for the next generation of therapies for effective management of acute pain in orthopaedic practice.

References

1. Chung F, Ritchie E, Su J: Postoperative pain in ambulatory surgery. *Anesth Analg* 1997;85:808-816.

2. Cousins MJ: Pain: The past, present, and future of anesthesiology? *Anesthesiology* 1999;91:538-551.

3. Tong D, Chung F: Postoperative pain control in ambulatory surgery. *Surg Clin North Am* 1999;79:401-430.

4. Carr DB, Goudas LC: Acute pain. *Lancet* 1999;353:2051-2058.

5. Woolf CJ, Salter MW: Neuronal plasticity: Increasing the gain in pain. *Science* 2000;288:1765-1769.

6. Samad TA, Moore KA, Sapirstein A, et al: Interleukin-1-mediated induction of COX-2 in the CNS contributes to inflammatory pain hypersensitivity. *Nature* 2001;410:471-475.

7. Praemer A, Furner S, Rice DP: *Musculoskeletal Conditions in the United States.* Rosemont, IL, American Academy of Orthopaedic Surgeons, 1999.

8. Liu SH, Jason WJ: Lateral ankle sprains and instability problems. *Clin Sports Med* 1994;13:793-809.

9. Liu SH, Nguyen TM: Ankle sprains and other soft tissue injuries. *Curr Opin Rheumatol* 1999;11:132-137.

10. Cherry DK, Burt CW, Woodwell DK: *National Ambulatory Medical Care Survey: 2001 Summary: Advance Data from Vital and Health Statistics No. 337.* Hyattsville, MD, National Center for Health Statistics, 2003.

11. Safran MR, Benedetti RS, Bartolozzi AR III, Mandelbaum BR: Lateral ankle sprains: A comprehensive review: Part 1. Etiology, pathoanatomy, histopathogenesis, and diagnosis. *Med Sci Sports Exerc* 1999;31(suppl 7):S429-S437.

12. McLemore T, Lawrence L: Plan and operation of the National Survey of Ambulatory Surgery. *Vital Health Stat 1* 1997;37:1-124.

13. Frank CB, Jackson DW: The science of reconstruction of the anterior cruciate ligament. *J Bone Joint Surg Am* 1997;79:1556-1576.

14. Duc TA: Postoperative pain control, in Conroy JM, Dorman BH (eds): *Anesthesia for Orthopedic Surgery.* New York, NY, Raven Press, 1994, pp 355-365.

15. Rawal N, Hylander J, Nydahl PA, Olofsson I, Gupta A: Survey of postoperative analgesia following ambulatory surgery. *Acta Anaesthesiol Scand* 1997;41:1017-1022.

16. Sinatra RS: Acute pain management and acute pain services, in Cousins MJ, Bridenbaugh PO (eds): *Neural Blockade in Clinical Anesthesia and Management of Pain,* ed 3. Philadelphia, PA, Lippincott-Raven, 1998, pp 793-835.

17. Sinatra RS, Torres J, Bustos AM: Pain management after major orthopaedic surgery: Current strategies and new concepts. *J Am Acad Orthop Surg* 2002;10:117-129.

18. Stephens J, Laskin B, Pashos C, Pena B, Wong J: The burden of acute postoperative pain and the potential role of the COX-2-specific inhibitors. *Rheumatology* 2003;42:(suppl 3): 40-52.

19. Hartmann CW, Goldfarb NI, Kim SS, Nuthulaganti BR, Seifeldin R: Care management for persistent pain: An introduction. *Dis Manag* 2003;6:103-110.

20. Moulin DE, Clark AJ, Speechley M, Morley-Forster PK: Chronic pain in Canada: Prevalence, treatment, impact and the role of opioid analgesia. *Pain Res Manag* 2002;7:179-184.

21. Kehlet H, Rung GW, Callesen T: Postoperative opioid analgesia: Time for reconsideration? *J Clin Anesth* 1996;8:441-445.

22. Cousins M, Power I: Acute and postoperative pain, in Wall PD, Melzack R (eds): *Textbook of Pain,* ed 4. Philadelphia, PA, WB Saunders, 1999, pp 447-491.

23. Fine PG, Ashburn MA: Functional neuroanatomy and nociception, in Ashburn MA, Rice LJ (eds): *The Management of Pain.* New York, NY, Churchill Livingstone, 1998, pp 1-16.

24. Modig J, Borg T, Karlstom G, Maripuu E, Sahlstedt B: Thromboembolism after total hip replacement: Role of epidural and general anesthesia. *Anesth Analg* 1983;62:174-180.

25. Craig DB: Postoperative recovery of pulmonary function. *Anesth Analg* 1981;60:46-52.

26. Gold BS, Kitz DS, Lecky JH, Neuhaus JM: Unanticipated admission to the hospital following ambulatory surgery. *JAMA* 1989;262:3008-3010.

27. Basbaum AI, Jessell TM: The perception of pain, in Kandel ER, Schwartz JH, Jessell TM (eds): *Principles of Neural Science,* ed 4. New York, NY, McGraw-Hill, 2000, pp 472-491.

28. Scholz J, Woolf CJ: Can we conquer pain? *Nat Neurosci* 2002;(suppl 5):1062-1067.

29. Levine JD, Reichling DB: Peripheral mechanisms of inflammatory pain, in Wall PD, Melzack R (eds): *Textbook of Pain,* ed 4. New York, NY, Churchill Livingstone, 1999, pp 59-84.

30. Wajima Z, Hua XY, Yaksh TL: Inhibition of spinal protein kinase C blocks substance P-mediated hyperalgesia. *Brain Res* 2000;877: 314-321.

31. Yaksh TL, Hua XY, Kalcheva I, Nozaki-Taguchi N, Marsala M: The spinal biology in humans and animals of pain states generated by persistent small afferent input. *Proc Natl Acad Sci USA* 1999;96:7680-7686.

32. Chery N, de Koninck Y: Junctional versus extra-junctional glycine and GABA(A) receptor-mediated IPSCs in identified lamina I neurons of the adult rat spinal cord. *J Neurosci* 1999;19:7342-7355.

33. Okano K, Kuraishi Y, Satoh M: Involvement of spinal substance P and excitatory amino acids in inflammatory hyperalgesia in rats. *Jpn J Pharmacol* 1998;76:15-22.

34. Hua XY, Chen P, Marsala M, Yaksh TL: Intrathecal substance P-induced thermal hyperalgesia and spinal release of prostaglandin E2 and amino acids. *Neuroscience* 1999;89:525-534.

35. Ma QP, Woolf CJ: Involvement of neurokinin receptors in the induction but not the maintenance of mechanical allodynia in rat flexor motoneurones. *J Physiol* 1995;486:769-777.

36. Woolf CJ, Thompson SW: The induction and maintenance of central sensitization is dependent on N-methyl-D-aspartic acid receptor activation: Implications for the treatment of post-injury pain hypersensitivity states. *Pain* 1991;44:293-299.

37. Merskey H, Bogduk N (eds): Task Force on Taxonomy of the International Association for the Study of Pain, in *Classification of Chronic Pain: Descriptions of Chronic Pain Syndromes and Definitions of Pain Terms.* Seattle, WA, IASP Press, 1994.

38. Burns JW, Hodsman NB, McLintock TT, Gillies GW, Kenny GN, McArdle CS: The influence of patient characteristics on the requirements for postoperative analgesia: A reassessment using patient-controlled analgesia. *Anaesthesia* 1989;44:2-6.

39. Preble LM, Guveyan JA, Sinatra RS: Patient characteristics influencing postoperative pain management, in Sinatra RS, Hord AH, Ginsberg B, Preble LM (eds): *Acute Pain: Mechanisms and Management.* St Louis, MO, Mosby-Year Book, 1992, pp 140-150.

40. Loeser JD, Melzack R: Pain: An overview. *Lancet* 1999;353:1607-1609.

41. Kehlet H, Wilmore DW: Multimodal strategies to improve surgical outcome. *Am J Surg* 2002;183:630-641.

42. Kehlet H: Acute pain control and accelerated postoperative surgical recovery. *Surg Clin North Am* 1999;79:431-443.

43. Peck CL: Psychological factors in acute pain management, in Cousins MJ, Phillips GD (eds): *Acute Pain Management*. New York, NY, Churchill Livingstone, 1986, pp 251-274.

44. Bonica JJ: History of pain concepts and pain therapy. *Mt Sinai J Med* 1991;58:191-202.

45. Samad TA, Sapirstein A, Woolf CJ: Prostanoids and pain: Unraveling mechanisms and revealing therapeutic targets. *Trends Mol Med* 2002;8:390-396.

46. Expert WHO: Committee on Cancer Pain Relief and Active Supportive Care. *Cancer Pain Relief and Palliative Care*. Geneva, Switzerland, World Health Organization, 1986.

47. National Health and Medical Research Council: (Australia): *Acute Pain Management: Scientific Evidence*. Canberra, Australia, 1999.

48. Royal College of Surgeons of England: College of Anaesthetists Commission on the Provision of Surgical Services: *Report on the Working Party on Pain After Surgery*. London, England, Royal College of Surgeons, 1990.

49. Carr DB, Jacox A: *Acute Pain Management: Operative or Medical Procedures and Trauma: Clinical Practice Guideline*. Rockville, MD, Agency for Health Care Policy and Research, Public Health Service, US Department of Health and Human Services, AHCPR publication no. 92-0032, 1992.

50. Ready LB, Ashburn M, Caplan RA, et al: Practice guidelines for acute pain management in the perioperative setting: A report by the American Society of Anesthesiologists Task Force on Pain Management, Acute Pain Section. *Anesthesiology* 1995;82:1071-1081.

51. Wilson PR, Caplan RA, Connis RT, et al: Practice guidelines for chronic pain management: A report by the American Society of Anesthesiologists Task Force on Pain Management, Chronic Pain Section. *Anesthesiology* 1997;86:995-1004.

52. National Pharmaceutical Council Website: Joint Commission on Accreditation of Healthcare Organizations: Pain: Current understanding of assessment, management and treatments: December 2001. Available at: http://www.npcnow.org/resources/PDFs/pain-monograph.pdf. Accessed February 19, 2004.

53. Rosenquist RW, Rosenberg J: United States Veterans Administration: Postoperative pain guidelines. *Reg Anesth Pain Med* 2003;28: 279-288.

54. Rowlingson JC, Rawal N: Postoperative pain guidelines: Targeted to the site of surgery. *Reg Anesth Pain Med* 2003;28:265-267.

55. Campbell J: Pain: The fifth vital sign. Presidential address. Los Angeles, CA: American Pain Society; November 11, 1995. Available at: http://www.ampain-soc.org/advocacy/fifth.htm. Accessed November 12, 2003.

56. Joint Commission on Accreditation of Healthcare Organizations (JCAHO): New clinical practice guidelines standards. *Jt Comm Perspect* 1999;19:6-8.

57. Acute Pain Management Guideline Panel: *Acute pain management: Operative or medical procedures and trauma: Clinical practice guideline*. Rockville, MD: US Department of Health and Human Services, Public Health Service, Agency for Health Care Policy and Research. 1992.

58. Ashburn MA, Caplan RA, Carr DB, et al: Practice guidelines for acute pain management in the perioperative setting: A report by the American Society of Anesthesiologists Task Force on Acute Pain Management. Available at: http://www.asahq.org/publicationsAndServices/pain.pdf. Accessed February 23, 2004.

59. Bodian CA, Freedman G, Hossain S, Eisenkraft JB, Beilin Y: The visual analog scale for pain: Clinical significance in postoperative patients. *Anesthesiology* 2001;95:1356-1361.

60. American Pain Society Quality of Care Committee: Quality improvement guidelines for the treatment of acute pain and cancer pain. *JAMA* 1995;274:1874-1880.

61. O'Brien CP: Drug addiction and drug abuse, in Hardman JG, Limbird LE, Molinoff PB, Ruddon RW, Gilman AG (eds): *Goodman & Gilman's The Pharmacological Basis of Therapeutics*, ed 9. New York, NY, McGraw-Hill, 1996, pp 557-577.

62. Vane JR: Inhibition of prostaglandin synthesis as a mechanism of action for aspirin-like drugs. *Nat New Biol* 1971;231:232-235.

63. Hemler M, Lands WE: Purification of the cyclooxygenase that forms prostaglandins: Demonstration of two forms of iron in the holoenzyme. *J Biol Chem* 1976;251:5575-5579.

64. Xie WL, Chipman JG, Robertson DL, Erikson RL, Simmons DL: Expression of a mitogen-responsive gene encoding prostaglandin synthase is regulated by mRNA splicing. *Proc Natl Acad Sci USA* 1991;88:2692-2696.

65. Needleman P, Isakson PC: The discovery and function of COX-2. *J Rheumatol* 1997;24(suppl 49):6-8.

66. Chandrasekharan NV, Dai H, Roos KL: COX3, a cyclooxygenase-1 variant inhibited by acetaminophen and other analgesic/antipyretic drugs: Cloning, structure, and expression. *Proc Natl Acad Sci USA* 2002;99:13926-13931.

67. Nichols ML, Allen BJ, Rogers SD, et al: Transmission of chronic nociception by spinal neurons expressing the substance P receptor. *Science* 1999;286:1558-1561.

68. Woolf CJ, Chong MS: Preemptive analgesia: Treating postoperative pain by preventing the establishment of central sensitization. *Anesth Analg* 1993;77:362-379.

69. Kissin I: Preemptive analgesia. *Anesthesiology* 2000;93:1138-1143.

70. Reisine T, Pasternak G: Opioid analgesics and antagonists, in Hardman JG, Limbird LE, Molinoff PB, Ruddon RW, Gilman AG (eds): *Goodman & Gilman's The Pharmacological Basis of Therapeutics*, ed 9. New York, NY, McGraw-Hill, 1996, pp 521-555.

71. Inturrisi CE: Clinical pharmacology of opioids for pain. *Clin J Pain* 2002;18(suppl 4):S3-S13.

72. Brooks P, Emery P, Evans JF, et al: Interpreting the clinical significance of the differential inhibition of cyclooxygenase-1 and cyclooxygenase-2. *Rheumatology (Oxford)* 1999;38:779-788.

73. Oates JA, FitzGerald GA, Branch RA, Jackson EK, Knapp HR, Roberts LJ II: Clinical implications of prostaglandin and thromboxane A2 formation (1). *N Engl J Med* 1988;319:689-698.

74. Simon RA: Oral challenges to detect aspirin and sulfite sensitivity in asthma. *Allerg Immunol (Paris)* 1994;26:216-218.

75. Cryer B, Feldman M: Cyclooxygenase-1 and cyclooxygenase-2 selectivity of widely used nonsteroidal anti-inflammatory drugs. *Am J Med* 1998;104:413-421.

76. Simon LS: Actions and toxicity of nonsteroidal anti-inflammatory drugs. *Curr Opin Rheumatol* 1996;8:169-175.

77. Dynastat: (parecoxib sodium for injection): Summary of product characteristics: Pfizer Global Pharmaceuticals, 2003. Available at: http://www.emea.eu.int/humandocs/Humans/EPAR/dynastat/dynastatM.htm. Accessed December 8, 2004.

78. Collantes E, Curtis SP, Lee KW, et al: The Etoricoxib Rheumatoid Arthritis Study Group: A multinational randomized, controlled, clinical trial of etoricoxib in the treatment of rheumatoid arthritis [ISRCTN25142273]. *BMC Fam Pract* 2002;3:10.

79. Leung AT, Malmstrom K, Gallacher AE, et al: Efficacy and tolerability profile of etoricoxib in patients with osteoarthritis: A randomized, double-blind, placebo and active-comparator controlled 12-week efficacy trial. *Curr Med Res Opin* 2002;18:49-58.

80. Ding C, Jones G: Lumiracoxib (Novartis). *IDrugs* 2002;5:1168-1172.

81. Bensen WG, Fiechtner JJ, McMillen JI, et al: Treatment of osteoarthritis with celecoxib, a cyclooxygenase-2 inhibitor: A randomized controlled trial. *Mayo Clin Proc* 1999;74:1095-1105.

82. Bensen W, Weaver A, Espinoza L, et al: Efficacy and safety of valdecoxib in treating the signs and symptoms of rheumatoid arthritis: A randomized, controlled comparison with placebo and naproxen. *Rheumatology (Oxford)* 2002;41:1008-1016.

83. Kivitz AJ, Moskowitz RW, Woods E, et al: Comparative efficacy and safety of celecoxib and naproxen in the treatment of osteoarthritis of the hip. *J Int Med Res* 2001;29:467-479.

84. Kivitz A, Eisen G, Zhao WW, Bevirt T, Recker DP: Randomized placebo-controlled trial comparing efficacy and safety of valdecoxib with naproxen in patients with osteoarthritis. *J Fam Pract* 2002;51:530-537.

85. Singh G, Fort JG, Triadafilopoulos G, Bello A: Abstract: SUCCESS-1: A global osteoarthritis (OA) trial in 13,274 randomized patients: Celecoxib provides similar efficacy to diclofenac and naproxen while providing significantly improved UGI safety. *Arthritis Rheum* 2001;44(suppl):496.

86. McKenna F, Borenstein D, Wendt H, Wallemark C, Lefkowith JB, Geis GS: Celecoxib versus diclofenac in the management of osteoarthritis of the knee. *Scand J Rheumatol* 2001;30:11-18.

87. Emery P, Zeidler H, Kvien TK: Celecoxib versus diclofenac in long-term management of rheumatoid arthritis: Randomised double-blind comparison. *Lancet* 1999;354:2106-2111.

88. Simon LS, Weaver AL, Graham DY: Anti-inflammatory and upper gastrointestinal effects of celecoxib in rheumatoid arthritis: A randomized controlled trial. *JAMA* 1999;282:1921-1928.

89. Bingham CO III: Development and clinical application of COX-2-selective inhibitors for the treatment of osteoarthritis and rheumatoid arthritis. *Cleve Clin J Med* 2002;69(suppl 1):SI5-SI12.

90. Ekman EF, Fiechtner JJ, Levy S, Fort JG: Efficacy of celecoxib versus ibuprofen in the treatment of acute pain: A multicenter, double-blind, randomized controlled trial in acute ankle sprain. *Am J Orthop* 2002;31:445-451.

91. Gimbel JS, Brugger A, Zhao W, Verburg KM, Geis GS: Efficacy and tolerability of celecoxib versus hydrocodone/acetaminophen in the treatment of pain after ambulatory orthopedic surgery in adults. *Clin Ther* 2001;23:228-241.

92. Daniels SE, Desjardins PJ, Talwalker S, Recker DP, Verburg KM: The analgesic efficacy of valdecoxib vs. oxycodone/acetaminophen after oral surgery. *J Am Dent Assoc* 2002;133:611-621.

93. Camu F, Beecher T, Recker DP, Verburg KM: Valdecoxib, a COX-2-specific inhibitor, is an efficacious, opioid-sparing analgesic in patients undergoing hip arthroplasty. *Am J Ther* 2002;9:43-51.

94. Desjardins PJ, Shu VS, Recker DP, Verburg KM, Woolf CJ: A single preoperative oral dose of valdecoxib, a new cyclooxygenase-2 specific inhibitor, relieves post-oral surgery or bunionectomy pain. *Anesthesiology* 2002;97:565-573.

95. FitzGerald GA, Patrono C: The coxibs, selective inhibitors of cyclooxygenase-2. *N Engl J Med* 2001;345:433-442.

96. Bombardier C, Laine L, Reicin A, et al: VIGOR Study Group: Comparison of upper gastrointestinal toxicity of rofecoxib and naproxen in patients with rheumatoid arthritis: Vigor Study Group. *N Engl J Med* 2000;343:1520-1528.

97. Silverstein FE, Faich G, Goldstein JL, et al: Gastrointestinal toxicity with celecoxib vs nonsteroidal anti-inflammatory drugs for osteoarthritis and rheumatoid arthritis: The CLASS study: A randomized controlled trial: Celecoxib Long-term Arthritis Safety Study. *JAMA* 2000;284:1247-1255.

98. Goldstein JL: on behalf of Class Investigators: Abstract: Gastrointestinal (GI) event rates in the CLASS study: 6-month vs longer-term follow-up analyses. *Gastroenterology* 2002;122:469-482.

99. Simon LS, Lanza FL, Lipsky PE, et al: Preliminary study of the safety and efficacy of SC-58635, a novel cyclooxygenase 2 inhibitor: Efficacy and safety in two placebo-controlled trials in osteoarthritis and rheumatoid arthritis, and studies of gastrointestinal and platelet effects. *Arthritis Rheum* 1998;41:1591-1602.

100. Goldstein JL, Kivitz AJ, Verburg KM, Recker DP, Palmer RC, Kent JD: A comparison of the upper gastrointestinal mucosal effects of valdecoxib, naproxen and placebo in healthy elderly subjects. *Aliment Pharmacol Ther* 2003;18:125-132.

101. Solomon DH, Schneeweiss S, Glynn RJ, et al: Abstract: The relationship between selective COX-2 inhibitors and acute myocardial infarction. *Arthritis Rheum* 2003;48:S697.

102. Cheng JC, Siegel LB, Katari B, Traynoff SA, Ro JO: Nonsteroidal anti-inflammatory drugs and aspirin: A comparison of the antiplatelet effects. *Am J Ther* 1997;4:62-65.

103. Leese PT, Hubbard RC, Karim A, Isakson PC, Yu SS, Geis GS: Effects of celecoxib, a novel cyclooxygenase-2 inhibitor, on platelet function in healthy adults: A randomized, controlled trial. *J Clin Pharmacol* 2000;40:124-132.

104. Leese PT, Talwalker S, Kent JD, Recker DP: Valdecoxib does not impair platelet function. *Am J Emerg Med* 2002;20:275-281.

105. Leese PT, Recker DP, Kent JD: The COX-2 selective inhibitor, valdecoxib, does not impair platelet function in the elderly: Results of a randomized controlled trial. *J Clin Pharmacol* 2003;43:504-513.

106. Noveck RJ, Laurent A, Kuss M, Talwalker S, Hubbard RC: Parecoxib sodium does not impair platelet function in healthy elderly and non-elderly individuals. *Clin Drug Invest* 2001;21:465-476.

107. Homoncik M, Malec M, Marsik C, et al: Rofecoxib exerts no effect on platelet plug formation in healthy volunteers. *Clin Exp Rheumatol* 2003;21:229-231.

108. Bannwarth B, Netter P, Lapicque F, et al: Plasma and cerebrospinal fluid concentrations of paracetamol after a single intravenous dose of propacetamol. *Br J Clin Pharmacol* 1992;34:79-81.

109. Willoughby DA, Moore AR, Coleville-Nash PR: COX-1, COX-2, and COX-3 and the future treatment of chronic inflammatory disease. *Lancet* 2000;355:646-648.

110. Simmons DL: Variants of cyclooxygenase-1 and their roles in medicine. *Thromb Res* 2003;110:265-268.

111. Botting R: COX-1 and COX-3 inhibitors. *Thromb Res* 2003;110:269-272.

112. Lewis KS, Han NH: Tramadol: A new centrally acting analgesic. *Am J Health Syst Pharm* 1997;54:643-652.

113. Schnitzer T: The new analgesic combination tramadol/acetaminophen. *Eur J Anaesthesiol* 2003;20(suppl 28):13-17.

114. Ultram (package insert). Raritan, NJ, Ortho McNeil Pharmaceutical, 2001.

115. McClellan K, Scott LJ: Tramadol/paracetamol. *Drugs* 2003;63:1079-1088. Erratum in: *Drugs* 2003;63:1636.

116. Liu SS, Mulroy MF: Neuraxial anesthesia and analgesia in the presence of standard heparin. *Reg Anesth Pain Med* 1998;23(suppl 2):157-163.

117. Omote K, Iwasaki H, Kawamata M, Satoh O, Namiki A: Effects of verapamil on spinal anesthesia with local anesthetics. *Anesth Analg* 1995;80:444-448.

118. Johnson A, Bengtsson M, Soderlind K, Lofstrom JB: Influence of intrathecal morphine and naloxone intervention on postoperative ventilatory regulation in elderly patients. *Acta Anaesthesiol Scand* 1992;36:436-444.

119. Horlocker TT, Benzon HT, Brown DL, et al: Regional anesthesia in the anticoagulated patient: Defining the risks. American Society of Regional Anesthesia and Pain Medicine; 2002. Available at: http://www.asra.com/items_of_interest/consensus_statements/index.iphtml. Accessed February 23, 2004.

120. Besson JM: The neurobiology of pain. *Lancet* 1999;353:1610-1615.

121. Collins SL, Moore RA, McQuay HJ, Wiffen PJ, Edwards JE: Single dose oral ibuprofen and diclofenac for postoperative pain. *Cochrane Database Syst Rev* 2000;2:CD001548.

122. Edwards JE, Loke YK, Moore RA, McQuay HJ: Single dose piroxicam for acute postoperative pain. *Cochrane Database Syst Rev* 2000;4:CD002762.

123. Reynolds LW, Hoo RK, Brill RJ, North J, Recker DP, Verburg KM: The COX-2 specific inhibitor, valdecoxib, is an effective, opioid-sparing analgesic in patients undergoing total knee arthroplasty. *J Pain Symptom Manage* 2003;25:133-141.

124. Hubbard RC, Naumann TM, Traylor L, Dhadda S: Parecoxib sodium has opioid-sparing effects in patients undergoing total knee arthroplasty under spinal anaesthesia. *Br J Anaesth* 2003;90:166-172.

125. Malan TP, Marsh G, Hakki SI, Grossman E, Traylor L, Hubbard RC: Parecoxib sodium, a parenteral cyclooxygenase 2 selective inhibitor, improves morphine analgesia and is opioid-sparing following total hip arthroplasty. *Anesthesiology* 2003;98:950-956.

126. Rasmussen GL, Steckner K, Hogue C, Torri S, Hubbard RC: Intravenous parecoxib sodium for acute pain after orthopedic knee surgery. *Am J Orthop* 2002;31:336-343.

127. Gan TJ, Joshi G, Viscusi E, et al: Preoperative parenteral parecoxib and follow-up oral valdecoxib reduces length of stay and improves quality of patient recovery following laparoscopic cholecystectomy surgery. *Anesth Analg* 2004;98:1665-1673.

128. Zhao S, Gan T, Joshi G, et al: Abstract: Reduction of opioid use and related side effects after laparoscopic cholecystectomy surgery (LCS): Another benefit of IV parecoxib sodium and oral valdecoxib in postoperative pain management. *J Pain* 2003;4(suppl 1):A925.

129. Joshi GP, Viscusi ER, Gan TJ, et al: Effective treatment of laparoscopic cholecystectomy pain with intravenous followed by oral COX-2 specific inhibitor. *Anesth Analg* 2004;98:336-342.

130. Kehlet H, Dahl JB: The value of "multimodal" or "balanced analgesia" in postoperative pain treatment. *Anesth Analg* 1993;77:1048-1056.

131. McQuay HJ, Edwards JE, Moore RA: Evaluating analgesia: The challenges. *Am J Ther* 2002;9:179-187.

132. Aida S, Yamakura T, Baba H, Taga K, Fukuda S, Shimoji K: Preemptive analgesia by intravenous low-dose ketamine and epidural morphine in gastrectomy: A randomized double-blind study. *Anesthesiology* 2000;92:1624-1630.

133. Aida S, Fujihara H, Taga K, Fukuda S, Shimoji K: Involvement of presurgical pain in preemptive analgesia for orthopedic surgery: A randomized double blind study. *Pain* 2000;84: 169-173.

134. Moiniche S, Kehlet H, Dahl JB: A qualitative and quantitative systematic review of preemptive analgesia for postoperative pain relief: The role of timing of analgesia. *Anesthesiology* 2002;96:725-741.

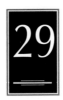

Venous Thromboembolism After a Total Hip Arthroplasty: Prevention and Treatment

Daniel J. Berry, MD

Abstract

The prevention and treatment of venous thromboembolic disease after total hip arthroplasty is a controversial issue that is important to orthopaedic surgeons and their patients. Important considerations include current risk factors, the efficacy and safety of preventive agents, the optimal duration of treatment with prophylaxis, the value of routine screening, and treatment recommendations after total hip arthroplasty.

Along with catastrophic cardiopulmonary problems, venous thromboembolism is the most likely complication that can lead to death after elective total hip arthroplasty (THA). Patients are at risk for venous thromboembolism after THA because vessel occlusion caused by kinking during surgery and postoperative inactivity may result in venous stasis, local trauma to veins may cause intimal injury, and a hypercoaguable postoperative state may result from surgery or other patient conditions. The risk of venous thromboembolism can be reduced with optimal perioperative management along with specific prophylactic treatment.

The use of prophylactic treatment after THA is controversial for many reasons, including the infrequency of clinically symptomatic events and the existence of contradictory literature on the subject. Studies are difficult to compare and interpret because of differing patient inclusion criteria, the use of tests of differing sensitivities to diagnose venous thromboembolism,[1] the establishment of differing criteria for a positive finding of thromboembolism, and differing definitions for complications resulting from prophylactic treatment regimens.

Rate of Occurrence of Venous Thromboembolism After THA

Early studies of THA indicated a high risk of symptomatic venous thromboembolic disease resulting in a mortality rate of 2% or greater when no specific prophylactic measures were used.[2,3] Recent studies show that the death rate from venous thromboembolism after THA has decreased markedly as a result of improvements in anesthesia, surgical technique,

rehabilitation of patients after surgery, and the common use of thromboembolism prophylaxis.[4-6]

Controversy concerning the current rate of occurrence of clinically significant venous thromboembolic disease has led to debate among orthopaedic surgeons about the use of aggressive venous thromboembolism prophylaxis that itself creates a risk of bleeding complications.[7-11] Although many studies identify a high rate of venous thromboembolism after THA, especially when sensitive detection tests are used, the clinical importance of many clots identified by these tests is questionable. Clots in the leg have a finite risk of progression to symptomatic deep venous thrombosis (DVT) or pulmonary embolism, but strict correlation between the sensitive surrogate end points used in most studies with clinically relevant thromboembolism has been difficult to establish.[12,13] The risk of fatal pulmonary embolism appears to be less than 0.3%, which is lower than reported in early THA studies. The level of risk reduction related to improved perioperative treatment compared with the level of reduction related to the use of prophylactic agents is uncertain. Recent evidence suggests the long-term risk of chronic venous insufficiency, even in patients with positive postoperative tests for DVT, is low in THA patients.[14,15] Some consensus panels have recommended effective pharmacologic prophylaxis after THA, whereas other authors believe that the rate of occurrence of venous thromboembolism is sufficiently low that aggressive pharmacologic prophylaxis may not be warranted.[6,16-19] Most orthopaedic surgeons in North America currently believe that some form of effective thromboembolic prophylaxis is justified after THA; the best agent for use is debatable.

Some measures available to reduce the risk of thromboembolism can be used to treat many THA patients, with little additional risk. Evidence shows that regional anesthesia is associated with a lower rate of venous thromboembolic disease.[20] Expeditious surgery and minimizing the time the hip is in a dislocated position reduces the risk for venous stasis. Prompt postoperative mobilization of the patient and calf exercises performed while in bed may help reduce the risk for thromboembolism.[21] Elastic stockings commonly are used, although their value has been questioned.[22] Factors associated with an increased risk of thromboembolism may be identified before surgery and include a prior history of the disease and specific molecular markers, which have been identified in recent studies.[23-27] For high-risk patients, a more vigorous prophylactic regimen often is recommended.[6]

Prophylactic Agents for the Treatment and Prevention of Venous Thromboembolic Disease

Many prophylactic agents, including oral pharmacologic agents, injectable pharmacologic agents, and mechanical agents, can be used for venous thromboembolism prophylaxis. Each of the currently available prophylactic agents has advantages and disadvantages in terms of effectiveness, risks for complications, and simplicity of administration that must be considered by the orthopaedic surgeon.

Warfarin

The advantages of warfarin include oral administration and a proven clinical track record.[28] Its disadvantages include delayed onset of anticoagulation, unpredictable dose response, and the need for regular monitoring.[29,30] Several studies have demonstrated that Coumadin (trademark name for warfarin sodium preparation, DuPont Pharmaceuticals, Wilmington, DE) is an effective agent to reduce venous thromboembolism. Lieberman and associates[31] studied 1,099 THAs treated with Coumadin within a mean of 15 days after THA. The fatal pulmonary embolism rate was 0.1% and major bleeding occurred in 2.9% of patients. In a recently published meta-analysis, Freedman and associates[32] concluded that Coumadin provided the best efficacy and safety of the available therapeutic agents.

Low-Molecular-Weight Heparins

The main advantage in using low-molecular-weight heparins (LMWHs) is predictable dose response, resulting in ease of administration and proven efficacy.[33] Disadvantages in using LMWHs include the risk for bleeding complications and the need for injection of the prophylaxis. Colwell and associates[34] reported on a 1994 study of LMWH used in 194 THAs which resulted in a deep venous thromboembolism rate of 5% and eight major episodes of bleeding. The optimal dosage and timing of LMWH administration is not definitive. In North America, most protocols begin within 6 to 24 hours postoperatively; in Europe, many patients receive a lower dose prior to surgery.[35-38] Indwelling epidural catheters should be avoided when LMWHs are used because of a risk of epidural hematoma.[39]

Several studies have compared the use of LMWHs with Coumadin.[40] In a study that used a venogram end point, no statistical difference in deep venous thromboembolism rates and no difference in bleeding rates between LMWH and Coumadin was shown.[41] Francis and associates[42] reported no statistically significant difference in the proximal deep venous thromboembolism rates between Coumadin and LMWH; however, results showed a significantly higher rate of bleeding in the group given LMWH in the early postoperative period. Colwell and associates[43] reported on 3,011 hips treated with either Coumadin or LMWH, with results of the study showing no statistically significant difference between the groups in rates of deep venous thromboembolism or pulmonary embolism; however, fewer bleeding complications occurred in the Coumadin group. These studies show that Coumadin and LMWH are approximately equally effective in preventing DVT after THA and that the bleeding complication rate appears to be slightly increased with the use of LMWH; this risk for bleeding complications can be reduced if LMWH is not administered early in the postoperative period.[39]

Aspirin

The most important advantages of aspirin are its low rate of adverse effects and ease of administration. However, it is uncertain whether aspirin reduces venous thromboembolism after THA as effectively as other agents.[6] In a 1994 study, Lieberman and associates[44] recommended that aspirin not be used as the sole agent for prophylaxis after THA.[44] Although the use of aspirin is controversial, good results have been reported. In one study, aspirin was shown to reduce the risk of venous thromboembolism by at least one third.[45] Sarmiento and associates[46] used aspirin and elastic stockings or mechanical compression in 1,492 THAs and reported a fatal pulmonary embolism rate of 0.13% and a nonfatal pulmonary embolism rate of 1%. Aspirin may provide some additional benefit by reducing the risk of myocardial infarction in the postoperative period.

Intraoperative Intravenous Heparin

Intraoperative intravenous heparin acts at the time most emboli presumably form, providing a low risk of venous thromboembolism when used with a comprehensive protocol of hypotensive epidural anesthesia or postoperative aspirin and early ambulation.[47,48] Proper intraoperative dosing is essential for safety.

Mechanical Prophylaxis Devices

Mechanical prophylaxis devices are safe and easy to use;[49] however, their relative efficacy when used as the sole prophylactic agent, compared with pharmacologic measures, is uncertain. In addition, patients do not always wear these devices regularly. Several studies have reported success with intermittent pneumatic compression. Hooker and associates[50] studied 502 patients treated with thigh-high intermittent pneumatic compression devices after THA. Using an ultrasound end point, they found a 5% deep venous thromboembolism rate, no fatal pulmonary emboli, and the occurrence of a pulmonary embolism in 0.6% of patients. Woolson[51] reported on 289 hips treated with thigh-high compression boots and found a 4% proximal deep venous thromboembolism rate (using an ultrasound end point) and no clinically evident pulmonary emboli. In this series, high-risk patients were treated with Coumadin.

New Prophylactic Agents

New prophylactic agents are being developed.[52] Fondaparinux, a synthetic pentasaccharide and factor Xa inhibitor, recently has been reported to be an effective prophylactic agent after THA.[53] Hirudin, an oral thrombin inhibitor, has proved successful in European trials.[54] It is hoped that newer agents may improve efficacy, reduce risks of complications, improve ease of administration, and reduce the need for patient monitoring.[54]

Consensus

At present, no single prophylactic agent has proved the most effective for all patients. Surgeons must consider the risks and benefits when choosing a prophylaxis method. The American College of Chest Physicians Consensus Panel recently published an evaluation of the different prophylactic agents for perioperative use after total joint arthroplasty.[6] Both Coumadin and LMWHs received the best (1A) ratings for elective THA. Adjusted-dose heparin was considered acceptable but more complex to use. Low-dose unfractionated heparin, aspirin, dextran, and intermittent pneumatic compression were considered less effective when used alone, and such usage was not recommended.[6] Mechanical prophylaxis can be added to any regimen without additional risk.

Duration of Venous Thromboembolism Prophylaxis

Thromboembolism after THA frequently occurs after hospital discharge.[55-57] The optimal duration of venous thromboembolism prophylaxis after THA is controversial and may depend on the postoperative regimen and patient factors.[28,58-62] A mean of 15 days of treatment with Coumadin was proven to be effective in one study.[31] Leclerc and associates[63] showed a low risk of venous thromboembolism in a large cohort of patients treated for a mean of 9 days after arthroplasty. Recent studies have suggested that prolonged outpatient prophylaxis with LMWH can further reduce the rate of venous thromboembolism,[36,64-69] although the magnitude of the reduction has been questioned.[59] At present, most surgeons prefer to administer prophylactic agents to hospitalized patients and many patients continue the use of a prophylactic agent for several days or weeks after discharge. One recent consensus panel recommended prophylactic treatment with an effective agent for at least 10 days,[70] and another recommended treat-

ment for at least 7 to 10 days.[6] For patients at high risk for venous thromboembolism, more prolonged prophylaxis (usually 6 weeks after surgery) is recommended.[6]

Screening for Venous Thromboembolism

Routine screening for venous thromboembolism after THA was popularized by the development of accurate noninvasive screening methods. The advantages of screening include the ability to identify and optimally treat any patients with clots and the opportunity to exclude patients without clots from the risks of longer prophylaxis.[71] Although screening is attractive in theory, a recent large prospective randomized trial comparing hospital discharge ultrasound with sham ultrasound showed no advantage to screening.[72] The value of screening depends on the accuracy of screening methods[73] and the risks of either continuing or discontinuing prophylaxis in a specific patient population and practice setting.[60] A recent consensus panel did not endorse routine screening.[6]

Treatment of Venous Thromboembolism After THA

If DVT or pulmonary embolism occurs after THA, an internist may become involved in the treatment; however, it is important that the orthopaedic surgeon participate in treatment decisions. Orthopaedic surgeons can best understand the relative risks of various methods of venous thromboembolic treatment in the acute postoperative patient. The early administration of intravenous heparin after THA carries a heightened risk of bleeding complications.[74] Bleeding complications are particularly common if a patient receives heparin presumptively without a proven diagnosis of venous thromboembolism.[75] The diagnosis should be confirmed with a reliable test before potentially risky treatment protocols (such as the administration of full-dose intravenous heparin) are instituted early in the postoperative period.

Symptomatic venous thromboembolism that occurs more than 1 week after THA usually is treated with heparin followed by warfarin. However, if venous thromboembolism is diagnosed in the first week after arthroplasty, decisions concerning the proper management should balance the risks of more aggressive treatment, which could lead to major bleeding problems, versus the risks of less aggressive treatment, which could risk pulmonary embolism.[76,77] Treatment options include: (1) observation and continued use, at the same dosage level, of the prophylactic agent already in use coupled with careful monitoring; (2) more intense anticoagulation treatment with either intravenous heparin or LMWH; or (3) placement of an inferior vena cava filter.[78] The most appropriate treatment depends on the specific patient circumstances.

Summary

A number of prophylactic agents are available to reduce the risk of venous thromboembolism after THA. The risk of venous thromboembolism after THA appears to have decreased with modern surgical and perioperative care; therefore, prophylactic agents must be chosen with an advantageous risk/benefit profile. A prophylactic agent that can be administered effectively and safely in a specific hospital and practice setting should be chosen. If a venous thromboembolic event occurs after surgery, participation by the orthopaedic surgeon in the treatment plan is important to reduce the risk of further complications.

References

1. Warwick D, Samama MM: The contrast between venographic and clinical endpoints in trials of thromboprophylaxis in hip replacement. *J Bone Joint Surg* 2000;82:480-482.

2. Johnson R, Carmichael JHE, Almond HGA, Loynes RP: Deep venous thrombosis following Charnley arthroplasty. *Clin Orthop* 1978;132:24-30.

3. Coventry MB, Nolan DR, Beckenbaugh RD: "Delayed" prophylactic anticoagulation: A study of results of complications in 2012 total hip arthroplasties. *J Bone Joint Surg Am* 1973;55:1487-1492.

4. Clarke MT, Green JS, Harper WM, Gregg PJ: Screening for deep venous thrombosis after hip and knee replacement without prophylaxis. *J Bone Joint Surg Br* 1997;79:787-791.

5. Warwick D, Williams MH, Bannister GC: Death and thromboembolic disease after total hip replacement: A series 1162 cases with no routine chemical prophylaxis. *J Bone Joint Surg Br* 1995;77:6-10.

6. Geerts WH, Heit JA, Clagett GP, et al: Prevention of venous thromboembolism. *Chest* 2001;119:132S-175S.

7. Fender D, Harper WN, Thompson JR, Gregg PJ: Mortality and fatal pulmonary embolism after primary total hip replacement: Results from a regional hip register. *J Bone Joint Surg Br* 1997;79:896-899.

8. Gillespie W, Murray D, Gregg PJ, Warwick D: Risks and benefits of prophylaxis against venous thromboembolism in orthopaedic surgery. *J Bone Joint Surg Br* 2000; 82:475-479.

9. Mcgrath D, Dennyson WG, Rolland M: Death rate from pulmonary embolism following joint replacement surgery. *J R Coll Surg Edinb* 1996;41:265-266.

10. Prentice CR: Thromboprophylaxis: Which treatment for which patient? *J Bone Joint Surg Br* 2000;82:483-485.

11. Thomas DP: Whither thromboprophylaxis after total hip replacement? *J Bone Joint Surg Br* 2000;82:469-472.

12. Oishi CS, Grady-Benson JC, Otis SM, Colwell CW Jr, Walker RH: The clinical course of distal deep venous thrombosis after total hip and total knee arthroplasty, as determined with duplex ultrasonography. *J Bone Joint Surg Am* 1994;76:1658-1663.

13. Pellegrini VD Jr, Clement D, Lush-Ehmann C, Keller GS, Evarts CM: The John Charnley Award: Natural history of thromboembolic disease after total hip arthroplasty. *Clin Orthop* 1996;333:27-40.

14. Ginsberg JS, Turkstra F, Buller HR, MacKinnon B, Magier D, Hirsh J: Postthrombotic syndrome after hip or knee arthroplasty: A cross-sectional study. *Arch Intern Med* 2000;160:669-672.

15. Warwick D, Perez J, Vickery C, Bannister G: Does total hip arthroplasty predispose to chronic venous insufficiency? *J Arthroplasty* 1996;11:529-533.

16. Clagett GP, Anderson FA Jr, Geerts W, et al: Prevention of venous thromboembolism. *Chest* 1998;114:531S-560S.

17. Consensus Conference: Prevention of venous thrombosis and pulmonary embolism. *JAMA* 1986;256:744-749.

18. Murray DW, Britton AR, Bulstrode CJ: Thromboprophylaxis and death after total hip replacement. *J Bone Joint Surg Br* 1996;78:863-870.

19. Murray DW, Carr AJ, Bulstrode CJK: Pharmacological thromboprophylaxis and total hip replacement. *J Bone Joint Surg Br* 1995; 77:3-5.

20. Westrich GH, Farrell C, Bono JV, et al: The incidence of venous thromboembolim after total hip arthroplasty: A specific hypotensive epidural anesthesia protocol. *J Arthroplasty* 1999;14:456-463.

21. McNally MA, Cooke EA, Mollan RA: The effect of active movement of the foot on venous blood flow after total hip replacement. *J Bone Joint Surg Am* 1997;79:1198-1201.

22. Hui AC, Heras-Palou C, Dunn I, et al: Graded compression stockings for prevention of deep vein thrombosis after hip and knee replacement. *J Bone Joint Surg Br* 1996;78:550-554.

23. Arcelus JI, Caprini JA, Reyna JJ: Finding the right fit: Effective thrombosis risk stratification in orthopedic patients. *Orthopedics* 2000;23:S633-S638.

24. Cofrancesco E, Cortellaro M, Corradi A, Ravasi F, Bertocchi F: Coagulation activation markers in the prediction of venous thrombosis after elective hip surgery. *Thrombosis Haemostasis* 1997;77:267-269.

25. Corradi A, Lazzaro F, Cofrancesco E, et al: Preoperative plasma levels of prothrombin fragment 1+2 correlate with the risk of venous thrombosis after elective hip replacement. *Acta Orthop Belg* 1999;65:39-43.

26. Lindahl TL, Lundahl TH, Nilsson L, Andersson CA: APC-resistance is a risk factor for postoperative thromboembolism in elective replacement of the hip or knee: A prospective study. *Thrombosis Haemostasis* 1999;81:18-21.

27. Phillipp CS, Dilley A, Saidi P, et al: Deletion polymorphism in the angiotensin-converting enzyme gene as a thrombophilic risk factor after hip arthroplasty. *Thrombosis Haemostasis* 1998;80:869-873.

28. Paiement GD, Wessinger J, Hughes R, Harris WH: Routine use of adjusted low-dose Warfarin to prevent venous thromboembolism after total hip replacement. *J Bone Joint Surg Am* 1993;75:893-898.

29. Messieh M, Huang Z, Johnson LJ, Jobin S: Warfarin responses in total joint and hip fracture patients. *J Arthroplasty* 1999;14:724-729.

30. Schuringa P, Yen D: Home prophylactic warfarin anticoagulation program after hip and knee arthroplasty. *Can J Surg* 1999;42:360-362.

31. Lieberman JR, Wallaeger J, Dorey F, et al: The efficacy of prophylaxis with low dose warfarin for prevention of pulmonary embolism following total hip arthroplasty. *J Bone Joint Surg Am* 1997;79:319-325.

32. Freedman KB, Brookenthal KR, Fitzgerald RH Jr, Williams S, Lonner JH: A meta-analysis of thromboembolic prophylaxis following elective total hip arthroplasty. *J Bone Joint Surg Am* 2000;82:929-938.

33. Warwick D, Bannister GC, Glew D, et al: Perioperative low-molecular-weight heparin: Is it effective and safe? *J Bone Joint Surg Br* 1995;77:715-719.

34. Colwell CW Jr, Spiro TE, Trowbridge AA, et al: Enoxaparin clinical trial troup: Use of Enoxaparin, a low-molecular-weight heparin, and unfractionated heparin for the prevention of deep venous thrombosis after elective hip replacement: A clinical trial comparing efficacy and safety. *J Bone Joint Surg Am* 1994;76:3-14.

35. Hull RD, Brant RF, Pineo GF, Stein PD, Raskob GE, Valentine KA: Preoperative versus postoperative initiation of low-molecular-weight heparin prophylaxis against venous thromboembolism in patients undergoing elective hip replacement. *Arch Intern Med* 1999;159:137-141.

36. Hull RD, Pineo GF, Francis C, et al: Low-molecular-weight heparin prophylaxis using dalteparin extended out-of-hospital vs in-hospital warfarin/out-of-hospital placebo in hip arthroplasty patients: A double-blind, randomized comparison. North American Fragmin Trial Investigators. *Arch Intern Med* 2000;160: 2208-2215.

37. Hull RD, Pineo GF, Francis C, et al: Low-molecular-weight heparin prophylaxis using dalteparin in close proximity to surgery versus warfarin in hip arthroplasty patients: A double-blind, randomized comparison. The North American Fragmin Trial Investigators. *Arch Intern Med* 2000;160:2199-2207.

38. Hull RD, Pineo GF, MacIsaac S: Low-molecular-weight heparin prophylaxis: Preoperative versus postoperative initiation in patients undergoing elective hip surgery. *Thrombosis Res* 2001;101:V155-V162.

39. Shaieb MD, Watson BN, Atkinson RE: Bleeding complications with enoxaparin for deep venous thrombosis prophylaxis. *J Arthroplasty* 1999;14:432-438.

40. Hull RD, Raskob G, Pineo G, et al: A comparison of subcutaneous low-molecular-weight heparin with warfarin sodium for prophylaxis against deep vein thrombosis after hip or knee implantation. *N Engl J Med* 1993;329:1370-1376.

41. RD Heparin Arthroplasty Group: RD heparin compared with warfarin for prevention of venous thromboembolic disease following total hip or knee arthroplasty. *J Bone Joint Surg Am* 1994;76:1174-1185.

42. Francis CW, Pellegrini VD Jr, Totterman S, et al: Prevention of deep vein thrombosis after total hip arthroplasty: Comparison of warfarin and dalteparin. *J Bone Joint Surg Am* 1997;79: 1365-1372.

43. Colwell CW, Collis DK, Paulson R, et al: Comparison of enoxaparin and warfarin for the prevention of venous thromboembolic disease after total hip arthroplasty. *J Bone Joint Surg Am* 1999;81:932-940.

44. Lieberman JR, Geerts WH: Prevention of venous thromboembolism after total hip and knee arthroplasty. *J Bone Joint Surg Am* 1994;76:1239-1250.

45. Anonymous: Prevention of pulmonary embolism and deep vein thrombosis with low dose aspirin: Pulmonary embolism prevention (PEP) trial. *Lancet* 2000;355:1295-1302.

46. Sarmiento A, Goswami AD: Thromboembolic prophylaxis with use of aspirin, exercise, and graded elastic stockings or intermittent compression devices in patients managed with total hip arthroplasty. *J Bone Joint Surg Am* 1999;81:339-346.

47. DiGiovanni CW, Restrepo A, Gonzalez Della Valle AG, et al: The safety and efficacy of intraoperative heparin in total hip arthroplasty. *Clin Orthop* 2000;379:178-185.

48. Nassif JM, Ritter MA, Meding JB, Keating EM, Faris PM: The effect of intraoperative intravenous fixed-dose heparin during total joint arthroplasty on the incidence of fatal pulmonary emboli. *J Arthroplasty* 2000;15:16-21.

49. Warwick D, Harrison J, Glew D, Mitchelmore A, Peters TJ, Donovan J: Comparison of the use of a foot pump with the use of low-molecular-weight heparin for the prevention of deep-vein thrombosis after total hip replacement. *J Bone Joint Surg Am* 1998;80:1158-1166.

50. Hooker JA, Lachiewicz PF, Kelley SS: Efficacy of prophylaxis against thromboembolism with intermittent pneumatic compression after primary and revision total hip arthroplasty. *J Bone Joint Surg Am* 1999;81:690-696.

51. Woolson ST: Intermittent pneumatic compression prophylaxis for proximal deep venous thrombosis after total hip replacement. *J Bone Joint Surg Am* 1996;78:1735-1740.

52. Eriksson BI, Ekman S, Kalebo P, et al: Prevention of deep vein thrombosis after total hip replacement: Direct thrombin inhibition with recombinant hirudin: CGP 39393. *Lancet* 1996;347:635-639.

53. Turpie AG, Gallus AS, Hoek JA: Pentasaccharide investigators: A synthetic pentasaccharide for the prevention of deep-vein thrombosis after total hip replacement. *N Engl J Med* 2001;344: 619-625.

54. Eriksson BI, Ekman S, Lindbratt S, et al: Prevention of thromboembolism with us of recombinant hirudin: Results of a double-blind, multicenter trial comparing the efficacy of desirudin (Revasc) with that of unfractionated heparin in patients having a total hip replacement. *J Bone Joint Surg Am* 1997;79:326-333.

55. Dahl OE, Gudmundsen TE, Haukeland L: Late occurring clinical deep vein thrombosis in joint-operated patients. *Acta Orthop Scand* 2000;71: 47-50.

56. White RH, Gettner S, Newman JM, Trauner KB, Romano PS: Predictors of rehospitalization for symptomatic venous thromboembolism after total hip arthroplasty. *N Engl J Med* 2000;343:1758-1764.

57. White RH, Romano PS, Zhou H, Rodrigo J, Bargar W: Incidence and time course of thromboembolic outcomes following total hip or knee arthroplasty. *Arch Int Med* 1998;158:1525-1531.

58. Davidson BL: Out-of-hospital prophylaxis with low-molecular-weight heparin in hip surgery: The Swedish study. *Chest* 1998;114(suppl 2): 130S-132S.

59. Heit JA: Low-molecular-weight heparin: The optimal duration of prophylaxis against postoperative venous thromboembolism after total hip or knee replacement. *Thrombosis Res* 2001;101:V163-V173.

60. Paiement GD: Prevention and treatment of venous thromboembolic disease complications in primary hip arthroplasty patients. *Instr Course Lect* 1998;47:331-335.

61. Svensson PJ, Benoni G, Fredin H, et al: Female gender and resistance to activated protein C (FV:Q506) as potential risk factors for thrombosis after elective hip arthroplasty. *Thrombosis Haemostasis* 1997;78:993-996.

62. Beuhler KO, D'Lima DD, Petersilge WJ, Colwell CW Jr, Walker RH: Late deep venous thrombosis and delayed weightbearing after total hip arthroplasty. *Clin Orthop* 1999;361:123-130.

63. Leclerc JR, Gent M, Hirsh J, Geerts WH, Ginsberg JS: The incidence of symptomatic venous thromboembolism during and after prophylaxis with enoxaparin: A multi-institutional cohort study of patients who underwent hip or knee arthroplasty. Canadian Collaborative Group. *Arch Intern Med* 1998;158:873-878.

64. Bergqvist D, Venoni G, Bjorgell O, et al: Low molecular weight heparin (enoxaparin) as prophylaxis against venous thromboembolism after total hip replacement. *N Engl J Med* 1996;335:696-700.

65. Comp PC, Spiro TE, Friedman RJ, et al: Enoxaparin Clinical Trial Group: Prolonged enoxaparin therapy to prevent venous thromboembolism after primary hip or knee replacement. Enoxaparin Clinical Trial Group. *J Bone Joint Surg Am* 2001;83:336-345.

66. Eikelboom JW, Quinlan DJ, Douketis JD: Extended duration prophylaxis against venous thromboembolism after total hip or knee replacement: A meta-analysis of the randomized trials. *Lancet* 2001;358:9-15.

67. Hull RD: New insights into extended prophylaxis after orthopaedic surgery: The North American Fragmin Trial Experience. *Haemostasis* 2000;3(suppl 2):95-100.

68. Nilsson PE, Bergqvist D, Benoni G, et al: The post-discharge prophylactic management of the orthopedic patient with low molecular weight heparin: Enoxaparin. *Orthopedics* 1997;20(suppl):22-25.

69. Planes A, Vochelle N, Darmon JY, Fagola M, Bellaud M, Huet Y: Risk of deep venous thrombosis after hospital discharge in patients having undergone total hip replacement: A double-blind randomized comparison of enoxaparin versus placebo. *Lancet* 1996;348:224-228.

70. Hirsh J: Evidence for the needs of out-of-hospital thrombosis prophylaxis: Introduction. *Chest* 1998;114(suppl 2):113S-114S.

71. Beuhler KO, D'Lima DD, Colwell CW Jr, Otis SM, Walker RH: Venous thromboembolic disease after hybrid hip arthroplasty with negative duplex screening. *Clin Orthop* 1999;361:168-177.

72. Robinson KS, Anderson DR, Gross M, et al: Ultrasonographic screening before hospital discharge for deep venous thrombosis after arthroplasty: The post-arthroplasty screening study: A randomized controlled trial. *Ann Intern Med* 1997;127:439-445.

73. Garino JP, Lotke PA, Kitziger KJ, Steinberg ME: Deep venous thrombosis after total joint arthroplasty: The role of compression ultrasonography

and the importance of the experience of the technician. *J Bone Joint Surg Am* 1996;78:1359-1365.

74. Patterson BM, Marchand R, Ranawat C: Complications of heparin therapy after total joint arthroplasty. *J Bone Joint Surg Am* 1989;71:1130-1134.

75. Lawton RL, Morrey BF: The use of heparin in patients in whom a pulmonary embolism is sus-pected after total hip arthroplasty. *J Bone Joint Surg Am* 1999;81:1063-1072.

76. Della Valle CJ, Jazrawi LM, Idjadi J, et al: Anticoagulant treatment of thromboembolism with intravenous heparin therapy in the early postoperative period following total joint arthro-plasty. *J Bone Joint Surg Am* 2000;82:207-212.

77. Della Valle CJ, Steiger DJ, CiCesare PE: Thromboembolism after hip and knee arthro-plasty: Diagnosis and treatment. *J Am Acad Orthop Surg* 1998;6:327-336.

78. Bicalho PS, Hozack WJ, Rothman RH, Eng K: Treatment of early symptomatic pulmonary embolism after total joint arthroplasty. *J Arthroplasty* 1996;11:522-524.

Index